METHODS OF
VITAMIN ASSAY

METHODS OF VITAMIN ASSAY

Fourth Edition

Edited by

Jorg Augustin, Ph.D.
Food Research Center
University of Idaho

Barbara P. Klein, Ph.D.
Department of Foods and Nutrition
University of Illinois

Deborah Becker, B.S.
SCI-TEK Laboratories

Paul B. Venugopal, Ph.D.
Vedal, Inc.

**For the Association
of Vitamin Chemists**

A Wiley-Interscience Publication

JOHN WILEY & SONS

New York / Chichester / Brisbane / Toronto / Singapore

Library of Congress Cataloging in Publication Data:
Main entry under title:

Methods of vitamin assay.

   "A Wiley-Interscience publication."
   Rev. ed. of: Methods of vitamin assay / Association of
Vitamin Chemists. 3rd ed. 1966.
   Includes bibliographies and index.
   1. Vitamins——Analysis. I. Augustin, Jorg. II. Association
of Vitamin Chemists. Methods of vitamin assay.

RS190.V5M48   1984   641.1'8   84-7335
ISBN 0-471-86957-0

Printed in the United States of America
10 9 8 7 6 5 4 3 2 1

Contributors

RAYMOND BERRUTI, B.S., Heterochemical Corp., 111 East Hawthorne Avenue, Valley Stream, NY 11580.

KENNETH J. CARPENTER, PH.D., Department of Nutritional Sciences, University of California, Berkeley, CA 94720.

C. O. CHICHESTER, PH.D., Department of Food Science and Technology, University of Rhode Island, Kingston, RI 02881.

HENRY B. CHIN, PH.D., National Food Processors Association, 1950 6th Street, Berkeley, CA 94710.

NEVILLE COLMAN, M.D. PH.D., Hematology and Nutrition Laboratory, Veterans Administration Medical Center, 130 West Kingsbridge Rd., Bronx, NY 10468.

INDRAJIT D. DESAI, PH.D., Division of Human Nutrition, University of British Columbia, Vancouver, B.C., VGT 1W5 CANADA.

SELWYN DE SOUZA, PH.D., Department of Food Science, University of Georgia, Athens, GA 30601.

JONATHAN W. DEVRIES, PH.D., James Ford Bell Technical Center, General Mills, Inc., 9000 Plymouth Avenue North, Minneapolis, MN 55427.

JANET A. DUDEK, M.S., National Food Processors Association, 1401 New York Avenue, N.W., Washington, DC 20005.

DAVID C. EGBERG, PH.D., James Ford Bell Technical Center, General Mills, Inc., 9000 Plymouth Avenue North, Minneapolis, MN 55427.

RONALD R. EITENMILLER, PH.D., Department of Food Science, University of Georgia, Athens, GA 30601.

EDGAR R. ELKINS, B.S., National Food Processors Association, 1401 New York Avenue, N.W., Washington, DC 20005.

WAYNE C. ELLEFSON, M.S., Hazleton Raltech, Inc., Box 7545, Madison, WI 53707.

JESSE F. GREGORY, III, PH.D., Department of Food Science and Human Nutrition, University of Florida, Gainesville, FL 32611.

R. GAURTH HANSEN, PH.D., Department of Nutrition and Food Science, Utah State University, Logan, UT 84322.

VICTOR HERBERT, M.D., J.D., Department of Medicine, Hahnemann University School of Medicine, Philadelphia, PA 19102.

ALAN J. JOHNSON, M.S., Systems Validation, Eli Lilly & Co., 1200 South Kentucky Ave., Indianapolis, IN 46221.

PAMELA M. KEAGY, PH.D., Western Regional Research Center, U.S. Department of Agriculture, 800 Buchanan, Berkeley, CA 94710.

LAWRENCE J. MACHLIN, PH.D., Research Division, Hoffmann-LaRoche, Inc., Nutley, NJ 07110.

R. A. MOFFITT, M.S., Analytical Services, Carnation Co., 8015 Van Nuys Boulevard, Van Nuys, CA 91412.

R. J. NOEL, PH.D., Department of Biochemistry, Purdue University, West Lafayette, IN 47907.

D. B. PARRISH, PH.D., Department of Biochemistry, Kansas State University, Manhattan, KS 66506.

OMER PELLETIER, PH.D., Laboratory Center for Disease Control, Health Protection Branch, Health and Welfare Canada, Ottawa, Ontario, K1A OL2 CANADA.

MARILYN M. POLANSKY, M.S., Vitamin and Mineral Nutrition Laboratory, Human Nutrition Institute, U.S. Department of Agriculture, Building 307, Base East, Beltsville, MD 20705.

ROBERT D. REYNOLDS, PH.D., Vitamin and Mineral Nutrition Laboratory, Human Nutrition Institute, U.S. Department of Agriculture, Building 307, Beltsville, MD 20705.

J. SCHEINER, M.S., Roche Chemical Division, Hoffmann-LaRoche, Inc., Nutley, NJ 07110.

JITENDRA J. SHAH, M.S., M.B.A., SGS Control Services, Memphis, TN 38118.

KENNETH L. SIMPSON, PH.D., Department of Food Science and Technology, University of Rhode Island, Kingston, RI 02881.

LAXMAN SINGH, PH.D., Vitamins, Inc., 200 East Randolph Drive, Chicago, IL 60601.

WON O. SONG, PH.D., Department of Food Science and Human Nutrition, Michigan State University, East Lansing, MI 48824.

KENT K. STEWART, PH.D., Department of Food Science and Technology, Virginia Polytechnic Institute and State University, Blacksburg, VA 24061.

J.N. THOMPSON, PH.D., Nutrition Research Division, Health and Welfare Canada, Ottawa, Ontario, K1A 0L2 CANADA.

SAMPSON C.S. TSOU, Asian Vegetable Research and Development Center, Box 42, Shanhua Tainan, Taiwan 741 REPUBLIC OF CHINA.

JOSEPH T. VANDERSLICE, PH.D., Nutrition Composition Laboratory, U.S. Department of Agriculture, Human Nutrition Research Center, Beltsville, MD 20705.

PAUL B. VENUGOPAL, PH.D., Vedal Inc., 6705 Trenton, Darien, IL 60559.

MICHAEL N. VOIGT, PH.D., Biochemistry Department, Memorial University, St. John's, Newfoundland, A1B 3X9 CANADA.

JOAN H. WALSH, PH.D., R.D., Department of Family Practice, San Joaquin General Hospital, Stockton, CA 95201.

BONITA W. WYSE, PH.D., R.D., Department of Nutrition and Food Science, Utah State University, Logan, UT 84322.

Preface

Methods of Vitamin Assay of the Association of Vitamin Chemists has become a classic in its field. The third edition, which is now out of print, was published seventeen years ago in 1966. Since then, several events occurred that have exerted a major impact on the field of vitamin analysis. The most important of these were the advent of nutritional labeling of foods and the increased interest of consumers in nutrition. These in turn, created a rash of investigations of the nutrient content, including vitamins, of foods, as well as studies of vitamin metabolism. Recently, more interest has been generated regarding the impact of vitamins, not only on nutritional status or health, but also on the effects of vitamins on disease prevention. The result has been a sharply increased demand on vitamin assay.

All these events led to two major developments with regard to vitamin analysis: (1) the increased analytical workload led to the development of automated analysis systems which allow the handling of a several-fold increase in sample numbers when compared to existing manual methods, and (2) the increased exposure of analysts and researchers to vitamin analysis made them aware of shortcomings of existing methods, leading to the development of new methods with higher sensitivity and greatly increased accuracy and precision. An example of new methodology that is emerging is high-performance liquid chromatography. This system offers the opportunity for the simultaneous determination of more than one vitamin, but even more importantly, it permits the chemical analysis of such vitamins as vitamin D in biological systems that previously could only be determined by animal assays.

The fourth edition constitutes an update to the state of the art in the field of vitamin analysis. Not only are the methods outlined in the chapters covering individual vitamins updated, but just as importantly, the new edition contains four additional chapters. Of these, three cover novel analytical systems, that is, chromatographic assays, radioimmunoassays, and automated assays. Because today's analysts are constantly faced with new technology, and since many are engaged in methods development, the editors considered it opportune to touch on some of these problems in a separate chapter.

In the formative stages of the fourth edition, the editors, in agreement with the Association of Vitamin Chemists, decided to assign chapter responsibilities to individual contributors. We believe this approach to be the most effective way to convey expert information in the various areas of vitamin assay to the analyst. In addition, more background on each vitamin was included to provide an historical perspective of the importance of each nutrient.

The methods described in this edition under individual vitamins are, in some instances, very similar to those in the previous edition. Where necessary, they were updated; if no longer in use, they were deleted. The decision to include or exclude any method was left up to the contributors and the editors, rather than a committee, as was the case with the earlier editions. The ultimate criterion for inclusion or exclusion of a method was the current extent of its usage, signifying that the new edition covers only those in present use. In addition, an effort was made in each chapter to acquaint the reader with new analytical developments for a particular vitamin. Thus, the scope of the book has expanded from a manual of analytical procedures to a reference source for new techniques.

We have attempted to maintain the spirit of the previous edition of *Methods of Vitamin Assay* in the presentations. However, those familiar with the third edition will find some changes in format and delivery among the chapters. Among the changes is the provision of a list of abbreviations used, as well as an overall list of suppliers for special equipment and chemicals for the assay procedures. We hope that the old and new users of *Methods of Vitamin Assay* will find the fourth edition as helpful as the previous editions.

JORG AUGUSTIN
BARBARA KLEIN
DEBORAH BECKER
PAUL B. VENUGOPAL

Moscow, Idaho
Urbana, Illinois
Northbrook, Illinois
Darien, Illinois

July 1984

Contents

METHODS OF VITAMIN ASSAY

1 Method Choice and Development

Kent K. Stewart

INTRODUCTION

The field of vitamin determination is undergoing rapid change. No longer are analysts limited to a few slow biological assays or to chemical methods that are of limited usefulness due to their lack of sensitivity and selectivity. The analyst today is faced with a dazzling array of methods for the determination of vitamins. There are methods using liquid chromatography, gas chromatography, mass spectrometry, infrared, visible, and ultraviolet spectroscopy, enzymes, flow injection analysis, and many others. Recently, there have been an increasing number of methods that use more than one technique, the so-called hyphenated methods, for example, the combination of gas chromatography and mass spectrometry. The problem is that the choice of the appropriate method can become very difficult since most analysts do not have the expertise to evaluate all the available techniques. It is often difficult to assess the appropriateness of any one method even if no others are available. Since most method development studies are not done under the conditions associated with the particular problems of the individual analyst, it is common that analysts will be required to do some method development or modification to solve their current problems.

Successful selection of the appropriate method, the successful development of a new method, or the successful modification of an existing method requires considerable insight into the nature of the problems and a careful use of the available resources. There are very few overviews that suggest the appropriate strategy for the selection and development of methods. Most of these are a few

1

lines or pages in general textbooks on analytical chemistry (see, e.g., references 1 and 2). Yet obviously such strategies are needed for those who do vitamin determinations. It is quite likely that the recent surge in new method development will continue for some years, and that the analysts of the future will be faced with an even more perplexing array of assay methods.

It was not always so. In the early days of vitamin assay, the methods used were mostly biological in nature. Growth rates or the lack of a pathological response were common assay techniques. The elucidation of the chemical structures and the metabolic pathways of the vitamins led to the discovery that given biological responses could be stimulated by several chemical compounds. As a result, the general concept was established that a given vitamin activity was associated with a number of chemically closely related compounds. The class of chemically similar compounds that elicited the same qualitative biological response has been called vitamers; for example, the vitamers of vitamin B_6 are pyridoxine, pyridoxal, pyridoxamine, and their respective phosphate esters. The discovery that sometimes even if the vitamers were present, the biological response was absent or was limited, led to the development of the concept of biological availability. Furthermore, it soon became apparent that while vitamers elicit the same qualitative biological response, often the quantitative responses differed with the animal species with the different chemical isomers of a vitamin. Measurement of a given vitamin activity with one species did not necessarily measure its activity in another. Obviously, more effective assay systems were needed. Fortunately, the potential for such systems was available.

Modern bioanalytical chemistry can be said to have started with the development of gas chromatography by Martin and James (3) and the amino acid analyzer by Spackman et al. (4). Since the invention of these powerful new techniques in the 1950s, the analytical chemistry of the vitamins has expanded explosively. There is now a large literature of new techniques for the assay of different vitamins and vitamers. No attempt to review the current literature will be made since it has been well covered by the other chapters in this book. Today many analysts use modern separation techniques and are determining the concentration of each separate vitamer in a sample. When the vitamin activity is needed, the quantity of each vitamer is multiplied by its biological potency for the species in question, and then the total activity is obtained by summing the individual activities as exemplified by the work of Slover et al. (5) with vitamin E assays. Presently, good methods are available for many of the vitamers in most matrices. Table 1.1 has an update of a recent evaluation of the state of the methods for vitamin assay in most matrices (6). The criteria for the evaluation of the methods were: If a qualified analyst used the best of the current methods, would the vitamin be accurately and precisely determined in food matrices?

The potential sources of errors in today's assays are many and varied. An idealized method can be flow charted as is shown in Figure 1.1 (7). Errors can enter at any place in the flow chart, and any error in any part of the assay can result in an incorrect final answer. If the wrong sample is taken, then no matter how careful the analyst is in performing the determination, the answer will

TABLE 1.1   State of Methodology for the Determination of Vitamins in 1982

Sufficient	Substantial	Conflicting	Fragmentary
	Niacin	Folacin	Biotin
	Riboflavin	Pantothenic acid	Choline
	Thiamin	Vitamin A	Vitamin K
	Vitamin C	Vitamin B_6[a]	
		Vitamin B_{12}[a]	
		Vitamin D	
		Vitamin E[a]	

[a]New methods look very promising.

probably be wrong. If the samples are improperly homogenized, then the aliquot taken will probably not be representative of the whole sample. If the extraction processes do not completely extract the vitamer(s), or if the vitamer(s) are partially or completely destroyed during the extraction, then the result will be too low. If the vitamers are not separated from each other or from interfering compounds, the results may be either low or high, depending upon the char-

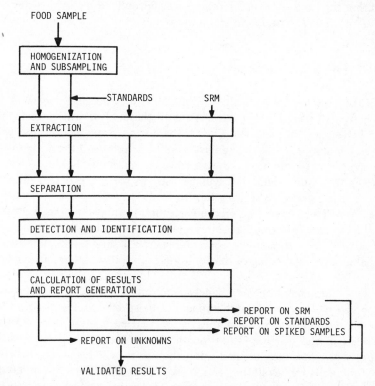

FIGURE 1.1   Flow chart for an ideal analytical method for the vitamin analysis of foods. Taken from reference 7. Reprinted by permission of Association of Official Analytical Chemists.

acteristics of the detection system. If the detection system is not selective, lacks sensitivity, is nonlinear, drifts, or measures compounds other than those desired, then the results will probably be incorrect.

Unfortunately it is often true that the calculation of the results is a major source of error. The development and preparation of the final reports from the results is another. Errors made at these stages are just as damaging as those made elsewhere. Since many assays are relative in nature, internal standards are often used to calibrate the assay systems. Errors made in the choice of these internal standards cause errors throughout the entire assay. Since ANY error can invalidate the assay, it becomes incumbent upon the analyst to ensure that the proper quality control systems are utilized. Evaluation of existing methods and development of new methods must ensure that these quality control systems exist.

It is the purpose of this chapter to present a systematic means of evaluating the critical aspects of assay techniques so that the readers may examine their existing methods, and other methods, and so that the appropriate new methods may be developed that meet the needs of the individual analyst. The concepts presented here are those of the ideal situation, and it is recognized that many of today's methods do not totally meet these standards. However, the author believes that the concepts presented here are appropriate goals for the evaluation and development of methods for vitamin assays.

CHOICE OF A METHOD

What is the best method? In all likelihood there is no single method for the determination of a specific vitamin. Usually the analyst will have to make a choice between several methods. Even if there is only one method for the assay of a given vitamin, it is still the analyst's job to determine if the assay is suitable for the specific determination. Analytical assay methods should be considered to be tools to acquire data that will be used to solve a problem or resolve a conflict. It is important to select a tool to fit the job rather than selecting a job to fit the tool. The first step in method selection is an evaluation of the external features of the situation which requires analytical determinations. These external factors are [1] general problem characteristics, [2] sample characteristics, and [3] available resources. Some of the common external factors are shown in Table 1.2.

Problem characteristics vary widely. The method used to make the determination will have a considerable impact on the specific usefulness of the results and their interpretation. It is for this reason that an analyst should ALWAYS be included in the original definition of the problem. The needed accuracy, precision, selectivity, etc., depend upon the use to which the data will be put. The best methods for regulatory actions will most likely be quite different from those used for quality control or research. Teaching methods need to be very simple and rugged. Regulatory methods need to meet the special requirements

TABLE 1.2   Factors in Problem Evaluation

General Problem Characteristics:
    End use of data
    Vitamin concentration range of importance to problem solution
    Required accuracy and precision
    Opportunity for duplicate determinations
    Documentation required
    Necessity for back-up samples
    Data validation requirements
    Method validation requirements
    Need for agreement between analysts
    Need for agreement between laboratories
    Necessity for peer acceptance of data
Sample Characteristics:
    Fragility of samples
    Maximum range of vitamin concentrations in samples
    Range of concentrations found in "routine" samples
    Needed sensitivity
    "Natural" variability of samples
    Availability of sample
    Cost of sample
    Quantity of sample that can be used for each determination
    Homogeneity of sample
    Probability of sample contamination
    Probability of interfering materials in samples
    Particle size of sample
    Toxicity of sample
    Probability of vitamer modifications with processing of the sample
    Stability of the vitamer in the sample matrix
    Use of sample after assay
Available Resource Characteristics:
    Money
    Equipment
    Computer facilities
    Training of personnel
    Space

of the law, as well as those of science. Quality control methods have special requirements of cost, speed, and the ability to be performed on site. Research methods often require very high sensitivity and can often tolerate the use of highly trained analysts. The duration of the entire project can be important. Often a careful evaluation must be made of: the implications of the effect of incorrect answers; the effects of no answers versus wrong answers; the usefulness of relative values versus absolute values; and the evaluation of the need to check for purity versus the need for quantification. These are not easy questions to address, and each problem will need to be evaluated individually. However, the analyst must face these questions if the results obtained are to meet the needs for the job. Thoughtful consideration of these and similar topics are the mark of a professional analyst.

Only after an analyst has defined the problem is it appropriate to start the detailed method selection. As in almost all scientific enterprises, the first place to go is to the scientific literature. Probably the best place to start is a broad review of the current status of the assays for the vitamer in question. This book has some excellent reviews. There are a number of other good reviews of the current methods and status of vitamin assays (6, 10–19). The food, nutrition, and biochemical literature often carry good current reviews of vitamin assays. The Association of Official Analytical Chemists (AOAC) methods manual (20) is a particularly important source of methods that have undergone thorough interlaboratory collaborative studies. For those who wish to look at the more recent studies, the abstracting journals such as Chemical Abstracts and Food Science and Technology Abstracts usually cover the greatest portion of the scientific literature pertaining to vitamin assays. The chemical, biochemical, and clinical chemical literature can be especially useful when exploring the intricacies of a chemical or biochemical method that is being considered for adaptation to a vitamin assay. Commercial and government publications should also be monitored. There are a number of good assays that have only been published in this literature. There are a number of articles that deal with the general problems of method evaluation, development, and data validation. Some recommended readings on these topics are found in references 21–30.

Novices in the field may have a tendency to only turn to the literature to find out what methods are suitable. This certainly is a sound approach and is quite often suggested in texts dealing with such matters. Nonetheless, there is an alternative, a way that is rarely mentioned in textbooks, and a way that often provides answers more quickly and more efficiently, that is, to get in touch personally with fellow analysts, be it from regulatory agencies, industry, academia, and/or suppliers. Talking with such sources, either by phone or at professional meetings, generally results in more complete information, since it is easier to provide it in this manner than by lengthy and time-consuming letter writing. Depending on the source, some caution should be exercised regarding this type of information.

Whether selecting a method from a set of existing methods or if developing a new method, the analyst needs to consider several criteria of the methods themselves to ensure that the appropriate selection is made. Method characteristics that are almost always important in method selection are given in Table 1.3.

A.   Accuracy and Precision

Usually, the most important parts of any assay are its accuracy and precision. Since these terms are commonly misunderstood, and it is important that they be properly used, it is useful to define them. The accuracy of an answer is the

TABLE 1.3   Method Characteristics

Accuracy
Precision
Sensitivity of method
Fragility of method
Method validation
Data validation
Cost factors
Peer acceptance
Safety features
Time factors

nearness it has to the correct answer. If more than one determination is made, then the accuracy of the mean value would usually be used to test the accuracy of the results. The precision of a series of results is the reproducibility of the measurements. One can have a very precise series of measurements, that is, very little variation between measurements of the analyte concentration in the same sample, and still have an inaccurate answer (for example if there was an incorrect constant term used for the calculations). Likewise, it is possible to have imprecise measurements yield an accurate result. For example, the mean of a large number of imprecise individual determinations can be an accurate value. Inaccuracies can come from many sources. Common sources are the systematic errors. These are produced by the measurement system by such factors as drift, improper calibration and calculation, and report generation errors. Errors introduced by interfering compounds are also quite common. The usual result of the presence of interfering compounds is to obtain values that are too high. This type of error is quite common in vitamin assays, obvious examples being the frequent high results obtained with the fluoresence assays for riboflavin and thiamin in cooked foods. Less frequent, but still common, are the low values obtained when some compound inhibits the response; an example would be the microbiological assay of vitamers in foods that have appreciable concentrations of antimicrobial activity. Recent work (8) has demonstrated that special problems of inaccurate answers can result from working at very low signal-to-noise ratios.

Imprecisions usually come from sample inhomogeneity, improper extraction procedures, instrument sources, and the analyst's technique or lack thereof. In evaluating the precision of an assay, particular attention must be paid to the homogenization and the extraction steps. Assay of the vitamin content of any new matrix should begin with a testing of the homogenization procedure. Instrumentation noise and drift are also common sources of imprecision. The contribution of these sources can usually be limited by making measurements with high signal-to-noise systems. The imprecision may not be due to the method, and could be a measure of the naturally occurring variability of the samples themselves. This is particularly true of the vitamin contents of fresh fruits and vegetables. In the evaluation of any given method, the analyst should immediately determine the accuracy and precision of the method over the concentration range of interest for the problem. If they are acceptable over this range, it is of only academic interest that the method is inaccurate or imprecise at concentrations outside that range.

It is usually necessary to develop a series of experiments to evaluate the accuracy and precision of the assay under the conditions to be used for the routine determinations. It is quite important that the accuracy and precision be determined with real samples and the entire assay procedure be tested. At a minimum, the analyst should check the accuracy by assaying a series of spiked samples containing a series of known different levels of the vitamer. The precision should be checked with at least several sets of pool samples containing low, medium, and high levels of the analyte. The use of pure standards to check the accuracy and precision is not a sufficient evaluation of most methods. Care should be taken that the spikes have the same chemical structure as the vitamin occurring in the sample. If there is more than one vitamin or vitamer in the sample, there should be a series of spikes for each vitamer found in the sample. The slope of the standard curve should be the same as the slope of the results of the spiked samples. Utilization of results generated from systems in which the slopes differ in pure solution from those of the spiked samples is rather dangerous.

Chromatographic assay systems should, if possible at all, include an internal standard both for calibration and quality control purposes. Internal standards should elute between the various vitamers and not at the beginning or the end of the chromatogram. They should be chemically similar to the vitamers being assayed so that factors that destroy or alter the vitamers will also affect the internal standard in the similar manner. When internal standards are used, they should be added at the earliest step possible in the assay and be carried through the entire assay procedure.

B.   Fragility of a Method

Some methods yield excellent accuracy and precision in one laboratory and very poor accuracy and precision in another. In some cases, good precision can be obtained on one day but not the next, even when the same analyst performs the determinations. In the evaluation of a method, it is quite useful to know what variation can be expected on a day-to-day basis, an analyst-to-analyst basis, or on a laboratory-to-laboratory basis. Methods that yield the same results no matter who the analyst is, or what day it is, or what laboratory does the work can be said to be rugged. Those that do not, can be called fragile. Methods vary in their fragility. While some can yield good results day in and day out with even poorly trained technicians, others are very fragile and require immense care, training and patience of very experienced analysts. In choosing a method the analyst should look at its sensitivity to the time of day, week, month, or year, check to see if the same precision and accuracy can be obtained day in and day out, and examine the reproducibility and accuracy from analyst to analyst and from laboratory to laboratory. A little time spent in such evaluation can save an enormous amount of time later.

C. Method Validation

Validation is one of the most neglected parts of method evaluation and development. Unfortunately, many authors, and even some journals, do not insure that each new or improved method has been validated both internally and by reference to another established method.

First, each method should be validated by the study of spike recoveries. A series of studies should be run that demonstrate that each vitamer of interest can be totally recovered from spiked samples. The spikes should be present at concentrations normally found in routine samples. Optimally, the slope of the response curve should be identical to the slope of the standard curve run in the absence of sample matrix. When these experiments yield the proper responses, then a series of experiments should be run demonstrating that another assay method based on a different principal yields the same answers with the same samples, preferably standard reference materials. Validation of a new method by comparison with a previously established method is a convenient manner to convince one's self and one's peers that the new method gives accurate answers. Unfortunately, agreement does not insure accuracy; both methods could be wrong. Likewise, disagreement does not necessarily indicate that the new method yields inaccurate results. It is very difficult, if not impossible, to prove the accuracy of a method. All that can be said is that two methods give comparable results, or that they do not. Probably the safest assurance of accuracy is when two different methods, based upon different chemical principals, yield the same results, then the methods have a reasonable probability of being accurate. Finally, the method should be validated by interlaboratory collaborative studies. Introduction of new methods that have not been validated can cause a great deal of confusion among today's vitamin analysts. The effort needed to validate a method is more than worthwhile when the cost of incorrect answers and/or conflicting results is considered.

D. Data Validation

Method validation is not sufficient to produce believable data. Any analyst can make a mistake even when using a validated method for vitamin determinations. Thus, to produce believable results, it is necessary to validate the individual sets of data. The data validation is accomplished most easily by using the proper quality control procedures. Today's analyst should require that a regular systematic quality control program is routinely included in any modern assay procedure.

Figure 1.1 gives the flow chart of an idealized method for vitamin determinations. With each set or batch of assays, the analyst should include AT A MINIMUM a set of pure standards and a zero sample blank. When the assays are being run as any part of any long-term study, then a pool sample or a Standard Reference Material should be included in each set of samples to be assayed. Each of these standards fulfills a different purpose. The use of pure standards insures that any change in the response of the system will be seen and thus can be taken into account when the calculations are done. The zero sample blank provides a check for baseline drift. The pool samples and/or the standard reference materials provide a means for checking for drifts due to the matrix effects. Careful workers will often include a series of spiked samples with different concentrations of added analyte to insure that the total response factor is the same for each set of samples. In those cases where it is important that the precision of the assay remain within rather tight bounds, it becomes useful to run a series of standards or spiked samples of identical concentration with each set of samples to monitor the lot-to-lot variation of the precision. Careful quality control provides validation of data and can save the analyst many painful and embarrassing moments. The time spent in developing and utilizing such procedures will usually provide ample payback.

The key to quality information is the consideration of the assay as a whole. Common problem points of assays are often left out of quality control procedures. Contamination, improper homogenization, and improper calculation procedures are common sources of error. It is not uncommon for quality control procedures to fail to catch such problems. If these procedures cannot be tested by quality control procedures, then special care has to be taken in the method development. For example, the size of the particles in a sample has a direct affect on the required sample size for homogenization. If it is impossible or impractical to have pool samples with the same particle size as the "real" samples, then special care needs to be taken with the original method development and validation to insure that the proper sample size is used for the sample homogenization. Similar care needs to be taken in other areas.

E.   Cost Factors

The key to the evaluation of the cost of an assay system is the evaluation of whether or not the results of the assay will be worth the effort and resources expended on it. Questions that need to be answered are: those that deal with the cost of the physical facilities of the laboratory; those that deal with the direct cost of the instrumentation, chemicals, and supplies; those that deal with the cost of personnel; those that deal with the computation and report generation; and those that deal with the maintenance costs.

Some of the areas that need to be addressed on the costs for physical facilities include the need for humidity and temperature control, the need for special air-handling facilities, the evaluation of the adequacy of electrical system, and an evaluation of whether or not the facility is clean enough to permit the assay to achieve the required accuracy and precision. The question of whether the installation of safety features will be required should be addressed, as should the questions about adequate lighting and adequate antivibration facilities. If a computer will be a part of the system, the analyst should check to be sure that it can be operated reliably in the laboratory. Many problems in computer operations result from dirt, vibration, moisture, the lack of proper grounds, and electrical noise. An astounding number of pieces of equipment generate electrical spikes that interfere with computer operations. The analyst should also check to be sure that the required facilities are available for sample storage, homogenization, and extraction.

Some of the questions that need to be answered about direct instrument cost include whether or not new equipment will need to be purchased or whether the existing equipment can be used. If new equipment is needed, can it then be used for other determinations? Maintenance cost should be carefully estimated. The costs of reagents need to be considered. The analyst should look at the cost of sample and reagent disposal which can be appreciable with some types of assays. The purchase costs of computational and report generation systems are often overlooked when the cost of a system is being assessed. Many modern assay systems require high-speed computer facilities with rather large memory capacities. The costs of these systems can be considerable, and there are times that their lack will cripple the productivity of the laboratory. Early evaluation of the required reports, their distribution, and archiving is also a part of the method consideration. Report generation systems can often be coupled with the computation systems, but must be included in the overall evaluation. Often these costs can be shared between several projects.

The costs of the personnel performing the assays are usually the single greatest cost of an assay system. It is extremely important that these costs be considered carefully and evaluated realistically. Careful attention needs to be paid to the degree of technical training and competence required for an assay system. Systems that require a Ph.D. as an operator will obviously be more expensive than those that only require a high school graduate. It is often the case that further specialized training is required and the cost and time required for this training should be considered. If the assay will be done over a period of time, consideration should be given to providing training for more than one analyst in order to avoid shutdown if the primary analyst leaves or becomes incapacitated. When considering personnel time, the time required for maintenance and equipment updating should also be considered. An evaluation of the expected repair and maintenance frequency is quite useful. Repair personnel often have to travel to the site of your laboratory to repair the instrumentation and computer facilities required for the assay. Estimations should be made not only on the minimum and average cost per visit, but also of the normal delay period before the repair person appears. A careful evaluation of the potential economics associated with an increase in the scale of an operation should be considered. Some assay systems can demonstrate considerable reduction in unit costs if the number of samples per batch or the number of samples per unit time can be increased. However, such savings do not always result from such scale-up and each system should be evaluated on its own merits.

F. Peer Acceptance

As is the case in many areas, appearances in vitamin assays can be as important as the facts. In many cases, it is as important that the analytical result be believed, as that it is accurate. This is quite often the case with vitamin assays. Since the vitamin assays are usually performed in response to health-related questions, an assay producing a result that is not believed by the users might as well not be done. Two requirements for producing believable data are [1] the peer acceptance of the method and [2] the validation of the data.

Peer acceptance of a method usually requires that the basic method be accepted by the analytical chemistry community. To achieve acceptance by this community requires that an adequate theoretical basis exist for the assay system, that the method has been sufficiently documented in the scientific literature (9), that the method has been given sufficient exposure for peer acceptance, and that the specific method observes the published restraints for the general assay. These requirements are obviously the same as those for the acceptance of any scientific theory or observation. The path is the same: Develop the theory, do the experiment, publish, and talk, talk, talk.

G.   Safety Features

The safety features of all laboratory procedures are receiving much more attention as modern analysts become more and more aware of hazards in the work place and of the fragility of our environment. The safety features of any assay should be carefully evaluated for the potential danger to the analyst, to other members of a laboratory, and to the environment and the general public. The dangers of radioactive material are well known and laboratories using these materials must be licensed. Other hazards are not as well known. Many compounds that are used as reagents or are by-products of an assay are carcinogenic; for example, a common product of hydrolytic enzyme assays, 6-naphthalamide, is a potent carcinogen. Some of the modern chromatographic system solvents are toxic; for example, acetonitrile is almost as toxic as hydrogen cyanide. Some compounds are explosive; for example, the commonly used bacteriostat sodium azide forms very explosive compounds in copper pipes. Many modern analytical systems use high-voltage electrophoresis; these systems have caused several deaths. Unfortunately, some analysts feel that they have done their bit for safety if they have adequate hoods or if they flush the materials down the drain. Most of these materials are as toxic in the general environment as they are in the laboratory, and care usually needs to be taken with their disposal. Unfortunately, disposal of chemical wastes has become very expensive. However, the failure to properly dispose of these compounds is even more expensive in the long run.

H.   Time Factors

The nature of the time factors of an assay is often important and can be crucial. When selecting a method, the time requirements of the problem must be met by the time attributes of the assay. The total time it will take to implement an assay once it is chosen needs to be estimated, including sufficient time for receipt of the instrumentation, the reagents, modification of the facilities, the analyst training, and the set-up and maintenance times. When evaluating the time features of an assay, the total time required for the assay needs to be determined. For kinetic or quality control operations, it is often important to know the speed of repetitive assays. For operations requiring large numbers of assays per day, it is important to know how many determinations can be made per hour. Remember when evaluating the time features of an assay to be sure to calculate the total time required for the assay. All too often analysts only include the measurement step in an assessment of the time required. Functions such as sampling, homogenization, and calculations are often more time consuming. Care taken in evaluating the time aspects of a method can save considerable time during the life of the assay.

METHOD DEVELOPMENT

It is quite common that even after a method has been chosen it will be necessary for the analyst to make some further modifications in the procedure. This is due to the difference in the problem, samples, or resources associated with the original technique and those associated with the analyst's current situation. Sometimes the analyst will conclude that no existing method will suffice and a new method will be needed. If either an improvement or a new method is needed, then the analyst needs to consider carefully the problem characteristics so that the new method's characteristics will be suitable.

The entry point into the development of a new or modified method depends upon the state of the field, the nature of the problem, and the expertise and wishes of the analyst. Figure 1.2 (7) is a flow chart for the development of an ideal analytical method. As can be seen, there are many entry points. This flow

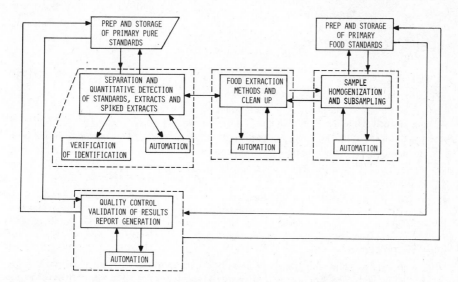

FIGURE 1.2   Flow chart for the development of an ideal analytical method. Taken from reference 7. Reprinted by permission of the Association of Official Analytical Chemists.

chart also demonstrates the interdependence of the different parts of the method and its development. All aspects of the quality control procedure are built right into the method development. This is as it should be for optimal method development. Quality control procedures can rarely be tacked onto a method after it has been completely developed. The flow chart also implies that the automation of a method should proceed right along with the method development as a whole. Automation development done during the method development can lead to a better method and often to more rapid method development. The automation and the quality control procedures are utilized in all parts of the method.

SUMMARY

The evaluation and development of analytical methods for vitamin determinations is a complex problem that requires careful evaluation of the problem at hand, the attributes of the available methods, and the resources available to the analyst. Careful consideration of these features can prevent costly errors and time delays. Proper method evaluation and development should lead to the production of believable data that will aid in the solution of the problem that originally generated the request for the assays.

ACKNOWLEDGMENTS

The author is grateful to W. R. Wolf, J. T. Vanderslice, and G. R. Beecher for penetrating discussions on various aspects of this topic.

LITERATURE CITED

1. Pickering, W. F. *Modern Analytical Chemistry.* Marcel Dekker, New York, 23–30, 37–53 (1971).

2. Christain, G. D. *Analytical Chemistry.* Xerox, Waltham, Mass. 463–469 (1977).

3. James, A. T. and Martin, A. J. P. "Gas-liquid partition chromatography: A technique of the analysis of volatile minerals." *Analyst* 77, 915 (1952).

4. Spackman, D. H., Stein, W. H., and Moore, S. "Automatic recording apparatus for use in the chromatography of amino acids." *Anal. Chem.* 30, 1190 (1958).

5. Slover, H. T., Lanza, E., and Thompson, R. H., Jr. "Lipids in fast foods." *J. Food Sci.* 45, 1583 (1980).

6. Stewart, K. K. "Problems in the measurement of organic nutrients in food products: An overview." In S. A. Margolis, Ed., *Reference Materials for Organic Nutrient Reference Materials.* Proceedings of a workshop held at the National Bureau of Standards, Gaithersburg, Md., October 23, 1980. N.B.S. Special Publication 635, National Bureau of Standards, Washington, D.C., 18–24 (1982).

7. Stewart, K. K. "Nutrient analysis of foods, the state of the art for routine analysis." In K. K. Stewart, Ed., *The State of the Art for Routine Analysis in 1979.* Proc. Symp. AOAC, October 15–18, 1979. Association of Official Analytical Chemists, Washington, D.C., 1–19 (1980).

8. Harnly, J. M. and Wolf, W.R. "Quality Assurance for Atomic Spectrometry" in *Analysis of Foods and Beverages—Modern Technique,* G. Charalambous. Ed, Academic Press, NY, 483–504 (1984).

9. Chalmers, R. A. "The analysis of a paper on analytical chemistry." In E. Wanninen, Ed., *Essays on Analytical Chemistry.* 551–557 (1977).

10. Hertz, H.S., and Chester, S.N. (Eds.) *Trace Organic Analysis: A New Frontier in Analytical Chemistry.* Proc. 9th Mater. Res. Symp., April 10–13, 1978. NBS Special Publication 519, National Bureau of Standards, Washington, D.C. (1979).

11. King, R. D. *Developments in Food Analysis Techniques—1.* Applied Science, London (1978).

12. Osborne, P. R. and Voogt, P. *The Analysis of Nutrients in Foods.* Academic Press, New York (1978).

13. Joslyn, M. A. (Ed.) *Methods in Food Analysis, 2nd ed. Academic Press, New York (1970).*

14. Pearson, D. *The Chemical Analysis of Foods,* 7th ed. Chemical, Publishing Co. Inc., New York (1977).

15. Pearson, D. *Laboratory Techniques in Food Analysis.* Butterworth, London (1973).

16. Lees, R. *Food Analysis: Analytical and Quality Control Methods for the Food Manufacturer and Buyer.* CRC Press, Cleveland (1975).

17. Macleod, A. J. *Instrumental Methods of Food Analysis.* Wiley, New York (1973).

18. *Methods in Enzymology.* Many volumes, Academic Press, New York.

19. Pomeranz, Y. and Meloan, C. E. *Food Analysis,* Rev. ed. Avi, Westport, Conn. (1978).

20. Association of Official Analytical Chemists. *Official Methods of Analysis,* 13th ed. Washington, D.C. (1980).

21. Seward, R. W. (Ed.) *Standard Reference Materials and Meaningful Measurements.* Proc. 6th Mater. Res. Symp., October 29–November 2, 1972. NBS Special Publication 408, National Bureau of Standards, Washington, D.C. (1975).

22. Youden, W. J. and Steiner, E. H. *Statistical Methods of the AOAC.* Association of Official Analytical Chemists, Washington, D.C. (1975).

23. LaFeur, P. D. (Ed.) *Accuracy in Trace Analysis: Sampling, Sample Handling, Analysis,* Vol. 1. Proc. 7th Mater. Res. Symp., October 7–11, 1974. NBS Special Publication 422, National Bureau of Standards, Washington, D.C. (1976).

24. DeVoe, J. R. (Ed.) *Validation of the Measurement Process.* ACS Symposium Series 63, American Chemical Society, Washington, D.C. (1977).

25. Massart, D. L., Dijkstra, A., and Kaufman, L. *Evaluation and Optimization of Laboratory Methods and Analytical Procedures.* Elsevier, Amsterdam (1978).

26. Inhorn, S. L. (Ed.) *Quality Assurance Practices for Health Laboratories.* American Public Association (1978).

27. Moss, M. K. and Golden, B. M. "An integrated laboratory sample/data management system." *Food Technol.* **33**(3), 46–49 (1979).

28. Garfield, G. M., Palmer, N., and Schwartzman, G. (Eds.) *Optimizing Chemical Laboratory Performance Through the Application of Quality Assurance Principles.* Proc. AOAC Symp., October 22–23, 1980. Association of Official Analytical Chemists, Washington, D.C. (1980).

29. Kateman, G. and Pijpers, F. W. *Quality Control in Analytical Chemistry.* Wiley, New York (1981).

30. Lundell, G. E. F. "The chemical analysis of things as they are." *Ind. Eng. Chem., Anal. Ed.* **5**(4), 1 (1933).

2 Biological Assays

Kenneth J. Carpenter

Biological assays with animals have been indispensable in the development of vitaminology for the isolation, purification, and identification of individual vitamins from natural sources. Physical and chemical assays determine accurately the total amounts of vitamins in food or feed samples but are valid only if the results can be related to biological activity. Traditional biological assays measure the effect on an animal's physiological processes such as reproduction, growth, storage in liver, and so on, of adding supplements to a diet lacking in only one vitamin. Other different criteria may now be used, based on the specific roles of these vitamins in metabolic reactions such as energy transfer, regulation of structural units, and so on. Biological assays are inevitably expensive and imprecise and are directly relevant only to the species used and to the dietary conditions in the assay procedure, but they do provide positive evaluations of vitamin potency and bioavailability. The bioassay is still used as a check against all other methods.

GENERAL CONSIDERATIONS

Commercially synthesized vitamins are used for supplementing or enriching both foods and feeds. Chemical assays and microbiological assays are employed to check the potency of commercial vitamin concentrates and to measure the vitamin content of foods. (The term "food" will be used to cover both foods and feeds.) The large amount of data obtained has been applied to the development of diet recommendations, and has resulted in part from studies of the effects of processing and cooking procedures, which lead to serious loss of some vitamins.

The accumulation of this data has been of great use, and has led to identification of problems in both human and livestock feeding. However, it is increasingly clear that these chemical and microbiological assays cannot answer all the questions concerned with the vitamin potency of foods.

Most vitamins exist in several different chemical forms (i.e., "vitamers"), and the proportional activities of different molecules may not be the same for the microorganism used in microbial assays as they are for humans or the other species.

The chemical differences between the various forms may appear quite small, as in the pyridoxine series: pyridoxine, pyridoxal, and pyridoxamine. In the series of compounds with vitamin K activity, these differences can be much larger: Menadione (K_3), phylloquinone (K_1), and the K_2 series where

$$-CH_2-CH=\overset{\overset{\displaystyle CH_3}{\displaystyle |}}{C}-CH_2-$$

occurs in multiples in the side chain.

There are several isomers for a single chemical form; among the tocopherols, the α-form is more potent as a vitamin than the δ-form, which has the most antioxidant activity.

Some provitamins may be of quite low, and even variable, activity as vitamin precursors in meeting the vitamin needs of man and animals. β-Carotene stands out in this respect as the main precursor in the vegetable kingdom for vitamin A. Sensitive chemical assay procedures measure accurately individual vitamers and isomers but not in terms of biopotency. However, biopotency can be calculated on the basis of the established knowledge on the chemistry and metabolism of these vitamers and isomers. Biological assays can serve as independent measures of vitamin activity and thereby confirm these estimates.

Bioavailability of vitamins from foods depends on the occurrence in free or bound forms, release in the digestive tract from the bound forms, and eventual absorption. Other components in foods may interfere with absorption, for example, phytols, isophytols, and squalene interfere with vitamin A and vitamin E absorption. Vitamin supplements usually contain vitamins mixed or dissolved in a lipid carrier medium, or stabilized with other material, or coated with protective agents to prevent potency loss during food processing. The carrier medium can lower the absorption; for example, most of the vitamin A present in a solution of vitamin A in mineral oil is not absorbed, because of the poor absorption of mineral oil that carries much of the vitamin through the digestive tract into the feces. Unless the protective coating agent is removed in the digestive tract, the coated vitamin will not be fully available for absorption. Chemical assay procedures do not duplicate the digestive process and only an animal assay will determine the availability.

Usually for a vitamin bioassay, groups of animals are first depleted of the vitamin by withholding its intake. Then known amounts of the vitamin are fed or administered, at a series of levels, to different groups of depleted animals. A standard response curve is prepared from either the response in growth or other appropriate criterion. Paralleling the groups fed known levels of vitamin, other comparable groups are fed correspondingly increasing amounts of test sample material, and the responses of the animals are recorded. The vitamin potency of the test sample is estimated by comparing this response of the animal with the standard response curve. These assays are based on the assumption that, under these comparable conditions, animals will respond similarly to equal amount of the vitamin.

Some of the various responses measured in the past are:

1. Growth rate in rats and chicks—vitamin A, pantothenic acid, riboflavin, pyridoxine, niacin, biotin, and folacin.
2. Radiographic or line test of leg bone (tibia) in rats or bone ash of leg bone (femur) in rats or center toe of one foot in chicks—vitamin D.
3. Liver storage tests in rats and chicks—vitamins A and E.
4. Resorption and gestation in female rats: number of living fetuses from dams with four or more implantation spots—vitamin E.
5. Restoration of normal cornification of the vagina in deficient female rats—vitamin A (1).
6. Correction of bleeding tendency or deficient blood coagulation in chicks—vitamin K.
7. Susceptibility of red blood cells from deficient rats to hemolysis in the presence of dialuric acid or hydrogen provide—vitamin E.
8. Percentage cure of polyneuritis in pigeons and restoration of bradycardia in rats—thiamin (2).

Both curative and prophylactic (preventive) assays are done, depending upon available facilities. However, the response, which gives the greatest precision for a given use of time and resources, is preferred.

ANIMAL ASSAYS

In the growth rate assay for vitamin A in rats, the weanling rats may have enough tissue reserves of vitamin A; so curative assay is done after feeding the animals a vitamin A-free diet for a depletion period. The index of depletion is either cessation of weight gain for a certain period or no more than a 1-g gain over a period of 4 days.

One assay where weight gain has not been the common response measure, even in fairly recent studies, has been that for vitamin D activity; the only rat bioassay still remaining in the AOAC's current edition of the Official Methods of Analysis is for vitamin D (16). Vitamin D extracted from the food is used in the assay, not the whole food, to minimize the effect of calcium and phosphorus (and presumably of any other factors affecting the availability of these minerals) present in the food, on the results. This is a curative assay with weanling rats transferred to a vitamin D-deficient diet for 18–25 days. When signs of rickets, that is, wobbly gait and enlarged joints, appear, the rats are randomized to either a standard or test treatment. The animals are sacrificed after either 7 or 10 days, and the end of a selected long bone (tibia, radius, or ulna) is cut through in a longitudinal median section and stained with silver nitrate. The degree of calcification of the metaphysis in each bone is scored by visual assessment on a scale from 0 to 12.

With one level each of standard and test material, the conclusion can only be whether or not the response to the test material is as good as that of the standard. The assay is considered invalid if the variance exceeds a certain maximum. The potency can be calculated by modifying the assay and including more than one level of both standard and test material.

Another response is based on the ash content of the rat's bones, usually the femur or humerus (3). To measure this response, a prophylatic assay is preferred with constant dosing of test material throughout the 3–6-week test period. Any exposure of the test animals to ultraviolet light results in synthesis of the vitamin under the surface of the skin; so exposure to light should be uniform for all animals.

Vitamin E deficiency in rats is characterized by a failure of the females to produce live young, and the correction of this has proved a more useful measure of vitamin E activity than has weight gain (4).

Vitamin K deficiency is characterized by a defect in blood clotting. Attempts to use this as a basis for an assay with rats have been frustrated by the influence of other variables, including protein source and coprophagy (5). These problems are not encountered with chicks (6).

With a folic acid-deficient diet, rats will not, in general, become depleted of the vitamin because of intestinal synthesis and coprophagy, but the addition of 1–2% of a sulfonamide drug such as succinylsulfathiazole to a purified diet, results in deficiency, characterized by weight loss and severe leukopenia after 3–4 weeks (7,8). The potency of test materials has been assayed either by measuring the growth response of depleted animals that are then fed the supplement continuously for a further 5 weeks (8) or by giving a succession of different doses to a single rat and comparing the maximum response to each over the following 5 days (9). The change in leukocyte count used as a second response measure does not improve the precisions of the assay.

Sulfa drugs are not effective in inhibiting the microbial synthesis of biotin in the intestines of rats. Biotin deficiency is developed by including in the diet, raw egg white as a source of avidin, a protein that binds biotin. The biological activity of pure biotin and biotin analogs can be determined by injecting these compounds subcutaneously (10). Therefore this method is not useful for the assay of biotin in foods. Chicks require dietary biotin and are used in the conventional growth assay for different sources of biotin (11,12).

Weight gain is not a satisfactory response in the biological assay of vitamin C using guinea pigs. Most assays are based on changes in the growth rate or other characteristics of their teeth. The preferred method is based on sectioning and staining incisor teeth and measuring the length of the odontoblast cells (13).

Methods now used in the biological assay of these vitamins are listed in Table 2.1 with references. In some cases, these references do not contain description of rigorous assays that could be used to measure the precision of the values. It should be easy to modify the procedures to test for linearity of response and for variability.

HUMAN ASSAYS

Despite satisfactory results from small-animal assays, it would be wrong to presume that the results must also apply to humans. Bioassay with humans is limited and we cannot deliberately induce a vitamin deficiency in subjects just to measure the relative curative effect of dietary supplements, although such experiments have been done in the past and provide unique information (34,35).

TABLE 2.1 Animal Assay Procedures to Measure Vitamin Activity of Foods and Pharmaceuticals

Vitamin	Species: Response Measured	Reference
Vitamin A	Depleted rats: weight gain	14,15
Vitamin D	Depleted rats: bone calcification	16
	Normal rats: bone ash	3
	Chicks: bone ash, alkaline phosphatase	17,18,19
Vitamin E	Rats: fetal resorption	4,20
Vitamin K	Chicks: prothrombin times	6
Ascorbic acid (Vitamin C)	Guinea pigs: length of odontoblast cells in incisor teeth	13
Thiamin	Rats: weight gain and enzyme activity	21
Riboflavin	Depleted rats: weight gain	22
	Chicks: weight gain	23
Pantothenic acid	Rats: weight gain	24,25
	Chicks: weight gain	26
Pyridoxine (Vitamin B_6 complex)	Rats: weight gain and enzyme assay	27,28
	Chicks: weight gain	23
Niacin	Rats: weight gain	29
Biotin (Vitamin H)	Rats: weight gain (chemicals given by injection only)	10
	Chicks: ordinary weight gain assay	11,12,30
Folacin (Pteroylglutamic acid)	Rats: weight gain	8,9
	Rats: levels of vitamin in liver	31
	Chicks: weight	23
Cobalamin (Vitamin B_{12})	Depleted mice: weight gain	32
	Depleted chicks: weight gain	33

Currently, a combination of physicochemical methods is used to measure the urinary excretion of vitamins and their metabolites, and/or blood vitamin levels to establish the bioavailability (36).

For many water-soluble vitamins, urinary excretion of the vitamin or its metabolites reflects the subject's nutrient status with regard to that vitamin (37). In other words, a depleted subject shows little excretion but this increases with dosing of the vitamin or any of its precursors, such as tryptophan in the case of niacin. If the vitamin is given in a form that cannot be absorbed or metabolized, there will not be any corresponding increase in urinary excretion. The response to a test dose is so rapid that the same subject can be used for a succession of tests.

Urinary analysis could, in theory anyway, miss a vitamin that was as biologically active as the one that was being measured, or it could be that the chemical procedure was not as specific as had been thought and was also measuring a biologically inactive analog of the vitamin. This approach is therefore not as satisfactory in principle as an assay measuring a physiological response, such as weight gain, which is quite independent of any assumptions about the chemistry of the vitamin, or the validity of an analytical procedure.

A study on the bioavailability of vitamin B_6 from an average American diet (38) gave the following results in summary:

Study period	Diet	Vitamin B_6 Intake (μg/day)	Vitamin B_6 Urinary Excretion (μg/day)
1. 36 days	Formula	1100	48
2. 36 days	Average American	2300	87
3. 36 days	Formula	2700	130

Six adult subjects were used and 24-hr samples of urine were collected. The vitamin content of urine and the diets were estimated by microbiological assay with *Saccharomyces carlsbergensis*. The extract of the food was used after it had been autoclaved in dilute acid. Urine collected during the latter half of each period was used in the assay. Pyriodoxine hydrochloride was used to supplement the purified formula diets.

By interpolation, the authors estimated that for a resulting urinary excretion of 87 μg/day the intake from a purified diet would be about 1860 μg/day. Since the actual daily intake on the American diet was 2,300 μg, they estimated that its availability was approximately 80% of that for the pure vitamin. This a simplification of the actual calculations, for which the reader is referred to the original paper (38).

No estimate of the standard error of this estimate was calculated, only the range when values for each subject were calculated separately. It was not possible to calculate a valid estimate of error because the treatments were not allocated at random, that is, each subject received the three treatments in the same order.

A similar procedure was used for measuring the bioavailability of pantothenic acid (38).

In studies on the bioavailability of different forms of folacin, it was found necessary to "saturate" the subjects with daily doses of the pteroylmonogluta-mate form of the vitamin. Then, when a single test dose of 0.5–1.0 mg of folacin in different form was given at breakfast, the urinary response was complete within 24 hr. For pteroylmonoglutamate, the recovery was about 25%. *Lactobacillus casei* was used in the assay of urines, which were not treated with conjugase enzyme (39).

There are many shortcomings in these assays which depend on chemical or microbiological procedures to measure the subjects' response.

BASIC FEATURES IN BIOLOGICAL ASSAYS

To ensure reproducible results, biological assays should be designed carefully to use the most appropriate response and to minimize elements of systematic error. The basic feature in conducting efficient and successful biological assays are:

1. Experimental design.
2. Environment and equipment.
3. Experimental animals—choice and care.
4. Basal and experimental diets and test material.

These features have been reviewed in earlier publications (40–42) and are still valid for biological assays with small animals.

A. Experimental Design

An appropriate biological response and the most suitable animal species are chosen for the assay of the specific vitamin. This response should increase or decrease with a change in dose or log dose of the vitamin. Measurement of this response and the number of animals used in the assay should be adequate for statistical evaluation and interpretation of results. Random errors are so much larger in bioassays for vitamins than in chemical analyses that it is essential to choose conditions that minimize these errors. These aspects are discussed with suitable examples.

The range of response of the animals to dosage with different levels of the vitamin being studied should be as large as possible in relation to the between-animal variability in response to the same level of vitamin. For assays with a "linear response" the appropriate measure is "within-treatment standard deviation of response: range of response over the range of doses used." Finney in section 8.6 of his book (43), discusses the quantity "$s/b_s X$" without attaching a symbol to it. The author calls it the κ (kappa) value (29), and these data from a niacin assay illustrate its use:

	After 14 Days	After 20 Days
Wt. gain/cage on basal diet (g)	11	12
Wt. gain/cage on highest vitamin level (g)	74	122
Range of response (g)	63	110
Within-treatment standard deviation of gain per cage	9.6	11.4
Kappa values	0.152	0.104

The kappa value should be kept as small as possible.

The standard deviation of the rats' weight gain was higher after 20 days than after 14 days, but the increase in range of response was proportionally greater still, so that the k value was less. The assay will therefore be more efficient at 20 days than at 14 days.

Similar comparisons can be made of the efficiency of using one or another response when both have been tested in the same assay. For example, the data below are for a chick assay in which both plasma calcium levels and "% bone ash" have been measured (19).

	Plasma Ca (mg/100 mL)	Bone Ash (%)
Value of Basal diet	4.92	4.16
Value on highest standard	6.05	7.66
Range of response	1.13	3.50
Within-treatment standard deviation	0.19	0.14
Kappa value	0.168	0.041

The kappa value for the "bone ash" procedure is only one-quarter that for the "plasma calcium" procedure. Obviously precision can also be improved by using more animals, that is, greater replication, but only in proportion to the square root of the number. Thus, it would take 16 times as many chicks to obtain the same degree of precision using plasma calcium as the response measure. Another way to increase precision is to choose doses of test material to give, as nearly as possible, the full range of linear response obtained with the standard. For a given design and number of replications, this will give the minimum "coefficient of variation" (c.v.) of potency estimate.

Under many assay conditions, the response to stepwise increments in vitamin dosage shows a gradual decrease at higher levels, and the lower range in which the response is linear is too small for an efficient assay. Under these conditions, it has been found useful to express the doses of standard and test material on a logarithmic basis. The "log dose" values should then be plotted against response. An example of data plotted with and without the doses being converted to logarithms is given in Figure 2.1.

Typically, the use of logarithms puts a higher portion of the response curve into a linear relationship, but the common blank is unusable. Also, on a logarithmic plot the test and standard responses are not exactly linear on a log scale. The curves should lie parallel to each other at a constant distance apart in the direction of the x axis, and it is the distance that gives the ratio of activities of test and standard. It is for this reason that they are named "parallel line assays." Standard deviation or λ (lambda) measures the relative efficiency of different assay conditions; λ is roughly equivalent to the κ value already discussed for slope-ratio assays. Since increments on the log scale do not have a dimension, λ can be expressed as s/b, where s is the standard deviation of the response within a treatment level and b is the mean increase in response per unit increment in dose.

To determine the shape of the dose-response curve, 5–6 graded levels of vitamin should be administered to similar but individual groups of animals and the response used to develop the curve. But once the limits for obtaining a linear response (either as a straight or logarithmic plot) have been determined, it appears that having two levels of both test and standard is most efficient, with a blank added only if it is a slope-ratio assay linear through the blank (43). If there is considerable doubt about the likely potency of a test material it may, of course, be useful to use a wider spread of doses, while realizing that the only usable results will be those for which the responses come within the limits of the responses to the standards. Accordingly the number of animals required for the assay will be determined. The experimental design is then set up with the required number of animals, dose levels of standard vitamins and assay samples, and the measurement of most suitable and precise response. Statistical methods in bi-

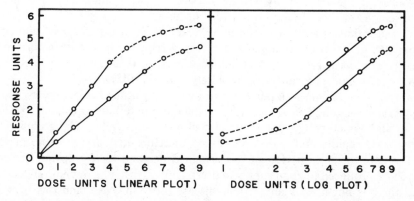

FIGURE 2.1 Response of increase in dosages of vitamins plotted with and without doses being converted to logarithims.

ological assay of vitamins, and the validity and meaning of biological assays have been reviewed (44–47).

B. Environment and Equipment

Animal room facilities should be adequate to keep the experimental animals comfortable and healthy. It will be advantageous to maintain these facilities conforming to the regulations of the Good Laboratory Practices of the U.S. Food and Drug Administration. Separate space should be available for feed mixing, equipment cleaning, waste disposal, autopsy, etc. Experimental animal rooms should be temperature controlled between 70°F and 75°F, with an optimum relative humidity of about 45% and with a range between 40–70%. Ventilation should be adequate with a flow rate of 0.25 ft³ fresh or purified air per animal with minimal drafts over the animals. Lighting should be adequate, uniform, and shut off for an 8-hr period during nights. Sanitation procedures should be adequate and should vary depending upon the animal species. Different species should be housed in different rooms.

Animal cages can be selected from any of the many commercial manufacturers. The size of the cage depends on the animal species, age of experimental animals, and the number of animals caged together. Experimental rats are housed individually in screen floored cages with individual feeders and watering devices; this minimizes coprophagy. Chick assays are conducted in group cages, but each cage can only provide one independent unit for statistical analysis.

C. Experimental Animals—Choice and Care

The choice of experimental animals is limited to the species best suited for the specific vitamin; depending on the response measured, more than one species can be used. Rats, mice, chicks, and guinea pigs are commonly used. It is more advantageous to obtain animals from commercial sources than to maintain breeding colonies. Good, healthy, parasite- and pathogen-free animals are needed. Commercial sources will provide the necessary genetic information, as well as the average weights of animals at different ages.

Conscientious attention to the needs and health of experimental animals is as important as strict compliance with assay requirements. Satisfactory maintenance of records regarding food intake, temperature and humidity conditions, and experimental procedures is absolutely essential (48).

When there has been opportunity to use any of a number of species, the rat has usually been the first choice. It is reasonably small, but big enough to handle easily and tame enough not to require gloves or special catching equipment. Rats breed rapidly and with large litters, therefore they are cheap to produce and to care for and, in view of the sustained demand for them, they are commercially produced in good supply in inbred lines. Although not entirely disease-free, there is not usually any serious disease problem. Also, and this is crucial in nutritional studies, rats show remarkably similar calorie intakes when offered different diets ad libitum containing a wide variety of individual foods.

Mice are even cheaper than rats and breed even faster. But they have some disadvantages. Technically, it is more difficult to measure their food consumption. They are generally less tame, and more difficult to handle. Last, a mouse colony has a strong smell and laboratory workers can absorb this smell on their clothes. Mouse assays were used on a large scale in elucidating the "animal protein factor," vitamin B_{12} (33).

Because of their slow reproduction rate and the requirement of a fairly high-roughage diet, guinea pigs are used for biological assays only when there is no possibility of using rats or mice. In practice, this restricts their use to assays for vitamin C for which guinea pigs alone, amongst available small animals, have a requirement.

The use of dogs is very expensive, and monkeys even more so, though these have been used on occasions in the belief that these are a closer model for humans than rodents are.

Poultry are obviously the species of choice when materials are being assayed for their potency in poultry diets. Chick bioassays continue to be used for vitamin D, and the different procedures have been reviewed (17,18,19). It is known that the first compound (vitamin D_2 or calciferol) produced on a large scale by irradiation of ergosterol and distributed as a potent source of vitamin D activity was almost inactive for chicks, although it was as active as the naturally occurring vitamin D_3 for the rat and for humans. Chicks have been used for the assay of biotin, pantothenic acid, vitamin B_{12}, other B vitamins, and vitamin K (6,23,26,30,34,49).

Laboratory workers have sometimes been afraid of using the chick as a test animal, assuming that broiler production-type housing will be needed. In fact, chicks can be kept in raised wire cages similar to those used for rats, but with a slot in the front panel through which the birds can reach a feed container fitted outside. Such cages have been illustrated (50). Chicks grow more uniformly if housed two or three together rather than if kept singly, but do not require to be in larger groups. Males from egg-laying strains can be bought very cheaply when day old. These birds are then best kept for a minimum of 4 days in a large group to learn feeding from a container and to allow elimination of weaklings. The growth potential is then even greater than that of the young rat, and an efficient experiment can be performed in relatively short period. The only hardship for attendants is that, when chicks are in open cages, the room temperature must be as high as 80°F for the first 10 days.

D. Basal and Experimental Diet

Biological assays for vitamins depend upon a suitable basal diet that is nutritionally complete except for one experimental variable, which is the vitamin to be assayed; this basal diet will be different for each animal species used in the assay. In the past, purified natural products were used; but interaction amongst the nutrients, such as the sparing action of tocopherols in repressing the oxidation of carotenoids and retinols in the digestive tract, and the influence of calcium, and phosphorus and vitamin D requirement, led to the formulation of semisyn-thetic diets.

Each basal ration consists of three major ingredients, carbohydrate, protein, and fat, and a suitable mixture of vitamin supplements and minerals, including essential trace metal salts. The basal diet must be from the same batch for all comparable test groups.

During the depletion period, the diet contains all nutrients except the vitamin to be assayed; the vitamin will be added to the diet of control group of animals and the test material will be added to the diet of experimental animals.

E. Animal Suffering and Human Ethics

It is difficult to maintain a sense of proportion on this subject; persons working with animals must face up to the issue sometime or other. Persons totally opposed to any kind of experimentation with animals accuse the vitamin analysts of being "vivisectionists" ready to commit any cruelty in the name of science. The vitamin researchers tend to ignore this issue, since vitamin assays do not literally involve vivisection. However, the methods that involve induction of deficiency states such as rickets or scurvy do result in some suffering to animals. So an efficient assay with the smallest number of required animals should be done within the shortest time period possible, and only after making sure that other analytical methods are not available. Animal house technicians should be trained to handle animals with care, avoiding needless suffering to these animals.

F. U.S. Government Regulations

Although the regulations under the Good Laboratory Practices for nonclinical studies do not generally apply to these types of biological assays, the regulatory agencies may audit the procedures if the results from the above assays are submitted in support of any petition. Therefore, it is advisable to conform to these regulations (51).

A TYPICAL ANIMAL ASSAY—NIACIN

A typical biological assay for niacin is presented here, taking into account basic features discussed previously. Chemical study of most cereal foods (whole wheat, rice, maize meal, etc.) indicates that the niacin (i.e., nicotinic acid and nicotin-amide) is present in bound forms that are only released by refluxing the foods under either acid or alkaline conditions. Maximum values for the niacin content of these foods are obtained by first autoclaving them with a solution of calcium hydroxide. There is controversy as to whether or not these "maximum" values best reflect the nutritional values of foods as a source of niacin because it is uncertain whether or not the bound forms are available to humans and animals. This can only be studied by a biological assay (29).

A. Choice of Animal Species

Chicks, rats, and mice are all cheap to use and can all be made niacin-deficient. The chick is farthest from humans on the evolutionary scale and therefore less desirable, other things being equal. Rats were chosen because it is found to be easier to measure their food consumption.

There are some differences in niacin nutrition between rats and humans. Deficient rats do not show the characteristic dermatitis and intestinal changes seen in human pellagra. Deficiency in the young rat shows up only as depressed growth and a rather nonspecific nervousness and roughness of coat. Another difference is the readiness with which tryptophan can be metabolized to nicotinamide. Most vertebrates metabolize a small proportion of free tryptophan, present in the tissues to niacin. Therefore a dietary deficiency of niacin can be compensated by increasing tryptophan levels in the diet. The extent of this tryptophan-niacin conversion at a given tryptophan level (expressed in relation to total dietary intake) differs in different species. Other amino acids influence this conversion; the higher the levels of these amino acids, the lower the conversion. When the tryptophan intake is relatively low, rats are able to obtain the niacin requirements from this source much better than humans. These differences do not seem to affect niacin availability and weight gain can be used as the response measure.

These species differences need not invalidate a rat assay provided that the test diets do not differ to any significant extent in the content of both tryptophan and other amino acids that might influence tryptophan metabolism.

B. Formulation of a Niacin-Deficient Diet

All the test materials and the protein sources chosen for the basal diet were analyzed for tryptophan content; literature values were used for the other amino acids and for the digestibility of the protein in each material. The diets were balanced in terms of digestible nutrients rather than total nutrients.

Deciding on the level of tryptophan for the test diets was a problem since it is needed for the growth of lean tissue (i.e., to permit weight gain) but, as discussed above, a generous intake will remove the need for dietary niacin. The diet shown in Table 2.2 was selected (52).

Casein and gelatin were chosen as the protein sources for the basal diet because these are easily obtained, reasonably priced, fairly constant in composition, and free from suspicion of toxicity. Free amino acids were added to meet the full requirements of the rat at the chosen protein level. The rest of the diet was formulated to contain at least the full requirement for young rats of each nutrient other than tryptophan and niacin. The levels of vitamins and minerals were taken from a review dealing with the requirements of laboratory animals (53). Most early assay experiments were done with vitamin and mineral mixes that are now known to lack some essential nutrients such as zinc, selenium, and folacin. In most cases, this probably made no difference because the animals

TABLE 2.2 Composition of the Basal Diet Used for the Assay of Niacin with Rats

Constituent	Amount (g/kg)
Casein (vitamin-free)	70
Gelatin	65.5
Corn oil	30
Amino acid supplement[a]	15.9
Vitamin supplement[b] (niacin-free)	5
Major mineral mix[c]	52
Trace mineral mix[d]	3
Sucrose	to 1000

[a]This consisted (in g) of the following L-amino acids: tryptophan, 0.21 (bringing the total level in the diet to 0.97 g/kg); lysine, 0.03; methionine, 1.56; cystine, 2.42; isoleucine, 1.65; leucine, 2.52; phenylalanine, 2.69; tyrosine, 1.34; histidine, 0.27; threonine, 2.08; and valine, 1.11.

[b]This was made up (in mg) of a retinyl palmitate concentrate (25,000 IU/g), 30.0; a Dl-α-tocopheryl acetate concentrate (500 IU/g), 120; menadione, 2.0; choline chloride, 1000; calcium pantothenate, 12.0; thiamin HCl, 4.0; riboflavin, 5.0; pyridoxine HCl, 9.4; folic acid, 2.0; a cobalamin premix (0.1% in mannitol), 20; and corn starch to 5000 mg.

[c]This was made up (in g) of KH_2PO_4, 17.4; $CaCO_3$, 11.5; $CaHPO_4$, 4.83; NaCl, 12.7; $MgSO_4$, 2.5; and corn starch to 52 g.

[d]This was made up (in mg) of $CuSO_4 \cdot 5H_2O$, 24.0; NaF, 1.0; ferrous citrate, 300; KIO_3, 0.4; $MnSO_4 \cdot 4H_2O$, 224; ZnO, 23.0; Na_2SeO_3, 0.09; and corn starch to 3000 mg.

had reserves to carry them through a short experiment; intestinal microbial synthesis and coprophagy could also provide some vitamins. It seems poor practice still to include chemicals such as inositol and p-aminobenzoic acid, which are not needed for higher animals.

Rats grow well on purified-type diets of widely varying fat content. Their requirement for essential fatty acids will be fully supplied by 3% of vegetable oils rich in polyunsaturated fatty acids, for example, cottonseed, corn, soy, or peanut oil. Including a somewhat higher level reduces the dustiness of diets and also leaves a margin of substitution. Thus, if the material under test contributes a significant amount of lipid, the level of standard oil can be reduced to keep the total lipid content constant. One upper limit to the level of fat is that liquid oils tend to settle out from a mix at a level of over 15%, and fats that are solid at room temperature tend to form lumps during diet mixing. An unstable oil may also oxidize quite rapidly when in contact with constituents of the mineral mix. The rancid products may reduce palatability of the diet and also its digestibility. Thus, the diets cannot be stored for long periods and, in some cases, the addition of an antioxidant (such as ethoxyquin) to the fat may be advantageous.

The choice of carbohydrate in the diet can also be important. Monosaccharides, particularly, give rise to high osmotic values in the fluid contents of the stomach and can reduce voluntary food intake. Lactose is poorly digested by the weaned rat and causes diarrhea and other problems when fed at a high level. Where test materials are likely to contribute high levels of carbohydrate to some diets, it would seem best to have similar carbohydrates in the basal diet so that, by substitution, there will be little difference in the final carbohydrate content of the different diets.

Sucrose was used in this study, and it would have been better to use a mixture of sucrose, cooked starch, and some 5% of cellulose as a source of fiber.

C. Testing the Response to the Pure Vitamin

Before beginning to assay test materials, optimal dose levels at which the test animals give a clear-cut linear response to the pure vitamin must be established. Wistar male rats, 21 days old, were used. There was no special reason for using male rats rather than females, except that males grow slightly faster and were available in the quantities required. If both sexes were to be used, then these would be allocated in a balanced design across all treatments, requiring a more complicated statistical analysis.

Niacin is one of the vitamins that is not stored to any great extent so that a deficiency condition appears in young rats within a few days of their being put on to a deficient diet. Figure 2.2 shows growth curves of rats that were transferred immediately on arrival to the basal diet and then, after 4 days, given various levels of supplementary nicotinic acid. It is conventional to refer to such figures as "growth curves" even though what is measured is body weight rather than length, the usual measure of human growth.

The results indicate the wide spread of growth rates with a diet containing 0.097% tryptophan from very little gain with no vitamin supplement to an average of 3.0 g/day with the highest supplement. The potential growth rate of young rats of this strain on this diet is 4–5 g/day. As the added nutrient level approaches the optimum, a standard increment gives only a smaller extra response.

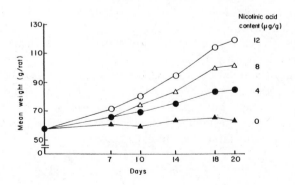

FIGURE 2.2 Growth rates of rats receiving the basal diet with different levels of supplementary nicotinic acid for 20 days.

D.   Formulation of Test Diets

After establishing satisfactory assay conditions and a linear growth response over a range of supplementation from 0 mg/kg to 12 mg/kg niacin, diets containing the test materials, were formulated. It is necessary to test each material at two levels at least. If the material contains a toxic, growth-depressant factor, there is no way of knowing that a small response to a single level of supplementation is due to this. With two levels of feeding, it would be detected because the higher level would not give a proportionally greater response due to the increasing effect of the toxic factor.

Common beans (*Phaseolus vulgaris*) and corn were two test materials; both were cooked in water and freeze-dried; the niacin content of each by chemical procedure was about 20 mg/kg. Test diets contained 215 g and 430 g beans or corn per kg. The protein present in the test materials contributes significant quantities of tryptophan and other amino acids. Hence isonitrogenous amounts of casein were removed from test diets containing beans/corn and the diets were rebalanced with free amino acids; each diet contributed the same amount of each essential amino acid. Two other test materials were also tested.

The assay will be valid only if the responses to the test materials are within the range of responses to the standard vitamin levels.

E.   Conduct of the Assay

The experiment required 96 rats; 104 were purchased to allow for elimination of any that were abnormal or extreme in weight. On arrival, the rats were placed in individual wire cages, 18 (height) $\times$ 25 (depth) $\times$ 18 (width) cm, suspended in racks so that feces and urine fell through the wire floor to sawdust-covered trays some 2 in. below. Each cage was fitted with an inverted water bottle from which the rat could drink by licking the nipple. A food pot containing the dry, powdered basal diet was placed on the floor of the cage. The pot had a lid with a large hole in it that allowed the rat to put in its head to eat, but made it more difficult for him to scrape out the food in search of something different at the bottom. Where possible, a rat that spilt a significant amount of food at this stage was eliminated from the experiment.

After 4 days, the rats were weighed individually to the nearest gram. More precise weighing is pointless because of hour-to-hour fluctuations in live weight with defecation, urination, and feeding. The balance needs to be well damped as the animals will make some movements even if held in a box. A digital, electronic balance is ideal but expensive and not essential. After eliminating any that looked abnormal, the number was reduced to 96 by removing those of extreme weight. Due to limitations in cage accommodation, two rats were put in each cage.

From the 96 rats, the 24 heaviest were first allocated at random to the 12 cages on the top level of the frame for holding the cages. The 12 diets were then allocated to them, again at random, from a table of random numbers. The next

24 heaviest were distributed in the next layer of cages and so on. Other methods of randomization could have been used but the essential points are:

1. The cages for a particular treatment are not all together in one portion of the rack. The animals could possibly be more subject to infection or some other stimulus, such as light or air currents than those on some other treatments.

2. The rats on one treatment cannot, even inadvertently, have been chosen with any kind of bias. This has been known to occur when people have put a hand into a group of animals to take out first all the animals of one treatment. The ones remaining for the last treatments are then the best "dodgers" and may well also be unrepresentative in other ways.

The "stratification" or "blocking" by starting weight was used in this experiment because the weights varied from 40 g to 60 g. It can never be wrong to stratify in this way when one can distinguish some variable that may possibly influence performance in the assay. In this present example, the final statistical analysis showed no influence from the combined effects of cage level and initial weight, but nothing had been lost. When animals of both sexes have to be used, it would certainly be appropriate to balance the experiment by "blocking" for sex, that is, insuring that each treatment had the same proportion of males and females assigned to it.

After recaging, the rats were reweighed as a check and then given the test diets. These were again provided ad libitum, that is, always available so that each rat could eat all it wished. It has been a matter of continuing debate as to whether or not ad libitum feeding experiments give valid comparisons of the nutritional value of different diets, rather than a combination of nutritional value and palatability. Because of the obvious effect of food intake on growth it is customary to measure "weight gain per g food eaten" rather than "weight gain" alone in ad libitum experiments. Even this measure, sometimes called "food efficiency" (FE), would fail with severely depressed food intake. However, the rat is less discriminating than most species, and on most diets its calorie intake is closely proportional to its metabolic size (body weight to the power $^{2}/_{3}$). This can be checked by calculation of "appetite quotients" for different diets (54). Where this rule holds true it means that rats growing less will also eat less, but that the lower food intake is the result of the rats remaining smaller rather than the cause of it.

Where food consumption is being measured, there has to be a way of measuring the spilt food. One sometimes sees a rat battery where food from a high cage is actually falling into a lower cage; this creates a double problem. In this study, food consumption was measured every 2 days, with more diet being added to the pots at those times. The rats were weighed twice a week. The intermediate weighings were not used in any final calculations but they provide early warnings of any potential problem. The practice also ensures that every rat is handled regularly and that any abnormality such as an infected eye is quickly spotted.

A common problem is a stoppage in a water bottle that deprives a cage of water for 1 or more days. This should, of course, be prevented daily by inspection of the animals and the water bottles.

On day 20 of the test period, the animals were weighed, put back in their cages, and then independently reweighed to eliminate any recording error of a single observation. The food pots were removed overnight before the final weighing to minimize the effect of variable gut fill on body weight.

F.   Analysis of the Results

After tabulating the results for weight gain and food consumed, food efficiency was calculated and the results graphed in the way shown in Figure 2.3. There has been a progressive response to increasing levels to the standard and of the test materials; the response to the latter has been within the range of responses to the standards, and the responses to increasing levels of each supplement were essentially linear.

The data were subjected to an ordinary two-way analysis of variance. There had been no significant effect of stratification of the rats on their subsequent response. It also showed that treatment differences were highly significant and that the pooled estimate of the standard error of each treatment mean was 0.18 g/day.

Since the responses appeared to be linear, the final potency was calculated according to Finney's slope-ratio procedure (43). The calculation was in this case carried out on a specially written computer program and the analysis

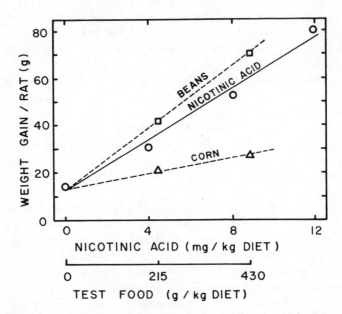

FIGURE 2.3   Graph showing relation of results for weight gain and food consumed.

indicated that all the criteria were satisfied. The potencies of the test materials were then calculated from the ratio of their regression slopes of "response against dose" to the slope of the response to the pure vitamin. Thus, the beans gave a slope ratio of 0.135 g/g of beans in 1 kg of diet, whereas pure niacin gave a slope of 5.38 g/mg niacin in 1 kg of diet. From the ratio of these two, the calculated potency of the beans is 25 mg niacin/kg. The standard error of this estimate was 1.8 mg/kg, calculated according to Equation 7.21 in Section 7.6 of Finney's book (43). For the corn, the calculated potency was 6 mg/kg.

Professional statistical advice was obtained for carrying out these calculations. Rough calculations of potency were done from graphed results. These provided a simple check for some types of computation error, such as putting the dose levels into the computer with a decimal point in the wrong position.

G. Overall Conclusions From the Study

Results summarized in Table 2.3 from a series of assays indicate that mature grains cooked at neutral pH gave rat assay values significantly lower than their total niacin content determined chemically. This confirms earlier studies, that niacin, found mostly in chemically bound forms in these foods, is of low availability to the rat. The results with foods in which the niacin is present largely as nicotinic acid and nicotinamide, indicate that the rat assay can provide data

TABLE 2.3   Rat Bioassay Values for Niacin in Relation to Chemical Analyses for Both "Free" and "Total" Niacin

	Niacin Values (Expressed as nicotinic acid) (mg/kg)			
	Chemically Free	Total (Free + Bound)	Rat Bioassay	Availability of Bound Form(s)[a]
Cereal foods				
Boiled milo	ND[b]	46	16	0.35
Boiled wheat	ND	57	18	0.32
Concentrate from wheat bran	ND	2800	480	0.17
Boiled rice	17	71	29	0.22
Boiled corn	1	19	6.8	0.32
Tortillas	12	13	14	—
Noncereal foods				
Baked potatoes	18	65	26	0.17
Baked liver	297	306	321	—
Freeze-dried instant coffee	315	597	417	0.36

[a]The ratio is calculated on the assumption that the free niacin portion is fully available. Thus, for boiled rice the ratio is calculated as $(29 - 17)/(71 - 17)$.

[b]ND means "not detected."

comparable to chemical analysis. The slightly higher bioassay values for beans may reflect a recognized problem in the colorimetric analysis of this material using the König reaction.

A TYPICAL HUMAN ASSAY—NIACIN

In studying the bioavailability of the "bound niacin" in different foods, it is important to establish that a material which had its niacin in a form of low availability for rats also had a low availability for humans (55). The material chosen was a concentrate of soluble, "bound niacin" prepared from wheat bran. Fed at a low level, this concentrate would contribute only negligible quantities of protein, requiring no adjustment to the basal diet.

Three subjects were used for 40 days; the subjects were scientists continuing their normal activities. Three materials were tested on each subject, using the "urinary metabolite" type of assay.

As with the rat assay, the basal diet must provide a constant daily intake of available niacin and also of trypophan and the other essential amino acids. A level of 20 mg niacin equivalent intake (i.e., niacin + 'tryptophan ÷ 60') per day was chosen. This just met the U.S. Recommended Dietary Allowance and was also expected to correspond to a point on the dose-response curve for urinary metabolites where, with an additional intake of available niacin, a large proportion would be recovered in the urine.

The diets were chosen to be as palatable as possible and excluded items that could be sources of variation of "niacin equivalent" intake. Thus, meat and fish were omitted and bread was made from special nonenriched white flour. The midday meal consisted of "formula" drink that served as a vehicle for providing supplementary minerals and vitamins (other than niacin). Only water could be drunk in addition to the diet. Coffee, in particular, can be a significant source of the vitamin.

Test doses contained niacin, which was still within the normal range of total daily intake. Large supplements could disrupt the normal mechanisms for absorption and metabolism. One portion of the concentrate was mixed with corn starch and water and baked at neutral pH, as for most cereal foods, and another portion was given the same treatment but with added calcium hydroxide (as in the production of Mexican and Central American tortillas). The second treatment resulted in the niacin being released from its bound form(s) and served as one positive control. The third test material was pure nicotinic acid.

From the literature and from a short preliminary test, it was found that a 14-day preliminary period of the basal diet should bring urinary excretion down to a plateau level; and so 24-hr urines were collected from day 6 on. Exactly 10% of each voiding was collected in plastic bottles containing two drops of an antimicrobial agent; each 24-hr period ended with the first morning voiding at 7 A.M. The final volumes in the bottles were then measured in the laboratory and the samples frozen until analyzed.

On days 14 and 15, each subject received one of the test doses spread over the 2 days, each total dose containing 35 mg niacin (except for the pure nicotinic acid which was only 24 mg). Urine continued to be collected each day. It was expected that the urinary response to the doses would be complete in 4–5 days and that excretion would return to plateau levels after that. The subjects were then given their second dose on days 22–23 and their third dose on days 30–31. The doses were given in a different order to each subject.

Each sample of urine was then analyzed in duplicate for the two main niacin metabolites, N^1-methylnicotinamide and N^1-methyl-2-pyridone-5-carboxamide and the total of the two calculated as niacin equivalents. A typical set of results for one subject is shown in Figure 2.4. The above-plateau response summed for the 6 days following each dose is set out in Table 2.4. The differences between treatments were significant. However, when the urines were analyzed for their creatinine content and the daily excretion of metabolites expressed "per mg creatinine," the residual variability was reduced and the treatment differences became highly significant. Presumably this must reflect the existence of collection errors such as errors in taking 10% fractions, or the morning collections going occasionally into the next day's bottle rather than the previous day's bottle.

Since the response to the bound niacin preparation was equivalent to only 24% of the dose and the average response to the two doses containing only free niacin was 76%, it was concluded that the phenomenon of "bound niacin" in a variety of foods, being of low availability to rats, could be duplicated in humans. Since there was no graded response curve to different levels of standard vitamin, it was not possible to calculate a statistically valid bioassay value. Nor did this

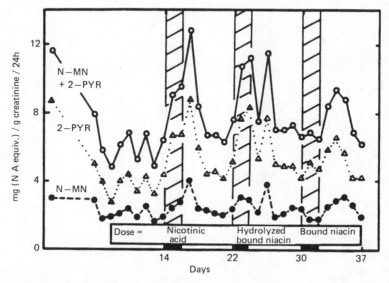

FIGURE 2.4 Excretion of the niacin metabolites N^1-methylnicotinamide (N-MN) and N^1-methyl-2-pyriodone-5-carboxamide (2-PYR) in relation to creatinine excretion with intermittent test doses containing niacin in different forms.

TABLE 2.4 The Mean Additional Excretion of Niacin Metabolites, Expressed As Nicotinic Acid Equivalents, Over the Six Days Following Test Doses Spread Over Two Days[a]

	Test Dose			Statistical Analysis	
	35 mg "Bound Niacin"	35 mg "Bound Niacin" Hydrolyzed with Lime	24 mg Pure Nicotinic Acid	Pooled Residual S.E. of Treatment Means	F Ratio for Treatment: Residual Variances
A. mg Metabolite/Subject					
N^1-methyl nicotinamide (N-MN)	2.2	3.2	3.8	±0.65	1.57
N^1-methyl-2-pyridone-5-carboxamide (2-Pyr)	6.0	18.2	17.1	±.71	15.5
N-MN + 2-Pyr	8.3	21.5	21.0	±2.19	12.1
B. Daily mg Metabolite/g Creatinine					
N-MN + 2-Pyr	6.3	16.6	15.9	±0.92	39.4

[a]There were 3 subjects each of whom took the three doses in different orders. The F ratios needed to be significant at the 5% and 1% levels, respectively, are 6.94 and 18.0.

study provide evidence that all the niacin assay values obtained with rats are applicable to humans.

LITERATURE CITED

1. Pugsley, L. I., Wills, G., and Crandall, W. A. "The biological assay of vitamin A by means of its influence on the cellular contents of the vagina of the rat." *J. Nutr.* **28**, 365 (1944).

2. Birch, T. W. and Harris, L. J. "Bradycardia in the vitamin B₁-deficient rat and its use in vitamin B₁ determinations." *Biochem. J.* **28**, 601 (1934).

3. Coward, K. H. *The Biological Standarization of the Vitamins,* 2nd ed. Bailliere, Tindall and Cox, London (1947).

4. Leth, T. and Sndergaard, H. "Biological activity of vitamin E compounds and natural materials by the resorption-gestation test, and chemical determination of the vitamin E activity in foods and feeds." *J. Nutr.* **107**, 2236 (1977).

5. Griminger, P. "Biological activity of the various vitamin K forms." *Vitamins Hormones* **24**, 605 (1966).

6. Frost, D. V., Perdue, H. S., and Spruth, H. C. "Vitamin K activity of menadione sodium bisulfite in chickens. *J. Nutr.* **59**, 181 (1956).

7. Spicer, S. S., Daft, F. S., Sebrell, W. H., and Ashburn, L. L "Prevention and treatment of agranulocytosis and leukopenia in rats given sulfanilyguanidine or succinylsulfathiazole in purified diets." *Publ. Health Repts.* **57**, 1559 (1942).

8. Asenjo, C. F. "Pteroylglutamic acid requirements of the rat and a characteristic lesion observed in the spleen of the deficient animal." *J. Nutr.* **36**, 601 (1948).

9. Kodicek, E. and Carpenter, K. J. "Experimental anaemias in the rat—2. The effect of various sulfonamides in producing a pteroylglutamic acid deficiency and the pteroylglutamic acid activity of test substances." *Blood,* **5**, 540 (1950).

10. Axelrod, A. E., Pilgrim, F. J., and Hofman, K. "The activity of *dl*-oxybiotin for the rat." *J. Biol. Chem.* **163**, 191 (1946).

11. McCoy, R. H., Felton, J. R., and Hofmann, K. "Biological activity of oxybiotin in the chick." *Arch. Biochem.* **9**, 141 (1946).

12. Moore, P. R., Luckey, T. D., Elvehjem, C. A., and Hart, E. G. "Biological activity and metabolism of dl-O-heterobiotin in the chick." *Proc. Soc. Exptl. Biol. Med.* 61, **185** (1946).

13. Crampton, E. W. "The growth of the odontoblasts of the incisor tooth as a criterion on the vitamin C intake of the guinea pig." *J. Nutr.* **33**, 401 (1947).

14. Davies, A. W. and Moore, T. "Vitamin A and carotene. 15. The influence of vitamin A reserve on the length of the depletion period in the young rat." *Biochem. J.* 31, **172** (1937).

15. Lakshamanan, M. R., Jungalwala, F. B., and Cama, H. R. "Metabolism and biological potency of 5,6-monoepoxyvitamin A aldehyde in the rat." *Biochem. J.* **95**, 27 (1965).

16. Association of Official Analytical Chemists. *Official Methods of Analysis,* 13th ed., Washington, D.C., 770 (1980).

17. Campbell, J. A. and Emslie, A. R. G. "Studies on the chick assay for vitamin D—3. The variability of chicks and the estimation of error from replicated group data." *Poultry Sci.*. **24**, 296 (1945).

18. Campbell, J. A., Migicovsky, B. A., and Emslie, A. R. G. "Studies on the chick assay for vitamin D—2. A comparison of four criteria of calcifications." *Poultry Sci.* **24**, 72 (1945).

19. Rambeck, W. A., Weiser, H., Haselbauer, R., and Zucker, H. "Vitamin D activity of different vitamin D₃ esters in chicken, Japanese quail and in rats." *Internat. J. Vit. Nutr. Res.* **51**, 353 (1981).

20. Ames, S. R. "Biopotencies in rats of several forms of alpha tocopherol. *J. Nutr.* **109**, 2198 (1979).

21. Gibby, W. A. and Gubler, C. J. "Biological activity of 1,N^6-Ethenothiamin, a fluorescent analog of thiamin, in rats." *J. Nutr.* **110**, 2117 (1980).

22. Lambooy, J. P. "Growth promoting properties of 6-3thyl-7-methyl-9-(1'-D-ribityl) isoalloxazine and 6-methyl-7-ethyl-9-(1'-D-ribityl) isoalloxazine." *J. Nutr.* **75**, 116 (1961).

23. Coates, M. E., Ford, J. E., Harrison, G. F., Kon, S. K., Shepheard, E. E., and Wilby, F. W. "The use of chicks for the biological assay of members of the vitamin B Complex—2. Tests on natural materials and other assays." *Brit. J. Nutr.* **6**, 75 (1952).

24. Lih, H., King, T. E., Higgins, H., Baumann, C. A., and Strong, F. M. "Growth-promoting activity of bound pantothenic acid in the rat." *J. Nutr.* **44**, 361 (1951).

25. Sarett, H. P. and Barboriak, J. J. "Inhibition of D-pantothenate by L-pantothenate in the rat." *Amer. J. Clin. Nutr.* **13**, 378 (1963).

26. Latymer, E. A. and Coates, M. E. "The availability to the chick of panthothenic acid in foods." *Brit. J. Nutr.* **47**, 131 (1982).

27. Gregory, J. F. and Kirk, J. R. "Assessment of roasting effects on vitamin B_6 stability and bioavailability in dehydrated food systems." *J. Food Sci.* **43**, 1585 (1978).

28. Gregory J. F. "Bioavailability of vitamin B_6 in nonfat dry milk and a fortified rice breakfast cereal product." *J. Food Sci.* **45**, 84 (1980).

29. Carter, E. G. A. and Carpenter, K. J. "The available niacin values of foods for rats and their relation to analytical values." *J. Nutr.* **112**, 2091 (1982).

30. Anderson, P. A., Baker, D. H., and Mistry, S. P. "Bioassay determination of corn, barley, sorghum and wheat." *J. Animal Sci.* **47**, 654 (1978).

31. Keagy, P. M. and Oace, S. M. "Development of a folacin bioassay in rats." *J. Nutr.* **112**, 87 (1982).

32. Bosshardt, D. K., Paul, W. J., O'Doherty, K., Huff, J. W., and Barnes, R. H. "Mouse growth assay procedures for the 'animal protein factor'." *J. Nutr.* **37**, 21 (1949).

33. Coates, M. E., Harrison, G. F., and Kon, S. K. "The chick assay of vitamin B_{12} and the animal protein factor." *Analyst. Lond.* **76**, 146 (1951).

34. Goldsmith, G. A., Rosenthal, H. L., Gibbens, J., and Unglaub, W. G. "Studies on niacin requirement in man. II. Requirements on wheat and corn diets low in tryptophan." *J. Nutr.* **56**, 371 (1955).

35. Goldsmith, G. A., Gibbens, J., Unglaub, W. G., and Miller, D. N. "Studies on niacin requirement in man—3. Comparative effects of diets containing lime-treated and untreated corn in the production of experimental pellagra." *Amer. J. Clin. Nutr.* **4**, 151 (1956).

36. Sauberlich, H. E., Dowdy, R. P., and Skala, J. H. *Laboratory Test For the Assessment of Nutritional Status.* CRC Press, Cleveland (1974).

37. Melnick, D., Hochberg, M., and Oser, B. L. "Physiological Availability of the vitamins I. The Human bioassay technic." *J. Nutr.* **30**, 67 (1945).

38. Tarr, J. B., Tamura, T., and Stokstad, E. L. R. "Availability of vitamin B_6 and pantothenate in an average American diet in man." *Amer. J. Clin. Nutr.* **34**, 1328 (1981).

39. Tamura, T. and Stokstad, E. L. R. "The availability of food folate in man." *Brit. J. Haematol.* **25**, 513 (1973).

40. Bliss, C. I. and Gyorgy, P. "The animal vitamin assay." In P. Gyorgy, Ed., *Vitamin Methods,* Vol. 2. Academic Press, New York (1951).

41. Guerrant, N. B. "General aspects of small animal experimentation." In P. Gyorgy, Ed., *Vitamin Methods,* Vol. 2. Academic Press, New York (1951).

42. Bliss, C. I. and Gyorgy, P. "Animal assay for vitamins." In P. Gyorgy and W. M. Pearson, Eds., *The Vitamins, Chemistry, Physiology, Methods,* Vol. 6. Academic Press, New York, 1 (1967).

43. Finney, D. J. *Statistical Method in Biological Assay*, 2nd ed. Charles Griffiths & Co., London (1964).

44. Finney, D. J. "The choice of a response metameter in bioassay." *Biometrics* **5**, 261 (1949).

45. Jerne, N. K. and Wood, E. C. "The validity and meaning of the results of biological assays." *Biometrics* **5**, 273 (1949).

46. Gridgeman, N. T. "On the errors of biological assays with graded responses and their graphical derivation." *Biometrics* **7**, **220** (1951).

47. Bliss, C. I. and White, C. "Statistical methods in biological assay of vitamins." In P. Gyorgy and W. N. Pearson, Eds., *The Vitamins, Chemistry, Physiology, Methods*, Vol. 6. Academic Press, New York, 21 (1967).

48. U.S. Dept. Health and Human Services, Public Health Service. *Guide for the Care and Use of Laboratory Animals*. Nat. Inst. Health, Publ. No. (NIH) 79–23, Washington, D.C. (1978).

49. Coates, M. E., Kon, S. K., and Shepheard, E. E. "The use of chicks for biological assay of members of the vitamin B complex—1. Tests with pure substances." *Brit. J. Nutr.* **4**, 203 (1950).

50. Carpenter, K. J., March, B. E., Milner, C. K., and Campbell, R. C. "A growth assay with chicks for the lysine content of protein concentrates." *Brit. J. Nutr.* **17**, 309 (1963).

51. Federal Register, Non-Clinical Laboratory Studies, Good Laboratory Practice; Requirements Established 41 51206 (1976).

52. Manson, J. A. and Carpenter, K. J. "The effect of a high level of dietary leucine on the niacin status of chicks and rats." *J. Nutr.* **108**, 1883 (1978).

53. Newberne, P. M. Bieri, J. G., Briggs, G. M., and Nesheim, M. C. "Control of diets in laboratory experimentation." *Inst. Lab. Resources News* **21**, A1 (1978).

54. Carpenter, K. J. "The concept of an appetite quotient for the interpretation of ad libitum feeding experiments." *J. Nutr.* **51**, 435 (1953).

55. Carter, E. G. A. and Carpenter, K. J. "The bioavailability for humans of bound niacin from wheat bran." *Amer. J. Clin. Nutr.* **36**, 855 (1982).

3 Microbiological Assays

Michael N. Voigt
and Ronald R. Eitenmiller

GENERAL CONSIDERATIONS

Microbiological methods of vitamin determination are based on the nutritional requirement of a microorganism for a certain vitamin. This allows the formulation of a basal medium that provides all of the growth requirements for the organism except for the vitamin to be assayed. When aliquots of the sample containing the vitamin being quantitated are added to the initially transluscent medium, followed by inoculation with the test organism, the organism reproduces in proportion to the vitamin content, which can be measured photometrically, or the metabolic products can be monitored. Over a defined concentration range, the method response will be directly proportional to the amount of vitamin present, and within this range, the sample and reference solutions can be compared accurately.

Compared with biological assay methods using animals, microbiological techniques possess the advantages of minimal requirements of space, labor, materials, and time. Although it is essential that a test organism has a requirement for the vitamin being assayed, this does not ensure that it is appropriate for employment. Many microorganisms can synthesize a vitamin from precursors, derivatives, or breakdown products that would not occur in the metabolism of animals or humans.

Simple and reliable procedures require the test organisms to possess the following characteristics: specifically require the vitamin forms that are biologically active in higher animals, be genetically constant during prolonged response, have a rapid growth cycle, have a growth response that is not easily influenced by neutralization salts or other substances that may be present in an extract of a sample and be nonpathogenic. Traditionally, the lactobacilli have been most widely employed, although yeasts, molds and protozoa are used. The lactobacilli and yeasts grow rapidly under facultatively anaerobic conditions, as in test tubes, producing sufficient cellular numbers and/or metabolic products to permit incubations of less than 24 hr. Molds and protozoa require about 3–5 days of incubation to attain the stationary or S phase of growth. Protozoa, viz. *Tetrahymena, Euglena, Ochromonas*, and *Poteriochromonas*, have more evolved ingestive and digestive systems than bacteria and yeasts that allow them to respond to conjugated forms of the vitamins, for example, thiamin pyrophosphate and folic acid polyglutamates. When using protozoan organisms, fewer problems are encountered with nonspecific stimulation, for example, fatty acid stimulation of the *Lactobacillus casei* assay for riboflavin or the sparing of the vitamin B_{12} requirement of *L. leichmannii* by deoxyribosides (1), and they possess a more mammalian-like response to the various forms of the vitamins that occur in natural materials 1,2).

   Tetrahymena thermophila, previously *T. pyriformis* WH_{14}, ATCC 30008, is a heterotrophic protozoan that requires thiamin, riboflavin, vitamin B_6, niacin, pantothenic acid, and lipoic acid (3). Generally, *T. thermophila* is as capable as the rat or chick in using conjugates of the water-soluble vitamins (4). *Tetrahymena* does not require vitamin B_{12}, ascorbic acid, and the fat-soluble vitamins (5). A few clones require biotin and choline. The inhibitory effect of visible light on the growth of *Tetrahymena* is due to the photodecomposition of thiamin, riboflavin, vitamin B_6, and folic acid. *Tetrahymena* obtains nutrients by diffusion through the cell membrane, pinocytosis, and phagocytosis (3). Ingested food particles collect in food vacuoles which contain glycosylases, deoxyribonuclease, ribonuclease, proteases, and conjugase.

   Poteriochromonas stipitata, formerly *Ochromonas malhamensis* ATCC 11532, *O. danica*, and *Euglena gracilis* are photoflagellates that obtain energy by a hetereotrophic and photoautotrophic combination. *P. stipitata* requires both light and complex nutrients for growth. Photosynthesis in this organism is low and does not compensate for respiration. There is a net consumption of oxygen. Carbon dioxide, starch, saccharides, and glycerol can serve as carbon sources, while ammonia is sufficient as a nitrogen source. Thiamin, biotin, and vitamin B_{12} complete its requirements, except for trace minerals (3). *O. danica* requirements are similar, except that it does not require vitamin B_{12}. *Ochromonas, Poteriochromonas*, and *Euglena* obtain nutrients by diffusion through the cell membrane, pinocytosis, and phagocytosis. Since *O. danica* can ingest and digest complex forms of vitamins, it can release and utilize biotin from biocytin and other peptide-bound biotins (6). Lactobacilli and yeasts do not possess these capabilities. The kinetics of cell division for phytoflagellates progressing through vitamin deficiency contain transient plateaus with the S phase of the cell cycle being differentially extended under vitamin deficiency (7,8).

METHODOLOGY

1. *Cultures for Vitamin Assays.* Ten organisms used for assaying the water soluble vitamins are listed in Table 3.1. Only the test organisms that have been shown to be reliable and specific for the physiologically useful forms of a given vitamin are listed. Media for maintenance of each culture and basal media for the corresponding vitamin assay, as well as incubation temperatures are also listed in Table 3.1. Lactic acid bacteria are usually maintained as stab inoculated cultures in a fastidious agar medium with granules of calcium carbonate added to each tube to increase the buffering capacity. All media should be held at 2–4°C in the dark to prevent inactivation of vitamins. Maintenance media may be dispensed in 10-mL portions into 16-mm or 18-mm test tubes and sterilized at 121°C for 10 min. For the growth of *Tetrahymena, Ochromonas,* and *Poteriochromonas* cells, 25-mm tubes should be used for inoculation of vitamin assays. Lactobacilli are stored at 2–4°C after an initial incubation of 30–37°C to produce a visible line of growth after 18–48 hr. *Neurospora* and *Saccharomyces* are carried on agar slants, while *Tetrahymena* is maintained on an agar slant immersed in H_2O. Transfer of all cultures in maintenance media is made at biweekly intervals. Lyophilization or liquid nitrogen freezing (9) may be used to preserve various cultures for later use as inoculum. Cultures are activated before the initiation of an assay by a minimum of three consecutive transfers, allowing 24 hr between each transfer for the lactobacilli and *Saccharomyces,* but 72 hr for the *Tetrahymena, Ochromonas, Poteriochromonas,* and *Neurospora.*

It is desirable that a minimal quantity of vitamin be transferred with the inoculum to the assay tubes. Any such carry-over results in high blanks and a shortening of the usable portion of the standard curve. To reduce the vitamin content of the inocula, it is necessary to centrifuge cultures and resuspend the packed cells into a medium devoid of vitamin. To further reduce growth of the test organism in the blank, the suspension of a test organism is diluted. If insufficient dilution is made, slight differences in the size of the drop of culture used as inoculum may introduce variations in the amount of growth in the assay tubes that is unrelated to the amount of vitamin present in the material being assayed.

Table 3.1 indicates the number of washings that need to be provided to the harvested cells of the test organisms, the solutions to be used for cell washings, and also the dilutions to which the cells should be diluted to prepare the inocula. An alternate way of reducing carry-over of the test vitamin from the inoculum to the assay medium is to grow the inoculum in the assay medium, which is fortified with a limited amount of the test vitamin.

Except for the basal media for the *Tetrahymena* tests, the basal media for vitamin assay can be prepared as described in the references cited in Table 3.1. Modifications to the original medium cited by Baker and Frank (1) for the *Tetrahymena* tests are given in the Reagent section of this chapter. Procedures for the preparation of the other media are also given in the Reagent section. To

TABLE 3.1   Conditions for the Microbial Assay of Water-Soluble Vitamins

Vitamin Assay	Culture Dilution[a]	Reagent Number[b]	Incubation Temperature (°C)	References
Thiamin				
Lactobacillus viridescens ATCC 12706	1:99	28,29;23	30	18,19
Ochromonas danica ATCC 30004	1:6.5	13,30;20	30	1,17
Riboflavin				
Lactobacillus casei ATCC 7469	1:19	28,29;24	37	19,24
Tetrahymena thermophila ATCC 30008	1:9	10,11,12;15	30	1
Vitamin B_6				
Saccharomyces uvarum ATCC 9080	1:1	31,32;25	30	19,24
Tetrahymena thermophila ATCC 30008	1:6,5	10,11,12;16	30	1
Kloeckera brevis ATCC 9744	—	28;25	30	26,27
Vitamin B_{12}				
Lactobacillus leichamannii ATCC 7830	1:1	28,29;27	37	19,24
Poteriochromonas stipitata ATCC 11532	1:6,5	13,30;18	30	1
Biotin				
Lactobacillus plantarum ATCC 8014	1:99	28,29;9	37	19
Ochromonas danica ATCC 30004	1:6.5	13,30;20	30	1,17
Niacin				
Lactobacillus plantarum ATCC 8014	1:99	28,29;9	37	19,24
Tetrahymena thermophila ATCC 30008	1:6.5	10,11,12;15	30	1
Pantothenate				
Lactobacillus plantarum ATCC 8014	1:99	28,29;9	37	19,24
Tetrahymena thermophila ATCC 30008	1:6.5	10,11,12;15	30	1
Choline				
Neurospora crassa ATCC 9277	1:50	22;21	25	19,28
Folate				
Lactobacillus casei ATCC 7469	1:99	28,29;26	37	19

[a]Wash and diluting solutions: saline for bacteria and yeast, water for protozoa and mold. Number of times resuspended: four with lactobacilli, once for yeast and Ochromonas, none for Tetrahymena.

[b]Maintenance media are the first media (weekly, monthly transfers), assay medium follows semicolon.

ensure a basal medium of uniform composition and to minimize the time consumed in media preparation, media should be prepared in bulk and stored at −20°C to suppress deterioration. Suitable dehydrated basal media for certain vitamin assays are available from several bacteriological supply firms.

2. *Assay Procedure.* Basal media are either thawed or rehydrated, the pH adjusted to the assay pH with the acids and bases listed in Table 3.2, and the medium is diluted so that the final concentration is twice that desired in the assay tubes. Into a series of 13-mm test tubes (lactobacilli, *Saccharomyces*), 25-mL Erlenmeyer flasks (*Tetrahymena, Ochromonas, Poteriochromonas*) or 50-mL Erlenmeyer flasks (*Neurospora*), as many as 10 levels of standard vitamin solution (Table 3.3) in triplicate and as many as five extract aliquots of sample (0.25, 0.5, 0.75, 1.0, and 1.25 mL or in multiples up to 2.5 mL) in duplicate are dispensed. Volumes are brought to 2.5 mL (5 mL for the choline test) with H_2O and then mixed with an equal volume of double-strength basal medium. A cover of aluminum foil fitting over an entire rack can be employed for assays conducted in test tubes. Individual glass caps are used for the *Ochromonas* and *Poteriochromonas* tests, whereas either glass or aluminum caps are employed for the *Tetrahymena* and *Neurospora* tests. The tubes are autoclaved at 121°C for the time recommended for each medium, which is usually 5 min. The *Saccharomyces* medium is steamed for 10 min. The mild sterilization conditions are used to minimize loss of nutrients and to avoid browning reactions. The sterilized tubes are allowed to cool until the temperature is uniform throughout all the assay vessels, a precaution that is necessary because even slight differences in initial temperature influence the growth either through stimulation, suppression, or cell injury. The cooled assay vessels are inoculated with one drop of inoculum from a 1-mL disposable pipette and incubated at a suitable temperature (Table 3.1). Constancy of temperature throughout the tubes of a given assay is ensured by employing a water bath. Incubation times for the lactobacilli and *S. uvarum* are 18–24 hr, whereas vitamin assays using *Tetrahymena, Ochromonas,* and *Neurospora* are incubated 5–7 days. Vitamin assays using *Ochromonas* or *Poteriochromonas* are incubated in a chamber illuminated with three 40-watt fluorescent "warm-tone" lamps, supplemented with two 25-watt tungsten lamps suspended about 1 m above a white surface and against a white background (1). After incubation, all assays are autoclaved at 121°C for 5 min. Except for the *Neurospora* test, absorbance, % transmission or turbidity of the assay solutions are measured at 620 nm against an uninoculated control. Mycelium from the *Neurospora* test is collected by filtration and weighed after drying at 110°C for 24 hr. Two separate runs should be completed to validate the analytical data.

3. *Extraction Methods.* Essentially all assays of vitamin contents in natural materials require the vitamin to be extracted from the sample in water-soluble form and in a state utilizable by the test organism. The task of sample preparation or extraction does not possess a generalized protocol. The exact conditions to obtain optimal extraction must be predetermined by experiment for each type of sample. The amount and concentration of the extracting agent must be

TABLE 3.2   Acids and Bases Showing the Least Effect on Various Microbial Assays and Recommended Assay pH Values.[a]

Vitamin Assay	Assay pH	Acid	Base
Thiamin			
L. viridescens	6.0	Hydrochloric	Potassium hydroxide
O. danica	5.5	Hydrochloric	Sodium hydroxide
Riboflavin			
L. casei	6.8	Hydrochloric	Potassium hydroxide
T. thermophila	6.1	Sulfuric	Sodium hydroxide
Vitamin B_6			
S. uvarum	4.5	Hydrochloric	Potassium hydroxide
T. thermophila	6.1	Acetic	Sodium hydroxide
Vitamin B_{12}			
L. leichmannii	6.1	Hydrochloric	Sodium hydroxide
P. stipitata	5.5	Hydrochloric	Sodium hydroxide
Biotin			
L. plantarum	6.8	Sulfuric	Sodium hydroxide
O. danica	5.5	Hydrochloric	Sodium hydroxide
Niacin			
L. plantarum	6.8	Sulfuric	Sodium hydroxide
T. thermophila	6.1	Sulfuric	Sodium hydroxide
Pantothenate			
L. plantarum	6.7	Sulfuric	Sodium hydroxide
T. thermophila	6.1	Sulfuric	Sodium hydroxide
Choline			
N. crassa	5.5	Sulfuric	Sodium hydroxide
Folate			
L. casei	6.8	Hydrochloric	Sodium hydroxide

[a]Voigt *et al.* (10), except for choline (Luecke and Pearson, 28). Acids evaluated were hydrochloric, sulfuric, citric, phosphoric, and acetic. Bases evaluated were potassium and sodium hydroxides.

sufficiently large to ensure complete extraction, but the procedure should not contribute significant quantities of interfering agents, such as neutralization salts (10), which would affect the growth of the test organism. Table 3.2 lists acids and bases that form salts showing the least effect on various microbial assays.

The physiological activity of the forms of the vitamin should also not be altered. Milder acid and alkali treatments are required when enzymatic digestion is incorporated into the extraction procedure. Enzymes can be employed to hydrolyze starches, proteins, and other conjugated complexes to facilitate physical operations, such as filtration and centrifugation, and also to release bound forms of vitamins. Enzyme preparations usually used are crudely purified natural materials and may contain appreciable amounts of vitamins. Blank determinations must be completed to allow for the correction of the vitamin content contributed by the enzyme preparation. Natural materials that have not been heat-treated may themselves contain enzymes capable of releasing vitamins from

TABLE 3.3 Concentrations of Water-Soluble Vitamins for Standard Assays[a]

Tube No.	Thiamin B[b]	Thiamin P[b]	Riboflavin B[b]	Riboflavin P[b]	B_6 B[c]	B_6 P[c]	B_{12} B[b]	B_{12} P[b]	Biotin B[b]	Biotin P[b]	Niacin B[b]	Niacin P[d]	Pantothenate B[b]	Pantothenate P[b]	Folate B[b]	Choline F[b]
1	0	0	0	0	0	0	0	0	0	0	0	0	0	0	0	0
2	0.2	0.1	5	1	0.1	0.1	5	0.3	3	3	0.1	1	2	3	10	10
3	0.5	0.3	10	1.5	0.2	0.3	7	1	5	10	2	2	4	5	20	10
4	1	0.5	15	2	0.4	0.5	10	3	7	15	3	3	6	10	30	40
5	1.5	1	20	5	0.6	1	15	10	10	20	5	5	8	15	50	100
6	2	2	30	10	0.8	1.5	20	20	15	30	10	10	10	20	100	200
7	3	3	40	15	1.2	2	25	30	20	40	15	15	12	25	150	400
8	4	4	50	20	1.6	2.5	30	50	30	60	20	30	14	30	200	800
9	5	5	60	30	2	3	70	70	40	100	30	50	16	50	250	1000
10	10	10	75	90	4	5	100	100	100	250	40	100	20	100	300	1500

[a] ng/mL, except B_{12}, folate, and biotin (pg/mL).

[b] B = bacterial or yeast assay; P = protozoan assay; F = fungal assay. Corresponding cultures are listed in Table 3.2.

[c] B (pyridoxol), P (pyridoxol, -al, -amine; equal proportion each isomer). For B, use pyridoxol as standard. For P, use equal proportions of pyridoxol, pyridoxal, and pyridoxamine.

[d] Use equal proportions of nicotinic acid and nictinamide for P.

the enzyme preparation used for extraction and may complicate the correction procedure. Such samples should be steamed for 10 min before adding the extracting enzyme. Certain natural materials contain inhibitors for the hydrolases, thereby necessitating the use of larger quantities of enzyme to release the vitamin, for example, in the analysis of yeast extract for folic acid. Bacterial action during the enzymatic digestion may be avoided by the addition of distillable bacteriostatic agents, such as those listed under Reagent 34.

Specific extraction methods for the vitamins are given in the chapters covering the individual vitamins. In each procedure, an aliquot of a sample estimated to contain a vitamin level within the sensitivity range of the assay method (Table 3.3) is weighed or pipetted into a suitable container. If a given amount of sample contains a concentration of vitamin greater than the range of the assay method, the extract is diluted with water or suitable buffer. At the completion of the extraction procedure, the solutions are adjusted to the optimal pH of the vitamin assay procedure (Table 3.1) followed by adjusting to the desired volume. Suspended particles are removed from the final extracts by centrifugation and, if necessary, by filtration.

EQUIPMENT

Equipment and glassware are those generally associated with the operation of microbiological laboratories. In addition, all laboratories designed for microbial vitamin analyses require the availability of the following:

1. *Incubators.* Capable of operating at temperatures ranging between 30 and 40°C within a limit of ± 0.5°C. Circulatory water baths or forced draft incubators are used with lactobacilli. A shaking forced-air incubator is needed when *Saccharomyces uvarum* is the test organism. Force-draft cabinet incubators either illuminated for *Ochromonas, Poteriochromonas,* and *Euglena* or nonilluminated for *Tetrahymena* and *Neurospora* are used. An illumination system is described in the procedures section and further details are provided by Baker and Frank (1).

2. *An Autoclave.* Of sufficient capacity (minimum 1 m³) to admit all trays or flasks or racks of tubes from a given assay (i.e., standards and samples).

3. *Culture Tube Racks.* To support 16-mm tubes (6 $\times$ 12). Metal trays (ca. 30 $\times$ 45 cm) with perforations to provide drainage are used to support assays employing flasks (*Tetrahymena, Ochromonas, Neurospora*).

4. *Screw-cap Culture Tubes 18 $\times$ 150 mm and 25 $\times$ 150 mm.* For maintaining and activating cultures are satisfactory. Lipless, disposable tubes 16 $\times$ 150 mm are needed for the lactobacilli and *Saccharomyces* tests, whereas 25-mL and 50-mL flasks with glass caps are used for the protozoan and *Neurospora* tests, respectively. Glass caps may be obtained by cutting 4-dram vials.

5. *Tube Mixer.* Such as a Vortex-Genie® (Fisher Scientific Products).

6. *Spectrophotometer or Nephelometer.* For measuring the absorbance or

turbidity optical density of the assay solutions at 620 nm, for example, Spectronic 20 (Bausch and Lomb).

7. *A Minimum of 1 m³ of Each Refrigeration and Frozen Storage Space for Media and Stock Cultures.*

8. *Clinical-Type Centrifuge.* With adapters to hold 18-mm culture tubes.

9. *Analytical Balances.* For preparing solutions and weighing *Neurospora* mycelium.

10. *Drying Oven.* For drying and sterilizing purposes.

11. *A Self-Refilling and Adjustable Apparatus for Pipetting Media and Water.* This is a useful timesaver (e.g., Cornwall Continuous Pipetting Outfit 2, 5 and 10 mL).

REAGENTS

The basal medium is the principal reagent and is either rehydrated if a commercially prepared medium is available, or it is prepared by mixing a number of stock solutions and chemicals. A distillable organic preservative, (for example, Reagent 34), is useful in preventing microbial growth in stock solutions. Precautions must be taken to hold all solutions in the dark and to conduct all operations in subdued light. The use of red or yellow fluorescent light is suitable. The stock solutions and reagents listed below are those used in several of the microbiological procedures. Additional reagents that are specific for any one assay method are described under that method.

Some of the reagents listed below contain compounds at the mg or below level. An alternative to weighing these compounds in their specified minute amounts is to prepare corresponding aqueous solutions and to pipet appropriate amounts into the formula solution.

1. *Acid Hydrolyzed Casein.* Stir 100 g of "vitamin-free" casein twice with 250 mL of 95% ethanol for 15 min and filter with suction. The alcohol treatment may be omitted if the casein is not to be employed in the niacin assay.

Transfer the alcohol-washed casein into a round-bottomed flask of at least 1 L capacity, preferably a flask having two necks ground to a standard taper. Mix well with 500 mL 6 N HCl. Fit the flask with a glass stopper and a water-cooled condenser and reflux over a low heat for 8–12 hr. Since casein tends to froth during the initial stage of hydrolysis, heat carefully and gradually. Mix the contents of the flask occasionally by shaking and have a wet towel available to cool the flask if the reaction becomes too vigorous.

After refluxing, fit the flask with a condenser and receiving flask suitable for vacuum distillation, and then remove as much HCl as possible by concentrating the hydrolyzate to a thick paste under reduced pressure. Air introduced through a bleeder tube placed at the bottom of the flask will serve to minimize bumping during the final stages of the concentration. The temperature at which the distillation is completed should not exceed 100°C. Temperatures of 70–80°C are recommended. To obtain rapid and complete distillation at this temperature range, it is necessary to reduce the pressure considerably. This may not be achieved with a water aspirator unless high water pressure is available. Care should be taken to trap the hydrochloric acid fumes, especially when using a vacuum pump.

It is advisable to redissolve the paste in approximately 200 mL H_2O and repeat the concentration to remove additional amounts of HCl; however, a satisfactory hydrolyzate can be attained with a single concentration to a thick paste. The acid concentration attained should be low enough so that subsequent neutralization will not yield sufficient salt to retard bacterial growth in the basal medium.

Dissolve the hydrolyzate paste in around 700 mL H_2O and adjust the pH to 3.5 with 40% NaOH. Decolorize by stirring with 20 g of activated charcoal (e.g., Norit A or Darco G-60) at room temperature. Stir until the filtrate of a test aliquot is light straw-colored. Depending on the charcoal used, this may take from 5 min to 60 min. This step also removes any residual niacin and folic acid that may have remained in the ethanol-washed casein. Filter through either a large fluted filter or by suction. Adjust the pH to 6.8, dilute to 1 L, and store refrigerated under toluene/chloroform or dry under vacuum. A precipitate of tyrosine may form in the solution on standing. Therefore, it is good practice to mix the solution before using. The insoluble material will dissolve when the entire medium is prepared. If the acid-hydrolyzed casein is to be used in the biotin assay omit the decolorization step. After adjustment of the pH to 3.5, add 15 ml of 30% hydrogen peroxide and allow the solution to stand for 24 h at 20-25°C. Adjust the pH to 7.0 with sodium hydroxide and add 10 g powdered manganese dioxide. Stir mechanically until oxygen is no longer evolved (ca 15 min). Filter as described above and dilute to 1 liter. The peroxide treatment destroys traces of biotin present in the vitamin-free casein.

Commercial casein hydrolyzates may be purchased, but their cost is high. These are available both as acid or enzyme hydrolyzed products. Either is satisfactory, although the enzyme hydrolyzate promotes more rapid growth of most test organisms. A procedure for the preparation of a vitamin-free enzyme hydrolyzed casein has been described by Roberts and Snell (14). Details are outlined on page 452.

2. *Cystine-Tryptophan Solution.* Suspend 4.0 g L-cystine and 1.0 g L-tryptophan or 2 g DL-tryptophan in 700–800 mL H_2O, heat to 70–80°C, and add 20% HCl dropwise with stirring until the solids are dissolved with about 12 mL of 20% HCl. Cool to 20–25°C and bring to 1 L with H_2O.

3. *Adenine-Guanine-Uracil Solution.* Heat 0.1 g each of adenine sulfate, guanine hydrochloride, and uracil in a 250-mL Erlenmeyer flask containing about 75 mL H_2O and 2 mL concentrated HCl. Cool after all the solids have dissolved. If a precipitate forms, add a few additional drops of concentrated HCl and heat. Repeat until no precipitate forms on cooling and then transfer to a 100-mL volumetric flask and bring to volume with H_2O.

4. *Vitamin Solution.* Weigh 20 mg riboflavin, 10 mg thiamin hydrochloride, 10 mg *p*-aminobenzoic acid, and 40 mg pyridoxine hydrochloride. Transfer to a 1-L volumetric flask and dilute to the mark with 0.02 N acetic acid.

5. *Pantothenate Solution.* Weigh 54.4 mg calcium pantothenate and transfer to a 500-mL volumetric flask. Dilute to the mark with 50% ethanol and store at 2–4°C. This solution contains 100 μg pantothenic acid/mL.

6. *Biotin Stock Solution.* Weigh 25.0 mg of anhydrous D-biotin (free acid), dilute to 500 mL with 50% ethanol, and store at 2–4°C.

7. *Niacin Stock Solution.* Weigh 50.0 mg of anhydrous niacin (dried over P_2O_5 or H_2SO_4 in a vacuum desiccator for 24 hr), dilute to 500 mL with 25% ethanol, and store at 2–4°C.

8. *Metals Mix A.* The following salt solution is incorporated into the basal media for the lactobacilli tests: 10 g $MgSO_4\cdot7H_2O$, 1.0 g KCl, 0.5 g $MnSO_4\cdot4H_2O$, 0.5 g $FeSO_4\cdot7H_2O$, and 23 mL 85% H_3PO_4 are dissolved in H_2O and diluted to 500 mL. The acidity of the solution prevents the precipitation of iron phosphate.

9. *Lactobacillus plantarum Basal Medium.* To prepare basal media for 100 pantothenic acid, biotin, or niacin tests, mix the following reagents: 25 mL casein hydrolyzate (Reagent 1), 25 mL cystine-tryptophan (Reagent 2), 5 mL adenine-guanine-uracil (Reagent 3), 5 mL vitamin solution (Reagent 4), 5 mL metals mix A solution (Reagent 8), 5.0 g glucose, 5.0 g sodium acetate, 125 mL H_2O, and omitting only the vitamin to be determined and adding the remaining necessary vitamins. Mix thoroughly, adjust to pH 6.8 with 40% NaOH using a pH meter or bromothymol blue as an external indicator (about 1 mL alkali), and bring to 250 mL. Some workers have obtained better growth when the concentrations of glucose or both glucose and sodium acetate are doubled. Satisfactory dehydrated media for the assay of these vitamins is available from Difco.

10. *Tetrahymena Medium (15).* The pH of a medium composed of the following is adjusted to 7.2 before autoclaving: 5.0 g proteose-peptone, 5.0 g tryptone, 0.2 g K_2HPO_4, and H_2O to bring to 1 L. Use 10 mL per 18-mm screw cap tube. Subculture every 7–10 days at 25°C.

11. *Hasken's Agar for Tetrahymena (15).* The following components are brought to 1 L after adjusting the pH to 7.2–7.4: 8 g dextrin, 0.6 g sodium acetate, 5.0 g yeast extract, 0.6 g liver extract, 5.0 g tryptone, and 16.0 g agar. Dispense 5-mL amounts into 18-mm screw cap tubes, autoclave and slant in long slopes. After setting, aseptically overlay with 2 mL sterile distilled H_2O. Subculture every 30 days at 18°C.

12. *Tetrahymena Maintenance Medium (16).* The following two solutions are autoclaved separately and combined, and then 10-mL amounts are aseptically dispensed into 25-mm screw cap tubes: Solution 1 consists of 10 g proteose-peptone dissolved in 900 mL H_2O with pH adjusted to 7.0, whereas Solution 2 consists of 10.0 g glucose and 1 mL 0.1 N H_2SO_4 brought to 100 mL with H_2O. Subculture every 7–10 days at 25°C.

13. *Ochromonas and Poteriochromones Maintenance Medium (1, 17).* 1 g BBL trypticase or Difco tryptone, 1 g Difco yeast autolyzate, 50 mg NBC liver 1:20 liver extract concentrate, 5.0 g sucrose, and 2.5 g glycerol are dissolved in H_2O, pH adjusted to 5.0 with 0.1 N KOH for *O. danica* or pH 6.5 for *P. stipitata*, brought to 500 mL with H_2O, dispensed in 10-mL amounts into 18-mm screw cap tubes, and autoclaved 15 min. Subculture every 7–10 days at 28–32°C under illumination.

14. *Metals Mix B.* Essential trace elements for the *Tetrahymena* tests are provided by finely grinding the following: 6.9 g $ZnSO_4 \cdot 7H_2O$, 4.2 g $MnSO_4 \cdot H_2O$, 7.8 g $Fe(NH_4)_2(SO_4)_2 \cdot 6H_2O$, 730 mg $CoSO_4 \cdot 7H_2O$, 170 mg $CuSO_4 \cdot 5H_2O$, 120 mg $(NH_4)_6Mo_7O_{24} \cdot 4H_2O$, 80 mg $Na_3VO_4 \cdot 16 H_2O$, and 80 mg H_3BO_3.

15. *Tetrahymena thermophila Niacin, Riboflavin, and Pantothenate Assay Medium (1, 17).* The following components are dissolved by heating at 100°C: 12.0 g Difco vitamin free casamino acids, 200 mg KH_2PO_4, 4 g $MgSO_4 \cdot 7H_2O$, 100 mg metals mix B (Reagent 14), 1 mL of 25.0 g $CaCO_3$ dissolved in minimal HCl and brought to 100 mL with H_2O, 200 mg citric acid monohydrate, 400 mg L-tryptophan, 200 mg DL-methionine, 400 mg diacetin, 1 mg thiamin hydrochloride, 10 µg biotin, 200 µg folic acid, 200 µg oxidized DL-thioctic acid, 600 µg pyridoxine hydrochloride, 600 µg pyridoxal hydrochloride, 600 µg pyridoxamine hydrochloride, 400 mg glycine, 1.2 g sodium acetate, 400 mg Sigma guanosine 2′ + 3′ monophosphoric acid mixed isomer, 50 mg Sigma adenosine 2′ + 3′ monophosphoric acid mixed isomers, 60 mg cytidylic acid, 200 mg uracil (the previous four items are dissolved by boiling with a few drops of 10% KOH, and then added to the other constituents), 100 mg adenine, 20 mg thymidine, 3.0 g glucose, and 550 mL H_2O. Upon cooling, the pH is adjusted to 6.1 with H_2SO_4 or NaOH. Basal media for niacin, riboflavin, or pantothenate estimation includes 2 mg each of nicotinic acid and nicotinamide, 1 mg of sodium riboflavin-5-phosphate, and 2 mg of calcium pantothenate per L. The vitamin being assayed is omitted from the medium. Vitamins are added from stock solutions. Riboflavin, biotin, folic acid, and thioctic acid solutions are stored frozen. Volatile preservative is added to refrigerated solutions. After pH adjustment to 6.1, 400 mL of a 5% soluble starch (Eastman) solution are added to the cold basal medium to bring the final starch concentration to 20 g/L. The starch solution is prepared by autoclaving a 5% (w/v) suspension for 10 min. The final volume is brought to 1 L.

16. *Tetrahymena thermophila B_6 Assay Medium (1,17).* The following components are dissolved by heating at 100°C: 12.0 g vitamin free casamino acid (Difco), 200 mg KH_2PO_4, 4.0 g $MgSO_4 \cdot 7H_2O$, 200 mg citric acid, 100 mg metals mix B (Reagent 14), 1 mL 2.5% $CaCO_3$ solution (see Reagent 15), 1 g sodium acetate, 400 mg diacetin, 100 mg adenine, 400 mg guanosine 2′ + 3′ monophosphate mixed isomers (Sigma), 200 mg uracil, 20 mg thymidine, 20 mg cytidine, 400 mg L-tryptophan, 400 mg glycine, 2.0 g DL-asparagine, 40 mg hypoxanthine, 3.0 g glucose, 2 mg thiamin, 20 µg biotin, 200 µg folic acid, 200

μg oxidized DL-thioctic acid, 1 mg sodium riboflavin phosphate, 2 mg nicotinic acid, 2 mg nicotinamide, 2 mg calcium pantothenate, 100 mg Tween 80, and H_2O to 500 mL. Upon cooling, the pH is adjusted to 6.7 with NaOH. 20 g soluble starch is added from a 5% solution (see Reagent 15) before bringing volume to 1 L.

17. *Metals Mix C.* Trace elements for the *Poteriochromonas* B_{12} test consists of bringing the following to 1 L with H_2O: 17.6 g $ZnSO_4 \cdot 7H_2O$, 12.4 g $MnSO_4 \cdot H_2O$, 1.4 g $Fe(NH_4)_2(SO_4)_2 \cdot 6H_2O$, 0.4 g $CuSO_4 \cdot 5H_2O$, 0.24 g $CoSO_4 \cdot 7H_2O$, and 3.0 g citric acid monohydrate.

18. *Poteriochromonas stipitata B_{12} Assay Medium (1).* The following constituents are dissolved by heating at 100°C: 2 g dibasic ammonium citrate, 300 mg $CaCO_3$, 6.0 g L-glutamic acid, 600 mg K_3PO_4, 800 mg $MgCO_3$, 1 g L-histidine hydrochloride monohydrate, 2.0 mg thiamin hydrochloride, 100 μg biotin, 20 mL metals mix C (Reagent 17), 200 mg $MgSO_4 \cdot 7H_2O$, 800 mg L-arginine hydrochloride, 2 mL 180 mg $(NH_4)_6Mo_7O_{24} \cdot 4H_2O$ in 1 L H_2O, 24.0 g sucrose, 600 mg $KHCO_3$, 800 mg DL-methionine, 4 mL 92 mg $Na_3VO_4 \cdot 16H_2O$ dissolved into 1000 mL H_2O with NaOH, then readjusted to pH 7.0 with HCl and brought to 1 L with H_2O, 10.0 g Hycase SH (acid hydrolyzed casein, Sheffield Chemical Co.), 2 g DL-asparagine, 200 mg L-tryptophan, 2.5 mg p-aminobenzoic acid, 4 mg NaCN, and H_2O to 900 ml. Upon cooling, the pH is adjusted to 5.5 with NaOH and then the volume is brought to 1 L with H_2O. A *Poteriochromonas Ochromonas* B_{12} basal medium is also available from Difco.

19. *Metals Mix D.* Trace minerals for the *Ochromonas* thiamin and biotin tests are supplied by finely grinding the following: 6.51 g $Fe(NH_4)_2(SO_4)_2$, 2.07 g $ZnSO_4 \cdot 7H_2O$, 0.75 g $MnSO_4 \cdot H_2O$, 0.15 g $CuSO_4 \cdot 5H_2O$, 0.23 g $CoSO_4 \cdot 7H_2O$, 0.27 g H_3BO_3, 40 mg $(NH_4)_6Mo_7O_{24} \cdot 4H_2O$, and 40 mg $Na_3VO_4 \cdot 16H_2O$.

20. *Ochromonas danica Biotin and Thiamin Assay Media (1,17).* Two mg of thiamin hydrochloride are added to the following cold basal medium when assaying for biotin, or 0.02 mg of biotin when assaying for thiamin: 400 mg nitrilotriacetic acid (Eastman), 600 mg KH_2PO_4, 0.8 g $MgCO_3$, 100 mg $CaCO_3$, 20 mg metals mix D (Reagent 19), 1 g NH_4Cl, 2 g $MgSO_4 \cdot 7H_2O$, 6 g L-glutamic acid, 800 mg L-histidine hydrochloride monohydrate, 800 mg L-arginine hydrochloride, 20.0 g glucose and H_2O to 900 mL. Upon cooling, adjust to pH 5.0 with NaOH, then add 24 mL of a 10% solution to Tween 80 and bring to 1 L with H_2O.

21. *Choline Assay Medium (19).* The medium for the *Neurospora crassa* test consists of the following: 40 g sucrose, 2 g NH_4NO_3, 10 μg biotin, 11.4 g ammonium tartrate, 2 g KH_2PO_3, 1 g $MgSO_4$, 0.2 g NaCl, 0.2 g $CaCl_2$, 700 μg $Na_2B_4O_7$, 500 μg $(NH_4)_6Mo_7O_{24}$, 1.1 mg $FeSO_4$, 300 μg $CuCl_2$, 110 μg $MnSO_4$, 180 μg $ZnSO_4$, dissolve, and adjust to pH 5.5 and bring volume to 1 L with H_2O.

22. *Neurospora Agar (19).* The maintenance medium for *N. crassa* consists of: 5 g yeast extract, 5 g proteose-peptone No. 3 (Difco), 40 g maltose, 15 g agar, 900 mL H_2O, heat to 100°C to dissolve, cool, adjust to pH 6.7, bring to

1 L, dispense 10 mL per tube, autoclave 10 min at 121°C, and slant before cooling.

23. *Thiamin LV Medium (19,20).* The basal medium for the *L. viridescens* assay for thiamin is composed of: 10 g thiamin-free yeast extract (prepare by suspending 10 g yeast extract into 100 mL 0.5 N NaOH, autoclave 30 min at 121°C, neutralize with acetic acid, autoclave an additional 10 min, and filter), 20 g tryptone, 20 g dextrose, 10 g sodium citrate, 10 g K_2HPO_4, 10 g NaCl, 1.6 g $MgSO_4 \cdot 7H_2O$, 280 mg $MnCl_2 \cdot 4H_2O$, 80 mg $FeSO_4$, 2 g Tween 80, 900 mL H_2O, adjust to pH 6.0 (HCl or KOH), and bring to 1 L. A dehydrated medium is available from Difco.

24. *Riboflavin LC Medium (19,24).* Basal medium for the *L. casei* test for riboflavin consists of: 22 g photolyzed peptone (prepare by dissolving 25 g peptone into 157 mL H_2O plus 12.5 g NaOH in 157 mL H_2O). The solution is dispensed into a glass dish of sufficient diameter to result in a maximum depth of no more than 2 cm. The solution is then exposed to a 100-watt lamp equipped with a reflector at about 30 cm from the surface of the solution for 8 hr at less than 25°C with occasional stirring. Then 4.5 g sodium acetate is added, the pH adjusted to 6–6.5, brought to 1 L and filtered if not clear, 2.0 g yeast supplement (prepare by dissolving 2 g yeast extract into 10 mL H_2O), add 3 g lead acetate in 10 mL H_2O, mix, filter, adjust to pH 10 with NH_4OH, filter, and readjust to pH 6.5 with acetic acid. Precipitate lead by passing hydrogen sulfide gas through the solution. Hydrogen sulfide may be generated by adding ferric sulfide to dilute sulfuric acid. Filter and dilute the solution to 20 mL, 20 g dextrose, 1.8 g sodium acetate, 0.2 g L-cystine, 1 g K_2HPO_4, 1 g KH_2PO_4, 400 mg $MgSO_4 \cdot 7H_2O$, 20 mg NaCl, 20 mg $Fe_2(SO_4)_2$, 20 mg $MnSO_4$, 900 mL H_2O, adjust to pH 6.8 (HCl or KOH), and bring to 1 L with H_2O. A dehydrated medium is available from Difco. An alternate medium, which is described on page 370, has also worked satisfactorily.

25. *Pyridoxine Y Medium (19-22).* The *S. uvarum* test employs a medium consisting of: 4 g asparagine, 20 mg L-histidine hydrochloride, 40 mg DL-methionine, 40 mg DL-tryptophan, 40 mg DL-isoleucine, 40 g DL-valine, 40 g dextrose, 400 μg thiamin hydrochloride, 400 μg Ca pantothenate, 400 μg nicotinic acid, 8 mg biotin, 20 μg riboflavin, 5 mg inositol, 200 μg H_3BO_3, 3 g KH_2PO_4, 1 g $MgSO_4$, 4 g $(NH_4)_2SO_4$, 490 mg $CaCl_2$, 200 μg KI, 40 μg $(NH_4)_6Mo_4O_{24}$, 80 μg $MnSO_4 \cdot H_2O$, 90 μg $CuSO_4$, 80 μg $ZnSO_4$, 500 μg $FeSO_4$, 900 mL H_2O, adjust to pH 4.5 (HCl or KOH), and bring to 1 L. A dehydrated medium is available from Difco. An alternate medium, which is described on page 423, has also worked satisfactorily.

26. *Folic Acid Casei Medium (19).* Basal medium for the *L. casei* test is prepared from the following: 10 g charcoal-treated Casitone (Difco Casitone dissolved in 100 mL H_2O plus 2 g activated charcoal, stir 30 min, and filter), 40 g dextrose, 40 g sodium acetate, 1 g K_2HPO_4, 1 g KH_2PO_4, 0.2 g DL-tryptophan, 0.6 g L-asparagine, 0.5 g L-cysteine hydrochloride, 10 mg adenine sulfate, 10 mg guanine hydrochloride, 10 mg uracil, 20 mg xanthine, 100 mg

Tween 80, 5 mg glutathione (reduced), 0.4 g $MgSO_4$, 20 mg NaCl, 20 mg $FeSO_4$, 15 mg $MnSO_4$, 1 mg riboflavin, 2 mg p-aminobenzoic acid, 4 mg pyridoxine hydrochloride, 400 μg thiamin hydrochloride, 800 μg calcium-pantothenate, 800 μg nicotinic acid, 20 μg biotin, 800 mL H_2O, adjust to pH 6.8 with HCl and/ or NaOH, and bring to 1 L with H_2O. A dehydrated medium is available from Difco. An alternate medium, which is described on page 453, has also worked satisfactorily.

27. *B_{12} LL Assay Medium (19).* Basal medium for the *L. leichmannii* test for vitamin B_{12} consists of: 15 g vitamin-free casamino acids (Difco), 40 g dextrose, 200 mg L-asparagine, 20 g sodium acetate, 4 g ascorbic acid, 400 mg L-cystine, 400 mg DL-tryptophan, 20 mg adenine sulfate, 20 mg guanine hydrochloride, 20 mg uracil, 20 mg xanthine, 1 mg riboflavin, 1 mg thiamin hydrochloride, 10 μg biotin, 2 mg niacin, 2 mg p-aminobenzoic acid, 1 mg calcium pantothenate, 4 mg pyridoxine hydrochloride, 4 mg pyridoxal hydrochloride, 800 μg pyridoxamine hydrochloride, 200 μg folic acid, 1 g KH_2PO_4, 1 g K_2HPO_4, 400 mg $MgSO_4$, 20 mg NaCl, 20 mg $FeSO_4$, 20 mg $MnSO_4$, 2 g Tween 80, 900 mL H_2O, adjust to pH 6.1, and bring to 1 L with H_2O. A dehydrated medium is available from Difco.

28. *Lactobacilli Broth (19, 23).* A medium for culturing lactobacilli may be prepared from: 15 g peptonized milk (Difco), 5 g yeast extract, 10 g dextrose, 100 mL tomato juice, 2.0 g KH_2PO_4, 1 g Tween 80, 800 mL H_2O, adjust to pH 6.7 with HCl and/or KOH, and bring to 1 L with H_2O. A dehydrated medium is available from Difco.

29. *Lactobacilli Agar (19).* Addition of 10 g agar to Reagent 28 yields a medium suitable for slants and stabs. A dehydrated medium is available from Difco.

30. *Fluid Thiogycollate Medium (16,19).* Maintenance media for the *Ochromonas* spp. may be prepared from 15 g Difco Casitone, 5 g yeast extract, 5.5 g glucose, 2.5 g NaCl, 0.5 g L-cystine, 0.5 g sodium thioglycollate, 0.75 g agar, 1 mg resazurin, 900 mL H_2O, adjust to pH 7.1 with HCl and/or NaOH, and bring to 1 L with H_2O.

31. *Malt Extract Broth (18).* A medium for the maintenance of *S. uvarum* is prepared from a 3% solution of malt extract (Difco) adjusted to pH 5.5 with HCl.

32. *Malt Extract Agar (18).* The semisolid complement of Reagent 31 is prepared by adding 1.5% agar to the malt extract broth.

33. *Physiological Saline Solution (0.9%).* Dissolve 9.0 g of NaCl into 1 L of H_2O. Transfer 10-mL amounts into tubes, cap, and autoclave.

34. *Volatile Preservative.* Stock solutions and fluids awaiting analysis may be protected against microbial action by the following preservative, which is removed by steam distillation during autoclaving: chlorobenzene/1,2-dichloroethane (ethylenedichloride)/n-butylchloride (1-chlorobutane) $(1 + 1 + 2)$. About 1 mL/L suffices. Overlayering the solution with a small amount of toluene plus

chloroform (0.5 and 1%, respectively) may also be used. Stock solutions of the vitamins may be prepared in 25% aqueous ethanol.

35. *1 N Sodium Hydroxide.* Since NaOH pellets are hygroscopic, amounts in excess of the calculated NaOH should be used. To prepare 18 L of 1 N NaOH, 720 g of NaOH are needed. From 1–15% in excess of this amount can be used, depending on the H_2O content of the NaOH pellets.

36. *0.1 N Sodium Hydroxide.* Determine the normality of Reagent 35 by titration against a standard acid and dilute to a concentration of 0.1 N NaOH with H_2O using proportions indicated by the following equation:

$$\text{mL Reagent 35 (Normality Reagent 35)} = 0.1 \text{ N (mL Reagent 36 Required)}$$

The alkali solution can also be standardized against potassium acid phthalate, H_2SO_4, or other acid of known concentration. This reagent is used in titrating the acid produced by the test organisms. Therefore, it is imperative that the normality of the solution either be exactly 0.1 N or close to it, in which case the exact normality has to be determined.

37. *Bromothymol Blue Solution.* Weigh 0.1 g of bromothymol blue indicator into a small beaker. Add 1.6 mL of 0.1 N NaOH and triturate with a stirring rod until dissolved. Dilute with H_2O to 250 mL.

PROCEDURES

The microbiological procedures for vitamin analyses require the use of properly activated cultures to achieve consistent results. Active stabs or broths of the stock culture, from 1–14 days old, are used for the preparation of the inoculum. The inoculum must be started three consecutive transfer periods before it is used in the assay, that is, 72 hr for lactobacilli and *Saccharomyces*, but 9 days for protozoa and *Neurospora*. If the acid produced in the lactobacilli tests is to be measured, the time of inoculation of the assay tubes should be chosen so that the titration can be completed 3 days later. The samples may be extracted and the standard and assay tubes set up and sterilized several days prior to inoculation provided contamination, thermo- and photodecomposition, and evaporation are prevented. The following techniques are common to microbiological assays.

1. *Preparation of Stock Culture and Inoculum.*

(a) Prepare stab or broth cultures in two or more subcultures using an appropriate medium from Table 3.1. Primary stock cultures should be maintained independently at two separate locations to avoid the accidental loss of a culture through contamination, incubator temperature fluctuation, or other unforeseen events.

(b) Transfer the culture through three consecutive incubations at the corresponding temperature indicated in Table 3.1. Inoculum should not be incubated longer than the transfer times indicated above because an organism tends to become attenuated and poor growth responses are encountered.

(c) Harvest and wash the cells through centrifugation at about 3000 $\times$ g for 10 min. An angle-head centrifuge layers cells so that decantation is facilitated. The cells are aseptically resuspended into 10 mL of sterile saline or water for washings and final culture dilutions as indicated in Table 3.1.

(d) Either a disposable 1-mL pipette or a sterile syringe may be used to dispense the resuspended cells. By pouring the resuspended cells into the open end of the syringe before inserting the plunger, the shear stress induced by drawing the cells through a 16–18-gauge needle can be avoided.

2. *Preparation of Samples.* Extract weighed samples, adjust pH (Table 3.2) and dilute to proper concentration (Table 3.3). Detailed instructions are provided under the analysis procedure given in the following chapters.

3. *Preparation of Standard Vessels.*

(a) In triplicate tubes or flasks, add aliquots of the working standard vitamin solution (Table 3.3). The required number of vessels for both the standard and samples should be placed in numbered racks or trays and identified by noting their positional arrangements.

(b) Add sufficient H_2O to bring the volume in each tube to 2.5 mL (5.0 mL for *Neurospora*).

(c) To each of these tubes add 2.5 mL (5.0 mL for *Neurospora*) of basal medium stock solution. The contents of the vessels are mixed using a vortex-type mixer. A continuous pipetting apparatus is a valuable time saver for dispensing H_2O and basal media.

4. *Preparation of Assay Vessels.*

(a) To duplicate or triplicate tubes or flasks, add three to five aliquots of the test solution. The test solution is used at several levels so that validity of the assay can be evaluated by comparing the calculated results at different test levels. AOAC procedures require that at least four sample aliquots be used (24). Some workers do not run duplicates at each level of sample, since each of the levels used already constitutes an independent observation.

(b) Add H_2O, basal medium, and mix as indicated for the standard vessels.

5. *Sterilization.* Except for steaming the *Saccharomyces* test for 10 min, autoclave the standard, and assay vessels at 121°C for 5 min. The vessels are removed immediately from the autoclave when atmospheric pressure is reached within the sterilization chamber. This avoids problems of growth suppression of test organisms induced by browning reaction products.

6. *Inoculation and Incubation.*

(a) Cool all the tubes to the incubation temperature. All tubes must be at the same temperature all the way through the rack. A water bath or convection incubator may be used for this purpose. This precaution is especially necessary when turbidimetric measurements are made, since in that procedure the rate of growth, rather than the extent of growth, is primarily being measured.

(b) Aseptically inoculate each tube with one drop of inoculum. It is convenient to use either a 1-mL or else a 5-mL pipette with a 5-mm tip bent at a 60° angle so that the pipette may be held almost horizontally while the drop is delivered vertically. A 5-mL or 10-mL syringe fitted with a 14–18-gauge needle may also be used.

(c) Incubate at the temperature indicated in Table 3.1. Tubes should be incubated in a water bath. All vessels for an assay must be maintained at exactly the same temperature. The lactobacilli and *Saccharomyces* tests are incubated 18–24 hr, while the remaining tests (protozoa and mold) are incubated 5–7 days. The lactobacilli tests are incubated 72 hr if acid is to be titrated.

7. *Turbidimetry and Acidimetry.*

(a) If turbidimetry is employed for measurement of yeast, bacterial, or protozoan growth, the absorbance, turbidity or percent transmission is measured against an uninoculated control. Mix well to suspend the organisms uniformly using a vortex mixer. For a valid assay, the AOAC requires that the percent T of the inoculated blank correspond to a dried cell weight of less than 0.3 mg/5 mL tube when read against the uninoculated blank (24). Generally, under proper conditions almost complete absence of growth will be found in the inoculated blank. AOAC procedure further states that the percent T observed at the highest level of standard must be equivalent to that of a dried cell weight of 0.625 mg/5 mL tube or greater. The turbidimetric method has the advantage of being more rapid and amenable to semiautomation. An automated technique for measuring the growth of organisms used in the analysis of vitamins has been described by Colvin et al. (25). The colorimeter used was interfaced with a microcomputer to allow the results to be reported in concentration. An example of the Elanco Autoturb® (Elanco Products Company, Indianapolis, Indiana) is shown in Figure 3.1.

(b) If acidimetry is used, transfer the contents of each tube to a 50-mL Erlenmeyer flask, and rinse the tube once with 5 mL water, adding the rinsing to the flask. Add about 0.1 mL 0.1% bromothymol blue, and titrate with 0.1 N sodium hydroxide to a green color, about pH 6.8. Hold a flask for a reference color for about 10–20 titrations and then substitute a new flask. The color in the reference flask changes on standing. The end point may be taken as where the yellow color changes to green or the green changes to blue, providing that all tubes are titrated identically. A glass electrode can be used for titrating, with the end point being pH 7.0. The procedure is rapid and may be automated. Colored extracts may be encountered in the assay of certain samples. Such colors may interfere by obscuring the end point and necessitate the use of another indicator or an electrometric titration. Titration in excess of 1.0 mL for the tubes containing 0.0 mL of the standard vitamin solution indicates an excessive amount of vitamin being present in the basal medium or from the inoculum, and thereby invalidates the assay. The remedy is to examine each constituent of the basal medium, the inoculum preparation

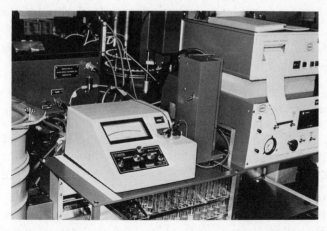

FIGURE 3.1 AUTOTURB® system for automated turbidity determination.

technique, and glassware preparation procedure to locate the source of the extraneous vitamin.

8. *Analysis of Data.* Examples of turbidimetric and titrimetric data are provided on pages 374 and 546–547, respectively. By whatever method growth is determined, a standard curve is prepared by plotting growth (turbidity, weight of mycelium, titratable acid) versus μg or ng of vitamin per tube. From the standard curve, the amount of vitamin in the various levels of test solutions is determined by interpolation. The sample assay is considered valid when there is no tendency for the vitamin values computed on a per mL sample extract basis to increase or decrease with the aliquot size used. Such a tendency is called drift. Various agents, for example, inhibitors and neutralization salts, can induce drift. When drift is due to the inadequacy of the medium, it may be corrected by supplementing the medium with the missing stimulator substances if these are known or can be found. Generally, this problem can be solved by modification of the method or elimination of the interfering substances.

When dealing with the analysis of unfamiliar biological systems, it is advisable to conduct a group of assays using different levels of sample concentration and comparing the results with those of the standard curve (see Chapter 18, Figure 18.1). Parallelism of the results with those of the standard curve indicates the test organism response to the particular vitamin of interest rather than to some other growth stimulant. It also signifies the absence of inhibitors in the test matrix.

The validity of microbiological assays is also shown by agreement of values on repeated assays, or on reassay with a different organism or animal. It is customary to assume that microbiological assays may be subject to an inherent error of 10–15% and to accept as identical, replicates that do not differ by more than that amount. Variability of this magnitude should be ascribed to inadequacies in the media used or to inadequate control of the factors associated with the assay, rather than to an innate variability of the test organism.

The sigmoidal dosage-response curves of microbial vitamin assays may be transformed into linear regressions by the logistic function. Validity of the test responses is then determined by evaluating sample and standard regressions for parallelism; that is, statistically, the null hypothesis tests whether the difference in slopes of the sample and standard curves equals zero. The student's t-test is employed at the 95% level to evaluate the null hypothesis. Confidence limits for the mean values are obtained by applying the likelihood function, as demonstrated by Schatzki and Keagy (11). Percent standard errors for each analysis may also be calculated, and ideally, they should be less than 10% (12). A computer software package has been developed and documented for evaluating microbiological vitamin assay data using the logistic transformation (13).

9. *Calculations.*

(a) Draw a standard curve for the assay by plotting either mL of 0.1 N NaOH titrated, absorbance or turbidity (ordinate) against concentration of vitamin per tube in the standard series.

(b) Determine the vitamin content of the vessels of the unknown sample series by interpolation of the values onto the standard curve.

(c) Calculate the vitamin content of the test material from the average of the values for 1 mL of test solution obtained from not less than three sets of these tubes which do not vary by more than 10% from the average using the following formula:

$$\mu g \text{ per g} = \frac{\text{average } \mu g \text{ per mL} \times \text{volume}}{\text{wt of sample}} \times \text{dilution factor}$$

AOAC procedures require that at least two-thirds of the original number of tubes used in the four levels of sample extract be included in the final mean (24). Since the accuracy claimed for microbiological assays is about $\pm 10\%$ of the mean, the results should be reported to two significant figures only. The reported data should also indicate the test organism used to determine the vitamin.

LITERATURE CITED

1. Baker, H. and Frank, O. *Clinical Vitaminology.* Interscience, New York (1968).
2. Baker, E. R., McLaughlin, J. J. A., Hutner, S. H., De Angelis, B., Feingold, S., Frank, O., and Baker, H. "Water-soluble vitamins in cells and spent culture supernatants of *Poteriochromonas stipitata, Euglena gracilis* and *Tetrahymena thermophila.*" *Arch. Microbiol.* **129**, 310 (1981).
3. Sleigh, M. *The Biology of Protozoa.* Elsevier, New York (1973).
4. Hutner, S. H. Ed. *Biochemistry and Physiology of Protozoa,* Vol. 3. Academic Press, New York (1964).
5. Hill, D. L. *The Biochemistry and Physiology of Tetrahymena.* Academic Press, New York (1972).

6. Baker, H. and Frank, O. "Vitamin analysis in medicine." In R. S. Goodhart and M. E. Shils, Eds., *Modern Nutrition in Health and Disease*, 5th Ed. Lea & Febiger, Philadelphia, 523–546 (1973).

7. Christopher, A. R., Dobrosielski-Vergona, Goetz, G., Johnston, P. L., and Carell, E. F. "Vitamin B_{12} and the macromolecular composition of Euglena—1. Kinetic analysis of the cell cycle and chloroplast replication." *Exptl. Cell Res.* **89**, 71 (1974).

8. Voigt, M. N., Eitenmiller, R. R., and Ware, G. O. "Vitamin assay by microbial and protozoan organisms: response to vitamin concentration, incubation time and assay vessel size." *J. Food Sci.* **43**, 1418 (1978).

9. Pearson, W. N. "Principles of microbiological assay," In P. Gyorgy, and W. N. Pearson, Eds., *The Vitamins*, Vol. 7, 2nd ed. Academic Press, New York (1967).

10. Voigt, M. N., Eitenmiller, R. R., and Ware, G. O. "Vitamin analysis by microbial and protozoan organisms: response to food preservatives and neutralization salts." *J. Food Sci.* **44**, 723 (1979).

11. Schatzki, T. F. and Keagy, P. M. "Analysis of nonlinear response in microbiological assay for folacin." *Anal. Biochem.* **65**, 204 (1975).

12. Bliss, C. and White, C. "Statistical methods in biological assay of the vitamins." In P. Gyorgy and W. N., Pearson, Eds., *The Vitamins*, Vol. 6, 2nd ed. Academic Press, New York, 23–138 (1967).

13. Voigt, M. N., Ware, G. O., and Eitenmiller, R. R. "Computer programs for the evaluation of vitamin B data obtained by microbiological methods." *J. Agric. Food Chem.* **27**, 1305 (1979).

14. Roberts, E. C. and Snell, E. E. "An improved medium for microbiological assays with *Lactobacillus casei.*" *J. Biol. Chem.* **163**, 499 (1946).

15. American Type Culture Collection. Catalogue of strains. ATCC, 12301 Parklawn Drive, Rockville, Md. 20852 (1974).

16. Conner, R. L. and Cline, S. G. "Iron deficiency and the metabolism of *Tetrahymena pyriformis.*" *J. Protozool.* **11**, 486 (1964).

17. Baker, H. and Frank, O. Departments of Preventive Medicine and Community Health and Medicine, New Jersey Medical School, East Orange, N.J. 07018. Private communication.

18. Strohecker, R. and Henning, H. M. "Vitamin Assay: Tested Methods." *Verlag Chemie*, GMBH, Weinheim/Bergstr, Germany (1966).

19. Difco Supplementary Literature. Difco Laboratories, Detroit, Michigan (1972).

20. Pennington, D., Snell, E. E., and Williams, R. J. "An assay method for pantothenic acid." *J. Biol. Chem.* **135**, 213 (1940).

21. Parrish, W. P., Loy, H. W., and Kline, O. L. "Further studies on the yeast method for vitamin B_6." *J. Assoc. Off. Agric. Chem.* **39**, 157 (1956).

22. Hurley, N. A. "Notes on the modification of the Atkin method for vitamin B_6 assays." *J. Assoc. Off. Agric. Chem.* **43**, 43–45 (1960).

23. Association of Official Analytical Chemists. "Changes in methods-microbiological methods for the B-vitamins." *J. Assoc. Off. Agric. Chem.* **41**, 61 (1958).

24. Association of Official Analytical Chemists. *Official Methods of Analysis*, 13th ed.,Washington, D.C. (1980).

25. Colvin, G., Gibson, G. L., and Neill, D. W. "Use of the 'Analmatic clinical system' in the microbiological assay of vitamin B_{12} and folic acid in serum." *J. Clin. Pathol.* **24**, 18 (1971).

26. Guilarte, T. R., McIntyre, P. A., and Tsan, Min-Fu. "Growth response of the yeasts *Saccharomyces uvarum* and *Kloeckera brevis* to the free biologically active forms of vitamin B_6." *J. Nutr.* **110**, 954 (1980).

27. Guilarte, T. R., Shane, B., and McIntyre, P. A. "Radiometric-microbiological assay of vitamin B_6: Application to food analysis." *J. Nutr.* **111**, 1869 (1981).

28. Luecke, R. W. and Pearson, P. B. "The determination of free choline in animal tissues." *J. Biol. Chem.* **155**, 507 (1944).

4 Chromatographic Assay of Vitamins

Jonathan W. DeVries

GENERAL CONSIDERATIONS

In nearly all vitamin laboratories routinely analyzing a large number and variety of samples for the content of the various vitamins, there has been a definite trend toward replacing labor-intensive manual wet chemical methods with mechanized procedures. Such mechanization often not only eliminates or reduces the amount of manual effort necessary to carry out a particular analysis, but also permits systems to be set up that can be run automatically with little or no operator interaction. When the analysis being done not only involves the quantitation for the analyte of interest, but also a separation of the analyte from what may be a complex matrix, chromatography is an excellent form of mechanization. Appropriate choices of apparatus, mobile phases, stationary phases, specific detectors, and data recorders provide systems with the potential to be rapid, sensitive, precise, and accurate in the operator-controlled, semiautomatic and automatic modes.

In 1905, Ramsey (1) first employed chromatography for the separation of mixtures of gases and vapors by selectively absorbing and desorbing them from solid substrates. The following year, Tswett (2, 3) separated colored plant pigments using a column technique, a process he called chromatography, color writing. After receiving relatively little attention for the next decade, the technique was popularized during the second to fifth decade of the 1900s by Palmer whose work in nutrition included a variety of studies involving vitamins or vitamin precursors (4–9).

In 1952, James and Martin (10) mechanized the separation process with the introduction of the gas-liquid chromatograph. Recognition of the potential simplicity, sensitivity, speed, and accuracy, along with dramatic advances in electronics and column technology which allow that potential to be realized, has resulted in widespread use of gas chromatography for a wide variety of analyses. However, because of the low volatility and thermal instability of the majority of vitamin compounds, its use in this area has been quite limited. One notable exception has been the separation and quantitation of the vitamin E vitamers, the tocopherols (11,12).

Mechanization of the liquid chromatography process to carry out difficult separations using liquids under high pressure flowing over beds of small sized particles (high-pressure liquid chromatography, HPLC) does not appear to have been brought about by an inventor or inventors per se, but rather to have evolved from classical liquid chromatography in the two decades beginning in the late 1950s.

Chromatography in its present form is the science of the separation and quantitation of closely related compounds. In both gas-liquid chromatography (GLC) and HPLC, the analyst can take advantage of the speed, selectivity, and sensitivity that these systems provide. In GLC, columns that are highly selective for the compounds of interest can be chosen and coupled with temperature programming techniques and physical property specific detectors to separate and quantitate volatile compounds of interest. In HPLC, highly selective column and solvent (mobile phase) combinations can be utilized with physical property specific detectors for the rapid separation and quantitation of nonvolatile compounds.

A.   Theory

Although it is not the purpose of this chapter to cover chromatographic theory in depth, a definition of the basic terms used in discussions and publications of chromatographic vitamin assays is necessary to aid the analyst starting in chromatography. Those analysts desiring a more thorough discussion of chromatographic theory are referred to *Basic Gas Chromatography* by McNair and Bonelli (13) and to *Introduction to Modern Liquid Chromatography* by Snyder and Kirkland (14).

A hypothetical chromatogram is shown in Figure 4.1, where:

T_r Retention time of component of interest. The retention time of a particular compound is essentially constant as long as all chromatographic variables such as stationary phase, mobile-phase composition and flow rate, temperature, and so on, are constant.

T_d System dead volume time. The time required for a compound unretained by the stationary phase to pass through the system.

T'_r Adjusted retention time. Adjusted retention time is equal to the retention time minus the system dead volume time. It is also equal

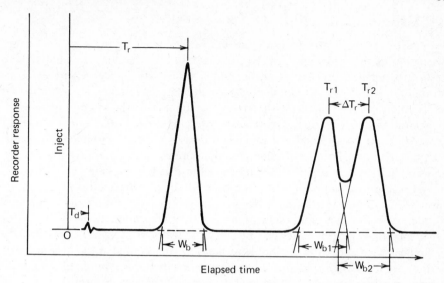

FIGURE 4.1 Hypothetical reconstruction of a typical chromatogram.

to the time spent in the stationary phase by the compound of interest.

W_b Width of peak at its base. Peak width is defined in the same time units as retention time and is measured at the intersection of lines drawn tangent to the sides of the peak curve and the chromatographic baseline.

N Number of theoretical plates in the column being used. The number of theoretical plates is an indication of the efficiency of the column, that is, its ability to maintain sharp narrow peaks as a function of retention time. It is calculated by the formula:

$$N = 16(T'_r / W_b)^2$$

HETP   Height equivalent of a theoretical plate. HETP is defined as:

$$\text{HETP} = L/N$$

where L equals the length of the column (usually in cm).

R Resolution. The ability of the stationary phase to separate two compounds of interest. Generally, the analyst can note the degree of resolution by observation. R can be calculated using the formula:

$$R = (T_{r1} - T_{r2})/[(W_{b1} + W_{b2})/2] = 2(T_{r1} - T_{r2})/(W_{b1} + W_{b2}) =$$

$$2\Delta T_r/(W_{b1} + W_{b2})$$

For $R = 1.5$, the two compounds will have less than 0.1% overlap.

B. Instrumentation

Since GLC finds relatively little use in routine vitamin analysis, no further discussion of that technique will be contained in this chapter. The analyst who wishes to pursue GLC for particular applications will find excellent basic information in *Basic Gas Chromatography* by McNair and Bonelli (13). Additional information can be obtained in references pertaining to the vitamin of interest.

For the analyst who carries out routine vitamin assays, HPLC offers numerous advantages over traditional wet chemical methods or other automated methods. Among these are simplicity, reduced sample preparation time, speed, accuracy, and simplicity. Of these, the one that can be most readily exploited by the analyst is that of reduced sample preparation time. By employing methods that utilize the HPLC column to its fullest extent as a tool for separating the compound of interest from other compounds, many of the purification steps necessary for other quantitation techniques can be eliminated. For truly routine analysis, the equipment used should be as simple as possible to accomplish the task at hand. In the case of HPLC, this means equipment that requires a minimal amount of operator time for setup, operation, maintenance, and service. For routine analysis, assembling of an optimum system of components, each meeting these criteria, and operating that system in the isocratic, that is constant mobile-phase composition mode will usually give the best results.

Although gradient elution, that is, the programmed change of mobile-phase composition from a weak eluting solvent to a strong eluting solvent, offers the advantage of being able to carry out certain complex separations and ion chromatographic separations, the advantages and disadvantages of gradient elution versus isocratic systems should be carefully considered.

The equipment necessary to carry out gradient elution is generally complex and expensive. In addition, gradient elution chromatographic separations usually require more time per sample to perform and need very high purity solvents to prevent baseline drift and ghost peaks. Isocratic elution offers the advantage of lower initial equipment investment and lower operating costs. Often two complete isocratic systems can be set up for approximately the same cost as a single complex gradient system. Operating costs are lower for isocratic systems due to less stringent solvent quality requirements and lower per sample analysis times. Optimum use of isocratic systems does, however, require that methods used for sample extraction and workup be carefully thought out.

A schematic of a typical HPLC system is shown in Figure 4.2. In addition to the components shown, a fraction collector could be added at the end of the system rather than allowing the eluent to go to waste. Although the components of the system could be discussed in any order, the order followed will be essentially that of the path followed by the mobile phase during operation.

1. *Solvent Reservoir.*   The mobile-phase reservoir used should meet the following criteria:

(a) Maintain the consistency of the mobile phase by minimizing evaporation and providing for stirring of the solution.

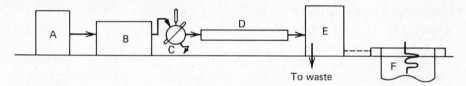

To waste

FIGURE 4.2   Schematic diagram of a typical high-pressure liquid chromatography system. A—solvent reservoir; B—precision flow pump; C—injector; D—column; E—detector; F—data recorder.

(b) Keep the solvent clean, particularly free of fine dust particles.

(c) Be easy to drain or change.

(d) Allow for the inclusion of an inert atmosphere over the mobile phase if necessary.

(e) Allow for degassing the mobile phase, if necessary, for proper operation of the chromatographic detector.

Usually an Erlenmeyer vacuum flask meets all of these criteria. In addition, this type of container is easy to stopper and store between uses.

2. *Pump or Pump System.*   The pump used to drive the mobile phase through the column should meet the following criteria:

(a) Exhibit precise flow characteristics. Although accurate flow of the mobile phase is not necessary for good HPLC results, that is 1.95 mL/min will work as well as 2.0 mL/min when the pump is set at 2.0 mL/min, both short-term (minute to minute and long-term (hour after hour) flow precision are necessary for vitamin quantitation. Pumping precision, as measured by retention shifts, should be better than $\pm 2\%$ relative standard deviation for most routine work. Because standard solutions are included in each run of a vitamin assay by HPLC, pumps that exhibit adequate precision but not necessarily good resettability, that is, the ability to be reset or returned to a previously determined flow rate provide excellent service for routine analysis.

(b) Operate with flow pulses that result in less detector noise than is inherent in the detector itself. Fluctuations in mobile-phase flow, if large enough, result in temporary baseline shifts or noise when they pass through the detector. The pumping system should minimize these fluctuations to the point that their effect is less than that of line voltage changes, detector electronic noise, or recorder electronic noise.

(c) Be made of materials that are chemically resistant to the mobile phase being used. Pumps that use stainless steel and polyfluorocarbons for the mobile-phase contact surfaces will generally meet this criterion for routine vitamin assay.

(d) Have flow and pressure capability adequate for the separations being carried out. With the back pressures generated by microparticulate columns, pressure capability of 0–5000 psi at flows of 0–5 mL/min is desirable.

(e) Require a minimal amount of operator attention. Pumps used for routine analysis should require little or no priming. Solvents should need no degassing for proper pump operation. Both procedures require a substantial amount of operator time which is usually at a premium in analytical laboratories.

(f) Be rugged in design and construction. Pumps of rugged construction reduce operator time involved in, and cost of, maintainence and service. In addition, in most vitamin assays, batches of samples requiring considerable analyst time are prepared for HPLC injection. Pump failure during the course of a run usually results in the loss of the prepared sample and the operators' time.

Although a wide variety of pump concepts and designs have been produced in the past, market forces dictated primarily by costs and laboratory requirements have essentially narrowed the range of commercially available pumps to three types, (1) the single piston reciprocating (pulse dampened and pulse compensated), (2) the multiple piston reciprocating, and (3) the diaphragm pump. Since it is not the purpose of this discussion to cover the mechanical details of the various systems, the reader desiring more information is referred to sources such as Snyder and Kirkland (14) or the various manufacturers' literature. With the wide variety of equipment and options available, the analyst can readily match a system to his needs. Less expensive rugged pumps that meet the criteria above can often be dedicated to one or several analyses. Because of their low cost, multiple systems can be set up to provide greater flexibility than can be achieved with more expensive systems featuring capabilities the analyst is unlikely to use.

3. *Sample Injectors.* The function of placing the standard solution or the sample solution on the chromatography column should be carried out using an injector that meets the following criteria:

(a) Minimizes band spreading of the compounds injected.

(b) Exhibits a high level of precision of the solution volume injected. Generally, loop-type injectors, where an appropriately sized loop is overfilled and a precise aliquot switched inline between the pump and column, exhibit better precision than those relying on operator-controlled microsyringe injections. The difficulties in filling and reading microsyringes results in greater injection variation.

(c) Be chemically inert to the solvents and samples being used.

(d) Be easy to operate. With the possible exception of the data system if used, the injector valve requires the greatest amount of operator interaction of the entire HPLC system and therefore simple, time-saving, operation is preferred.

(e) Be of rugged design and construction. Designs requiring minimal maintainence and service reduce costs and downtime. In addition, rugged seal materials in the moving parts of the valve improve injection precision and increase column life by reducing the amount of seal material sloughed onto the HPLC column.

4. *Automatic Sample Injectors.* Perhaps one of the greatest time-saving devices available to the laboratory that has large numbers of a particular analysis

or analyses to carry out is the autosampler. The capability of allowing the analyst to spend valuable laboratory time carrying out necessary sample preparations and allowing HPLC operations to continue unattended during nonworking hours can improve productivity tremendously. In addition to the criteria set up for injectors in general, the following also apply to autosamplers:

(a) The autosampler should have a level of precision adequate for the analysis being carried out and high enough to alleviate the need for addition of internal standards (these require additional sample preparation and quantitation time).

(b) No void space should be present above the sample in the sampler vial, or if present, should be able to be filled with an inert gas. This is particularly important when analyzing air-sensitive samples. Autosamplers that maintain the inert gas over the sample or carry out injections without allowing air to contact the solution allow air-sensitive samples to be rerun at a later time, should a change of some parameter such as mobile phase or detector attenuation be indicated as the result of the original unattended run.

(c) The autosampler should provide for exclusion of light from the sample holding area. Maintaining the lowest possible light level for light-sensitive vitamins, particularly on extended analytical runs, is desireable.

(d) The autosampler should be rugged and built as simply as possible, in light of operating requirements, to minimize cost and downtime.

5. *Column Hardware.* Column hardware, that is, not including packing, should meet the following criteria:

(a) Be made of chemically inert materials capable of withstanding the maximum pressure to be encountered during use.

(b) Have mirror smooth interior surfaces to minimize sample band broadening.

(c) Have zero dead volume, that is, be absent of voids containing no packing to minimize broadening of sample bands.

(d) Be equipped with end fittings that allow rapid interchange of columns and that are durable enough to withstand numerous column changes.

6. *Detectors.* The most common type of HPLC detectors used in vitamin analysis are the UV absorbance (single fixed, multiple fixed, and variable wavelength), the fluorometric (dual filter, monochromator-filter, and dual monochromator), and, to some extent, the electrochemical.

The following are the parameters that should be considered when selecting a detector:

(a) Signal-to-noise ratio. Selecting a detector with too low a signal-to-noise ratio for a particular application can result in imprecise quantitation of peaks. On the other hand, there is often a substantial price penalty associated with a detector having a higher than necessary signal-to-noise ratio.

(b) Drift. Selection of detectors with minimal upscale or downscale drift reduces the chance of loss of data during unattended analysis for those analysts considering automated HPLC vitamin analysis.

(c) Relative sample sensitivity. The ability of the detector, when combined with the rest of the HPLC system to detect the vitamin component at the level of interest. Obviously this ability is necessary for the analyst to carry out the analysis by HPLC.

(d) Linearity. Linear detector response over a wide range of concentrations of the vitamin of interest reduces the number of dilutions required or the need for complex calibration curves.

(e) Flow cell design. The flow cell of the detector should be designed to minimize band broadening and therefore recombination of the components separated in the column. In addition, inlet and outlet tubing connections to the flow cell should be designed to pass any gas bubbles out of the system.

(f) Provision for slight back pressure on the flow cell. The flow cell and connecting tubing should be able to withstand a minimum back pressure of 30–50 psi to minimize any outgassing of dissolved gases from the mobile phase in the detector cell.

(g) Convenience of operation, ruggedness, and minimal effect of external factors such as flow and temperature changes.

(1) Fixed-wavelength UV absorbance detectors. A schematic of a typical fixed wavelength detector is shown in Figure 4.3. Single fixed-wavelength units generally operate on the intense Hg wavelength at 254 nm, which provides excellent sensitivity for vitamins absorbing at 254. Because of their simplicity, they are relatively low in cost. This combination of cost and sensitivity makes this a good choice for many routine applications. One drawback of this detector system for vitamins in products such as foods is that many other compounds absorb at this wavelength as well. Additional selectivity can be achieved at relatively low cost by inserting

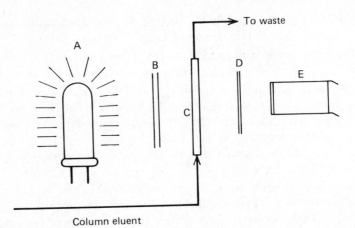

FIGURE 4.3 Schematic diagram of a typical fixed wavelength detector. Phosphors and filters can be changed as necessary to provide a variety of detection wavelengths. A—source lamp; B—phosphor; C—flow cell; D—filter (light); E—photo cell.

various filters and/or phosphors into the system, as shown in Figure 4.3. Using appropriate filter/phosphor combinations, the wavelengths 280, 295, 313, 340, 365, 405, 436, and 546 nm can readily be utilized. Many of these wavelengths, in particular 280, 295, and 313 nm, allow the detection of the vitamins of interest while giving little to no response to other sample components. With the addition of the increasingly popular zinc and cadmium source lamps and associated electronics and filters the wavelengths 214 nm and 229 nm can utilized as well. Additional filter combinations will likely provide additional wavelengths to use in the future.

(2) Continuously variable wavelengths UV-visible detectors. A schematic of a continuously variable wavelength detector is shown in Figure 4.4. Generally speaking, these detectors are capable of operating in the

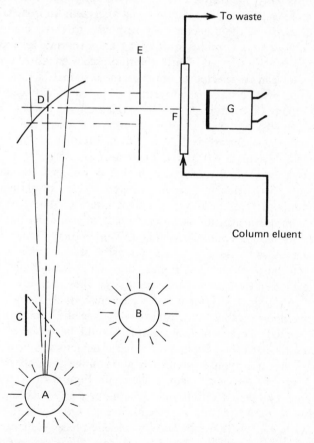

FIGURE 4.4 The monochromator system of a variable wavelength detector allows selection of any desired wavelength within the working range of the detector. A—deuterium source lamp; B—tungsten source lamp; C—source change mirror; D—grating monochrometer; E—monochrometer slit; F—flow cell; G—photo cell.

range of 190–800 nm. Because of the optics associated with this type of detector, they cost significantly more than their fixed multiple-wavelength counterparts. Maintainence and service costs tends to be higher due to the relatively short life of the deuterium lamp (approximately 1 year under normal use conditions) and the need to fine-tune the optics of the system. The variable-wavelength detector can be set to the absorbance maximum of the compound of interest for greatest sensitivity. In practice, due to the lower light intensity resulting from the monchromatic fractionation of the deuterium lamp output when compared with the intensity of filtered mercury lamp output, the sensitivity of the continuously variable UV detector at the absorbance maximum is often less than the sensitivity of the fixed wavelength detector using a wavelength near the maximum.

(3) Fluorometric detectors. In contrast to UV absorbance detectors which offer only one degree of specificity, namely the selection of appropriate wavelengths for the vitamin being analyzed, fluorometric detectors offer three. First, the detector only responds to those compounds that fluoresce. Second, an excitation wavelength appropriate for the compound of interest can be selected. Third, the fluorescent emission wavelength of the detector can be selected to optimize the response of the compound of interest. On some occasions, a fourth degree of specificity can be obtained by derivitizing the analyte. A schematic diagram of a fluorescence detector is shown in Figure 4.5. For most routine work where the excitation and emission wavelengths are well separated, a dual filter unit of proper design will provide adequate sensitivity. There are many models currently available with a wide variety of optical and flow cell systems, and it is wise to evaluate the particular detector being considered by actually analyzing the vitamin of interest at the levels of interest. Where excitation and emission maxima are not well separated, for example, vitamin E with excitation at 290 nm and emission at 330 nm, a dual monochromator unit may be necessary. Because of the intensity of the xenon lamp and the design of the flow cell and optics, dual monochromator units usually provide excellent sensitivity and specificity. They are, however, quite expensive. As with dual filter units, a particular dual monochromator fluorescence detector should be tested for the specific application for which it is intended. Three notes of caution should be observed when using fluorometric detectors. First, fluorometric detectors have a significantly narrower linear response to concentration range than absorbance detectors. A typical response curve is shown in Figure 4.6. As can be seen, care must be taken to dilute all samples properly to bring the analyte concentration into the linear response range. Otherwise order-of-magnitude errors can easily occur. Second, mobile phases that can quench the fluorescence of the sample should be avoided. Third, compounds coeluting from the HPLC column with the compound of interest and having a high absorbance at either the excitation or emission maxima may not fluoresce and therefore not show up on the chromatogram. They may, however,

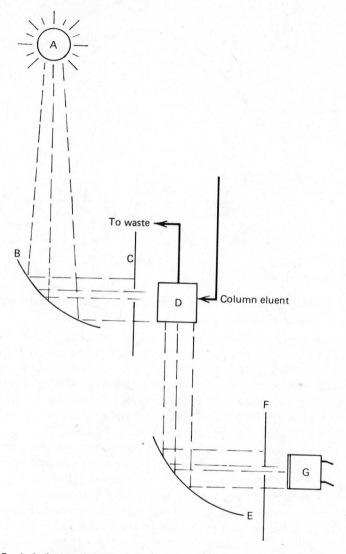

FIGURE 4.5 A dual monochromator detector incorporates a monochrometer system in both the excitation and emission light paths. In the dual filter fluorescence detector the monochromators are replaced by appropriate optical filters. A—source lamp (xenon); B—excitation monochrometer; C—excitation monochrometer slit; D—flow cell; E—emission monochrometer; F—emission monochrometer slit; G—photocell.

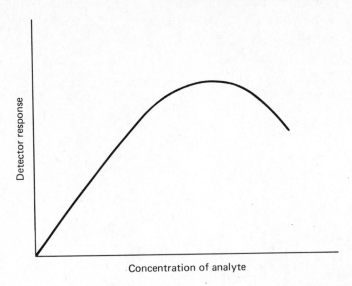

FIGURE 4.6 Output response curve of a fluorescence detector as a function of analyte concentration.

absorb some of the excitation or emission energy and therefore reduce the signal generated by the compound of interest.

7. *Intercomponent Connecting Tubing.*   All tubing and connections should be made of chemically resistant materials capable of withstanding the operating pressure of the system being used. All tubing used to connect the injector to the column and the column to the detector should be as short and of as narrow a bore as possible. In addition, all connections involved should be the zero dead volume type. This combination of tubing and connectors will minimize peak broadening, thereby increasing sensitivity and resolution. The analyst whose work requires frequent column changes or component rearrangement should select connecting fittings that will withstand repeated removal and insertion without leaking. For laboratories having a variety of HPLC components and wishing to maximize flexibility, a sturdy zero dead volume union (the compression screw type works very well) should be selected. All components including columns should then be outfitted to connect to these unions. Any combination of components can then be arranged.

8. *Component and/or System Control.*   With the advent of effective and moderately priced microprocessor technology, nearly all HPLC components and systems are microprocessor controlled. Individual component control offers excellent versatility for setting up optimized systems of various components. In addition, malfunctions in the controller of a single component can be corrected by swapping that component. On the other hand, complex system controllers can be used to carry out difficult procedures and often procedures for a number of different analyses can be stored in memory and recalled when needed. The

optimum component is one that can operate as a stand-alone unit for most routine work and still be readily coupled to a system controller should the need arise.

9. *Data Recording.* The permanent records of the analyses, the chromatograms, can be obtained using either strip chart recorders or a more advanced data processing system that can do post-run quantitation of the compounds of interest. Either instrument should have the following characteristics:

(a) Have a full-scale pen response time less than that of the detector being used.

(b) Have electronic noise levels equal to or lower than the noise levels of the HPLC system to which it is attached.

(c) Have a variable recording speed (0.5–10 cm/min) to conserve paper during routine analysis yet provide expanded traces should they be necessary for better viewing of poorly resolved peaks.

(d) Have input characteristics that match the output of the detector being used.

C. Column Packings

The column required for a particular separation is described by the mode of chromatography in which it operates. The three common types of columns (and modes) used for vitamin assay by HPLC are normal-phase, reverse-phase, and ion-exchange chromatography columns.

The normal phase, also termed liquid-solid chromatography, column separates compounds by an adsorption mechanism. The column packing is generally a high-surface-area silica or silica with a polar moiety chemically bonded to it. The packing preferentially adsorbs polar compounds over nonpolar ones and therefore elution order is based on compound polarity with the least polar compounds eluting first and the most polar last. Normal-phase columns have the advantage of being very efficient and providing excellent resolution, being easy to pack, and being lower in cost than other separation mode types. Normal-phase columns have the disadvantage of being easily contaminated by foreign compounds in the samples being analyzed and thereby suffering permanent loss of efficiency and resolution. A further disadvantage of normal-phase columns is the necessity of using solvents that are usually more expensive and difficult to handle than those used for ion-exchange or reverse-phase chromatography.

Reverse-phase chromatography derives its name historically from the fact that compounds are eluted in reverse order from that of adsorption chromatography. The mechanism of separation on reverse-phase columns, while not clearly understood, is believed to result from the preferential partitioning of nonpolar compounds into a bonded stationary phase from a polar mobile phase, usually water and a polar organic solvent. Reverse-phase packings are generally very durable and have substantially longer useful life than normal-phase columns. In addition, the mobile phase used, often primarily water, is less expensive. The disadvantages of reverse-phase packings are cost of manufacture and the fact that columns are more difficult to pack with them than with most other packings. This results in higher column prices which partly offset the savings achieved in solvent costs and greater durability.

Ion-exchange column packings, as the name implies, function by an ion-exchange mechanism. The packings are usually made by chemically bonding a moiety with ionic functionality to the outer surface of silica particles. The obvious advantage of ion-exchange columns is their ability to separate ion-exchangeable vitamins. A potential disadvantage of ion-exchange columns is the necessity of running gradient elution from a weakly ionic mobile phase to a strongly ionic mobile phase for many applications.

A number of general requirements are applicable to all column packings used in HPLC. They are:

1. Particles must be rigid enough to withstand the pressures at which the chromatographic mobile phase will be pumped without fracturing or compressing.

2. The packing must be insoluble in (and undegraded by) the mobile phase being used.

3. The packing should be of the smallest average particulate size compatible with the application and instrument being used to give the largest possible surface area and best resolution.

4. Particle size range should be as narrow as possible to permit easy column packing and to provide columns with high efficiency.

For additional information on these and other column-packing materials, the analyst is referred to *Introduction to Liquid Chromatography* by Snyder and Kirkland (14). After packing or purchasing a new column, it is advisable to test it with samples for which it will be used. A test chromatogram, along with a record of conditions, retention times, efficiency, and the resolution achieved for compounds of interest, should be filed for future reference.

D. Chromatographic Techniques

1. *Injection.* Injections of standard solutions and sample solutions should always be the same volume and in the same solvent to minimize differences in peak width between the standard and samples. The volume of the injection should be the smallest possible giving good precision and detection. Preferably the injection should be in a solvent that is of solvent strength equal to or less than that of the mobile phase (see Figure 4.7). In this case, the strong solvent in the chromatographic system (reverse-phase) is methanol. As can be seen, when the mixture being injected is dissolved in methanol, only the smallest of the injection volumes gives a chromatogram where the compounds are resolved at the baseline. On the other hand, when the mixture is dissolved in mobile

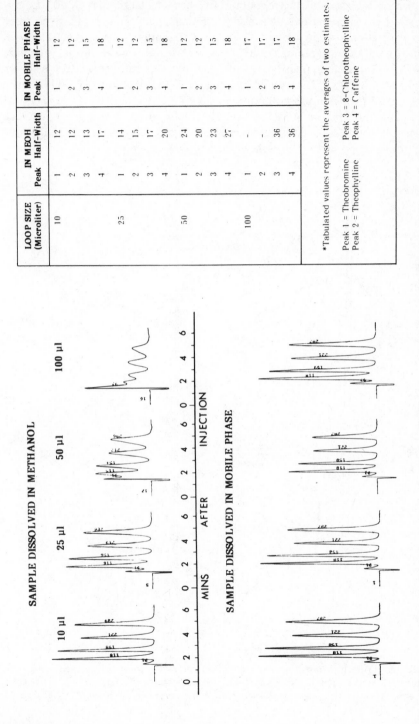

LOOP SIZE (Microliter)	IN MEOH		IN MOBILE PHASE	
	Peak	Half-Width	Peak	Half-Width
10	1	12	1	12
	2	12	2	12
	3	13	3	15
	4	17	4	18
25	1	14	1	12
	2	15	2	12
	3	17	3	15
	4	20	4	18
50	1	24	1	12
	2	20	2	12
	3	23	3	15
	4	27	4	18
100	1	–	1	17
	2	–	2	17
	3	36	3	17
	4	36	4	18

*Tabulated values represent the averages of two estimates.

Peak 1 = Theobromine   Peak 3 = 8-Chlorotheophylline
Peak 2 = Theophylline   Peak 4 = Caffeine

SAMPLE DISSOLVED IN METHANOL

10 µl   25 µl   50 µl   100 µl

MINS   AFTER   INJECTION

SAMPLE DISSOLVED IN MOBILE PHASE

FIGURE 4.7 Effect of varying injection size and injection solvent makeup on chromatographic efficiency and resolution. Instrument, SP 8000; column, 10µm RP-8, 4.6 × 250 mm; flow, 2 mL/min; mobile phase, 58 + 22 + 20 of 0.01 M sodium acetate + 1% acetic acid + methanol; detector, UV 270 nm. Each injection contains 500 ng of each of the four components dissolved in the volumes of injection solvent indicated. Figure courtesy of Spectra Physics (15).

phase before injection, injection volumes five times as large, that is, 50 μL, give chromatograms showing baseline resolution of all four components. Even when using an injection solvent that is the same as the mobile phase, resolution will be lost if the injection volume is too large as evidenced by the 100 μL injection of the mixture in mobile phase. An additional illustration of this effect is shown in Figure 4.8. Here, a mixture of five sugars is being chromatographed on a bonded phase propylamino column using 80 + 20 acetonitrile − H₂O as the mobile phase. In Figure 4.8a, 20 μL of a solution of 0.6 mg/mL of each component dissolved in water are injected. In Figure 4.8b, 4 mL of the 0.6 mg/ mL solution were diluted to 10 mL with acetonitrile giving a solution containing

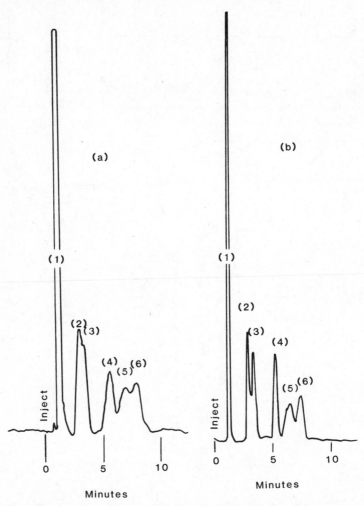

FIGURE 4.8 Effect of varying injection solvent on chromatographic efficiency and resolution. Instrument, various components; column, 10-μm bonded propylamino; flow, 1.5 mL/min; mobile phase, 80 + 20-acetonitrile + water; detector, RI @ 8x. (1) Water, (2) fructose, (3) glucose, (4) sucrose, (5) maltose, (6) lactose.

0.24 mg/mL of each component in 60 + 40 acetonitrile — H_2O. Without changing the detector attenuation or any other chromatographic conditions, 20 µL of this solution were injected. As can be seen, the chromatographic efficiency has improved so dramatically that the peak heights of the components in Figure 4.8b are equal to or greater than those of Figure 4.8a despite the fact that the concentration of each component is now only 40% of that of Figure 4.8a. As a result of this increased efficiency, the resolution between components has improved as well.

Analysts using injectors having restrictor bypass loops built into the injector system should exercise caution when analyzing sample solutions derived from samples of varying matrices. Even though the same injection solvent is used for the standards and the samples, large variations in sample components (i.e., foods) can often result in injection solutions of various viscosities. Bypass loop injectors depend on a constant ratio (1 + 5.5) of solvent flowing through the bypass loop compared with the sample loop during injection of the sample onto the column. If the sample solution being injected has a higher viscosity than the standard solution, the ratio between loops will increase and the sample injection will undergo greater dilution as it enters the column. This will result in peak widening and a decrease in peak height and often in inaccurate quantitation.

2. *Quantitation.* Quantitation of HPLC chromatograms can be done using either a peak height or peak area measurement. Because the HPLC detectors commonly used for vitamins are concentration and not mass dependent, peak height measurements generally provide more accurate data. This is due to the fact that poorly resolved peaks can be more accurately quantitated using the peak height method (14) and that concentration-dependent detector response is relatively unaffected by slight changes in flow rates. Calibration can be done using either external or internal standard techniques. Nearly all HPLC injection valves have adequate precision to eliminate the need for internal standard methods for accurate quantitation. This eliminates the extra sample preparation time involved with internal standard addition. Also eliminated is the need to find a compound with a retention time different from any components of the sample, that is chemically similar to the components of interest, that is not present in the original sample, is stable, and is readily available.

(a) Manual peak height measurement. Peak height measurements can readily be carried out to within ±1% relative standard deviation for a 10-cm peak using a metric ruler with 1-mm graduations. Generally speaking, when samples with a single component of interest are being manually injected, an analyst using a metric rule and an electronic calculator can perform measurements and calculations in the same amount of time that it takes to enter data and parameters into an electronic data system so that measurements and calculations can be performed electronically.

(b) Electronic data systems. Properly selected and programmed electronic data processors can save a great deal of analysts' time when automatic HPLC is performed on large batches of samples or when multiple components are being measured for each sample. When considering an electronic data processor, the following factors should be considered:

(1) Accuracy and precision with which unit carries out data measurement.

(2) Ease of data entry (i.e., sample weights, peak retention times) and programmability of processor unit. Units requiring excess time for data entry or for reprogramming will offset gains in time achieved over manual measurement and calculation.

(3) Ruggedness of unit. Excess unit failure results in high maintainence and service costs, as well as loss of data from analytical runs during which failure occurred.

(4) Versatility of unit. Units that can be connected to a variety of HPLC detectors and programmed for a variety of quantitation methods provide the greatest versatility. In addition, the ability to carry out postrun calculations specific to the analyst's needs is desirable. Care must be exercised in the utilization of the electronic data system to minimize quantitation errors. Proper operation of these units is dependent on the operator having a good understanding of the chromatography being carried out, as well as of the operating parameters of the data processor.

Accuracy of the measurements and postrun calculations performed by the data system depend on the operator setting the appropriate parameters. The most common data system errors result from the following parameters being improperly set:

(a) Peak width. A peak width setting that is too narrow results in broad, small peaks not being measured. A peak width setting that is too wide will result in narrow peaks being missed.

(b) Slope sensitivity. Too low a sensitivity setting results in small peaks being missed and the beginning of large peaks being detected too late. Likewise the end of large peaks will be detected too early. Too high a sensitivity results in the measurement of noise as peaks and in some cases the splitting of large peaks due to noise superimposed on that peak.

(c) Peak identification. Correct retention times and retention time windows must be set for the analysis being run.

(d) Scaling factors and sample weight. Scaling factors and sample weights are entered to correct for sample weights and sample dilution. Proper values must be entered.

(e) Detector zeroing. With certain data systems, improper detector zeroing is not readily apparent but results in improper measurement of the peaks in the chromatogram.

Before relying on electronic data processing to measure and calculate component quantities, the chromatographic parameters for a particular analysis should be worked out, a statistically significant number of samples run, and the results measured and calculated both electronically and manually. Standard statistical analysis should then show no significant difference between the two methods of quantitation. Once appropriate data system parameters have been established, quantitation errors during routine analysis can be minimized by incorporating the following practices:

(a) Always obtain a chromatographic trace with the data system printout, either from the data system plotter or from an attached strip chart recorder.

(b) Run appropriate standards and recalibrate system with each run or within the run if necessary.

(c) Observe the processing codes (and tic marks on the chromatogram) to assure that the data system is properly processing the detector signal it receives.

(d) Include a check sample in each analytical run whose analytical result can be compared with results obtained during previous runs.

3. *Peak Purity and/or Qualitative Analysis.* Reducing the probability that a foreign compound may be coeluting with the vitamin of interest is a concern of any analyst performing vitamin assay by HPLC. With the availability of appropriate high-efficiency columns, appropriate mobile phases, and function-selective detectors, this is generally not a problem for routine assay work. At times, however, there may be reason to question the purity of the compound as represented by the peak in the chromatogram. There are a number of techniques available to resolve such a question.

(a) Increase chart speed. Frequently coeluting peaks have retention times that differ only slightly, yet are sufficiently different so that a second peak becomes apparent on the leading or trailing edge of the main peak when the chart is run at high speed.

(b) Peak height ratioing. By passing the column eluent through two UV detectors set at two different wavelengths, the peak height ratio between detectors for the sample peak should match the ratio found for the standard peak. Similarly, one can apply the peak ratioing technique to two types of detectors, say a fluorescence detector and a UV detector in the case of fluorescent compounds.

(c) Continuous UV scanning. Detectors are available that provide on-the-fly scanning capability in the UV region during the chromatographic run. If the UV scans of the sample peak do not match those of the standard peak under the same conditions, coelution is occurring. Such instruments are expensive, however, and one can often purchase two less expensive detectors and do peak height ratioing. The second detector can also be used in another chromatographic system.

(d) Thin-layer chromatography (TLC). The detector eluent can be collected as the sample peak is eluting. The solution can then be spotted on a microscope slide TLC plate, the plate developed, and the thin-layer chromatogram observed for the presence of spots other than the vitamin of interest.

(e) Sample spiking. In cases where the vitamin of interest is the smaller contributor to a coelution peak, spiking the sample with a known amount of vitamin standard will often result in the coeluting peak being observed as a second peak on the leading or trailing edge of the vitamin peak. Obviously the recorder chart speed should be set as high as possible when using this technique.

METHODS AVAILABLE

Inasmuch as many of the chapters in this book relating to the individual vitamins contain methods for analyzing that vitamin by HPLC, the methods included here simultaneously analyze more than one vitamin. The method for simultaneously analyzing vitamins A and E is based on the work of Egberg et al. (16) and DeVries et al. (17). It has been used in the author's laboratory on a routine basis for over 4 years on a wide variety of samples. Minor modifications have been made where necessary to expand the method's capabilities for particularly difficult matrices, that is, to improve its universality. These modifications have been incorporated into the method as presented here.

The HPLC method for niacin, niacinamide, pyridoxine, thiamin, and riboflavin is based on an ion-pairing reverse-phase technique reported by Kirchmeier and Upton (18) and by Taillie et al. (19). The reported methods were modified somewhat for routine use with automated HPLC equipment. The wavelength of the detector was adjusted so as to allow all of the vitamins to be analyzed using a single response range for most multivitamin premixes and preparations. The ion-pairing reagent was changed from hexanesulfonate to pentanesulfonate to improve the resolution between thiamin and riboflavin and thus substantially reduce the analysis time per sample. The modified method has been used successfully for several years on a variety of multivitamin matrices such as premixes, capsules, and tablets. The reproducibility and recovery obtained over this time period agree with the published data (18). The method as described here applies primarily to vitamin concentrates. Methods of a similar nature have been applied to foods and urine (20-24). The reader is advised to survey original papers dealing with the matrix of his/her particular interest.

ANALYTICAL METHODOLOGY: SIMULTANEOUS ANALYSIS OF VITAMIN A AND VITAMIN E

A. Principle

Samples to be analyzed for vitamin A and vitamin E are saponified, neutralized, and diluted to volume. Two aliquots of the extract are analyzed using chromatographic conditions optimized for each vitamin. Although simultaneous quantitation of the two vitamins by a single HPLC injection in the isocratic mode or in the gradient elution mode is possible, experience has shown it to be much more practical to make separate injections of a single extract on two chromatographs. Chromatographic conditions are optimized for maximum efficiency, selectivity, and sensitivity with minimal analysis time for each vitamin. When two chromatographic systems are not available, the stability of the extract (less than 0.3% degradation in 4 hr when protected from light) allows a group of samples to be chromatographed first for one vitamin, then the other.

B. Reagents

1. *Vitamin A Acetate.* Prestandardized, encapsulated, equivalent to about 30 mg of retinol per g of oil (USP).

2. *Vitamin E Acetate.* α-Tocopheryl acetate No. 6679 (Eastman).

3. *Methanol.* Methanol should be of suitable purity for isocratic HPLC operation.

4. *Vitamin A Standard Solution.* (Equivalent to 30 μg of retinol/mL). Dissolve 100 mg of vitamin A standard oil in 10 mL acetone in a 100-mL amber volumetric flask. Dilute to volume with 95% ethanol. Prepare fresh daily.

5. *Vitamin E Standard Solution.* (Equivalent to 350 μg of α-tocopheryl acetate/mL). Dissolve 35 mg of α-tocopheryl acetate in 10 mL of acetone in a 100 mL-amber volumetric flask. Dilute to volume with 95% ethanol. Prepare fresh daily.

6. *Nitrogen Gas.* Equip a nitrogen gas cylinder with appropriate apparatus to provide a nitrogen atmosphere over the saponification mixture while refluxing is being carried out.

7. *Aqueous Potassium Hydroxide (0.5 g/mL).* Taking appropriate precautions, dissolve 50 g KOH in 50 mL H_2O. After bringing to room temperature, adjust the volume of the solution to 100 mL.

8. *Ethanolic Potassium Hydroxide (0.25 g/mL).* Taking proper precautions, dissolve 25 g KOH in 75 mL 95% ethanol. After bringing to room temperature, adjust volume to 100 mL. Prepare fresh daily.

9. *Acetic Acid Solution (0.125 g/mL).* Dissolve 125 g glacial acetic acid in 700–800 mL 95% ethanol in a 1 L volumetric flask. Bring to volume with 95% ethanol.

10. *Ethanol-Tetrahydrofuran Solution.* Combine equal volumes of 95% ethanol and tetrahydrofuran. Mix before using.

11. *Mobile Phase—Vitamin A.* Combine 87 parts of methanol (grade suitable for isocratic chromatography) with 13 parts H_2O.

12. *Mobile Phase—Vitamin E.* Combine 95 parts of methanol (grade suitable for isocratic chromatography) with 5 parts of H_2O. Adjust pH to 5.0 with acetic acid.

C. Equipment

1. *Saponification Flasks.*   Erlenmeyer flasks (125 mL, low actinic or amber) are equipped with reflux condensers. Provision should be made to provide an inert atmosphere such as nitrogen over the saponification mixture during heating.

2. *Pump.*   Constant flow capable of providing up to 3 mL/min at pressures up to 3000 psi.

3. *Injector.*   Loop injector, either manual or automated, capable of injecting 20 μL of solution.

4. *Column.*   For vitamin A: 10 μm, 25-cm × 3.2-mm Vydac ODS (No. 201 TPX, Separations Group). For vitamin E: 10 μm, 25-cm × 3.2-mm reverse phase C8 (850952706, Dupont).

5. *Detectors.*   For vitamin A: Variable wavelength UV set at 328 nm or multiple fixed wavelength set to operate 313 nm. For vitamin E: A dual monochromator fluorescence detector set for excitation 295 nm (10-nm slit) and emission 330 nm (10-nm slit).

D. Procedure

1. *Standard Preparation.*   Into a 125-mL amber Erlenmeyer flask pipette 10 mL of each of the vitamin A and vitamin E standard solutions. Add 10 mL 95% ethanol. To a second amber Erlenmeyer, pipette 5 mL of each of the vitamin A and vitamin E standard solutions. Add 20 mL 95% ethanol. Treat in the same manner as samples being analyzed beginning in step three.

2. *Sample Preparation.*   Grind all low moisture samples to pass a 40-mesh sieve. Mix all samples thoroughly to insure homogeneity. If samples cannot be analyzed immediately, protect from light and excess heat by storing in a cool dark place. Weigh a 3-g portion of the sample into a 125-mL Erlenmeyer flask. For high sugar samples, add 3 mL H_2O to form a slurry. Add 30 mL 95% ethanol to all low-fat samples and 22 mL to high-fat samples.

3. *Saponification.*   Add a pea-size piece (approximately 50 mg to serve as an antioxidant) of pyrogallic acid to each flask and swirl. Add 4 mL KOH solution (0.5 g/mL) to the standards and low fat samples. Add 8 mL of ethanolic KOH solution (0.25 g/mL) to the high-fat samples. Attach flasks to reflux condensers and nitrogen atmosphere and reflux with occasional swirling for 45 min. Cool to room temperature.

4. *Neutralization and Extraction.*   Add 25 mL of ethanolic acetic acid to each flask with swirling. Quantitatively transfer the contents of the flask to a 100-mL amber volumetric flask with ethanol-THF solution. Dilute to volume with ethanol-THF solution and mix well. Allow to stand for a minimum of 15 min to allow the fatty acid salts to precipitate and the solutions to clarify.

5. *Chromatography of Vitamin A.*   Using the Vydac ODS column and the vitamin A mobile phase, adjust the flow rate to 1.5 mL/min and allow the HPLC system to equilibrate for 30 min. Set the detector for 313 or 328 nm and

inject 20 μL of each of the standard and sample solutions. Typical chromato-grams are shown in Figure 4.9. Intersperse standards and samples as necessary to assure accurate quantitation (usually every 6–10 samples).

6. *Chromatography of Vitamin E.*   Using the Dupont C8 column and the vitamin E mobile phase, adjust the flow rate to 1.5 mL/min and allow 30 min for the system to equilibrate. Set the fluorometric detector to excitation of 290 nm (10-nm slit) and emission of 330 nm (10-nm slit) and inject 20 μL of each of the standard and sample solutions. Typical chromatograms are shown in Figure 4.10. Intersperse standards with samples as necessary (usually every 6–10 samples) to assure accurate quantitation.

7. *Quantitation.*   Measure the peak heights of the standards and samples either manually or electronically. Calculate the quantity of vitamin in each sample using the equation:

Vitamin A (IU/100 g) = $PH/W \times K \times 33300$

where PH = peak height of sample;

      W = weight of sample in grams;

   33300 = dilution factor times conversion from μg/g to IU/100 g;

      K = concentration of vitamin A (μg/mL) in saponified standard divided by its respective peak height. (Use the mean K value determined for the two standards).

Vitamin E (IU/100 g) = $PH/W \times K \times 0.10$

where PH = peak height of sample;

      W = weight of sample in grams;

   0.10 = dilution factor times conversion from μg/g to IU/100 g;

      K = concentration of vitamin E (α-tocopheryl acetate in μg/mL) divided by its respective peak height. (Use the mean K value determined for the two standards).

SIMULTANEOUS ANALYSIS OF NIACIN, NIACINAMIDE, PYRIDOXINE, THIAMIN, AND RIBOFLAVIN

A. Principle

This method applies to concentrated vitamin matrices such as multivitamin tablets, powder concentrates, and capsules. Inasmuch as the levels of these vitamins generally occur in the approximate ratio niacin or niacinamide-pyri-doxine-thiamin-riboflavin of 10+1+1+1, the standards are made up in these ratios and the UV absorbance detector is set at a wavelength to allow quantitation of all four vitamins in a single response range. The samples are extracted with aqueous acetic acid containing a pairing ion (an anion compatible with and capable of pairing with the cations of the vitamins being analyzed) in a heated ultrasonic bath. After cooling and dilution, the samples are separated and quantitated by ion-pairing reverse-phase liquid chromatography.

B.   Reagents

1. *Mobile Phase.*   Part A. Dissolve 2.0 g pentane sulfonic acid (sodium salt), and 20 mL acetic acid in approximately 1500 mL H_2O. Dilute to 2 L with H_2O. Part B. Dissolve 0.5 g pentane sulfonic acid (sodium salt), and 5 mL acetic acid in approximately 400 mL methanol of a grade suitable for isocratic HPLC. Dilute to 500 mL with methanol. Combine 800 mL Part A with 200 mL Part

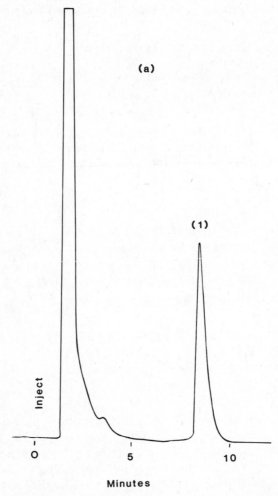

FIGURE 4.9   Chromatograms derived from HPLC assay of vitamin A. (a) Retinol standard after workup. (b) Extract from after workup. Peak 1, all-*trans*-retinol. Peak 2, 13-*cis*-retinol. Chromatographic conditions as described in procedure.

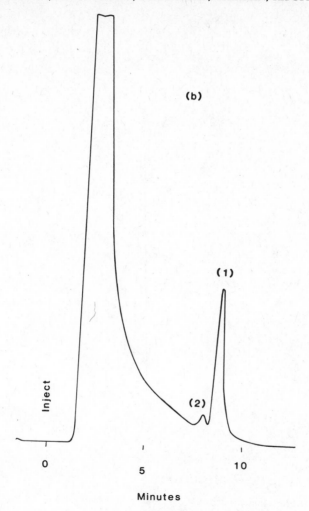

FIGURE 4.9 (*Continued*)

B. If greater resolution or longer retention times are necessary, increase the amount of Part A in the mobile phase.

2. *Extraction Solvent.* Use mobile phase Part A.

3. *Vitamin Stock Standard Solution.* (1 mg/mL niacin, 1 mg/mL niacinamide, 0.1 mg/mL pyridoxine HCl, 0.1 mg/mL thiamin HCl, 0.1 mg/mL riboflavin). Into a 1 L amber volumetric flask weigh to the nearest 0.0001 g, 1.000 g niacin, 1.000 g niacinamide, 0.100 g pyridoxine HCl, 0.100 g dried thiamin HCl, and 0.100 g riboflavin. Add approximately 800 mL mobile-phase Part A and place in ultrasonic bath heated to 50°C to aid solution. Cool to room temperature after a clear solution has been obtained and dilute to volume with mobile-phase Part A.

(a)

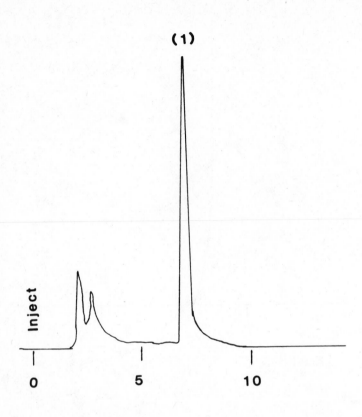

Minutes

FIGURE 4.10 Chromatograms derived from HPLC assay of vitamin E. (a) α-Tocopherol standard after workup. (b) Extract after workup. Peaks 1, 2, and 3 are α, β + γ, and δ tocopherol respectively. Chromatographic conditions as described in procedure.

4. *Working Standard Solution 1.*   (100 μg/mL niacin, 100 μg/mL niacinamide, 10 μg/mL pyridoxine HCl, 10 μg/mL thiamin HCl, 10 μg/mL riboflavin). Pipette 10 mL stock standard solution into a 100-mL amber volumetric flask. Dilute to volume with mobile-phase Part A.*

5. *Working Standard Solution 2.*   (50 μg/mL niacin, 50 μg/mL niacinamide, 5 μg/mL pyridoxine HCl, 5 μg/mL thiamin HCl, 5 μg/mL riboflavin). Pipette 5 mL stock standard into a 100-mL amber volumetric flask. Dilute to volume with mobile-phase Part A.*

*If a vitamin concentrate contains large amounts of a carrier substance such as $CaCO_3$, it should be added to the working standard solution as well. For example, if the concentrate contains 85% $CaCO_3$ and a 100 mg concentrate sample is being weighed, then 85 mg $CaCO_3$ should be added to the working standard solution.

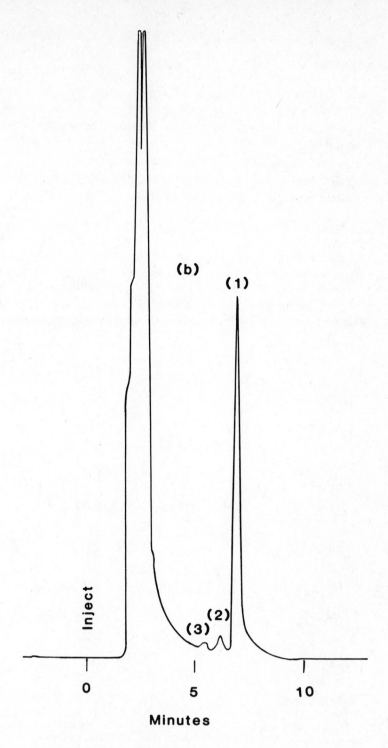

FIGURE 4.10 (*Continued*)

C. Equipment

1. *Pump.*   Constant flow capable of delivering up to 3 mL/min at pressures up to 3000 psi.

2. *Injector.*   Loop injector, either manual or automated, capable of injecting 20 μL of solution.

3. *Column.*   10 μm, 25-cm $\times$ 3.2-mm reverse-phase C18.

4. *Detectors.*   Variable wavelength UV set at 285 nm with a 4-nm bandwidth or fixed multiple wavelength detector set to operate at 280 nm.

D. Procedure

1. *Extraction.*   Weigh a portion of the homogeneous sample that will give individual component concentrations within the range of their respective standards, but never less than 20 mg, into a 100 mL-amber volumetric flask. Add a magnetic stirring bar to those samples that contain reduced iron. Add approximately 80 mL of mobile-phase Part A and place in an 50°C ultrasonic bath for

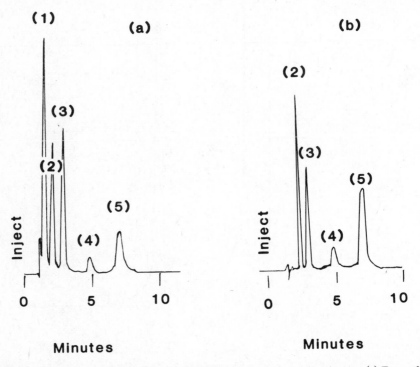

FIGURE 4.11 Chromatograms derived from HPLC assay of B-vitamin mixtures. (a) Trace of B-vitamin standards dissolved in mobile phase part A. (b) Trace of extract obtained from vitamin concentrate. Peaks 1, 2, 3, 4, and 5 are niacin, niacinamide, pyridoxine, thiamin, and riboflavin, respectively. Chromatographic conditions as described in procedure.

15 min. Remove magnetic stirring bar if used and rinse any extraction solvent into the flask with mobile phase Part A. Cool to room temperature and dilute to volume. Filter if necessary with GFA filter to clarify solution.

2. *Chromatography.* Adjust flow rate to 1.5 mL/min and allow system to equilibrate for 1–2 hr. (Ion-paired chromatography systems take significantly longer than other reverse-phase systems to reach equilibrium). Inject equal volumes of each standard and sample using injection volumes of 20 μL. A typical chromatogram is shown in Figure 4.11. Intersperse standards with samples as necessary to assure accurate quantitation (usually every 6–10 injections).

3. *Quantitation.* Measure the peak height of the standard and sample peaks either manually or electronically. Calculate the respective quantity of each vitamin using the equation:

$$\text{Vitamin content (\%)} = PH/W \times K \times 10$$

where
- PH = peak height of sample;
- W = weight of sample in mg;
- 10 = product of dilution, conversion from μg to mg and conversion to percent;
- K = concentration of respective vitamin in μg/mL in standard divided by its respective peak height. (Use mean K value from two standards).

LITERATURE CITED

1. Ramsey, W. "A determination of the amounts of neon and helium in atmospheric air." *Proc. Roy. Soc.* **A76**, 111 (1905).

2. Tswett, M. "Physikalisch-chemische studien uber das chlorophyll. Die adsorptionen." *Ber. Deut. Botan. Ges.* **24**, 316 (1906).

3. Tswett, M. "Adsorptionsanalyse und Chromatographische Methode. Anwendung auf die Chemie des Chlorophylls." *Ber. Deut. Botan. Ges.* **24**, 384 (1906).

4. Palmer, L. S. "Carotenoids as fat-soluble vitamins." *Science* **50**, 301 (1919).

5. Bechdel, S. I., Eckles, C. H., and Palmer, L. S. "Vitamin B requirement of the calf." *J. Dairy Sci.* **9**, 409 (1926).

6. Thurston, L. M., Eckles, C. H., and Palmer, L. S. "The role of the antiscorbutic vitamin in the nutrition of calves." *J. Dairy Sci.* **9**, 37 (1926).

7. Jones, I. R., Eckles, C. H., and Palmer, L. S. "The role of vitamin A in the nutrition of calves."*J. Dairy Sci.* **9**, 119 (1926).

8. Palmer, L. S. "The chemistry of vitamin A and substances having vitamin A effect." *J. Am. Med. Assoc.* **110**, 1748 (1938).

9. Jenness, and Palmer, L. S. "The vitamin A potency of creamery butter produced in Minnesota." *J. Dairy Sci.* **28**, 473 (1945).

10. James, A. T. and Martin, A. J. P. "Gas-liquid partition chromatography." *Analyst* **77**, 915 (1952).

11. Sheppard, A. J. and Hubbard, W. D. "Collaborative study of GLC method for vitamin E." *J. Pharm. Sci.* **68**(1), 115 (1979).

12. Association of Official Analytical Chemists. *Official Methods of Analysis,* 13th ed. 752–758, Washington, D. C. (1980).

13. McNair, H. M. and Bonelli, E. J. *Basic Gas Chromatography.* Varian Associates, Palo Alto, Calif. (1968).

14. Snyder, L. R. and Kirkland, J. J. *Introduction to Modern Liquid Chromatography,* 2nd ed. Wiley-Interscience, New York (1979).

15. Reece, P. A. and Cozamanis, I. "Injector loop sizes in HPLC." *Chromatogr. Rev.* **5,** 14, (1979).

16. Egberg, D. C., Heroff, J. C., and Potter, R. H. "Determination of all-trans and 13-cis vitamin A in food products by high pressure liquid chromatography." *J. Agric. Food Chem.* **25,** 1127 (1977).

17. DeVries, J. W., Egberg, D. C., and Heroff, J. C. "Concurrent analysis of vitamin A and vitamin E by reversed phase high performance liquid chromatography." In G. Charalambous, Ed., *Liquid Chromatographic Analysis of Food and Beverages,* Vol. 2. 477 (1979).

18. Kirchmeier, R. L. and Upton, R. P. "Simultaneous determination of niacin, niacinamide, pyridoxine, thiamin, and riboflavin in multivitamin blends by ion-pair high-pressure liquid chromatography." *J. Pharm. Sci.* **67,** 1444 (1978).

19. Taillie, S. A., Thornhill, R. A., and Toomay, T. L. "HPLC analysis of B vitamins in enrichment concentrates." Presented 61st annual meeting Amer. Assoc. of Cereal Chemists, (October 1976).

20. Toma, R. M. and Tabekhia, M. M. "High performance liquid chromatographic analysis of B-vitamins in rice and rice products." *J. Food Sci.* **44,** 263 (1979).

21. Kamman, J. F., Labuza, T. P., and Warthesen, J. J. "Thiamin and riboflavin by high performance liquid chromatography." *J. Food Sci.* **45,** 1497 (1980).

22. Roser, R. L., Andrist, A. H., and Harrington, W. H. "Determination of urinary thiamin by high pressure liquid chromatography." *J. Chromatogr.* **146,** 43 (1978).

23. Skurray, G. R. "A rapid method for selectively determining small amounts of niacin, riboflavin and thiamin in foods." *Food Chem.* **7,** 77 (1981).

24. Fellman, J. K., Artz, W. E., Tassinari, P. A., Cole, C. L., and Augustin, J. "Simultaneous determination of thiamin and riboflavin in selected foods by high-performance liquid chromatography." *J. Food Sci.* **47,** 2048 (1982).

5 Automated Vitamin Analysis

David C. Egberg
Omer Pelletier
Alan J. Johnson
James N. Thompson

GENERAL CONSIDERATIONS

A trend exists in modern analytical laboratories to employ automation whenever it can be economically justified. This would include not only automated data handling but mechanical systems that replace the standard manual steps characteristic of chemical or microbiological analytical methods. This chapter presents some tested automated vitamin methods, both chemical and microbiological. Although many automated chromatographic vitamin techniques could be categorized as automated vitamin methods, they are best handled in a separate section.

The automated methods described in this chapter have the common characteristic of mechanically replacing the manual steps used in vitamin analysis. These would include such steps as: pipetting, dialysis, distillation, timing reactions, solvent partitioning, and recording analytical response such as fluorescence, absorbance, or turbidity. Two general categories of automated hardware are available; these two categories would be flow and discrete sample analysis. With discrete sample automation, samples are separated from each other by nonfluid boundaries such as a cuvette and reagents are mechanically dispensed. After a predetermined time, a response (e.g., absorbance, fluorescence) is measured from which the concentration of the analyte is calculated. Flow analysis would be divided into continuous flow and stop-flow. With stop-flow automation, the sample and reagents are pumped into a cell, flow is stopped, and the response is measured. With continuous flow analysis, an aliquot of fluid sample is pumped through glass or inert plastic tubing. Sample aliquots are separated by portions of washing solvent. Analytical operations such as dialysis cleanup, solvent partitioning, reagent addition, and mixing can be performed on the sample aliquot before the analytical response is measured as the sample is pumped through a flow cell contained in a colorimeter or fluorometer. In spite of the dilution that occurs between sample and wash portions, the repeatability of the system affords excellent quantitation of analyte concentration. This improved repeatability over manual methods is characteristic of automation and is an additional benefit to cost savings realized upon implementation of automated methods. Continuous flow systems may be segmented with a gas, usually air, to decrease diffusion, or unsegmented, which has been called flow-inject analysis.

It will be noted that most of the automated chemical techniques reported in this chapter are of the segmented continuous flow variety. This is because this technique has been employed more frequently than unsegmented vitamin analysis. This popularity is most likely related to the variety of analytical steps that can be automated using this methodology and the commercial availability of the equipment.

The methods described in this chapter have been tested, some collaboratively, and found to be essentially identical to the time-tested manual methods. This is not surprising since automation allows the manual steps to be essentially duplicated and only labor has been removed from well-established chemical and microbiological methods; hence, the extraction and chemistry is essentially the same as that discussed in other sections of this book. The accuracy and generality of a method remains a function of the chemistry or microorganism used for quantitation and not automation per se.

Despite the obvious benefits to be realized from automation, it is not necessarily economical for every laboratory. There must be a certain minimum volume of samples before the time savings compensate for equipment investment costs and the fixed time necessary to get the automated system ready for use. Also, certain automated methods do not save much time because little labor has been automated. Careful examination of total potential time savings is recommended before addition of automated equipment.

It is the opinion of these authors, however, that if a sufficient analytical demand exists, that the quantity and quality of analytical data for thiamin, riboflavin, niacin, and ascorbic acid in complex biological matrices generated by automated techniques would be very difficult to match by any other analytical technique available at the time of this writing.

METHODS AVAILABLE

The methods that have been automated employ the basic chemical or microbiological techniques described in other sections of this book. Ascorbic acid has been automated by continuous flow using the reduction of 2,6-dichlorophenolindophenol (1–4), osazone formation with 2,4-dinitrophenyl hydrazine (5–7), quinoxaline formation with o-phenylenediamine (8–10) and reaction with diazotized 4-methoxy-2-nitroanaline (11).

Riboflavin analysis has been automated with continuous flow by taking advantage of its fluorescence, removing impurities with permanganate oxidation, and obtaining a blank after reducing the riboflavin with hydrosulfite (12–20). Frequently sample matrices allow omission of oxidative cleanup or blank determination. Both bisulfite (14) and hydroxylamine (19) have been successfully used to remove excess permanganate. A procedure using pyridine-butanol extraction has been reported (21,22) as well as a method employing discrete-sample automation (23). Microbiological determination of riboflavin has been automated (24).

Oxidation of thiamin to thiochrome with potassium ferricyanide followed by extraction of the thiochrome into isobutanol with fluorescence measurement has been automated using continuous-flow automation (21,22,25–29). A blank fluorescence is determined by omitting the ferricyanide oxidation step. The thiamin is extracted from the food matrix by acid hydrolysis followed by enzymatic hydrolysis with a phosphatase such as Clarase or Takadiastase. Adsorption-desorption cleanup using an ion-exchange system is required for accuracy in certain, but not all, food products (22). Because of the analogous extraction procedures, the same extract used for thiamin analysis may be used for riboflavin analysis with considerable labor savings. Automated analysis employing a discrete sampling technique has been reported (30) as well as automated microbiological methodology (24).

The colorimetric analysis of niacin is based on the reaction of a cyanogen halide, such as cyanogen bromide, with the pyridine nucleus of niacin giving rise to a chromophore upon further reaction with an aromatic amine. This chemistry has been subjected to continuous-flow automation (31–33). The niacin is extracted from a food matrix using base hydrolysis; during this step any amide derivatives are converted to nicotinic acid. These automated procedures have been compared with microbiological methods and manual methods by interlaboratory collaborative study (33,34). Discrete sample automated analysis has been reported (35) as well as automated microbiological methodology (24).

The standard colorimetric assays commonly used for vitamin B_6 analysis in pharmaceutical preparations are not sufficiently specific for use in food and feed analysis and these techniques have been only automated for pharmaceuticals (17,36,37). A fluorometric method has been reported for foods but requires prior chromatographic separation (38). Automated methods for vitamin B_6 in complex biological systems employ microbiological techniques (4,39,40). This is also the state of the art for folates, biotin, pantothenic acid, and vitamin B_{12}. The levels are so low and the matrices so complex in biological systems such as foods that satisfactory chemical methods amenable to automation simply do not exist.

Continuous flow has been used to automate a fluorimetric method for folic acid in vitamin tablets (41). Automated microbiological methods are most frequently reported (23,42–46) for this vitamin as well as pantothenic acid (23) and vitamin B_{12} (44,45,47,48); however, an automated spectrophotometric method (49) and an automated radioassay (50) technique have been used for fermentation broth and placental lactogen, respectively.

The effective use of chromatographic techniques for the determination of fat-soluble vitamins is perhaps the reason there exist few examples of the use of automation for these vitamins. Continuous-flow automation has been reported for the determination of vitamin A in milk (51,52), pharmaceuticals (53), serum (54), and cattle feeds (55) and for serum tocopherol (56).

DETERMINATION OF ASCORBIC ACID AND DEHYDROASCORBIC ACID (TOTAL VITAMIN C)

Of the numerous automated methods for the determination of ascorbic acid, the method reported by Pelletier et al. (5) employing osazone formation of oxidized ascorbic acid has the advantage of measuring ascorbic acid and dehydroascorbic acid, both of equivalent biological activity. Also, the method is not subject to the numerous interferences typical of the oxidative techniques such as 2,6-dichloroindophenol color reduction. Although this specificity is not necessary for certain applications such as analysis of pharmaceutical preparations, it is mandatory when a method is indiscriminately applied to a broad spectrum of biological matrices as is done in food analysis.

Another excellent method for the determination of total vitamin C is based on the reaction of dehydroascorbic acid with *o*-phenylenediamine to form a fluorescent quinoxaline derivative. Different modifications of this method have been reported in the literature (8–10) differing primarily in the technique used to oxidize ascorbic acid to the dehydro species. As with the osazone method, this technique is applicable to a broad spectrum of materials, and it has been shown that the biologically active hydrolysis product, diketogulonic acid, does not interfere in this fluorometric procedure (8). Interference by diketogulonic acid is also eliminated in the osazone methods described in the following section.

ANALYTICAL METHODOLOGY

I.   2,4-DINITROPHENYLHYDRAZINE DETERMINATION OF
      VITAMIN C IN FOODS WITH CONCENTRATIONS LARGER
      THAN 10 MG/100G

A.   Principle

The test reactions for determining ascorbic acid (AA) plus dehydroascorbic acid (DHAA) consist in (1) converting AA to DHAA by oxidation with 2,6-dichloroindophenol, (2) complexing DHAA with boric acid to prevent subsequent reduction of DHAA to AA upon addition of homocysteine, (3) forming osazones with 2,4-dinitrophenylhydrazine (DNPH) and developing the osazone color with nitric acid. Test blanks to evaluate background color and the formation of osazones with interfering materials are prepared by (1) reducing DHAA with homocysteine, (2) forming a complex of AA with boric acid to prevent its oxidation and thus eliminate the formation of osazone with DNPH, (3) allowing the DNPH and acid reactions.

Test reactions for the separate determination of AA are exactly as for AA plus DHAA, but test blanks differ from the test reactions only by omitting oxidation of AA with 2,6-dichloroindophenol to prevent the formation of osazones due to AA in these blanks. The only osazone formation in these blanks is due to DHAA and is subtracted from the test reaction.

B. Equipment

1. *Automated Sample Processor.*   The Analmatic Preparation Unit (Baird & Tatlock) available from Searle Analytical, Inc., or an equivalent instrument, is satisfactory. With the Analmatic processor, pipetting is accomplished by syringes mounted on removable plate assemblies and linked to a multiway change-over valve. Samples (picked up from cups) and reagents are delivered into test tubes in a tray capable of carrying batches of 100 test tubes. Each tube is processed at the rate of 12 sec per addition, some being done simultaneously. A complete cycle takes 20 min. A mini-mixer (No. 127-0090, Searle Instruments) insures automatic thorough mixing in each test tube.

2. *Double Beam Spectrophotometer or Colorimeter.*   The Bausch and Lomb Spectronic UV-200 equipped with a double micro flowthrough sample compartment (No. 39-20-15), two micro flowthrough cells (1-cm path length), and an interface cable (No. 34-31-55) or an equivalent interfaced instrument is satisfactory.

3. *Data Printer.*   Bausch and Lomb DP-100 No. 34-31-50, or other printer compatible with above or equivalent instrumentation.

4. *Waste System.*   Micro flowthrough system and waste jars (Bausch and Lomb No. 33-30-09 or the equivalent).

5. *Vacuum Pump.*   Bausch and Lomb 33-30-11 or the equivalent.

6. *Waterbath.*   Polystyrene water bath (100 L × 70 W × 15 H) maintained at 150°C with a refrigerating unit (Beckman, model 1888) and a circulating pump (Haake, model E51) or the equivalent.

7. *Sample Cups.*   Polystyrene 2-mL cups (Technicon No. 127-0090).

8. *Test Tubes.*   Disposable test tubes 15 × 85 mm (RTU, Becton and Dickinson Labware).

C. Reagents

The chemicals for preparing reagents are analytical reagent grade and the water is glass distilled and deonized.

1. *17% Metaphosphoric Acid Solution.* Without heating, dissolve 50-g pellets containing 34% HPO_3 and 59% $NaPO_3$ in H_2O and dilute to 100 mL. Store at 3°C and prepare weekly since HPO_3 in solution is slowly hydrolyzed to H_3PO_4.

2. *0.64% Metaphosphoric Acid Solution.* Dilute 37.6 mL 17% HPO_3 to 1 L with H_2O. Prepare fresh daily.

3. *0.1% 2,6-Dichlorophenolindophenol Solution.* Dissolve 200 mg 2,6-dichlorophenolindophenol (sodium salt) in approximately 150 mL hot H_2O, cool, and dilute with H_2O to 200 mL. Keep in the refrigerator when not in use. The solution is stable up to 2 weeks at 3°C.

4. *5% Boric Acid.* Dissolve 50 g H_3BO_3 in H_2O and dilute to 1 L. Prepare every 2 weeks and store at room temperature.

5. *1.5% 2,4-Dinitrophenylhydrazine.* Dissolve 15.0 g 2,4-dinitrophenylhydrazine in 9 N H_2SO_4 and dilute to 1 L with 9 N H_2SO_4. This solution is stable for 2 weeks if refrigerated.

6. *Ascorbic Acid Standard.* Dissolve 100 mg ascorbic acid (preferably U.S.P. Reference Standard) in 0.64% HPO_3 and dilute to 200 mL with the same solvent. Pipette 2, 4, 6, 8, and 10 mL respectively, in separate 100 mL volumetric flasks and dilute to volume with 0.64% HPO_3. These diluted standards contain 10, 20, 30, 40, and 50 $\mu g/mL$, respectively. Prepare fresh weekly and store at 3°C.

7. *45% Potassium Phosphate Dibasic Solution.* Dissolve 45 g K_2HPO_4 in H_2O and dilute to 100 mL. Prepare fresh weekly and store at room temperature.

8. *0.31% DL-Homocysteine Solution.* Dissolve 155 mg DL-homocysteine in H_2O and dilute to 50 mL. Prepare fresh daily.

9. *2.75% Boric Acid Solution.* Dilute 55 mL 5% H_3BO_3 to 100 mL with H_2O. This solution is stable for 2 weeks at room temperature.

10. *2,6-Dichloroindophenol and Boric Acid Solution.* Into a 100-mL volumetric flask, add 3.35 mL 0.1% 2,6-dichloroindophenol solution, 36 mL 5% H_3BO_3, and dilute to 100 mL with H_2O. Prepare daily and filter.

11. *Homocysteine Solution for Blanks.* Mix 24.3 mL 0.31% homocysteine with 34.3 mL H_2O, 30.0 mL 45% K_2HPO_4, and 2.9 mL 17% HPO_3. Prepare fresh daily and filter.

12. *Homocysteine Solution for Reactions.* Mix 24.3 mL 0.31% homocysteine with 30.0 mL 45% K_2HPO_4 and 2.9 mL 17% HPO_3. Prepare fresh daily and filter.

13. *0.68% 2,4-Dinitrophenylhydrazine plus 1.67% Thiourea.* Dissolve 3.34 g thiourea in 100 mL 9 N H_2SO_4, add 90 mL 1.5% 2,4-dinitrophenylhydrazine and dilute to 200 mL with 9 N H_2SO_4. Prepare daily and filter.

14. *Nitric and Citric Acid Mixture.* Dissolve 50 g citric acid in methanol to make 100 mL. To this solution, add slowly, while stirring, 150 mL concentrated HNO_3. Mix well. Let cool to room temperature before use. Use within 90 min after preparation.

D. Procedure

1. *Extraction.*

(a) Homogenize a representative portion for 3 min in a Waring Blendor in presence of sufficient 17% HPO_3 and H_2O to give a concentration of vitamin C ranging from 20 to 40 $\mu g/mL$ 0.64% HPO_3.

(1) Possible conversion of AA to DHAA is not considered a problem since metaphosphoric acid is known to prevent aerial oxidation of AA and, in any event, the primary purpose of the procedure is the measurement of total vitamin C (AA plus DHAA).

(b) Filter extracts through Whatman No. 2 filter paper. Extracts from samples containing much undissolved material (e.g., potatoes) are best filtered through glass wool.

2. *Determination.* Using the Analmatic processor, proceed as follows:

(a) Place aliquots of standards and samples in polystyrene cups for processing according to the following sequence, using one cup for each pair of test tubes placed in two subsequent rows, the first one being for test blanks: 0.64% HPO_3 (2 cups for reagents reference tubes), standard of 40 $\mu g/mL$ (used only for adjustment of the spectrophotometer when readings are taken directly in the concentration mode), first series of standards (10, 20, 30, 40, and 50 $\mu g/mL$), 0.64% HPO_3, second series of standards (as for the first series), 0.64% HPO_3, standard of 40 $\mu g/mL$, samples (series of 15), 0.64% HPO_3 and standard of 40 $\mu g/mL$. Other series of 15 samples are followed by 0.64% HPO_3 and a standard of 40 $\mu g/mL$.

(b) Syringes on the plate assemblies are arranged as follows to add in test tubes the required volumes of samples and reagents to the test tubes.

(1) To determine AA separately from DHAA, the syringes for the

Syringe Plates	Syringe Volumes (mL)	Reagent Number	Volumes Added (mL) Blanks	Volumes Added (mL) Reactions
A	1.0	Sample	0.2	—
	2.5	11	0.8	—
	1.0	Sample	—	0.2
	2.5	10	—	0.8
	1.0	12	—	0.5
B	1.0	9	0.5	—
	2.5	13	1.0	—
	2.5	13	—	1.0
C	5.0	14	2.0	—
	5.0	14	—	2.0

blanks must be the same as for the reaction, and the same reagent is used for the blanks as for the reaction, except for Reagent 10, which is modified for the blanks by diluting 36 mL 5% H_3BO_3 to 100 mL with H_2O without incorporating 2,6-dichloroindophenol.

(c) With the syringes in plate A, the samples are picked up from each individual cup and transferred consecutively to corresponding test tubes in the first row (test blanks) with homocysteine and K_2HPO_4 (Reagent 11) and simultaneously in the second row (test reactions) with 2,6-dichloroindophenol and H_3BO_3 (Reagent 10). While such additions are made simultaneously in the third and fourth rows of tubes, homocysteine and K_2HPO_4 (Reagent 12) are added in the second row. After additions from plate A are complete, the tubes are allowed to stand 90 min from the time of addition to the first tube.

(d) With the syringes in plate B, H_3BO_3 (Reagent 9) is added to the first row and subsequently, as it is added to the third row, the thiourea and dinitrophenylhydrazine (Reagent 13) are added to the first two rows. After the additions and mixing are completed the tubes are either kept at room temp for 3 hr or at 15°C for 17 hr.

(1) The latter is preferable because it increases the sensitivity by 30% and is theoretically less subject to interference from sugars. In practice however, a comparison of both modes showed no significant difference.

(e) With the syringes in plate C, the nitric and citric acid mixture (Reagent 14) is dispensed in the reactions and blanks tubes which are cooled at 15°C before the addition.

(f) After 30 to 90 min at room temp, adjust the spectrophotometer to zero absorbance at 520 nm with the reagent reference tubes and initiate the automatic measurement (reactions minus blanks).

3. *Calculations.* From the mean net absorbance (y) for each of the five consecutive levels of standards (x) in $\mu g/mL$, calculate the slope (b) and intercept (a) according to the following equation:

$$y = a + bx$$

Calculate the vitamin C concentration (x') in the diluted sample by the following formula:

$$x' = \frac{F(y' - a)}{b}$$

where y' represents the net absorbance of the sample (test reactions minus test blank) and a represents the intercept, b the slope of the standard curve, and F represents a correction factor for possible changes in sensitivity during the course of analysis.

$$F = 2\, As/(Ab + Aa)$$

where *As* is the absorbance of the 4th higher level of standard in the standard curve, and *Ab* and *Aa* represent the absorbance of the same standard placed before and after each group of samples.

II. 2,4-DINITROPHENYLHYDRAZINE DETERMINATION OF VITAMIN C IN FOODS WITH EXPECTED CONCENTRATIONS LESS THAN 10 MG/100 G

A. Principle

The method is based on the same principles as Method I, except that larger aliquots of sample extracts must be utilized because of the lower concentrations, and precautions must be taken in case of samples with relatively high sugar contents such as certain noncitrus fruits to remove possible moderate interference from these sugars. Since fructose and sucrose in concentrations higher than those expected from noncitrus fruits give a rather constant increase (8%) in vitamin C values, possible interference is eliminated by incorporating a mixture of these sugars in the solutions of standards and samples, but in such case the color development of osazones is made with sulfuric acid to avoid the turbidity formed by nitric acid. In other cases the nitric and citric acids solution can be utilized.

B. Equipment

All the equipment listed in Method I is required. In addition, a dispensing burette capable of dispensing 2 mL in 20 sec is required when using H_2SO_4 for the color development.

C. Reagents

Reagents 1, 3, 4, 5, 7, and 14 from Method I are required plus the following:

15. *0.85% Metaphosphoric Acid Solution.*   Dilute 50 mL 17% HPO_3 to 1 L with H_2O. Prepare fresh daily.

16. *10% Glucose Plus 5% Fructose.*   Dissolve 10 g glucose and 5 g fructose in 0.85% HPO_3 and dilute to 100 mL with 0.85% HPO_3. Prepare only when required for assaying samples with high sugar contents.

17. *Ascorbic Acid Standard.*   Dissolve 100 mg ascorbic acid (USP Reference) in 0.85% HPO_3 and dilute to 100 mL. Dilute 10 mL of the above to 100 mL with 0.85% HPO_3. Pipette 2, 4, 6, 8, and 10 mL, respectively, of this second dilution into separate 100-mL volumetric flasks and dilute to volume with 0.85% HPO_3. These diluted standards contain 2, 4, 6, 8, and 10 μg/mL. respectively. Prepare fresh weekly and store at 3°C.

  (a) For determining vitamin C in samples with a high sugar content add 10 mL of solution Reagent 16 per 100 mL final dilution of standards.

18. *3.33% Boric Acid Solution.*   Dilute 66.6 mL 5% H_3BO_3 to 100 mL with

H_2O. This solution is stable for 2 weeks at room temperature.

19. *2,6-Dichloroindophenol and Boric Acid Solution.*   Into a 100-mL volumetric flask, add 13.3 mL 0.1% 2,6-dichloroindophenol solution, 66.6 mL 5% H_3BO_3 and dilute to volume with H_2O. Prepare daily and filter.

20. *Homocysteine and K_2HPO_4 Solution.*   Dissolve 210 mg DL-homocysteine in 50 mL H_2O, add 85 mL 45% K_2HPO_4, and mix. Prepare fresh daily and filter.

21. *1.2% 2,4-Dinitrophenylhydrazine Plus 3% Thiourea.*   Dissolve 6 g thiourea in 100 mL 9 N H_2SO_4, add 160 mL 1.5% 2,4-dinitrophenylhydrazine, and dilute to 200 mL with 9 N H_2SO_4. Prepare daily and filter.

22. *85% Sulfuric Acid.*   Required only when solution Reagent 16 is utilized.

D. Procedure

1. *Extraction.*   Extract as in Section I.D.1 except that samples are diluted to give a final concentration of 4–8 µg vitamin C per mL 0.85% HPO_3. For samples with a relatively high concentration of sugars (e.g., noncitrus fruits), 10 mL of solution Reagent 16 is incorporated into each 100-mL final dilution.

2. *Determination.*

(a) Using the Analmatic processor, proceed generally as in Section I.D.2 but add 1.0-mL aliquots of appropriate solutions of standards and samples directly to the test tubes without utilizing cups.

(b) Syringes on the plate assemblies are arranged as follows to add the required volumes of reagents to test tubes:

Syringe Plates	Syringe Volumes (mL)	Reagent Numbers	Volumes Added (mL)	
			Blanks	Reactions
A	1.0	20	0.5	—
	1.0	19	—	0.5
	1.0	20	—	0.5
B	1.0	18	0.5	—
	2.5	21	1.0	—
	2.5	21	—	1.0
C	5.0	14	2.0	—
	5.0	14	—	2.0

(c) With the syringes in plate A, homocysteine and K_2HPO_4 (Reagent 20) are added in the first row of tubes (test blanks) while 2,6-dichloroindophenol and H_3BO_3 (Reagent 19) are added in the second row (test reactions). While such additions are made in the third and fourth row, homocysteine and K_2HPO_4 (Reagent 20) are added in the second row. After additions from plate A are complete, the tubes are allowed to stand 90 min from the time of addition to the first tube.

(d) With the syringes in plate B, H_3BO_3 (Reagent 18) is added to the first row and subsequently, as it is added to the third row, thiourea and 2,4-dinitrophenylhydrazine (Reagent 21) are added to the first two rows.

(1) The remainder of the determination is carried out exactly as described in Section I.D.2(d–f) except that when sulfuric acid is used for color development it must be dispensed slowly from a buret (2 mL in 20 sec) and in such cases, the spectrophotometric measurements are taken 75 min after the addition of H_2SO_4.

3. *Calculation.* See Section I.D.3.

III. FLUOROMETRIC DETERMINATION OF ASCORBIC ACID AND DEHYDROASCORBIC ACID (TOTAL VITAMIN C)

A. Principle

The ascorbic acid is extracted simultaneously from the matrix with methanolic metaphosphoric acid and oxidized to dehydroascorbic acid by activated charcoal. The dehydroascorbic acid in the filtrate reacts with *o*-phenylenediamine to form a fluorescing quinoxaline derivative. The blank fluorescence is determined by resampling the filtrate while boric acid is pumped into the flow scheme. The boric acid precludes formation of the dehydroascorbic acid-fluorescing derivative by complexing with dehydroascorbic acid.

Since ascorbic acid does not react with *o*-phenylenediamine without oxidation to the dehydro form, the amount of dehydroascorbic acid in a food product can be determined by omitting addition of activated charcoal and following the same procedure.

B. Equipment

1. *AutoAnalyzer II System.* Technicon equipped with the flow scheme shown in Figure 5.1 or equivalent.

2. *Fluorometer.* An Aminco Fluorocolorimeter with J4-7413 flow cell and J4-7125 4-watt lamp (SLM Instruments) or Technicon Fluoronephelometer equipped with a flow cell is used, with a primary filter (7-60), band pass 70% T at 365 nm, and secondary filter (Technicon 126-0077-01), band pass 40% T at 440 nm, or equivalent.

C. Reagents

1. *Brij 35 Solution.* Dissolve 35 g Brij (Technicon) in 65 g H_2O.

2. *Metaphosphoric Acid–Methanol HPO_3 Extraction Solvent (4% aqueous HPO_3·methanol).* Dissolve 80 g HPO_3 in 1 L H_2O and dilute to 2 L. Mix this solution with 667 mL methanol. Prepare fresh at least weekly.

3. *Wash Solution.* Add 1.5 mL Brij solution (Reagent 1) to 1 L of extraction solvent (Reagent 2) and filter.

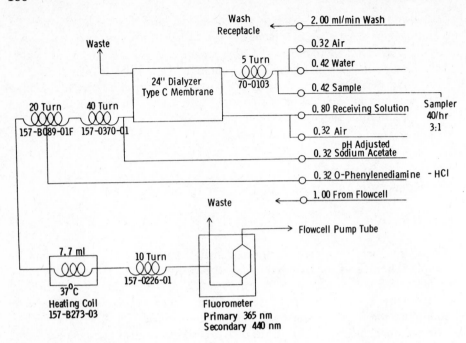

FIGURE 5.1 Flow scheme for automated analysis of ascorbic acid and dehydroascorbic acid (Method III).

4. *Dialysate Receiving Solution.* Add 1 L H_2O to 1 L wash solution (Reagent 3). Add 1.5 mL Brij solution (Reagent 1).

5. *Sodium Acetate Solution.* Dissolve 302 g anhydrous sodium acetate in H_2O and dilute to 1 L with H_2O. Add 1.5 mL Brij solution (Reagent 1) and filter.

6. *Boric Acid Solution.* Dissolve 5 g H_3BO_3 in 100 mL sodium acetate solution (Reagent 5). Prepare fresh daily.

7. *pH-Adjusted Sodium Acetate Solution.* Adjust the pH of sodium acetate solution (Reagent 5) to that of H_3BO_3 with HCl (pH 6.9).

8. *o-Phenylenediamine Dihydrochloride (0.5 mg/mL).* Dissolve 50 mg *o*-phenylenediamine hydrochloride and dilute to 100 mL with H_2O. Prepare fresh daily.

9. *Acid Washed Norit.* Add 1 L HCl solution prepared by adding 100 mL concentrated HCl to 900 mL H_2O, to 200 g Norit. Heat the mixture to boiling and filter using a suction flask. Place the cake of Norit in a beaker and add 1L H_2O, stir, and filter. Repeat this water washing step and dry 16 hr at about 120°C.

10. *Ascorbic Acid Standards.* Accurately weigh 100 mg ascorbic acid (stored in a desiccator) into a 100-mL volumetric flask, dissolve, and dilute to volume with extraction solvent (Reagent 2). Pipette 10 mL of above solution (which contains 1.0 mg ascorbic acid/mL) into 100 mL volumetric flask and dilute to

volume with Reagent 2. This solution contains 100 $\mu g/mL$. For working standards, pipette 2 mL, 10 mL, and 25 mL of 100 $\mu g/mL$ solution into three 100-mL volumetric flasks and dilute to volume with extraction solvent (Reagent 2). These contain 2, 10, and 25 $\mu g/mL$.

D. Procedure

1. *Standard Curve.* Weigh 0.20 g Norit into each of three plastic Falcon cups (Becton, Dickinson and Co.). Add 100 mL of each working standard (2, 10, and 25 $\mu g/mL$) and shake the cups in a mechanical shaker for 10 min. Filter a portion of this mixture through Whatman No. 2 filter paper and immediately transfer to filtrate from diSPO funnels to AutoAnalyzer sampler and pump through the instrument. Peak the recorder with the 25 $\mu g/mL$ standard. Standard and sample filtrates should be pumped through the system as soon as possible after oxidation to dehydroascorbic acid.

2. *Extraction.*

(a) Low moisture samples. Grind sample to pass a 40-mesh sieve. In addition to 0.20 g Norit, accurately weigh a portion of sample (maximum weight 5 g) containing about 1.5 mg ascorbic acid into a Falcon cup and dispense 100 mL extraction solvent (Reagent 2). Cap and shake the mixture for 10 min. Filter the extract and pump and filtrate through the AutoAnalyzer. Certain products that do not disperse upon shaking in a disposable Falcon cup are extracted more efficiently in a blender.

(b) High-moisture samples (fruits and vegetables). Grind sample in high-speed blender, such as Osterizer. Weigh a portion of this slurry (maximum weight 5 g) containing about 1.5 mg of ascorbic acid into a 100-mL volumetric flask and dilute to volume with extraction solvent (Reagent 2). Mix thoroughly and transfer the contents to a Falcon plastic cup containing 0.20 g Norit. Treat as described for low-moisture samples.

(c) Dehydroascorbic acid. Treat samples as described in previous steps (a,b) except omit the use of Norit.

3. *Blank Determination.* Replace the pH adjusted sodium acetate (Reagent 7) line with the boric acid solution (Reagent 6). Pump the standards and samples through the flow scheme to obtain blank values.

4. *Calculations.* Plot peak height standard minus blank versus concentration. Obtain the sample concentrations in $\mu g/mL$ by comparing the blank-corrected peak heights for each sample with the standard curve. Calculate the total vitamin C or dehydroascorbic acid level as follows:

$$\text{mg vitamin C}/100 \text{ g} = \frac{C}{W} \times 10$$

where C = concentration in $\mu g/mL$,
            W = sample weight in g,

and 10 is a combined factor taking into account 100 mL extract, level reported per 100 g, and conversion of μg to mg.

DETERMINATION OF RIBOFLAVIN

Riboflavin is quantitated by utilization of its natural fluorescence. For accurate results, it is necessary to oxidize certain interfering materials with permanganate. The blank fluorescence is determined by destroying the riboflavin. In one method the riboflavin is destroyed with light (21,22) and in the other method hydrosulfite is used (14). The same hydrolysate used for riboflavin analysis (hydrosulfite method) may be used for the automated thiamin procedure.

I. FLUOROMETRIC DETERMINATION OF RIBOFLAVIN (LIGHT DESTRUCTION METHOD)

A. Principle

Diastase digestion of foods converts the coenzyme forms of vitamin B_2 to free riboflavin. Except for fruits, it is necessary to hydrolyze foods with dilute HCl before enzymatic digestion to extract riboflavin completely. Riboflavin is measured fluorometrically after some of the interfering fluorescing compounds have been destroyed by oxidation, while others have been eliminated by extraction of riboflavin into a pyridine-butanol mixture. Correction is made for the remaining interfering compounds by using blanks in which riboflavin has been destroyed by light.

B. Equipment

1. *AutoAnalyzer System (Technicon).*   Use with the following modules: Sampler with a cam to run 40 tests per hour with sample-to-wash ratio of 2:1, proportioning pump, fluorometer with primary filter No. 110-831 (460 nm) and secondary filter No. 110-818 (510 nm), recorder, and plattered manifold (see Figure 5.2).

2. *Irradiation Apparatus (see Figure 5.3).*   Equipment comprises circular rack made from aluminum sheet, Hg Lamp (G.E. H400, A33-1, 76), ballast voltage regulator (G.E. 400), and timer (G.E. Time switch TSA-47).

3. Nylon 50-mL Tubes with Caps.

C. Reagents

1. *0.1 N Hydrochloric Acid Solution.*   Add 8.5 mL HCl to 1 L H_2O.

2. *Riboflavin Standard Solutions.*   Accurately weigh 20 mg USP Riboflavin Reference Standard that has been dried to constant weight over H_2SO_4 in a

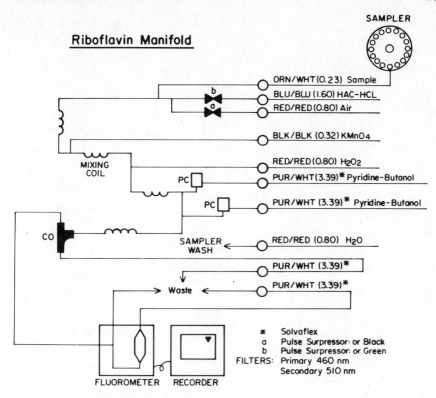

Riboflavin Manifold

SAMPLER

ORN/WHT (0.23) Sample
BLU/BLU (1.60) HAC-HCL
RED/RED (0.80) Air
BLK/BLK (0.32) KMnO4
RED/RED (0.80) H2O2
PUR/WHT (3.39)* Pyridine-Butanol
PUR/WHT (3.39)* Pyridine-Butanol
RED/RED (0.80) H2O
PUR/WHT (3.39)*
PUR/WHT (3.39)*

MIXING COIL
PC
PC
CO
SAMPLER WASH
Waste
FLUOROMETER   RECORDER

*   Solvaflex
a   Pulse Surpressor: or Black
b   Pulse Surpressor: or Green
FILTERS: Primary 460 nm
         Secondary 510 nm

FIGURE 5.2   Manifold diagram for riboflavin analysis (Method I).

vacuum desiccator. Dissolve in 1 L 0.1 N HCl and store in glass-stoppered light-resistant bottle under toluene at about 3°C. Dilute an aliquot of stock solution with 0.1 N HCl to a concentration of 2.0 μg/mL. Prepare fresh daily.

3. *Flavin Adenine Dinucleotide (FAD) Solutions.*   Accurately weigh a sample of FAD, dried in a vacuum desiccator over H_2SO_4, and equivalent to 20 mg riboflavin. Dilute to 1 L with 0.1 N HCl to a concentration equivalent to 20 μg riboflavin/mL. Store under toluene in a glass-stoppered light-resistant bottle at about 3°C. Dilute an aliquot of stock solution with 0.1 N HCl to a concentration of 2.0 μg riboflavin/mL. Prepare fresh daily.

4. *2.5 M Sodium Acetate Solution.*   Dissolve 205 g anhydrous sodium acetate in H_2O and dilute to 1 L.

5. *10% Takadiastase Solution.*   Dissolve 10 g Takadiastase (Pfaltz and Bauer) in H_2O and dilute to 100 mL. Prepare fresh daily.

6. *Acetic Acid–Hydrochloric Acid Mixture.*   Mix 45 mL glacial acetic acid with 55 mL 0.1 N HCl. *Careful, gas is produced.*

7. *1% Potassium Permanganate Solution.*   Dissolve 1 g $KMnO_4$ in 100 mL H_2O and filter. Prepare fresh daily.

8. *0.6% Hydrogen Peroxide Solution.*   Dilute 2 mL 30% H_2O_2 to 100 mL with H_2O. Prepare fresh daily.

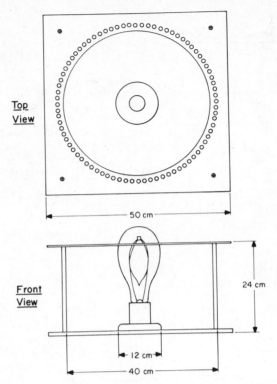

FIGURE 5.3 Irradiation apparatus for riboflavin determination (Method II).

9. *Pyridine and n-Butanol Mixture.*   Mix 8 volumes pyridine with 92 volumes *n*-butanol.

10. *Ethylene Glycol Monomethyl Ether.*

D. Procedure

1. *Preparation of Samples.*

(a) In case of nonhomogeneous food samples, grind representative portions with a food chopper (e.g., meat, fish and egg) or blend directly in a high-speed blender (e.g., fruit and vegetable). Dry cereal products to constant weight at room temperature, avoiding exposure to light, and grind to a fine powder.

(b) Place appropriate aliquots of samples on a fresh or "as is" basis into preweighed 50-mL nylon tubes and mix with a glass rod together with 10 mL 0.25 N HCl for most foods; for fish, meat, and dairy products, 0.4 N HCl is used. Add H_2O to make about 25 mL in each tube.

(1) Appropriate weights (g) of food depend on expected concentrations (mg/100 g) of thiamin (B_1) and riboflavin (B_2) as follows except that weight of starchy products should be less than 8 g:

Type of Food	Concentration (mg/100 g)	Weight (g)
Fruits, vegetables, juices and liquid dairy products	B_1 or B_2 < 0.05	11–15
	B_1 or B_2 = 0.05–0.1	6–9
	B_1 + B_2 > 0.1	4–5
Fish, meats, eggs, cereals, non-liquid dairy products, nuts and by-products	B_1 or B_2 < 0.1	5.5–6.5
	B_1 or B_2 = 0.1–0.2	4–5
	B_1 + B_2 > 0.1	2.5–3.5

(2) Exposure of samples to light must be avoided to prevent destruction of riboflavin.

(c) When acid hydrolysis is omitted (i.e., for fruits), add 2 mL 2.5 M sodium acetate (Reagent 4) and follow by 2 mL Takadiastase solution (Reagent 5). Mix the contents of each tube with a glass rod and rinse the rod into the tube with about 1 mL H_2O. Cover the tubes with caps and incubate for about 20 hr at 40°C.

(d) When acid hydrolysis is included before digestion (i.e., for all foods except fruits), cover the tubes with aluminum foil before autoclaving for 30 min at 121°C. Cool the samples and add sodium acetate and Takadiastase as described above.

(e) Following digestion, add H_2O to the tubes to a final content of 40 g; for fruits, 8 mL ethylene glycol monomethyl ether is added in place of H_2O. Heat tubes to which ethylene glycol monomethyl ether has been added for 10 min at 95°C and add H_2O to 40 g, mix each sample thoroughly, and filter through glass fiber filter paper (Whatman grade GF/A).

(1) Extract riboflavin from flour premixed by blending with H_2O at high speed for 5 min and diluted with H_2O to required concentration. A standard diluted with H_2O must be utilized for the calculations.

2. *Preparation of Standards and Control.*   Pipette 1, 2, 3, 4, or 5 mL riboflavin (2 μg/mL) standard solution, or 2 mL working FAD control solution into separate 50-mL nylon tubes. Add 0.1 N HCl to all tubes to make 25 mL and treat exactly as described for samples.

(1) It is not necessary to prepare a reagent blank (Takadiastase) when samples concentrations are read from a standard curve.

3. *Automated Analysis.*   Set the automated system according to the manifold diagram (Figure 5.2). Pump the acetic acid-HCl mixture (Reagent 6) and 0.6% H_2O_2 (Reagent 8) for 5 min before introducing the $KMnO_4$ solution (Reagent 7). Once the baseline has been established, adjust peak height to about 75 chart units with the standard of 0.25 μg riboflavin/mL. Run two sets of riboflavin standards (0.05–0.25 μg riboflavin/mL) placing a cup of H_2O after each set. Run a separate riboflavin (0.20 μg/mL), FAD, 10 samples, H_2O, and one more riboflavin standard (0.20 μg/mL). Repeat the same arrangement for each group of 10 samples. Determine the blank fluorescence corresponding to the above

determinations using 2-mL aliquots that have been irradiated for 3 hr in test tubes covered with aluminum foil.

(1) At all times during the analysis and the sample preparation, care must be taken to avoid destruction of riboflavin by light by utilizing low light intensity in the laboratory.

4. *Calculations.* Plot a standard curve by drawing a line of best fit of net fluorescence peak height (*H*) in chart units (minus blank) against riboflavin concentration in $\mu g/mL$. Read the concentration (*C*) corresponding to the net *H* (minus blank) of each sample. Correct for any drift by multiplying *C* by factor (*F*) which is calculated as follows:

$$F = \frac{\text{average } H \text{ for the two initial standards of } 0.2 \ \mu g/mL}{\text{average } H \text{ for the standards of } 0.2 \ \mu g/mL \text{ before and after 10 samples}}$$

II. FLUOROMETRIC DETERMINATION OF RIBOFLAVIN (HYDROSULFITE DESTRUCTION METHOD)

A. Principle

The riboflavin is extracted from the sample by acid hydrolysis followed by enzymatic hydrolysis. After pH adjustment, the extract is pumped into the flow scheme where it is subjected to dialysis and permanganate cleanup before the fluorescence is measured. The blank is determined by recycling the samples while dithionite (hydrosulfite) is pumped into the flow system. The hydrolysate used in this procedure may also be used in thiamin procedure (Thiamin Method I).

B. Equipment

1. *AutoAnalyzer II System (Technicon).* Use with the flow scheme shown in Figure 5.4 or equivalent.

2. *Technicon Fluoronephelometer.* Use equipped with LY-013-B008-01-C flow cell or Amino Fluoro-Colorimeter equipped with J4-7413 flow cell and J4-7125 4-watt lamp. The fluorometer should have a primary filter with band pass 50% T at 530 nm (Technicon No. 518-7004 or Wratten 47B), and secondary filter - sharp cut 37% T at 513-527 nm, 80% T at 557 nm (Technicon 518-7032, or 2A-12).

C. Reagents

1. *Brij 35 Solution.* Dissolve 35 g Brij (Technicon) in 65 g H_2O.

2. *0.1 N Hydrochloric Acid.*

3. *Metaphosphoric Acid.* Dissolve 15 g HPO_3 in 1 L H_2O and adjust the pH to 1.9 with sodium acetate. Add 30 g NaCl, 1 mL Brij solution (Reagent 1) and filter. Prepare the solution fresh weekly.

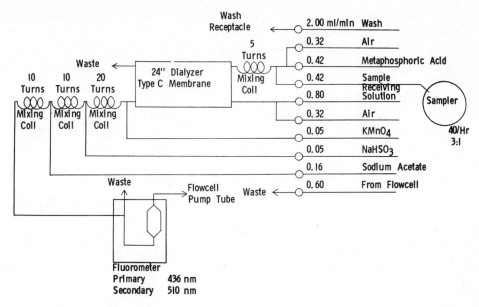

FIGURE 5.4   Flow scheme for fluorometric determination of riboflavin (Method II).

4. *1.25 N Sodium Acetate.*   Dissolve 345 g sodium acetate trihydrate in H₂O and dilute to 2 L.

5. *Metaphosphoric Acid Buffer (pH 4.3).*   Dissolve 15 g HPO₃ in 1 L H₂O and adjust the pH to 4.3 with crystalline sodium acetate. Prepare the solution fresh daily.

6. *Wash Solution.*   Adjust the pH of 2 L 0.1 N HCl to 4.3 using 1.25 N sodium acetate (about 240 mL). Add metaphosphoric acid buffer (Reagent 5) to make 4 L solution; add 4 mL Brij solution (Reagent 1). Prepare the solution fresh daily.

7. *Dialysate Receiving Solution.*   Mix equal volumes of Reagent 6 and Reagent 3.

8. *0.4% Sodium Acetate.*   Dissolve 4.0 g sodium acetate in H₂O and dilute to 1 L.

9. *Takadiastase Solution.*   Dissolve 1 g Takadiastase (Pfaltz and Bauer) in Reagent 5 and dilute to 100 mL. Use 8 mL of the Takadiastase solution for each of the samples and standards. Prepare fresh daily.

10. *1% Potassium Permanganate.*   Dissolve 2.0 g KMnO₄ in 200 mL H₂O by stirring for 30 min with a magnetic stirrer and filter the solution. Prepare the solution fresh weekly and store in a dark bottle.

11. *Sodium Bisulfite.*   Dissolve 1.1 g NaHSO₃ in 50 mL pH 7 phosphate buffer (4.55 g KH₂PO₄ and 9.45 g Na₂HPO₄ per liter H₂O). The sodium bisulfite level should be adjusted so that there is about a 10% excess over the amount required to reduce the permanganate. This can be done visually in the continuous-flow system. A large excess of bisulfite is to be avoided. Once the proper bisulfite

concentrate is detected, it is not necessary to repeat this procedure until the pump tubes are changed. Prepare the solution fresh daily.

12. *Sodium Hydrosulfite.* Dissolve 2.0 g $Na_2S_2O_4$ in 100 mL 0.4% sodium acetate solution (Reagent 8). Keep the solution in an ice bath while in use (stable about 2 hr).

13. *Riboflavin Standards.*

   (a) Stock, 50 μg/mL. Dissolve 50.0 mg riboflavin (stored in a dark desiccator) in 800 mL 0.1 N HCl (overnight magnetic stirring required) and dilute to 1 L with 0.1 N HCl. Store under toluene in the dark and prepare fresh every other week.

   (b) 10 μg/mL. Dilute 40 mL of (a) to 200 mL with 0.1 N HCl.

   (c) 1 μg/mL. Dilute 10 mL of (b) to 100 mL with 0.1 N HCl. Prepare (b) and (c) fresh daily.

   (d) Pipette X mL of (c) into a 100-mL amber volumetric flask and add 0.1 N HCl so that the volume is 50 mL. Autoclave and treat the standards exactly the same as samples.

X mL (c)	mL 0.1 N HCl	Concentration at 100 mL Final volume (μg/mL)
1	49	0.01
3	47	0.03
5	45	0.05
10	40	0.10
15	35	0.15

D. Procedure

1. *Sampling.* Grind a representative portion of the sample to pass a 40-mesh sieve. Grind high-moisture samples in a blender to a homogeneous consistency.

2. *Extraction.* Add an accurately weighed portion of ground material (1.5 g maximum) containing about 10 μg of thiamin or riboflavin into a 100-mL amber volumetric flask, followed by 50.0 mL 0.1 N HCl. Take care to wash the sides of the flask and disperse the sample. Cover the flasks with foil and autoclave for 30 min at 121°C; exhaust the autoclave slowly to prevent bumping.

   (a) Some products spatter during hydrolysis in a volumetric flask. These products should be hydrolyzed in an Erlenmeyer flask and the hydrolyzed material quantitatively transferred to a 100-mL volumetric flask and treated in the same manner as the other samples. Allow the samples to cool to room temperature. The samples can be stored overnight at this point.

3. *Sample Preparation.*   Adjust the dispensing unit so that when an aliquot (i.e., 6.0 mL) of sodium acetate (Reagent 4) is added to 50.0 mL 0.1 N HCl, the pH is 4.3 ± 0.1. To each sample, dispense the predetermined aliquot of 1.25 N sodium acetate (Reagent 4) with swirling, and add 35 mL of pH 4.3 metaphosphoric buffer (Reagent 4). Check the pH and adjust the pH of any sample hydrolysate differing from the standards by more than ±0.1 pH unit. If this extract is to be used for thiamin detection, add 8 mL Takadiastase solution (Reagent 9) and heat at 37°C overnight before diluting to volume. This enzymatic procedure will not have a significant effect on the riboflavin measurement. Make sure that Takadiastase (Reagent 9) is also added to the standards since the enzyme contains trace amounts of riboflavin. Dilute the samples to volume with metaphosphoric acid buffer (Reagent 5), add a drop of Brij 35 solution (Reagent 1) and filter through glass fiber filter paper (Whatman GF/A or equivalent shown not to absorb riboflavin).

4. *Fluorescence Measurement.*   Pump the high standard (0.15 μg/mL) through the system and set the recorder at 100% using the standard calculation adjustment on the fluorometer. Aspirate and pump the set of standards and samples through the system. After every 20 samples, aspirate a 0.10-μg/mL standard to correct for any drift. If a sample is more concentrated than the highest standard, dilute with wash solution until the peak height is within the set of standards.

5. *Riboflavin Blank Measurement.*   After the samples have been pumped through the system, replace the sodium acetate solution with the sodium hydrosulfite solution (Reagent 12). After observing a shift in the base line, adjust the recorder base line and resample the filtrates to obtain the blank value.

6. *Calculations.*   The set of standards provides a linear standard curve passing through the origin when plotting peak height in chart units versus concentration (μg/mL). Subtract the blank peak heights from the sample peak height. Obtain sample concentration in μg/mL by comparison of the sample peak height with the standard curve.

$$\text{Riboflavin, mg/100 g} = \frac{C_S \times 10}{W}$$

where C_S = concentration of sample, μg/mL
             W = sample weight (g).

The 10 is a combined factor taking into account 100 mL extract, level reported per 100 g, and conversion of μg to mg.

DETERMINATION OF THIAMIN

This method automates the standard thiochrome assay discussed in the thiamin chapter of this book (21,22,27). It has been shown that ion-exchange cleanup is required only for certain food products (22). This has also been observed in the author's laboratory. The hydrolysate used for thiamin analyses can also be used for riboflavin assay.

The automated method in this section is only applicable to substances that do not require an ion-exchange cleanup prior to analysis. A number of samples from a particular class of foods should be tested with and without ion exchange cleanup using the manual procedure described in the thiamin section of this book. If it is shown that the ion-exchange step is not required by establishing equivalent thiamin results either with or without ion exchange, this automated method may be used for these foods.

A. Principle

The thiamin is extracted from the sample by acid hydrolysis followed by enzymatic hydrolysis. An aliquot of the extract is pumped into a flow scheme where the thiamin is oxidized to thiochrome with alkaline potassium ferricyanide, the thiochrome is extracted into isobutyl alcohol and measured fluorometrically. The sample blank fluorescence is determined by sampling the filtrate with the potassium ferricyanide removed from the flow scheme. The hydrolysate used in this procedure may be used in the riboflavin procedure.

B. Equipment

1. *AutoAnalyzer II System.*   Technicon or equivalent with the flow scheme shown in Figure 5.5.

2. *Technicon Fluoronephelometer.*   Equipped with 365-nm excitation filter (Technicon FS-518-7000) and 440-nm (Technicon 126-0077-01) emission filter, or equivalent.

C. Reagents

1. *Brij 35 Solution.*   Dissolve 35 g Brij (Technicon) in 65 g H_2O.

2. *0.1 N Hydrochloric Acid.*

3. *Stock Metaphosphoric Acid.*   Dissolve 15 g HPO_3 in 1 L H_2O and adjust the pH to 1.9 with sodium acetate. Add 30 g NaCl and 1 mL Brij solution (Reagent 1) and filter. Prepare the solution fresh weekly.

4. *1.25 N Sodium Acetate.*   Dissolve 345 g sodium acetate trihydrate in H_2O and dilute to 2 L.

5. *Metaphosphoric Acid Buffer (pH 4.3).*   Dissolve 15 g HPO_3 in 1 L H_2O and adjust the pH to 4.3 with crystalline sodium acetate. Prepare the solution fresh daily.

6. *Wash Solution.*   Adjust the pH of 2 L 0.1 N HCl to 4.3 using about 240 mL Reagent 4. Add Reagent 5 to make 4 L solution; add 4 mL Brij (Reagent 1). Prepare the solution fresh daily.

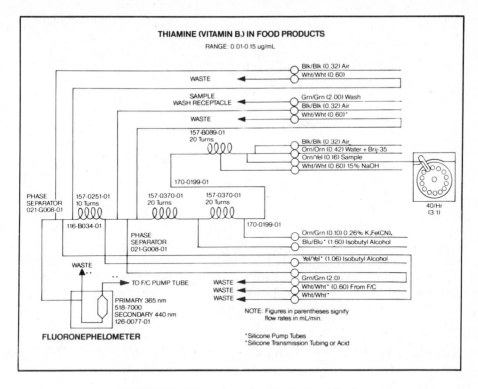

FIGURE 5.5   Flow scheme for thiamin determination.

7. *Takadiastase Solution.*   Dissolve 1 g Takadiastase (Pfaltz and Bauer) in metaphosphoric acid buffer (Reagent 5) and dilute to 100 mL with buffer. Use 8 mL Takadiastase solution for each of the samples and standards. Prepare fresh daily.

8. *15% Sodium Hydroxide Solution.*   Dissolve 300 g NaOH in H_2O and dilute to 2 L.

9. *0.25% Potassium Ferricyanide.*   Dissolve 0.25 g potassium ferricyanide in water and dilute to volume in a 100-mL amber flask. Prepare fresh daily.

10. *Thiamin Standards*:

(a) Stock, 50 $\mu g/mL$. Dissolve 50 mg thiamin hydrochloride in 800 mL 0.1 N HCl and dilute to 1 L with 0.1 N HCl. Prepare fresh biweekly.

(b) 10 $\mu g/mL$. Dilute 20 mL of (a) to 100 mL with 0.1 N HCl.

(c) 1 $\mu g/mL$. Dilute 1 mL of (b) to 100 mL with 0.1 N HCl. Prepare (b) and (c) Fresh daily.

(d) Pipette X mL of (c) into a 100-mL amber volumetric flask and add 0.1 N HCl so that the volume is 50 mL. Autoclave and treat the standards exactly the same as samples.

X mL (c)	mL 0.1 N HCl	Concentration at 100 mL Final Volume (μg/ mL)
1	49	0.01
3	47	0.03
5	45	0.05
10	40	0.10
15	35	0.15

D. Procedure

The procedure is the same as for Riboflavin Method II, except for step 5. For thiamin blank measurement, replace $K_3Fe(CN)_6$ solution (Reagent 9) with H_2O. Allow 30 min to wash excess $K_3Fe(CN)_6$ out of tubing. Reset the base line to zero and resample the filtrates. The calculation of thiamin content is done the same way as in the riboflavin determination.

COLORIMETRIC DETERMINATION OF NIACIN AND NIACINAMIDE

A. Principle

Niacin is extracted from biological materials by basic hydrolysis with calcium hydroxide. The amide and any amide derivative are hydrolyzed to the acid salt. Calcium hydroxide is effective because a minimum of hydrolysate darkening is observed. Colorimetric reaction with cyanogen bromide and sulfanilic acid is a common technique and is amenable to continuous flow automation. As in any automated vitamin method, certain steps such as extraction are conducted manually.

After hydrolysis with calcium hydroxide, the calcium hydroxide is dissolved with dilute hydrochloric acid and a phosphate buffer is added to the flask. The resulting mixture is filtered and the filtrate is pumped into the flow scheme where it is dialyzed, and reacted with cyanogen bromide and sulfanilic acid. The absorbance of the resulting color is measured continuously and used for quantitation. The blank absorbance is determined by recycling the sample through the system and replacing the cyanogen bromide with water.

B. Equipment

1. *AutoAnalyzer II System.*   Technicon with the flow scheme shown in Figure 5.6, or equivalent.

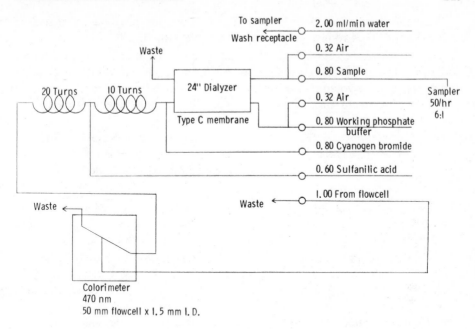

FIGURE 5.6   Flow scheme for colorimetric determination of niacin and niacinamide.

C.   Reagents

1. *Brij 35 Solution.*   Dissolve 35 g Brij in 65 g H_2O.

2. *Stock Buffer.*   Dissolve 130 g Na_2HPO_4 and 71 g KH_2PO_4 in about 900 mL warm H_2O. Cool solution to room temp and dilute to 1 L.

3. *Working Buffer (pH 6.7).*   Dilute 150 mL stock buffer (Reagent 2) to 1 L and add 1.5 mL Brij 35 solution (Reagent 2). Filter through Whatman 2V filter paper before using.

4. *Sample Buffer (pH 7.6).*   Dissolve 272 Na_2HPO_4 and 48 g KH_2PO_4 in about 1.8 L warm H_2O. Cool solution to room temperature and dilute to 2 L.

5. *Sulfanilic Acid.*   Add 100 g sulfanilic acid to 500 mL H_2O. Add concentrated NH_4OH (about 40 mL) with mixing until sulfanilic acid is dissolved. Adjust to pH 7.0 with HCl (1:3) and dilute to 1 L with H_2O. Filter solution and store in cool dark place. Prepare solution fresh every other week.

6. *1.5 N Hydrochloric Acid.*   Add 249 mL concentrated HCl to 2 L volumetric flask and dilute to volume.

7. *Cyanogen Bromide.*   Weigh approximately 50 g CNBr into beaker containing 300 mL warm (40°C) H_2O and stir to dissolve. Cool solution and dilute to 1 L. Prepare solution fresh every other week. CAUTION: WEIGH OUT CYANOGEN BROMIDE AND PREPARE THIS SOLUTION IN A FUME HOOD! CYANOGEN BROMIDE IS VERY POISONOUS.

8. *Sample Wash Solution.*   Dilute 3.0 mL Brij solution (Reagent 1) to 2 L with H_2O and filter resulting solution through Whatman 2V filter paper.

9. *Calcium Hydroxide Slurry.*   Add 22 g $Ca(OH)_2$ to 200-mL volumetric flask and add about 100 mL H_2O, shake to form slurry, and dilute to volume. Empty contents of volume into 250-mL beaker equipped with magnetic stirrer. When sampling from this slurry, make sure that mixing rate is sufficient to ensure homogeneity.

10. *Basic Solution for Waste Container.*   Dissolve 150 g NaOH in 300 mL H_2O contained in 4-L reagent bottle. Waste solution is pumped into this container. It is recommended that this container be placed in a fume hood.

11. *Niacin Standards:*

(a) Stock, 10 μg/mL. Weigh 50.0 mg nicotinic acid (stored in desiccator) into 500-mL volumetric flask, dissolve and dilute to volume with H_2O. Dilute 25 mL of this solution to 250 mL with H_2O. Prepare stock fresh each day.

(b) Working standards. Pipette X mL stock standard (a) to 100-mL volumetric flask containing 5 mL calcium hydroxide slurry containing 0.55 $Ca(OH)_2$ (Reagent 9). The calcium hydroxide (0.55 g) can be weighed into the flask or added by slurry. Add water to adjust volume to about 55 mL before autoclaving. Autoclave and treat standards exactly the same as samples.

X mL (a)	mL H_2O	Concentration at 100 mL Final volume (μg/mL)
30	20	3.0
20	30	2.0
10	40	1.0
5	45	0.5

D. Procedure

1. *Sampling.*   Grind representative portion of sample to pass 40-mesh sieve.

2. *Extraction.*   Add accurately weighed portion of ground material containing about 0.2 mg niacin to 100-mL volumetric flask. For products containing low niacin levels, do not use over 1.5 g of product. This assures maximum recovery of niacin present. Add 5 mL calcium hydroxide slurry (Reagent 9) using Rainin pipet or add 0.55 g calcium hydroxide. Add about 50 mL H_2O, cover with foil, swirl, and autoclave at 121°C for 2 hr.

(a) Some products spatter during hydrolysis. These products are hydrolyzed in a disposable Falcon plastic container with calcium hydroxide (Reagent 9) and 50 mL H_2O. Hydrolyzed material is quantitatively transferred to 100-mL volumetric flask and treated in the same manner as other samples.

3. *Sample Preparation.*   While solutions are still hot, add 10 mL 1.5 N HCl using an Oxford pipettor, and swirl to dissolve remaining $Ca(OH)_2$. Make sure all $Ca(OH)_2$ is dissolved. Let samples cool to room temperature. Samples may be stored at this point. Add 25 mL sample buffer (Reagent 4), 2 drops Brij solution (Reagent 1), and dilute to volume with H_2O. (A precipitate forms and final pH is about 6.7.) Shake mixture and filter through Whatman 2V filter paper. Disposable diSPo collection funnels are convenient.

4. *Colorimetric Measurement.*   Pump high standard (3.0 μg/mL) through system and set recorder at 100% using standard calibration adjustment on colorimeter. Aspirate and pump a set of standards and sample filtrates through system. After every 20 samples, aspirate a standard and allow pen to come to baseline to establish that instrument is functioning properly. If sample is more concentrated than highest standard, dilute with working buffer until peak height is within set of standards.

5. *Blank Measurement.*   After sample filtrates have been pumped through system, replace CNBr line with H_2O line and allow H_2O to pump for about 15 min. Resample filtrates to obtain blank value. A dual-channel system eliminates blank measurement for most food products.

6. *Calculations.*   The set of standards provides a linear curve passing through origin when standard peak height is plotted versus concentration is μg/mL. Subtract sample blank peak heights from sample peak heights. Determine sample concentration in μg/mL by comparison of blank corrected peak height of sample with the standard curve:

$$\text{Niacin, mg}/100 = \frac{C_S \times 10}{W}$$

where C_S = concentration of sample (μg/mL)
          W = sample weight (g).

The 10 is a combined factor taking into account 100 mL extract, level reported per 100 g, and conversion of μg to mg.

DETERMINATION OF VITAMIN A

A. Principle

It is most often the case, with the analysis of vitamin A in a biological material, that the extract requires chromatographic cleanup prior to determination by fluorescence or colorimetric determination with antimony trichloride. In certain situations, when chromatographic cleanup is not required, automation allows the facile analysis of large numbers of samples. Milk is an example of just such a situation.

This is an automated version (51) of a fluorometric method for determining vitamin A in whole milk, partially skimmed milk, skimmed milk, and chocolate milk (56). Naturally occurring and added retinol derivatives are measured, but not β-carotene. Milk is saponified to convert retinyl esters to retinol and to remove other fluorescent lipids. Retinol is extracted with hexane and is determined fluorometrically. The most difficult steps to automate are those in which the saponified milk is extracted and a clear solution of retinol is recovered for fluorometry. As the separation in the system is affected by the presence of milk, standards in the automated method are prepared in unfortified milk rather than in water (51).

B. Equipment

1. *AutoAnalyzer System (Technicon) with a Technicon Sampler IV.*   Remove one of the two teeth on a 20/hr (2:1) cam to make a 10/hr (1:2) cam and Technicon Pump III.

2. *Technicon Fluorometer II.*   With primary filters 110-810 (7-54) and 110-836 (34A) and secondary filter 110-828 (465 nm).

3. *Spectrophotometer.*

C. Reagents

1. *Water-dispersible Dry Vitamin A Palmitate Beadlets.*   Palma-Sperse Type 250-S (Hoffmann-La Roche Ltd.) containing about 250,000 IU vitamin A/g.

2. *Ethyl Ether.*   Redistill dry ether over reduced iron powder immediately before use.

3. *Hexane.*   HPLC quality, glass distilled.

4. *Potassium Hydroxide Solution.*   Dissolve 500 g KOH in H_2O and dilute to 1 L.

5. *95% Ethanol.*

D. Procedure

The laboratory should be feebly illuminated with tungsten lights. The automated equipment and all solutions containing vitamin A should be shielded from light.

1. *Analysis of Water-Dispersible Retinyl Palmitate (Palma-Sperse).*

(a) Weigh three 30-mg portions of Palma-Sperse in 100-mL Erlenmeyer flasks. To each add 25 mL H_2O and stir at 60°C for 10 min. Transfer to 250-mL separatory funnels, using 20 mL H_2O, followed by 20 mL diethyl ether to rinse flasks, and extract three times with 50-mL portions of diethyl ether. Wash pooled ether extracts with 50 mL H_2O, then add 50 mL hexane. Allow to stand and remove separated water. Transfer to 250-mL volumetric flasks and dilute to volume with hexane. Remove three 2-mL aliquots from each flask and dilute to 10 mL in separate volumetric flasks. Read in spectrophotometer at 326 nm and calculate the mean vitamin A content as retinol, using $E_{1m}^{1\%}$ 1820 (i.e., assume $^+\epsilon_{max}$ for retinyl ester is 52,200).

(1) Palma-Sperse should be stored at 5°C in a tightly sealed brown bottle. It has a uniform vitamin A content and it will retain its potency for several months. The bottle should be inverted several times before opening to mix the contents.

2. *Preparation of Vitamin A Standards in Milk.*

(a) Stir 1.5 L unfortified milk for 10 min using a magnetic stirrer. Weigh 30 mg of the analyzed Palma-Sperse and transfer to 250-mL volumetric flask. Add 50 mL milk and swirl for 30 sec. Make up to volume with milk, add a magnetic stirrer, and stir for 30 min. Dilute 10-mL, 8-mL, 4-mL, 2-mL, and 1-mL aliquots to 100 mL with milk. Use the milk alone as a blank.

(1) 30 mg Palma-Sperse usually contains the equivalent of about 2.5 mg retinol. The final dilutions should contain about 1, 0.8, 0.6, 0.4, and 0.2 μg retinol/mL from Palma-Sperse.

3. *Arrangement of Analytical System.*

(a) Assemble components as in Figure 5.7. Alkali and ethanol, which are preheated to 60°C in coils (B) in water bath, are mixed with milk from the sampler. The mixture, segmented with air bubbles, passes through a mixing coil (a) and a saponification coil (40 ft) in the same water bath at 60°C, for 10 min. After saponification, a portion is removed for extraction and the remainder is discarded at C through a DO separator (Technicon connector No. 116-0203-00) which is positioned so that the waste leaves downwards.

(1) A horizontal piece of Teflon tubing (5 cm long) is attached to the outlet to direct the flow to a beaker; it is important that this outlet should be short and free of obstructions, as small particles will sometimes be discharged.

(b) The major part of the saponified sample is blended with hexane in a coil of glass beads (D) placed close to the pump. Water and a new sequence of air bubbles are added and the organic and aqueous phases are allowed to separate first in a coil in a bath at 32°C (E) and then in a straight horizontal glass tube 35 cm long. The lower aqueous phase is removed using a BO separator (Technicon electrolyte trap No. 116-0100-00) and an inverted C5 debubbler (Technicon connector No. 116-0202 P05). Air is removed with a small amount of hexane before the debubbler in the flow-cell by a CO debubbler (Technicon connector No. 116-0202-P00) and the remaining hexane is passed through the flow cell. The arrangement of the three final separators is shown in Figure 5.8. All connections in this system that have contact with alkali are made with glass tubing joined with short pieces (1 cm) of Teflon tubing.

(1) The ends of the Teflon connectors will need to be widened with a blunt instrument before they are slipped over the glass tubes. The tubes

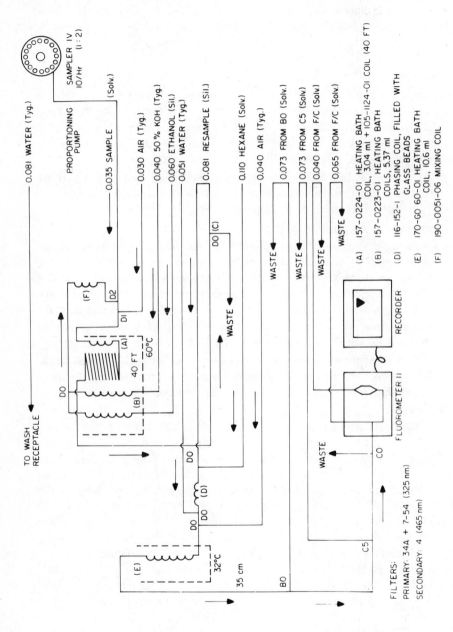

FIGURE 5.7 Automated equipment for determination of vitamin A.

124

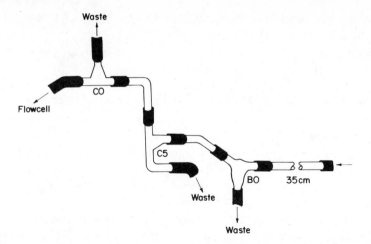

FIGURE 5.8   Arrangement of three separators for removal of aqueous phase and air.

should be pushed together inside a Teflon sleeve until they touch. If a connection fails and alkali spills and wets the surface of the connectors, it will be impossible to rejoin the parts unless all alkali is rinsed off and the connectors are dried with tissue. For this reason, it is preferable to assemble and test the system using water in place of the KOH solution. Once the system has been successfully assembled with Teflon connectors, it can be used for many months without need for replacements other than pump tubes.

4. *Operation of the Analytical System.*

(a) Disconnect the line to the fluorometer at the CO separator and let line run to waste. Pump reagents for at least 20 min to ensure that the system is equilibrated and that the hexane layer separates cleanly. Reconnect the flow cell.

(1) If water enters flow cell at this time or subsequently, the cell must be washed with alcohol. Disconnect the flow cell at the CO separator and place cell inlet line in a beaker of alcohol.

(b) Arrange standards and samples in sampler as follows: standards with 0, 0.2, 0.4, 0.6, 0.8, and 1.0 μg added retinol/mL; 10 samples followed by standards with 0 μg and 1.0 μg added retinol/mL. Repeat the latter sequence as required to complete the analyses.

(1) The system should be tested when first assembled to verify that the peaks attain steady-state values. Arrange a sequence of identical standards in the sampler (1.0 μg added retinol/mL) and when they have been taken up, place the inlet tube to the sampler in a beaker of the same standard for 5 min. The individual peaks should be at least 95% of the height of the plateau obtained with the continuous input (steady state). The level of the plateau will vary ±5%.

(2) The system will accept occasional chocolate milk samples but as particles usually remain after saponification, the system may block after

a long sequence. Chocolate milk samples should therefore always be separated by cups of H_2O.

5. *Maintenance of the Analytical System.*   When analyses are finished, disconnect the flow cell and draw KOH solution into the sample, hexane, and ethanol lines for 10 min. Finally place all the inlet lines in water for at least 30 min. Change the resample (0.081 Silicone) and hexane (0.11 Solvaflex) manifold tubes daily.

6. *Calculation.*

(a) Measure the peak heights. Deduct the height of the blank from those of the remaining standards and plot a graph of the increase in height (mm) against added vitamin A (μg retinol/mL). Read the vitamin A concentrations in the samples directly from this graph.

(1) The graph should be a straight line passing through the origin. Do not subtract the blank value from the values for the samples. The blank value represents the vitamin A already present in the milk used to dilute the standards.

(2) In routine analysis, the standard curve can be omitted and the response can be calculated from a blank and one standard (1 μg added retinol/mL) placed in the sampler tray after every 10 samples.

AUTOMATED MICROBIOLOGICAL VITAMIN ASSAY

The AUTOTURB® System (57,58) marketed by Elanco Products Co., a subsidiary of Eli Lilly and Company, is a semiautomated analytical system for turbidimetric microbiological analysis. The AUTOTURB® System provides automated performance of the time-consuming manual steps leaving the operator free to do the operations that are not practical to automate. The system consists of three basic components—the diluter module for dilution of standard and samples, the reader module for measuring and recording the turbidity of each assay tube, and a special water bath incubator designed for the assay tube module. The reader portion of this system can be readily interfaced with a variety of digital computers, ranging from desk-top calculators to large sophisticated computer systems. Most existing analytical microbiological procedures are easily adapted to the AUTOTURB® System resulting in greater efficiency, accuracy, and precision of analysis.

The diluter consists of two pneumatically activated metering valves and associated sample loops, a carousel carrier for standard and sample tubes on the upper portion of the instrument, and a rake and track underneath for advancing the assay tube module. A special dual syringe unit delivers the medium used as diluent. Vacuum, compressed air or tank nitrogen (45 psi), and electrical power are necessary for operation of the diluter. The diluter automatically removes a sufficient quantity of sample from each sample tube on the carousel to wash previous solutions from the sample loops and valves and to fill the "loops." The valves switch positions to deliver medium through the valves and loops washing the two samples into two empty assay tubes. Two 0.1-mL samples are diluted first with 9.9 mL medium (100-fold dilution) followed by two 0.15-mL portions similarly diluted (67-fold dilution) to provide the four assay tubes that represent each sample tube. Standards and samples are treated alike. An 80-tube test is diluted in 7.5 min and occupies one assay tube module.

The reader module consists of a spectrophotometer equipped with a flow cell on the upper portion of the instrument and the rake and track below as in the diluter unit. The reader automatically passes from 6 mL to 8 mL of incubated broth from each assay tube through the flow cell, measures turbidity of the cell suspension, and records it. Turbidity is measured to the nearest 0.1% T and is recorded on a paper tape or in a computer. The contents of 80 assay tubes are measured in about 14 min. The reader module requires vacuum source and electrical power.

The following is a general guide to be used to modify existing procedures for application to the AUTOTURB® System.

A. Principle

Same as for manual methods.

B. Equipment

The equipment listed in the chapters on specific vitamin procedures remains basically the same. However, it should be noted that an increase in precision will reduce the required replications. On the other hand, the increase in efficiency provided by automation will increase the number of determinations expected from a competent technician by two- to three-fold. Adjustments in amounts of existing equipment may be necessary for changes in work load with the addition of an AUTOTURB® System.

C. Reagents

The reagents listed in the chapters on specific vitamins remain the same with two exceptions:

1. *Basal Medium.* The basal medium will be the same except it must be further diluted 1:2 with water because the AUTOTURB® Diluter transfers the medium to culture tubes at the concentration at which it will be incubated.

2. *Working Standard Solution.* Since the AUTOTURB® Diluter measures constant volumes of solutions, the different concentrations of standards required for a standard line must be prepared by the technician. Four or five standard levels, including a zero concentration, generally are sufficient. These concentrations have an arithmetic spacing, that is, 0, 1, 2, 3----. These concentrations can be calculated by determining the actual standard concentration per culture tube

from the existing procedure and then multiplying by 10 to obtain the concentration per mL of the working standard solutions. These solutions should be prepared from the stock solution and used on the day of the assay. Glass pipettes should be properly used in preparing standards and samples. Details of operations that must be controlled to produce accurate assays are discussed by Kavanagh and Ragheb (59).

D. Sample Procedure for Pantothenic Acid

"Preparation of Standard Tubes," for the manual procedure, calls for 0.0, 0.5, 1.0, 1.5, 2.0, 2.5, 3.0, and 4.0 mL of a working standard solution at 0.05 μg of pantothenic acid activity per mL to be added to tubes resulting in standard concentrations of 0, .025, .05, .075, 0.1, 0.125, and 0.2 μg of pantothenic acid activity per tube. Multiply these concentrations by 10 and eliminate intermediate concentrations because the AUTOTURB® automatically makes an intermediate dilution. This results in standard solutions of 0, 0.25, 0.5, 1.0, and 1.5 μg of pantothenic acid/mL to be presented to the diluter. After automatic dilution, the final concentrations per tube are 0, 0.025, 0.0375, 0.05, 0.075, 0.1, 0.15, and 0.225 μg. These concentrations are similar to those of the manual curve. This example is presented as a workable guideline and may be altered to obtain different curve levels.

1. *Preparation of Stock Culture.*   Same as for manual methods.

2. *Preparation of Inoculum.*   Same as for manual methods.

3. *Preparation of Samples.*   Sample preparation is the same as outlined in the procedures for individual vitamins with the single exception of dilution of the sample. Concentration of the final sample (μg/mL) solution will have to be approximately 10-fold greater than that concentration (μg/tube) in the manual procedure.

4. *Preparation of Standard Tubes.*   None required.

5. *Preparation of Assay Tubes.*   Preparation of standard and sample assay tubes are automatically carried out by the AUTOTURB® Diluter once the sample and standard solutions are presented to the instrument. Ten to 15 mL of standard or sample solution are put into a sample tube which is then placed in the carousel. The loaded carousel is positioned on the diluter, the sample probed attached, and medium pickup lines put into the medium. When finished, the entire test is contained in an 80-tube module ready for autoclaving. Each sample tube of standard or sample results in four assay tubes, two at a dilution of 100 and two at a dilution of 67.

6. *Sterilization.*   Same as for manual methods.

7. *Inoculation.*   Same as for manual methods.

8. *Measurement of Turbidity.*   At this point of the assay, the AUTOTURB® System method differs from the manual method in that no titration is required. Six to eight milliliters of medium from each assay tube is automatically drawn through the flow cell of the spectrophotometer, and percent light transmittance of the flowing suspension of cells is measured and recorded.

9. *Calculations.* Since each loop produces a different standard line, the data must be sorted according to loop. For manual operations, the easy way is to mark the paper tape to include all four responses from a sample between two lines. The first response following a line will be loop number 1, the second being loop number 2, etc. Standard responses are used to construct four standard lines for plotting absorbance versus concentration on rectangular coordinate paper if absorbance is easily obtained. Otherwise, plot logarithm of transmittance against concentration on single decade log paper. Draw a smooth curve through the points.

Four lines are always used when interpolation is by means of any kind of digital computer, even the hand-held form (60,61,62). One reason for using a computer is to reduce the error of interpolation of potency from the standard line to a minimum. Interpolation error can be 2–3% when done manually.

If the two responses from a pair of loops are nearly identical, the mean of the responses can be used in constructing the standard line and in obtaining potencies from it without introducing significant, additional error in manual interpolation. A consistent difference between the two sample sizes indicates a problem to be investigated because such results show that potency is not independent of concentration as it must be for the assay to be valid (61).

Shape of vitamin standard lines range from nearly straight for vitamin B_{12} to strongly curved for folic acid. Fairly elaborate expressions have been used as interpolation formulae (62). Certain lines can be fitted by a quadratic equation, while others can be fitted over a portion of the curve by a straight line and over the curved part by a quadratic equation (62). The expression used depends upon the computational facilities and accuracy needed. When a high degree of accuracy is not required, interpolation from a graph may be adequate, requiring less effort than calculation in the absence of an efficient computer system.

Only a portion of the standard line may be usable as in the example shown in Figure 5.9. The portion above concentrations of standard greater than 2–3 μg should not be used because slope of the line is too small. The steeper the line, the more accurate is interpolation of potency from it. Values outside, on the low as well as on the high side of the proper range, are used only as a rough indication of potency to guide dilution for the subsequent assay.

Accuracy of assaying should be monitored continually. A good practice is to include in each assay a repeat of a concentration of the standard curve placed toward the end of the assay and a concentration between two points prepared as carefully as a standard concentration. The control samples test operations of the AUTOTURB® System, accuracy of dilution, and procedures for obtaining potency from the standard line. Potencies of these control samples should be very close to their true values. Most of the errors in assays with the AUTO-TURB® System are external to it. The most common error is inaccurate dilution of sample by the analyst.

Application of the AUTOTURB® System will be illustrated by an assay for pantothenic acid. The samples were either points of the standard line or solutions prepared from the standard solution. Concentrations of standards refer to those in the sample tubes in the diluter carousel. Responses as % T are given in Table

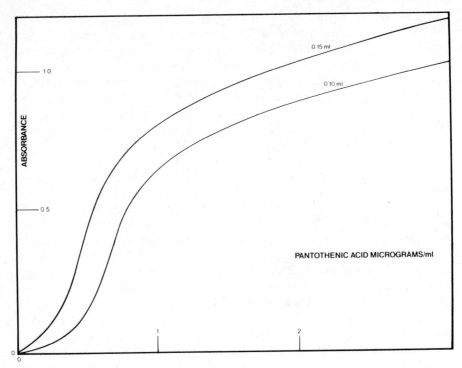

FIGURE 5.9   Standard curves for determining pantothenic acid using the AUTOTURB® analyzer.

TABLE 5.1   Typical Transmittance Values for Pantothenic Acid Assay after 20 Hr Incubation at 37°C

Standards (μg/mL)	Sample Volumes (mL)			
	0.1	0.1	0.15	0.15
0	99.70	99.64	99.73	99.75
0.2	90.70	92.17	88.10	89.86
0.4	84.40	85.22	57.67	61.49
0.6	59.72	61.10	26.63	30.71
0.8	31.80	33.23	20.01	21.07
1.0	22.66	24.11	16.80	17.34
1.2	20.29	20.40	14.30	14.71
1.4	17.49	19.00	12.46	13.44
Samples				
0.50	78.31	79.80	36.88	40.94
0.75	38.03	38.42	21.77	22.58
0.60	60.88	62.52	27.60	29.65
0.40	85.86	85.74	60.63	65.21

TABLE 5.2 Potencies for Samples in Table 5.1

Sample (μg/mL)	Sample Size (mL)				Mean Potency	RSD (%)
	0.1	0.1	0.15	0.15		
0.5	0.46	0.45	0.52	0.52	0.49	8
0.75	0.76	0.77	0.70	0.74	0.74	4
0.60	0.59	0.59	0.59	0.61	0.60	2
0.40	0.37	0.39	0.36	0.38	0.37	4

5.1. Potencies interpolated from the four standard lines are given in Table 5.2. These potencies were obtained from the four smooth curves drawn through the four sets of responses. Two of the lines are given in Figure 5.9. Only the region of the lines between 0.4 μg/mL and 0.8 μg/mL should be used in assaying because the portions outside are too strongly curved for accurate work.

Turbidimetric vitamin assays may be more variable than tubidimetric antibiotic assays. Part of the variation is caused by clumping of bacteria. Treatment with Thoral to break the clumps, as suggested by Tanguay (63) and Heed (64), improves replication of turbidity and should be used routinely for vitamin assays.

LITERATURE CITED

1. Egberg, D. C., Larson, P. A., and Honold, G. R. "Automated determination of vitamin C in some fortified foodstuffs." *J. Sci. Food Agric.* **24**, 789 (1973).

2. Sauberlich, H., Goad, W. C., Skala, J. H., and Waring, P. "Procedure for mechanized (continuous-flow) measurement of serum ascorbic acid (vitamin C)." *Clin. Chem.* **22**, 105 (1976).

3. Hoffman, M., Bar-Akiva, A., Tanhum, L., and Berkenstadt, Y. "Automated determination of ascorbic acid in orange and grapefruit juices." *Anal. Biochem.* **38**, 35 (1970).

4. Saindelle, A., Ruff, F., and Parrot, J. L. "Automation of the determination of ascorbic acid in whole blood, urine, and tissues." *Soc. Chim. Biol.* **51**, 621 (1969).

5. Pelletier, O. and Brassard, R. "Determination of vitamin C (L-ascorbic acid and dehydroascorbic acid) in food by manual and automated photometric methods." *J. Food Sci.* **42**, 1471 (1977).

6. Pelletier, O. and Brassard, R. "New automated method for serum vitamin C." *Adv. Autom. Anal. Technicon Int. Cong.* **9**, 73 (1972).

7. Aeschbacher, H. U. and Brown, R. G. "Automated vitamin C analysis." *Clin. Chem.* **18**, 965 (1972).

8. Egberg, D. C., Potter, R. H., and Heroff, J. C. "Semiautomated method for the fluorometric determination of total vitamin C in food products." *J. Assoc. Off. Anal. Chem.* **60**, 126 (1977).

9. Roy, R. B., Conetta, A., and Salpeter, J. "Automated fluorometric method for the determination of total vitamin C in food products." *J. Assoc. Off. Anal. Chem.* **59**, 1244 (1976).

10. Kirk, J. R. and Ting, N. "Fluorometric assay for total vitamin C using continuous flow analysis." *J. Food Sci.* **40**, 463 (1975).

11. Geller, M., Weber, O. W. A., and Senkowski, B. Z. "Automated determination of ascorbic acid in multivitamin preparations." *J. Pharm. Sci.* **58**, 477 (1969).

12. Roy, R. B., Buccafuri, A., and Salpeter, J. "Semiautomated fluorometric analysis of riboflavin in nutrient premixes containing reduced iron." *J. Assoc. Off. Anal. Chem.* **60**, 122 (1977).

13. Roy, R. B., Salpeter, J., and Dunmire, D. I. "Evaluation of urea-acid system as a medium of

extraction for B-group vitamins. Simplified automated analysis of riboflavine in food products." *J. Food Sci.* **41**, 996 (1976).

14. Egberg, D. C. and Potter, R. H. "Improved automated determination of riboflavine in food products." *J. Agric. Food Chem.* **23**, 815 (1975).

15. Kirk, J. R. "Automated method for the analysis of riboflavine in milk, with application to other selected foods." *J. Assoc. Off. Anal. Chem.* **57**, 1085 (1974).

16. Mellor, N. P. and Maass, A. R. "Automated fluorometric method for the determination of riboflavin in human urine." *Adv. Autom. Anal. Technicon Int. Congr.* **9**, 67 (1972).

17. Bryant, R., Burger, F. J., Henry, R. L., and Trenk, F. B. "Semiautomated simultaneous assay of thiamine, riboflavin, pyridoxine, and niacinamide in multivitamin preparations." *J. Pharm. Sci.* **60**, 1717 (1971).

18. Albright, B. E. and Degner, E. F. "Advances in automated vitamin analyses." *Automat. Anal. Chem., Technicon Symp.* **1**, 461 (1967).

19. Jacobson, B. S. "Hydroxylamine hydrochloride in automated and manual methods for riboflavin determination." *J. Assoc. Off. Anal. Chem.* **60**, 147 (1977).

20. Egberg, D. C. "Semiautomated method for riboflavin in food products: Collaborative study." *J. Assoc. Off. Anal. Chem.* **62**, 1041 (1979).

21. Pelletier, O. and Madere, R. "Automated determination of thiamin and riboflavin in various foods." *J. Assoc. Off. Anal. Chem.* **60**, 140 (1977).

22. Pelletier, O. and Madere, R. "Comparison of automated and manual procedures for determining thiamine and riboflavin in foods." *J. Food Sci.* **40**, 374 (1975).

23. Ramirez-Munoz, J. "Determination of riboflavin in pharmaceutical products by automatic discrete-sample analysis." *Anal. Chim. Acta* **72**, 407 (1974).

24. Berg, T. M. and Behagel, H. A. "Semiautomated method for microbiological vitamin assays." *Appl. Microbiol.* **23**, 531 (1972).

25. Ribbron, W. M., Stevenson, K. E., and Kirk, J. R. "Comparison of semiautomated and manual methods for the determinations of thiamin baby cereals and infant and dietary formulas." *J. Assoc. Off. Anal. Chem.* **60**, 737 (1977).

26. Kirk, J. R. "Automated method for the analysis of thiamine in milk with application to other selected foods." *J. Assoc. Off. Anal. Chem.* **57** (1974).

27. Pelletier, O. and Madere, R. "New automated method for measuring thiamine (vitamin B₁) in urine." *Clin. Chem.* **18**, 937 (1972).

28. Defibaugh, P. W., Smith, J. S., and Weeks, C. E. "Assay of thiamin in foods, using manual and semiautomated fluorometric and microbiological methods." *J. Assoc. Off. Anal. Chem.* **60**, 522 (1977).

29. Albright, B. E. and Degner, E. F. "Advances in automated vitamin analyses." *Automat. Anal. Chem., Technicon Symp.* **1**, 461 (1967).

30. Park, J. Y. "Comparative study of colorimetric and fluorometric determination of thiamine (vitamin B₁) by an automated discrete-sampling technique." *Anal. Chem.* **47**, 452 (1975).

31. Egberg, D. C., Potter, R. H., and Honold, G. R. "Semiautomated determination of niacin and niacinamide in food products." *J. Agr. Food Chem.* **22**, 323 (1974).

32. Van Gend, H. W. "Automated colorimetric method for the determination of free nicotinic acid in minced meat." *Z. Lebensm.-Unters. Forsch.* **153**, 73 (1973).

33. Gross, A. F. "Automated method for the determination of niacin and niacinamide in cereal products. Collaborative study." *J. Assoc. Off. Anal. Chem.* **58**, 799 (1975).

34. Egberg, D. C. "Semiautomated method for niacin and niacinamide in food products: Collaborative study." *J. Assoc. Off. Anal. Chem.* **62**, 1027 (1979).

35. Ramirez-Munoz, J. "Determination of niacin and niacinamide in pharmaceutical products by automatic discrete-sample analysis. *Anal. Chim. Acta* **71**, 321 (1974).

36. Pelletier, O. and Madere, R. "Automated and manual determination of pyridoxine in multivitamin preparations." *Can. J. Pharm. Sci.* **9**, 99 (1974).

37. Crockett, R., Mesnard, P., Grenie, D., and Dang, R. "Analytical study of a pyridoxine color reaction and its application in manual and automatic measurements of pyridoxine in pharmaceutical compounds." *Bull. Soc. Pharm. Bordeaux* **108**, 7 (1969).

38. Gregory, J. F. and Kirk, J. R. "Improved chromatographic separation and fluorometric determination of vitamin B_6 compounds in foods." *J. Food Sci.* **42**, 1073 (1977).

39. Davis, R. E., Smith, B. K., and Curnow, D. H. "Automated method for the microbiological assay of serum pyridoxal." *J. Clin. Pathol.* **26**, 871 (1973).

40. Smith, B. K. "Serum pyridoxal and a method for its measurement." *Austral. J. Med. Technol.* **4**, 133 (1973).

41. Samuelian, S. "Automated method for determination of folic acid in single tablets." *Adv. Autom. Anal., Technicon Int. Symp.* **169** (1974).

42. Tennant, G. B. "Continuous-flow automation of the *Lactobacillus casei* serum folate assay." *J. Clin. Pathol.* **30**, 1168 (1977).

43. Magnus, E. M. "Automated microbiological assay for folic acid." *Folic Acid, Proc. Workshop* **152** (1975).

44. Tennant, G. B. and Withey, J. L. "Assessment of work-simplified procedures for the microbiological assay of serum vitamin B_{12} and serum folate." *Med. Lab. Technol.* **29**, 171 (1972).

45. Colvin, G., Gibson, G. L., and Neill, D. W. "Use of the Analmatic clinical system in the microbiological assay of vitamin B_{12} and folic acid in serum." *J. Clin. Pathol.* **24**, 18 (1971).

46. Davis, R. E., Nicol, D. J., and Kelly, A. "Automated method for the measurement of folate activity." *J. Clin. Pathol.* **23**, 47 (1970).

47. Viola, L., Vianello, S., and Cavatorta, L. "Automation of the microbiological determination of tetracycline with *Bacillus cereus* and vitamin B_{12} with *Lactobacillus leichmannii*." *Farmaco, Ed. Prat.* **25**, 315 (1970).

48. Morisi, G. and Gualandi, G. "Automation in analysis. II. Automatic analysis of drugs containing vitamin B_{12}. *Ann. 1st Super Sanita* **4**, 351 (1968).

49. Secchi, N. and Valentini, L. "Automatic analysis of cobalamins in fermentation media." Fr. 2,083,992 (Cl. G Oln), 21 Jan 1972, Ita. Appl. 21,399 A/70,03 Mar 1970; 7 pp.

50. Ohman, J. and Fri, A. "Fast radioimmunoassay methods for human placental lactogen (HPL), insulin, and vitamin B_{12}. Simplification of sample preparation and data processing." *Recent Adv. Nucl. Med. Proc. World Congr. Nucl. Med. 1st,* **850** (1974).

51. Thompson, J. N. and Madere, R. "Automated fluorometric determination of vitamin A in milk." *J. Assoc. Off. Anal. Chem.* **61**, 1370 (1978).

52. Thompson, J. N., Erdody, P., Maxwell, W. B., and Murray, T. K. "Fluorometric determination of vitamin A in dairy products." *J. Dairy Sci.* **55**, 1077 (1972).

53. Kahan, J. "Automated fluorometric assay of vitamin A in pharmaceutical preparations." *J. Assoc. Off. Anal. Chem.* **57**, 1074 (1974).

54. Kahan, J. "Automated fluorometric assay of serum vitamin A." *Int. J. Vit. Nutr. Res.* **43**, 127 (1973).

55. Weil, A. and Regnier, J. M. "Automatic determination of vitamin A in inorganic compounds for cattle feeding." *Ind. Aliment. Agr.* **88**, 1539 (1971).

56. Gutteridge, J. M. C. and Stocks, J. "Automated colorimetric method for the determination of serum tocopherol." *Lab. Pract.* **25**, 25 (1976).

57. Kuzel, N. R. and Kavanagh, F. W. "Automated system for analytical microbiology I: Theory and design considerations." *J. Pharm. Sci.* **60**, 764 (1971).

58. Kuzel, N. R. and Kavanagh, F. W. "Automated system for analytical microbiology II: Construction of system and evaluation of antibiotics and vitamins." *J. Pharm. Sci.* **60**, 767 (1971).

59. Kavanagh, F. W. and Ragheb, H. S. "Microbiological assays for antibiotics and vitamins: Considerations for assuring accuracy." *J. Assoc. Off. Anal. Chem.* **62**, 943 (1979).

60. Kavanagh, F. W. "Automated system for analytical microbiology III: Computer interpolation of potency." *J. Pharm. Sci.* **60**, 1858 (1971).

61. Kavanagh, F. W. "Automated system for analytical microbiology V: Calibration lines for antibiotics." *J. Pharm. Sci.* **64**, 844 (1975).

62. Kavanagh, F. W. "Microbiological turbidimetric methods: Linearization of antibiotic and vitamin standard curves." *J. Pharm. Sci.* **66**, 1520 (1977).

63. Tanguay, A. E. "Improvement of the microbiological assay for Leucovorin." *Appl. Microbiol.* **18**, 1088 (1969).

64. Heed, E. J. "Improvements of microbial assays of vitamins." *Appl. Microbiol.* **24**, 286–287 (1972).

6 Sampling for Vitamin Analyses

Edgar R. Elkins and Janet A. Dudek

GENERAL CONSIDERATIONS

The purpose of this chapter is to convey to the analyst engaged in nutrient analysis the importance of sampling and sample preparation; to point out some of the problems that may be encountered; and to describe methods that may be used to overcome those problems. The natural variability of the nutrient content of foods is an accepted fact and cannot be avoided. Thus, the analyst must employ methods of sampling and sample preparation that will reduce the errors inherent in selecting and preparing the sample for analysis. It is self-evident that the results obtained by any test method can be no better than the sample on which tests were performed.

Ideally, the sample obtained should be small enough to be transported to the laboratory and still accurately represent the material being sampled, that is, a representative sample. The sample must be handled in such a way that no significant compositional changes occur due to exposure to detrimental conditions of temperature, light, or oxygen, for example. It is impossible to give methods that will cover all the conditions and problems in sampling and sample preparation; much will still remain with the judgement of the analyst.

The question of sampling and sample preparation procedures gained added attention in 1973 due to the nutritional labeling regulations established by the Food and Drug Administration (FDA) (1). The FDA spelled out in its regulation how sampling and sample preparation should be treated in compliance situations (2).

THE GENERAL PROBLEM

A representative sample must contain the relative proportions or concentrations of the vitamins that are in the food being examined. The more varied the material, the more complex are the manipulations involved in obtaining a representative sample. Sampling techniques will vary, but in general can be classified according to the types of material to be tested.

1. *Homogeneous Materials.*   Single-phase or well-mixed powders present the simplest case because each part is typical of all the others, and any portion of the original may be used as the analytical sample. It should be realized, however, that many materials that appear to be homogeneous are not, especially if large volumes are involved. As a rule, even solutions or powders should be mixed thoroughly immediately prior to sampling.

Small quantities of powders or solutions may be mixed by rotating and shaking them in a closed container, using a volume at least twice that of the sample size to be drawn. Mixing may also be accomplished by pouring the product from one container to another several times. Larger quantities of solutions contained in vats or large tanks can sometimes be mixed with a mechanical stirrer or large paddle.

Certain materials are easily oxidized, and aeration in the mixing is to be avoided. When mixing is impossible, geometric sampling described below must be used.

2. *Heterogeneous Materials.*   These require more complicated sampling techniques, and the difficulties increase in proportion both to the size of the lot to be analyzed and to the variations existing within it. The only procedure that can be relied upon to give a truly representative sample is to grind the entire lot to such a degree of fineness that, after thorough mixing, a degree of homogeneity approaching that of a solution is reached. Although such treatment is usually impractical, it must be recognized that any other procedure represents a compromise between practicality and accuracy. In each case, the technique employed must be based upon consideration of (1) the accuracy acceptable or attainable, (2) the degree of homogeneity in the lot, (3) the amount of time, labor, and money available, and (4) the purpose of the analysis.

With heterogeneous materials of great bulk or size, like a carload of grain or a shipment of feed, it is often necessary to prepare a succession of samples of progressively decreasing size before amounts are reached that are convenient for transport to or storage in the laboratory. These samples are designated primary, secondary, tertiary, etc. The analytical sample is finally prepared from the last of these. In order that each sample may be satisfactorily representative of the whole, the procedure known as geometric sampling is employed.

In geometric sampling, the lot is considered as some sort of regular geometric solid (e.g., cube, cylinder, or cone). This is divided, at least mentally, into a number of equal volumes and a subsample is withdrawn at random from each. All subsamples should be of equal size. When combined and thoroughly mixed, these constitute the primary sample. When the geometric technique is employed, it is essential that the division of the lot be such that portions are withdrawn from all parts, not merely from the surface or from one side. This type of sampling is the basis of most official procedures and must be employed whenever knowledge of the character of the lot is lacking.

If it is known that the lot is made up of several sublots of different origins (e.g., a carload of poultry feed supposedly of the same formula but produced on three different days), each sublot may be sampled (geometrically, if necessary) and a sublot sample obtained by mixing. Then a quantity of material is taken from each sublot sample, this quantity being proportional to the contribution of that sublot to the whole lot. These proportional quantities are combined into a grand composite representative of the total. For example, if a 100-lb lot is made up of sublots weighing 25, 35, and 40 lb, the primary sample might be prepared by taking 25-, 35-, and 40-g portions, respectively, from the different sublots. This type of sampling is, of course, restricted to materials in which there can be satisfactory mixing of the various subsamples. The Association of Official Analytical Chemists has established official sampling procedures for certain food commodities (3).

Unless the primary sample is a liquid or a finely divided solid, it must be put through some type of comminuting operation to reduce the particle size sufficiently to permit ready mixing. For dry materials, several types of grinders are available, such as Wiley Mills, burr mills, and hammer mills. A rolling pin is often sufficient to break up brittle material. A mortar and pestle may be used for small dry samples, such as tablets. Wet materials may be minced with a knife, ground through a food chopper, or blended with a high-speed rotary cutter such as the Waring Blendor, a food processor, or a homogenizer (e.g., Brinkman Polytron).

During all of these operations, changes in moisture content must be considered and prevented. Accidental losses of juices may change not only the vitamin content but also the vitamin concentration, since the vitamin concentration of the juice may differ from that of the remainder of the sample.

The primary sample must be thoroughly mixed before and after comminution. The secondary sample should then be taken geometrically, thoroughly mixed, and stored under conditions most conducive to retention of the vitamins. The assays should be conducted as promptly as possible, but if delays are necessary, samples may be preserved by refrigerating, freezing after the addition of a stabilizing medium, or freeze-drying. For small samples, immersion freezing in liquid nitrogen followed by frozen storage can be used. Dehydration is an acceptable storage procedure for products to be sampled for vitamins such as niacin and riboflavin, but folacin and ascorbic acid would be lost by this procedure.

Even the secondary, or laboratory sample is much larger than the amount needed in the actual assay. Accordingly, only a portion of the well-mixed sample need be taken for analysis. In many cases, either the entire sample or a portion of it is comminuted further in a Waring Blendor or other similar enclosed high-speed choppers. In such cases, it is common practice to add liquid so that a uniform slurry will result. If liquid is added, the material and liquid must both be added to the blender in known quantities so that the composition of the slurry bears a known relation to that of the material sampled.

A word of caution should be added. In industrial work, the primary sample is frequently taken by employees not connected with the laboratory. Reliable samples must not be expected unless these workers have been carefully trained and indoctrinated, and have frequent, nonperiodic inspection of their work. Without such precautions, the job is likely to seem an unnecessarily complicated nuisance which can be easily cut short without detection.

3. *Multivitamin Analysis.* A single extraction procedure is an ideal situation. These methods have not been perfected to the point of routine use, but some workers have reported satisfactory results with single-extraction procedures in preparation for determinations by high-performance liquid chromatography (4,5,6). Usually, these methods involve drying, freeze-drying, milling, addition of acid, and autoclaving. Samples are filtered before injection into the liquid chromatographic system. The sample preparation procedure outlined by Fellman et al. (6) permits the simultaneous determination of thiamin and riboflavin by HPLC.

4. *Individual Vitamins.* Specific sampling and sampling preparation problems as they pertain have been reviewed (7) and will be briefly addressed in this chapter. Special care must be taken to minimize the effects of enzymes and catalysts or to prevent undue exposure of the sample to oxygen or to light. Table 6.1 lists various conditions that may cause vitamin loss during sampling and sample preparation. Attention to these conditions will be helpful in preserving the vitamin during the sample preparation procedure. Vitamin A and pro-vitamin A (carotene) are sensitive to light and oxidation. Samples should be prepared in dim natural light or under a subdued light source (yellow incandescent light filters or gold fluorescent tubes) (7). Samples should be stored in brown or

TABLE 6.1. Potential Causes of Nutrient Loss During Sampling and Sample Preparation

Vitamin	Acid	Alkali	Heat	Light	Oxidation
Carotene				*	*
Thiamin (B$_1$)		*	*		*
Riboflavin (B$_2$)		*		*	
B$_6$				*	*
Pantothenic Acid	*	*	*		
Folacin			*	*	*
B$_{12}$		*			
Ascorbic acid		*	*		*
Niacin					
Vitamin D			*	*	*
Vitamin E		*	*	*	*

amber glass bottles after preparation. Riboflavin, vitamin B_6, folacin, vitamin D, and vitamin E are also sensitive to light and should be treated accordingly. The sample used for ascorbic acid analysis should be prepared immediately with the extracting acid used in the assay to prevent oxidation to dehydroascorbic acid and the biologically inactive form, ketogulonic acid.

Sample preparation problems with thiamin are due to the vitamin's sensitivity to heat and alkali. Care should be taken during grinding procedures so that a minimal amount of heat is generated, and samples that approach alkaline pH should be acidified.

In general, exposure of the sample to heat, light, moisture, or air, should be minimized or measurable losses will occur. Most vitamins are relatively stable in the dry state, so the water content should be reduced when possible. Another problem that may occur is vitamin loss during thawing. In many cases, samples can be extracted directly from the frozen state, in the stabilizing medium.

STATISTICS APPLIED TO SAMPLING

The accurate measurement of a nutrient in a food depends on the ability to assess the extent of natural variability and the analytical variation of the method used. Both are of the utmost importance. The procedural methodology used to determine methods variability is termed the "collaborative test." With some exceptions, very little data have been obtained on methods variability for specific foods at the various levels expected (8).

There are many excellent texts on statistical techniques and all include sampling (9–11). The following discussion will describe briefly the statistical design for the determination of sample variation along with definitions for various statistical terms. A brief description of the FDA's compliance procedures for nutrition labeling is included also.

The number of samples to test for estimating the mean and variability of a particular lot depends on the homogeneity of the lot, the size of the lot, and the risk one is willing to take on reaching a wrong conclusion. If all the items in a lot are nearly identical, then only a few samples need be tested. The less homogeneous the lot, the more samples are needed, that is, the chance that a value is near the lot average becomes less as the variability increases. The larger the lot, the greater the chance for variation if the lot is not homogeneous. One should, therefore, draw a larger number of test samples from larger lots than smaller lots. Lot homogeneity is more important than lot size in determining the sample size.

The variation within a lot of material or within any other series of analyses which it is desired to consider as a group (and for which a logical basis of grouping exists) is usually expressed in the form of a statistic known as the standard deviation. This statistic is also useful, as will be shown below, in estimating the reliability of an average and in estimating the number of subsamples necessary to attain a desired level of accuracy.

In a series of n observations, let x be the value of a single observation, $\bar{x}$ the mean of n observations, and d the deviation of any single observation from the mean, $d = x - \bar{x}$. The standard deviation is given by the equation $s_0 = \sqrt{\Sigma d^2/n}$. For example, assume the following values for the riboflavin content in μg per g of the milk from cans selected at random from a truck load of such cans: 1.79, 1.69, 1.58, 1.88, 1.78, 1.70, 1.75, 2.01, 1.71, 1.91. Then $\bar{x} = \Sigma x/n = 17.80/10 = 1.78$. The individual deviations from 1.78 are respectively 0.01, -0.09, -0.20, 0.10, 0.00, -0.08, -0.03, 0.23, -0.07, 0.13. The squares of these deviations are 0.0001, 0.0081, 0.0400, 0.0100, 0.0000, 0.0064, 0.0009, 0.0529, 0.0049, 0.0169. Then $\Sigma d^2 = 0.1402$ and $s_0 = \sqrt{0.1402/10} = 0.118$.

In most cases, as in this one of the riboflavin content of the cans of milk, the n observations made are a very small fraction of a much larger number N (all the cans of milk), which it is not feasible to analyze. The true mean, $m = \Sigma x/N$, and the true standard deviation of all samples $\sigma = \sqrt{\Sigma d^2/N}$, are not directly realizable.

The best estimate of m obtainable from n observations is $\bar{x} = \Sigma x/n$. In attempting to get the best of σ, the hypothetical standard deviation of all N samples from the limited number of n observations, it is found that in general s_0 is less than σ. This is because the value of σ is primarily determined by the largest deviations, and in a limited series of n observations one is less likely to encounter the largest deviations that would be found in a much larger number of N observations. Therefore, in arriving at the best estimate of σ, one arbitrarily chooses a value that is larger than $\sqrt{\Sigma d^2/n}$, and this is done by decreasing the denominator under the square root sign by 1. Experience has taught that $s = \sqrt{\Sigma d^2/(n-1)}$ is a better estimate of σ than is $s_0 = \sqrt{\Sigma d^2/n}$; and the former term s is defined as the estimate of the hypothetical standard deviation of all samples, or estimate of σ, and is used wherever σ is called for. In the data on the 10 cans of milk, $s = \sqrt{0.1402/(10-1)} = \sqrt{0.0156} \simeq 0.13$ (instead of 0.118 found previously for s_0).

It should be noted that the standard deviation, s, is in the same dimensions as the original measurements (x's). This is also true of the individual deviations (d's). It is frequently useful to consider the standard deviation not only as a measure of variation but also as a unit in terms of which any deviation may be expressed. A deviation from the mean in terms of this new unit is designated at t; in other words $t = d/s$. The expression of the deviations in terms of t values makes possible certain useful generalizations that apply with satisfactory accuracy to most variations normally encountered. One of the generalizations is Table 6.2, which shows that fraction of the lot sampled that varies from the mean in both directions by not more than the value of t shown.

It follows that one standard deviation ($t = 1$) represents that deviation on both sides of the mean (total range of $2s$) within which 68% of all observations will occur when the distribution is normal and the number of observations is sufficiently large; 95% of all observations will fall within $0.67s$ on either side of

TABLE 6.2 Fraction of Lot Which Deviates from the Mean by Not More Than t

t	Lot Fraction	t	Lot Fraction	t	Lot Fraction
0.1	0.080	0.8	0.576	1.8	0.928
0.2	0.159	1.0	0.682	2.0	0.954
0.4	0.310	1.2	0.770	2.6	0.9906
0.5	0.382	1.4	0.838	3.0	0.9973
0.67	0.500	1.6	0.890	4.0	0.9994

the mean (a total range of $1.34s$). A chemist would be inclined to express it thus: There is 95% chance that the error of a single observation will not exceed $2s$, a 68% chance that this error will not exceed s, and a 50% chance that this error will not exceed $0.67s$.

Experience teaches that in a small number of 10–20 observations, the range from the lowest to the highest is usually about $3s$, that is, three times the standard deviation. This is borne out in the above example of the riboflavin content of the cans of milk, where $s \simeq 0.13$, and the range $(2.01 - 1.58)$ is 0.43.

If, in sampling the truck load of milk, we had taken, not one collection consisting of 10 cans, but 10 collections, each consisting of 10 cans, and we had analyzed each can, we could calculate 10 means, each representing 10 cans of milk. These 10 means would not be identical but would show some degree of variation. Because each mean includes some high values and some low values that tend to compensate each other, there will be less variation in the means than was found in the individual cans.

Consider a series of means, r values of $\bar{x}$, with a mean of means $\bar{\bar{x}} = \Sigma \bar{x} / r$. Let $e = \bar{x} - \bar{\bar{x}} = $ the deviation of any mean from the mean of means. When r is sufficiently large, $\bar{\bar{x}}$ approaches m, the hypothetical true mean of all observations, and e is considered equal to $\bar{x} - m$. It follows that $s_0 = $ standard deviation of the means $= \sqrt{\Sigma(\bar{x} - \bar{\bar{x}})^2 / r} = \sqrt{\Sigma e^2 / r}$. It is possible to prove mathematically that, from n observations, the best estimate of s_0 may be obtained from the expression:

$$S = \text{estimate of } S_0 = s / \sqrt{n} = \sqrt{\Sigma d^2 / n(n - 1)}$$

This equation, like the previous one for $s = $ estimate of σ, will be accepted as a proposition that experience has shown to be valid and for which mathematical proof is available. It is to be noted that this is the standard deviation of means of n observations, but only one series of n observations is needed for its calculation. On our truck load of milk, for example, we do not need to take 10 collections of 10 cans each to calculate the standard deviation of means of 10 cans; we may estimate the standard deviation of such means with sufficient accuracy for our purpose from only one collection of 10 cans.

The deviations of means from the mean of means may be expressed in standard deviation units, just as in the case of deviations of individual values from their mean. The values given in Table 6.2 for the relation between t and the probability that any given value of x will lie within the range $(\bar{x} - d)$ and $(\bar{x} + d)$, hold also for the relation between t and the probability that the value of $\bar{x}$ will lie within the range of $(\bar{\bar{x}} - e)$ and $(\bar{\bar{x}} + e)$. In the latter case, we are dealing with the standard deviation of the means, $S = s/\sqrt{n}$, instead of simply s. Since S decreases as the square root of n increases, it follows that the magnitude of any error of $\bar{x}$ decreases as the square root of n increases. These ideas are illustrated by the following statements:

If	There Is a	That	Falls Within the Range
$n = 1$	68% chance	x	$m \pm s$
	95% chance	x	$m \pm 2s$
$n = 10$	68% chance	$\bar{x}$	$m \pm S = m \pm 0.316s$
	95% chance	$\bar{x}$	$m \pm 2S = m \pm 0.632s$
$n = 100$	68% chance	$\bar{x}$	$m \pm S = m \pm 0.1s$
	95% chance	$\bar{x}$	$m \pm 2S = m \pm 0.2s$
$n = 10,000$	68% chance	$\bar{x}$	$m \pm 2S = m \pm 0.01s$
	95% chance	$\bar{x}$	$m \pm 2S = m \pm 0.02s$
	99.7% chance	$\bar{x}$	$m \pm 3S = m \pm 0.03s$
	99.994% chance	$\bar{x}$	$m \pm 4S = m \pm 0.04s$

These ideas may be applied to the data previously given on the riboflavin content of the cans of milk. Here s was previously found to be 0.13, and we may now calculate the standard deviation of the means, $S = 0.13/\sqrt{10} = 0.04$. It follows that while, as previously shown, there is a 68% chance that any single observation will fall in the range 1.78 ± 0.13; there is also a 68% chance that the mean of 10 observations, 1.78, lies within ± 0.04 of m, the hypothetical true mean of all of the values; also a 95% chance that this mean of 10 observations, 1.78, lies with a range of $m \pm 2S = m \pm 0.08$, or a 99.7% chance that 1.78 lies within a range of $m \pm 3S = m \pm 0.12$. If we wished to increase the precision, or the confidence that we could have a given precision, we should increase the number of observations n. By making 100 observations instead of 10 we could decrease the standard deviation of the means to

$$S = 0.13/\sqrt{n} = 0.13/\sqrt{100} = 0.013$$

This new mean of 100 observations, x_{100}, would probably be slightly different from 1.78. There would be a 68% chance that the true mean is included in the range $\bar{x}_{100} \pm 0.013$; a 95% chance, in the range $\bar{x}_{100} \pm 0.026$, etc. Here, by taking 10 times as many observations the probable error is decreased to about one-third, more exactly to $1/\sqrt{10}$.

If the Allowable Error Is	And the Desired Confidence Is	The Number of Observations Required Is
s	68%	1
$0.316s$	68%	10
$0.1s$	68%	100
s	95%	4
$0.316s$	95%	40
$0.1s$	95%	400
s	99%	$(2.6)^2 = 6.8 \simeq 7$
$0.316s$	99%	68
$0.1s$	99%	680

The above-mentioned relations allow us to determine the probability that a single observation will have an error of a certain magnitude; also the probability by which the mean of no observations will have an error of a smaller magnitude. It follows that there is a relation between four quantities: *the number of observations,* the *standard deviation,* the *confidence* that one can have that the *error of the observed mean* will not exceed a certain magnitude. The relation of these four quantities is expressed by $t = e\sqrt{n}/s$. Solving the expression for n, $n = (ts/e)^2$. Here, n is the number of observations; t is the confidence or probability factor, since when $t = 1$, $pr = 68\%$; when $t = 2$, $pr = 95\%$, etc.; e represents the error, $e = m - \bar{x}$, or the difference between the observed means, $\bar{x}$, and the true mean, m. For a given series of observations, for example, the riboflavin content of a truckload of cans of milk s is reasonably constant, but S decreases as the square root of n increases, and the number of observations required increases with the square of the confidence factor t and decreases with the square of the allowable error e.

The following statements further illustrate the application of specific cases.

These ideas may be illustrated by application to the case of the riboflavin content of the truckload of cans of milk cited above. If we wished to have 95% confidence that the result for the entire truckload is accurate to within 10% ($\pm$), then $t = 2$ and the allowable error $= 10\%$ of $1.78 = 0.18 = e$. The number of cans required would be

$$n = (ts/e)^2 \simeq (2 \times 0.13/0.18)^2 = (1.44)^2 = 2.08 \simeq 3 \text{ cans.}$$

If we wished to have 99% confidence that the result is accurate to 5%, then t

$= 2.6$, the allowable error is 5% of $1.78 = 0.09$, and the number of cans required becomes $(2.6 \times 0.13/0.09)^2 = (3.41)^2 = 11.6 \simeq 12$ cans.

It should be emphasized that the precision that can be achieved in this type of calculation cannot exceed the precision of the analytical method. If the inherent error of the riboflavin method is 5%, then it is futile to attempt to increase the accuracy of the estimate of the truckload beyond 5% by taking a larger number of samples. We can calculate that, in order to have 99% confidence that our result is accurate to 1%, we should require $(2.6 \times 0.13/0.018)^2 \simeq 354$ cans; but since each riboflavin estimation is subject to a 5% error it is meaningless to attempt any accuracy better than 5%.

In ordinary analytical work, 99% confidence, $t = 2.6$, is the maximum confidence that has any useful significance; and more often a 95% confidence, $t = 2$, is considered satisfactory.

In routine analytical work, it is not expected that individual analyses of many portions of each lot will be made. Surveys along the lines indicated in the foregoing discussion will indicate the variability normally encountered in the material. If this variability (as measured by the standard deviation) is found to be reasonably uniform from lot to lot, subsequent sampling will normally be performed by sampling at the number of points calculated by the method described above and combining equal or suitably proportionate quantities of these portions to form a composite primary sample. This is the mechanical equivalent of obtaining the mean of the individual analyses, but, of course, by this procedure, the individual analyses are not available. With no basis for estimating the variation within the lot, therefore, the reliability of the assay is limited by the validity of the assumption that the variation is similar to that found in the lots surveyed when the sampling procedure was established. The risk involved is usually taken without hesitation because of the diminution in analytical work involved, but the fact that the assumption exists must be remembered to lead the way out of difficulties arising from its misapplication.

The FDA promulgated nutrition labeling regulations in 1973 (1). The compliance procedures have been thoroughly discussed (2) and can be obtained from FDA in pamphlet form (12). Compliance with nutrition label claims is evaluated by analyzing a 12-unit (retail size) composite sample made up of units randomly chosen from different cases within a production lot.

Composites rather than individual containers are analyzed in order to reduce the level of variability and analytical time. Naturally occurring nutrients can be no more than 20% below the labeled values. Added nutrients must be at least equal to the labeled value.

For naturally occurring nutrients (class-II nutrients), FDA has assumed a maximum standard deviation of 25% of the lot average. This level of variability is not a requirement of the compliance procedures but has merely been assumed to describe the chances of lot acceptance (2,12). FDA suggests that the more variable lots be labeled more conservatively to reduce the risk of noncompliance.

APPLICATIONS TO VARIOUS TYPES OF PRODUCTS

A.   Meat and Other Animal Tissues

1. *Fresh, Frozen, and Cured Meats.*   It is difficult to suggest one sampling technique to find the average vitamin content of a whole animal or several animals. Factors such as species, breed, and nutritional status affect the vitamin content. In addition, variations occur among individual muscles and organs. In sampling different cuts of meat or similar cuts from different animals, it is desirable to take a percentage of each piece, and these portions should be from different locations.

If a study is to be made of the change in vitamin content due to cooking, storage, or processing, it is advisable to sample one cut from one side of the carcass and a similar cut from the other side of the same carcass. This procedure has been described for pork and is applicable to other meats (13). A method to calculate true retention can be used to compare vitamin contents of cooked and raw samples (14). Percent true retention is calculated according to the following formula:

$$\% \text{ TR} = \frac{N_c}{N_r} \times \frac{W_c}{W_r} \times 100$$

where N_c = nutrient content per gram of cooked food;
   N_r = nutrient content per gram of raw food;
   W_c = weight in grams of food after cooking;
   W_r = weight in grams of food before cooking.

Due to the variability of meat and to prevent moisture loss, the primary sample should be large (5–10 lb) (3). This sample should be passed through a meat grinder or chopper. A subsample of this ground meat may be blended with a portion of water (or other extractant such as a buffer solution or 0.1 N HCl) and a portion taken for analysis. This sample should be withdrawn while the blender is running, and it is advisable to make several withdrawals rather than one. There is a tendency for fat to liquefy and separate if ground too finely. This can happen with hard sausages and sandwich meats in which the fat and other solids are coarsely intermingled (7).

An alternate to blending is to grind the meat three times, each followed by mixing to yield a pastelike sample. Ground samples should be kept in glass or containers with air and water tight covers. All determinations on fresh meat should be done promptly, but if this is not possible, chill sample to inhibit decomposition (3).

Frozen meats may be similarly handled after thawing at low temperature (40–50°F) to avoid enzymatic changes. It is reasonable to expect equalization of vitamin content in cured meat cuts due to diffusion of the curing solution. Some leaching of water-soluble factors into the curing solution may occur.

2. *Canned Meats.*   Canned meats are frequently solidly packed in cans and a somewhat longer heat process is required for sterilization. The meat near the periphery of the can is subjected to heat for a longer time than the meat near the center. The concentration of the heat-labile vitamins varies for this reason. The only recommended sampling procedure is to grind the entire contents of the can and remove subsamples for assay.

Variation can be expected from one cut to another and from one can to another. Since different packers use different retort temperatures and times, brand-to-brand variation can be expected. Other contributing factors are size of can and age of the sample.

3. *Dehydrated Meat.*   Dehydrated meat does not seem to present any unique sampling problems, but it is desirable to reconstitute with four volumes of water before blending.

4. *Seafoods.*   Fresh, frozen, and canned seafoods present sampling problems that are similar to meats. An additional consideration is the enzymatic destruction of thiamin in raw fish and fish products (15). The raw sample should be blended with an extractant such as 0.1 N HCl to prevent destruction of thiamin.

When sampling small fish (≤ 6 in) use 5–10 fish that have been cleaned, scaled, and eviscerated. In sampling large fish, from each of ≥ 3 fish, cut three cross-sectional slices 1-in thick, one slice from just back of the pectoral fins, one slice between the first slice and vent, and one slice just back of the vent. Grind or chop the sample three times, mixing thoroughly between each treatment (3). Canned fish products packed in brine or oil should be drained 2 min on a No. 8-12 sieve. Liquid may be analyzed separately, if desired, or discarded. Those products packed in sauce or broth should be drained and all liquid collected. Weights of meat and liquid should be determined and then proportionate amounts of meat and liquid should be recombined. Recombined portions should be blended until homogeneous (3).

Frozen fish should thaw at room temperature before blending, and drip should be discarded. Grind or chop the sample three times, mixing thoroughly after each treatment.

5. *Protein Concentrates for Animal Feeds.*   Meat meal, tankage, liver meal, etc., vary greatly from lot to lot. If the lot consists of several bags of a product, a sample may be prepared by withdrawing a portion from each bag. A representative number of bags should be sampled.

B. Pharmaceuticals

1. *Liquids.*   Mix thoroughly by inverting several times, taking care that any sediment is dispersed in the liquid. Viscous samples may require prolonged mixing.

2. *Powders.*   Powders such as yeast, liver concentrates and synthetic preparations may be sampled as described under 1.

3. *Tablets.*   Weigh at least 20 tablets, grind to a fine powder, mix thoroughly, and sample for analysis. Tablet sampling for quality control presents a problem because the number of tablets that can be conveniently drawn from each lot is limited. The granules from which the tablets are manufactured may be sampled and the analyses will indicate the degree of homogeneity before tablet formation. A homogeneous granulation does not mean that all tablets will be uniform, since the particle size of the granules will influence the flow rate into the tablet-forming machines. Therefore, the tablets themselves must be sampled from the production line at established intervals. These tablets should be mixed and a random sample of not less than 20 tablets selected. The sample is ground to a fine powder and an aliquot taken for analysis.

4. *Capsules, Dry Filled.*   Weigh at least 20 capsules, then open and empty the contents. Clean the shells of adhering powder, weigh the shells, and subtract this weight from the filled weight. Mix thoroughly and take an aliquot for analysis. For quality control of manufacturing practices, use procedure similar to that for tablets.

5. *Capsules, Soft Elastic.*   For capsules containing only oil, weigh at least 20 capsules, open, and empty the contents into a small beaker. Mix the oil and take an aliquot for analysis. Wash the shells several times with ether or acetone until they are free of oil. Allow shells to dry, weigh, and subtract weight of shells from the filled weight.

For capsules containing a mixture of water-soluble vitamins in oil, it is easiest to analyze the whole capsule if an aqueous extraction is employed. Select 20 capsules or more, add extractant, dissolve capsules, and proceed with extraction. If a nonaqueous reagent is used, the gelatin capsule should be dissolved in a small amount of water before extraction.

An alternate procedure is to open the capsules, wash the shells with organic solvent, and then rinse the shells with ice water to remove any water-soluble vitamins clinging to the shell. Following an acetone rinse, the shells are dried. This procedure should be used only if the water-soluble vitamins have not separated from the oil suspension.

C.   Cereals and Cereal Products and Mixed Feeds

1. *Whole Grains.*   The sample must be ground before attempting an extraction. Overheating during grinding must be avoided since many of the vitamins are heat labile. Burr mills and hammer mills are satisfactory when properly used, but laboratory mills tend to separate the bran from the remainder of the seed (7). Sieving of the ground sample will lead to fractionation of grain as well, and so should be avoided.

2. *Uncooked Cereals.*   Products such as farina, corn meal, and other un-

cooked cereals are often enriched. When the enriching material is granular, a primary sample of at least 1 lb should be ground and thoroughly mixed to evenly distribute the enriching material. If the enriching material is in powdered form, precautions should be taken to include the powder adhering to the inside of the container.

For products of this type, the primary sample should consist of at least 4 oz. Two to five grams can be used for analysis after grinding and mixing.

3. *Ready-to-Eat Cereals.*   Many ready-to-eat cereals are enriched, and the nutrients may be added to the grain early in the process or sprayed on the products just before packaging. Thiamin is unstable at the high temperatures encountered in cooking and toasting and is likely to be sprayed on the end product. The nutrient distribution in many of these enriched ready-to-eat cereals is not uniform, and when sampling for vitamin analysis, it is advisable to have a primary sample of at least 8 oz. If the primary sample is to be drawn from several lots, each portion making up the composite should weigh at least 8 oz.

4. *Flour and Mixed Feeds.*   Standard sampling techniques for flour have been established (3). To sample large lots of flour, sample a number of sacks equivalent to the square root of the number of sacks in the lot, but at least 10 sacks. From each sack to be sampled, draw a core from one corner of top diagonally to center of the sack by means of a cylindrical, pointed, polished metal trier ½ in. in diameter with a slit ≥ one-third of the circumference. Draw a second core from other top corner to one-half the distance to the center of the sack.

Place cores in a clean, dry, air-tight container and seal. Before sampling for analysis, alternately invert and roll container approximately 25 times to provide a homogeneous mixture.

5. *Baked Goods.*   Standard sampling techniques for bread are generally satisfactory for baked goods. Loaves should be weighed, and then cut into slices 2–3 mm thick. Slices are then spread on paper and dried in a warm room until sufficiently crisp and brittle to grind well in a mill. Sample should pass through a No. 20 sieve. Care should be taken so that no loss of solids can occur whereby loss would be considered moisture (3). Vitamin content may be markedly different between crust and crumb, and therefore, the primary sample must be carefully prepared.

6. *Macaroni, Egg Noodles, and Similar Products.*   Select enough pieces to assure a representative sample, break these into small fragments, and mix well. Grind 300–500 g in a mill until all materials pass through a No. 20 sieve. Keep ground sample in a sealed container to prevent moisture changes (3).

D.   Dairy Products

1. *Milk, Dried Milk, and Evaporated Milk.*   Thoroughly mix all liquids by pouring from one vessel to another, by plunging, or by mechanical stirring. If sampling evaporated milk or condensed milk, be sure to scrape adhering material from sides and bottom of container. Take subsample of ≥ 200 mL (3).

To sample dried milk, a tube should be passed through the powder at an even rate. Primary sample should be 300–500 g. Contents of at least one bore should be discharged directly into a clean, dry sample container, and container should be large enough to allow mixing by shaking (3).

2. *Butter.* Use butter triers long enough to pass diagonally to base of container. If sample is large, take ≥ two cores so that the minimum weight of the total sample is ≥ 200 g (3).

3. *Eggs—Liquid, Frozen and Dried.* For large lots of eggs, it is advisable to draw several samples for separate analyses because it is difficult to get one composite representative sample. Liquid eggs should be mixed thoroughly and 300 g taken for subsequent analyses. To sample frozen eggs, take boring diagonally across can from ≥ three widely separated parts, starting 2–5 cm in from edge and extending to opposite side as near to the bottom as possible. Pack tightly into sample jar and completely fill it to prevent partial dehydration of the sample. Before analyzing, warm sample in bath at < 50°C and mix well. To sample dried eggs, randomly select small amounts of sample totaling 300–500 g, mix three times through a domestic flour sifter to break up lumps. Store in cool place until analyzed (3).

E. Fruits and Vegetables

1. *Fresh Material.* Raw fruits and vegetables pose special sampling problems due to the ease of oxidative and enzymatic destruction of vitamins. When bruised, finely cut, or hot samples are assayed, conditions are favorable for destruction. Losses can be minimized by placing the primary sample directly into a stabilizing medium and blending or mixing the entire sample. The efficiency of the stabilizing medium may be increased by chilling.

An alternate treatment is to place the entire primary sample into a suitable receptacle containing dry ice and rapidly freeze the product. If the sample is kept in a frozen state, subsequent subdivision can be carried out before the final mixing or blending with the desired extractant or stabilizing medium.

When sampling for vitamins such as carotene, riboflavin, and vitamin B_6, it is advisable to prepare samples in subdued light, as these vitamins can be destroyed by intense light.

(a) Small Types (Berries, Corn, Peas). Mix primary sample without damaging the individual particles. Divide and subdivide until a portion suitable for grinding or blending remains. Blend the subdivided sample (usually 200–300 g) with the desired extractant or stabilizing medium and withdraw the assay aliquot.

It may be necessary to store the slurry for several days prior to analysis. Storage is not recommended in ascorbic acid work, but initial preparation using 6% metaphosphoric acid has been shown to prevent oxidation of ascorbic acid (16). For carotene, the sample can be stored if the slurry is prepared by blending the subdivided sample with 1% alcoholic KOH, followed by refrigeration. For B-complex work, add 1 ml chloroform to the mixture of sample and extractant (usually 0.2 N H_2SO_4 or 0.1 N HCl) during blending. Place the blended sample into a storage container and cover the surface with a thin layer of toluene to further inhibit microbial growth, and refrigerate. Heat the container in flowing steam for 10 min before withdrawing the assay sample to minimize the introduction of toluene with the sample.

(b) Large Types (Apples, Tomatoes, Cabbage, Carrots). To compensate for unit-to-unit variation, a large number of individual units should be selected. This primary sample is generally too large to grind and mix in available laboratory equipment, and it is necessary to select portions from each unit of the primary sample. The effect of variability within the unit can be minimized by taking sections from opposite sides. These sections should be immersed immediately in the extractant or stabilizing medium to prevent enzymatic action at the cut surfaces. The aliquot for analysis can be withdrawn from the blended slurries.

(c) Leaves and Shoots (Spinach, Asparagus, Broccoli). In subdividing, it is essential to take proportionate parts of each unit and proportionate amounts of each type of tissue in each unit. Sample by breaking or cutting the desired portions of each unit. Immerse the sample in a stabilizing medium to prevent enzymatic changes at the cut surfaces.

2. *Frozen Materials.* The thawing and refreezing of foods can lead to vitamin destruction, particularly destruction of ascorbic acid and carotene. When sampling a frozen fruit or vegetable, the product should be thawed until the individual pieces of fruit or vegetable can be separated. Commercial blanching conditions vary, and therefore, level of enzyme inactivation varies. A representative sample can be obtained by combining six packages of fruits or vegetables. An electric knife can be used to subdivide individual packages with a minimum of thawing. It is advisable to blend the frozen sample with an extractant or stabilizing solution to prevent oxidation or enzymatic destruction.

3. *Canned Materials.* A representative sample can be obtained by combining the contents of six consumer-size cans of small type, leafy or shoot materials, or 12 consumer-size cans of large-type materials. If No. 10 or larger cans are to be sampled, combine one to three cans. Empty the contents of each can onto a copper-free screen suspended over a pan and allow contents to drain 2 min. Combine solids from all cans and weigh. Combine the liquid from all cans and weigh. Mix each fraction, taking care not to rupture the skin of the solid particles. Take proportionate amounts of solids and liquid and mix or blend with the desired extractant or stabilizing medium.

LITERATURE CITED

1. "Nutrition labeling of foods." *Code of federal regulations*, 21, Food and Drugs, Section 101.9 (1982).

2. Roberts. H.R. "The statistics of nutrition sampling and analysis." *J. Assoc. Off. Anal. Chem.* **57**, 1181 (1974).

 3. Association of Official Analytical Chemists. *Official Methods of Analysis*, 13th ed. Washington D.C. (1980).

 4. Toma, R. B. and Tabekhia, M. M. "High performance liquid chromatographic analysis of B vitamins in rice and rice products." *J. Food Sci.* **44**, 263 (1979).

 5. Kamman, J. F., Labuza, T. P. and Warthesen, J. J. "Thiamin and riboflavin analysis by high performance liquid chromatography." *J. Food Sci.* **45**, 1497 (1979).

 6. Fellman, J. K., Artz, W. E., Tassinari, P. D., Cole, C. L., and Augustin, J. "Simultaneous determination of thiamin and riboflavin in selected foods by high-performance liquid chromatography." *J. Food Sci.* **47**, 2048 (1982).

 7. Aulik, D. J., "Sample preparation for nutrient analysis." *J. Assoc. Off. Anal. Chem.* **57**, 1193 (1974).

 8. Elkins, E. R. "Interlaboratory variability in nutrient analysis and two cooperative studies." *J. Assoc. Off. Anal. Chem.* **57**, 1193 (1974).

 9. *Laboratory Manual for Food Canners and Processors*, Vol. 2, 3rd ed. The National Canners Association. Avi, Westport, Conn. (1968).

10. Youden, W. J. *Statistical Methods for Chemists*. Wiley, New York (1951).

11. Steel, Robert G. O., and Torrie, J. H. *Principles and Procedures of Statistics*, McGraw-Hill, New York (1960).

12. "Compliance manual for nutrition labeling." Division of Mathematics BF110, Food and Drug Administration, Washington, D.C.

13. Cross, H. R., Moss, M. K., Ono, K., Tennent, I., Slover, H. T., Wolf, W., Thompson, R., Lanza, E., and Stewart, K. "Sampling of fresh pork for nutrient analysis." *J. Food Sci.* **46**, 1007 (1981).

14. Murphy, E. W., Criner, P. E., and Gray, B. C. "Comparison of methods for calculating retentions of nutrients in cooked foods." *J. Agric. Food Chem.* **23**, 1153 (1975).

15. Institute of Food Technologists' Expert Panel on Food Safety and Human Nutrition. "The effects of food processing on nutritional values." *Food Technol.* **28**, 77 (1974).

16. Vavich, M. G., Stern, R. M., and Guerrant, N. B. "Nutritive value of canned foods. Determination of ascorbic acid of fresh green peas." *Ind. Eng. Chem. Anal. Ed.* **17**, 531 (1945).

7 Vitamin A

D. B. Parrish, R. A. Moffitt, R. J. Noel, and J. N. Thompson

GENERAL CONSIDERATIONS

Recognition of the dietary requirement for vitamin A began with the observations of McCollum and Davis (1,2) and Osborne and Mendel (3) in 1913 that there was a factor in certain fats essential for growth of rats. Subsequently that factor was called "fat-soluble A" to distinguish it from "water-soluble B" that also was required for growth (4). Following a proposal by Drummond, the term vitamin A was adopted for "fat-soluble A" (5).

All vertebrates apparently required vitamin A for growth, life, reproduction, vision, and maintenance of differentiated epithelia and mucus secretion; vitamin A also is involved in the vision of invertebrates (6,7). The discovery, isolation, chemistry, and early studies on the nutritional role and metabolism of vitamin A are described elsewhere (5,8,9).

This chapter concerns analytical methods for vitamin A. Carotene is considered only where necessary to obtain the total vitamin A value in extracts of foods or other products containing preformed vitamin A.

A. Occurrence and Sources

Two groups of substances possess vitamin A activity: (1) retinol and derivatives of it, and (2) carotene and a number of other provitamin A carotenoids of plant origin. Vitamin A (retinol) occurs naturally only in animals. Some 90–95% of the total vitamin A reserves are usually in the liver in the form of retinyl esters. The esters are secreted into milk; retinol, however, is the predominant form of vitamin A in egg yolk. Provitamins A and other nonvitamin carotenoids of plant origin that are consumed in foods are absorbed and stored intact by certain mammalian species. The provitamins also are converted enzymatically to retinol in the intestinal wall (5,7–13).

Except in blood serum and egg yolk, most naturally occurring vitamin A exists as mixtures of long-chain fatty acid esters of retinol, predominently the palmitate (8,12,14). Fish livers normally contain large reserves of vitamin A and were formerly the commercial source of that vitamin. Today, however, synthetic vitamin A, first prepared over 35 years ago, is used in almost all vitamin A supplements and fortifications of foods and feeds (15–18).

B.   Definitions, Formulas, and Names

The nomenclature policy consistent with the IUPAC-IUB and American Institute of Nutrition recommendations for vitamin A and related compounds will be followed where appropriate (19). Vitamin A is the generic descriptor for all β-ionine derivatives, other than the provitamin A carotenoids, with the qualitative biological activity of all-*trans*-retinol (vitamin A alcohol). Provitamin A carotenoid is the generic descriptor of all carotenoids with the qualitative activity of β-carotene.

The formula for retinol is shown in Figure 7.1. Because of the double-bonded structure, stereoisomers are possible. Most natural vitamin A is in the form of all-*trans*-retinyl esters, but 13-*cis*-retinol (neo-vitamin A) is found in fish livers and some synthetic retinols. Small and variable amounts of *cis*-isomers may be found in other natural sources (8,20–22). The chemical properties of retinol isomers are similar, but the spectral properties and biological activities differ (Table 7.1).

Dehydroretinol (3-dehydroretinol, vitamin A_2) esters are found along with retinyl esters in fish-liver oils; they are much higher in the livers of fresh-water species (8,22,36). Small amounts of the aldehyde form of vitamin A, retinaldehyde, have been detected in egg yolk and some other materials (12,36). The 11-*cis*-retinaldehyde is an important intermediate in the visual process

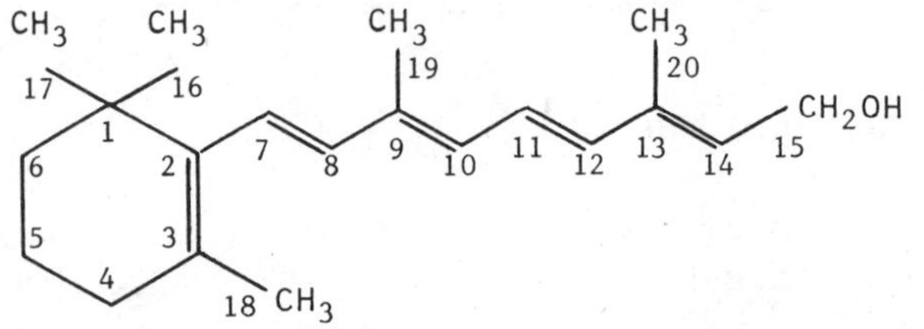

FIGURE 7.1   Structure of retinol (Vitamin A).

(7,14,37,38). Retinaldehyde has about 90% of the vitamin A activity of retinol (8,35).

C. Metabolism

When vitamin A esters are consumed as part of the diet, they are hydrolyzed in the intestinal lumen and mucosa to retinol and fatty acids. In absorption, the esters are reformed, predominantly as the palmitate, and carried in lymph chylomicrons to the liver, where they are stored in the parenchymal cells, from which retinol later can be mobilized for use by the body (6,12,14,37,39). Carotene (Figure 7.2) and other carotenoids may be absorbed and carried to the liver in some species, but a part of the provitamin A in those species and all absorbed by other species (e.g., swine) may be converted to vitamin A (8,12,13,36). In the conversion, a dioxygenase apparently catalyzes cleavage of the carotenoid at the 15–15′ position, with addition of oxygen to yield retinaldehyde. Then aldehyde reductase catalyzes formation of retinol, which is esterified and transported to the liver. Hydrolysis of esters and re-esterification may occur in the liver. A small amount of free retinol may be carried to the liver in the portal circulation (14,37,39).

To supply vitamin A required by body tissues and cells, retinyl esters in the liver are hydrolyzed. The water-insoluble retinol then is taken up by a retinol-binding protein (RBP), which is transported in the plasma as a retinol-RBP-prealbumin complex. It has not been determined how the target tissues take up the retinol, but they seem to have specific retinol- and retinoic acid-binding proteins that play a part in transfer of those substances from plasma to tissues (6,37,39–41).

If retinoic acid is absorbed, it is transported by the portal system. Trace amounts of retinoic acid also are formed in tissues by oxidation of retinol or retinaldehyde. Retinoic acid is not stored in the liver but is rapidly metabolized in the body. Retinoic acid, or some metabolite of it, may be the metabolically active form of vitamin A for some functions, because supplements of either retinol or retinoic acid are effective for growth and in preventing many overt signs of vitamin A deficiency. Retinoic acid also maintains egg production in birds and some reproductive functions in the avian male. There appears, however, to be an absolute requirement for retinol in vision and for reproduction in male and female mammals (7,12,36,37,39,42–44).

Except for the role of vitamin A in vision, the mode of action at the tissue or cellular level remains to be determined. Vitamin A may have roles in glycosylation reactions, and retinoids may be useful in chemoprevention of cancer (12,37–39,41,45).

Regardless of whether animals consume retinol, retinyl esters, retinaldehyde, or retinoic acid, vitamin A is excreted in urine and feces for the most part as metabolites of retinoic acid and other unidentified forms (14,42,46).

In repletion of vitamin A reserves following a deficient state, significant quantities of retinol esters are synthesized and stored in the liver only after the

TABLE 7.1 Properties of Some Forms of Vitamin A[a]

| | Vitamin A₁ | | | | Vitamin A₂ |
Property	All-trans-Retinol	13-cis-Retinol	trans-Retinyl Acetate	trans-Retinaldehyde	trans-Dehydroretinol
Empirical formula	$C_{20}H_{30}O$	$C_{20}H_{30}O$	$C_{22}H_{32}O_2$	$C_{20}H_{28}O$	$C_{20}H_{28}O$
Molecular weight	286	286	328	284	284
Crystalline form[b]	Pale yellow prisms	Pale yellow needles	Pale yellow prisms	Light orange prisms	Yellow crystals
Melting point (°C)	62–64	58–60	56–58	61–62	63–65
Optical activity	None	None	None	None	None
Solubility, H₂O	—	—	—	—	—
Solubility, fats, organic solvents	+	+	+	+	+
Fluorescence in UV, hexane solution	Yellow-green	Yellow-green	Yellow-green	Yellow-green	Brownish-orange[c]
λmax(nm), ethanol	324–325	328	325–326	381	351

	1832	1686	1560	1530	1450
$E_{1cm}^{1\%}$, ethanol	1832	1686	1560	1530	1450
ϵ_{max}, ethanol	52,480	48,300	51,180	43,400	41,300
λ_{max}(nm), isopropanol	324–326		324–326	1535	
$E_{1cm}^{1\%}$, isopropanol	1830		1530		
λ_{max}(nm), light pet.	325		324–326		
$E_{1cm}^{1\%}$, light pet.	1830				
SbCl$_3$ color	blue	blue	blue-green	blue-green	blue-green
λ_{max}(nm), SbCl$_3$ color	620	620	620	664	693
$E_{1cm}^{1\%}$, SbCl$_3$ color	4800		4580		
Relative bioactivity[d]	100	75	87	91	40–50[e]
IU/g[f]	3,330,000	2,495,000	2,900,000	3,030,000	1,330,000
SbCl$_3$ color, IU/g[g]	3,330,000	3,330,000	2,910,000		

[a] Data from references 21, 23–35, some of which contain additional data on these compounds and other isomers and derivatives; a few are authors' unpublished.

[b] Crystalline form and size varies with solvent and conditions of preparation.

[c] Fluorescence in liver tissue of fish.

[d] Activity relative to that of all-*trans*-retinol = 100.

[e] Lower value based on growth; higher on liver storage and vaginal smear tests.

[f] Defined biopotency of all-*trans*-retinol in IU or USP units; other values based on relative biopotency data.

[g] Based on color intensity relative to all-*trans*-retinol.

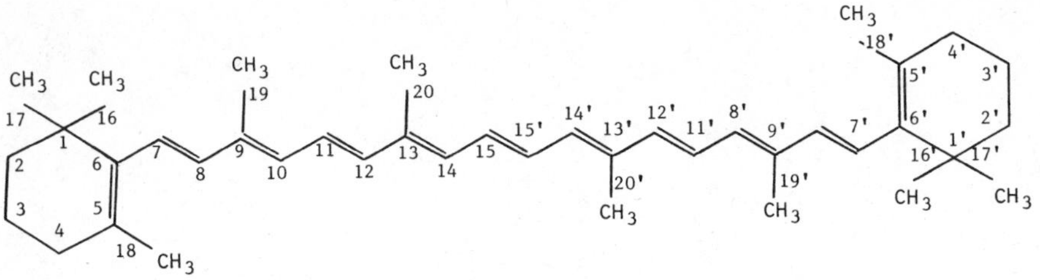

FIGURE 7.2   Structure of β-carotene, one of the provitamins A.

tissue subcellular or micellular sites have been filled (47). In hypervitaminosis A, the tissue sites holding vitamin A ester become filled and no more retinol-binding protein is available as a carrier, causing free retinol to circulate in plasma. At the tissue sites, the high concentrations of free retinol apparently degrade the extracellular matrix of tissues (12,40,48). Thus, excessive intakes of vitamin A are toxic.

D.   Vitamin Forms in Foods, Feed, and Pharmaceuticals

Natural forms of preformed vitamin encountered in vitamin A assays are primarily esters of retinol in liver oils, livers, other fatty animal tissues, and dairy products; however, protein-bound retinol is found in serum, tissues, and egg yolks, with minor quantities of retinaldehyde in egg yolk and possibly some other animal sources.

Synthetic vitamin A is used in pharmaceuticals, animal feed supplements, and for fortification of human foods, including margarine, low-fat milk, nonfat dried milk, some cereals, infant formulas, special dietary foods, snack and breakfast bars and rolls, drink mixes, and certain cereal products supplied for dietary aid programs. Synthetic vitamin A is commonly prepared in the form of retinol acetate or palmitate. These esters can be obtained in crystalline form, but for commercial purposes they are supplied as concentrates in oil, "soluble" emulsions, or in dry, stabilized powders or beadlets that consist of a gelatin, pectin, or similar matrix incorporating vitamin A along with emulsifiers, carbohydrates, antioxidants, etc. Some preparations are combinations of vitamin A and one or more other fat-soluble vitamins (17,18,49).

E.   Standards, Units, and Conversion Factors

A defined standard vitamin A for analytical purposes is the USP Reference Standard, a solution of vitamin A acetate (retinyl acetate) in cottonseed oil, obtained from the United States Pharmacopeial Convention, Inc., Rockville, MD. The vitamin A content is equivalent to about 30 mg retinol/g; the specific value is stated on each container. The standard is packaged in gelatin capsules containing about 250 mg of solution, 24 capsules per lot.

All-*trans*-retinol and all-*trans*-retinol acetate, both pale yellow crystalline products, supplied by Eastman Kodak Co. in 1 g ampules, also are used as standards. However, even the best commercially available crystalline products contain some impurities. It is difficult to protect the crystalline vitamin A once the ampule is opened. It must be promptly and properly resealed under pure nitrogen and protected from light and heat. An advantage of using the USP capsules as a standard is that they are relatively inexpensive and unused portions are discarded.

Present practices and regulations of official agencies require that the vitamin A value for pharmaceuticals and concentrates for food or feed manufacture be stated in USP or international units, which by definition are the same. However, the vitamin A activity of the USP Reference Standard and results by the USP assay method for vitamin A are stated in mg rather than USP units (50).

The USP vitamin A unit is defined as the specific biological activity of 0.3 μg of all-*trans*-retinol, but since the biological activity is not determined by the official assay, some confusion results. However, in the USP XX vitamin A assay method, a weight-to-USP unit relationship is introduced. It states that each mg of vitamin A alcohol (determined) represents 3333 USP units of vitamin A (50). That equivalence would apply only if the vitamin A determined is the all-*trans*-isomer, or if factors applied, such as in the USP method, properly correct for presence of other isomers (50,51).

Formerly the vitamin A activities of foods were stated in international units, where one IU was equivalent to 0.3 μg retinol or 0.6 μg β-carotene. The definition was unsatisfactory and required qualification when applied to human nutrition because of the apparent poorer conversion of carotene to retinol in man than in experimental animals. For that and other reasons, human vitamin A requirements and vitamin A values of foods have been restated in retinol equivalents (RE) (52-54). By definition, one RE is equivalent to 1 μg of retinol, 6 μg of β-carotene, and 12 μg of other provitamin A carotenoids. In terms of international units, one RE is recognized as equal to 3.33 IU of retinol or 10 IU of β-carotene (54).

The RE has not been adopted for stating vitamin A values of animal feeds. It has not yet been recognized by the FDA for the US-RDA values used for food labeling purposes (55), nor is it used in Canada.

F. General Analytical Procedures and Precautions

Interferences in colorimetric, spectrophotometric, fluorometric, or high-performance liquid chromatography (HPLC) determinations of vitamin A may arise from carotenoids, fats, waxes, compound lipids, steroids, other fat-soluble vitamins, isomers and oxidation products of vitamin A, and additives present in the material analyzed. If quantities of lipids or other interfering materials are relatively low (e.g., blood serum of swine or humans in the postabsorptive state), satisfactory results may be obtained by breaking the vitamin-protein complex by denaturation with alcohol, followed by simple solvent extraction of vitamin A. Even substantial amounts of lipid do not interfere seriously (e.g., in liver) if the level of vitamin A is relatively high; alkaline digestion is not required in such samples (3,56,57).

For many samples, alkaline hydrolysis (saponification) is required to convert retinyl esters to retinol so that saponifiable material may be discarded in the aqueous fraction. Alkaline digestion also breaks down the gelatin, pectin, or similar matrices of stabilized vitamin A products to free the retinol ester for hydrolysis and extraction. If the form of vitamin A present is unknown, or more than one form is present, alkaline hydrolysis is required. Dimethyl sulfoxide, warm water, glycerine, or phosphate solutions have been used to attempt to free vitamin A from stabilizing matrices, but recoveries generally have been less satisfactory than when alkaline hydrolysis was used (58).

If only relatively small amounts of carotenoids are present in a vitamin A sample extract, correction may be made for them in the colorimetric assay (8,59). Larger quantities of carotenoids should be removed by chromatography on alumnia, magnesia, or silica gel (60). Irrelevant fluorescent materials in the extract, such as the carotenoid phytofluene, could interfere with methods based on fluorometry. Steroids, other vitamins, and decomposition products interfere in spectrophotometric determinations; column chromatography does not always remove them satisfactorily (60). An advantage of HPLC assays is that vitamin A can be separated from many closely related substances by selection of one or more appropriate columns and solvent systems.

Presence of *cis*-isomers of retinol affects the vitamin A activity so that the true potency is not reflected by results of colorimetric or fluorometric assays. The spectrophotometric method for vitamin A in concentrates corrects for the 13-*cis* isomer but not for other isomers that may be present. A reaction with maleic anhydride may be used to estimate bioactivity of vitamin A (21,51). Although *cis*-isomers may be fairly high in certain samples of pharmaceuticals and fish liver oils, the contents are usually smaller and of less concern in foods and feeds, and a correction for their presence is generally unnecessary (51,60). However, retinol isomers can be separated and determined by HPLC. When separated, their contribution to total vitamin A activity, even if calculated only approximately, should not be overlooked.

When assaying for vitamin A in foods or feeds, we usually are interested in determining total vitamin A activity, which may include contributions from provitamin A sources. In foods or feeds where retinyl esters are the principal source of vitamin A activity, inclusion of a determination of carotene in the assay provides for a satisfactory estimate of total vitamin A activity. Margarine colored with carotene often has one-third or more of the vitamin A activity from carotene. If large quantities of yellow corn are included in animal feeds, crytoxanthin also should be determined. In products given a yellow color by adding carotenals, vitamin A activity from that source should not be overlooked (8,54,60,61). Methods for preformed vitamin A, even though they include a carotene assay, should not be used for plant products where provitamin A carotenoids are the source of vitamin A activity.

How samples are handled before and during an assay is important because vitamin A is unstable in the presence of unsaturated fats, air, light, heat, moisture, acids, heavy metallic ions, and other pro-oxidants. Samples should be preserved under dry conditions in closed containers in a freezer from the time of receipt until analysis; analysis should be performed as soon as possible. If it is necessary to grind the sample, it should be done just before the assay is started. The size of the analytical sample should be large enough so that it truly represents the vitamin A content of the lot. That is especially critical for samples containing stabilized vitamin A. Fats and solutions must be mixed thoroughly (8,58–60).

Assays should be done as rapidly as possible consistent with accuracy; avoid hold-over periods. Keep vitamin A in solution; expose to air or light as little as possible. Vitamin A is fairly stable for short periods of time at room temperature in neutral lipid films or good grades of hydrocarbon solvents. During an analysis some isomerization of vitamin A may occur from exposure to light, heat, or catalyst; or oxidation products may be formed. In colorimetry, color intensity is somewhat greater at cooler temperatures, but it is unnecessary to work in a cold room (59,60).

ANALYTICAL METHODOLOGY

I. COLORIMETRIC METHOD

A. Principle

The following references provide background information on this method (23,24,57,59,60,62–67). The assay is based on the measurement of the unstable blue color resulting from reaction of vitamin A and antimony trichloride (or other Lewis acids). Within certain limits, absorbance at 620 nm is a function of vitamin A concentration. The reading for the retinol moiety is essentially the same whether all-*trans*-retinol, retinol isomers, or retinyl esters are determined, but colors developed by retinaldehyde, dehydroretinol, and similar compounds absorb maximally at somewhat longer wavelengths. Carotenoids react more slowly than vitamin A, forming blue-green colors absorbing at somewhat shorter wavelengths. In the vitamin A determination, carotenoids must be removed or corrections made for them.

The method outlined is designed for simplicity, speed, and use of small volumes of costly, volatile, or noxious solvents, while still providing satisfactory results. Alternative procedures given in the method adapt it to a variety of products.

Some critical points of the method are: freedom from moisture (with $SbCl_3$ reagent); a photometer with well-dampened, direct-reading galvanometer and low-intensity radiation at 620 nm; subdued light conditions; and removal of carotenoids in the final extract before colorimetry, or correction for them.

B. Equipment

1. *Photoelectric Colorimeter.*   With 620-nm filter, or use simple spectrophotometer set at 620 nm that provides essentially a linear relationship to concentration of vitamin A within limits of about 0.07–0.7 absorbance (A). The deflection-type galvanometer must reach a pause point within 3 sec or less after the color reagent is added. To reduce color fading, uncertainty of pause point, and galvanometer drift, a constant, low-intensity light source is required (well-charged battery or voltage regulator). The light path should be relatively narrow and not pass near top or bottom of solution in tube. The Evelyn photoelectric colorimeter (Penn Airbourne Products Co.), the Spectronic 20 (Bausch & Lomb), or similar instruments are suitable. With some instruments, radiation intensity should be reduced by means of a rheostat (66).

2. *Colorimetric Absorption Tubes.*   Matched test tubes that project above top of instrument so that reagent can be added after tube containing vitamin A is placed in path of light beam. Mixing depends on turbulence of rapidly adding a 6- to 10-fold volume of reagent to vitamin A solution in the tube. Tube size should provide height of final blue solution 2 to 2.5 times i.d. of tube. Best readings are made with tubes of about 18-mm i.d., and final solution volume of 10 mL. Tube selected must fit tube holder snugly.

3. *Reagent Dispenser.*   All-glass automatic pipette, hypodermic syringe, or pipette and filler bulb (snapping bulb off to release solution) are satisfactory. For the latter item, cut off and recalibrate a 10-mL transfer pipette at 9 mL (or use other suitable volume).

4. *Long-Necked Ground-Glass Flasks and Stoppers and Air or Water Condensers.*   To fit 125, 250, or 500 mL as required for sample size. Calibrate flask in neck at a convenient marker, such as at 130, 260, 520 mL. Other flasks and cold-finger condensers may be used, but they will necessitate transfers and more time.

5. *Spin Bars.*   To help dispense solid samples by shaking—not for magnetic stirring, which is ineffective with some samples.

6. *Extraction Device.*   Heavy-duty centrifuge tube (50–60 mL), ground-glass stopper, or screw cap with Teflon liner. To extract larger volumes required when analyzing low-potency samples or those requiring chromatography, use 125-mL or 250-mL separatory funnels (no rubber stoppers).

7. *Centrifuge.*   With rotor size to carry extraction tubes.

8. *Evaporation Assembly.*   To remove solvent from extract transferred to colorimetric tube. Use U-shaped connecting tube. With a flexible hose, connect the single straight arm to back-flow safety bottle and to water aspirator. Insert a two-way stopcock in the system to open and close vacuum, a manometer or gauge to measure vacuum, and a condenser to collect solvent vapors (or use suitable hood). Attach stoppers to the two bent arms of the U-tube and cover them with Teflon tape. Connect, two at a time, colorimeter tubes containing

vitamin A extract to stoppers of the apparatus; heat in a 60–65°C water bath, shaking gently to speed evaporation (optionally evaporate under partial vacuum and nitrogen). Amount of solution in tubes must be small enough to prevent losses by bumping and frothing.

9. *Reagent Containers.* Amber glass of suitable sizes. Glass stoppers for chloroform and SbCl₃ reagents. Glass or Teflon closures for other solvents.

10. *Chromatographic Tube.* Glass tube (18 × 200 mm, ∼12-mm i.d.) sealed to 5 × 80-mm tube, fitted into a stopper; or 10 × 100-mm glass tube joined to a 20 × 40-mm reservoir on one end and a 5 × 70-mm tube fitted into a stopper on the other end. The smaller chromatographic tube requires less absorbent and solvent, but solvent flow is more difficult to control.

11. *Fraction Collector (68).* Special equipment fraction collector (Corning Glass Works, no. 912000), or side-arm distilling receiver (Lab-Glass, no. 6490, with three-way stopcock in vacuum line to break vacuum), or equivalent.

12. *Fraction Receivers.* Graduated or volumetric containers (10 mL and 25 mL).

13. *Simple 50-mL or 100-mL vacuum apparatus (68).* Or rotary evaporation apparatus, to concentrate aliquots of extract for chromatography.

14. *Ultraviolet Light.* Use *only* low-intensity long wave (360-nm) apparatus. UVL-22 (Ultra Violet Products, Inc.) or equivalent.

C. Reagents

1. *Hexane.* Commercial grades, clear and free of nonhydrocarbon contaminants, boiling point range 60–68°C.

2. *Alcohol.* 95% ethanol, SD 3A, 30, or USP, aldehyde-free by Schiff's test.

3. *Acetic Anhydride.*

4. *Pyrogallol Solution.* 1% (w/v) pyrogallic acid in alcohol (Section I.C.2). Prepare daily.

5. *Ether.* Diethyl ether. USP. Must be free of peroxides. Use Joressen's reagent test (69).

6. *Chloroform.* Clear and free of H₂O. If necessary, filter through adsorption alumina. Do not redistill unless used promptly because about 0.75% of alcohol is added as a preservative.

7. *Colorimetric Reagent.* All listed developed similar blue colors with vitamin A, but each should be used with a calibration curve developed for it alone.

(a) Antimony Trichloride (most stable). Product must not contain fluids or colored material, and crystals should separate when shaken. Weight ¼ lb, unopened bottle. Open and empty contents into wide mouth, glass-stoppered bottle containing 300 mL chloroform. Obtain weight of SbCl₃ by difference. Add chloroform to make a 22% (w/v) solution. Stopper. Dissolve crystals by slight warming and occasional swirling. Let settle and decant or filter rapidly into amber, glass-stoppered bottle. Add 3% acetic anhydride and mix. Reagent is stable at room temperature in tightly closed container. Discard after 2 months. Moisture forms insoluble white precipitates.

(b) *Trifluoroacetic Acid.* Add 1 volume trifluoroacetic acid (Eastman) to 2 volumes chloroform. Store as in (a). Some preparations develop less blue color on standing; discard after 1 week.

(c) *Trichloroacetic Acid.* A solution of trichloroacetic acid in chloroform (2 + 1, w/v). Protect from light. Reagent is unstable on standing; make fresh solution each time.

8. *To Clean Glassware Used For SbCl₃ Solutions.*   Rinse in 50% HCl, or soak in 10–15% Rochelle salt solution to which a small amount of detergent is added. Rinse and wash thoroughly in hot detergent solution.

9. *70% Potassium Hydroxide Solution.*   Make enough solution of free-flowing, reagent-grade KOH pellets in proportions of 1 g to 1 mL H_2O (70% w/v) for each determination. Do not store; may develop color on standing.

10. *Adsorption Alumina.*   Neutral alumina, activity grade 1, Woelm (ICN Pharmaceuticals), or Bio-Rad Laboratories. Adjust to 5% H_2O content. Place 5 g H_2O in a small bottle, add 95 g alumina, and mix by shaking until no lumps are observed. Cool ≥ 2 hr before use. Do not expose original or prepared alumina to air. Store in small, well-filled, tightly closed bottles.

11. *Sodium Sulfate, Anhydrous.*   Must not retain carotenoids dissolved in hexane.

12. *Vitamin A Standard.*   USP vitamin A reference solution. Store in refrigerator (p. 158-159).

13. *Carotene Standard.*   Crystalline β-carotene (Sigma Chemical Co.). Carotene is unstable. Open sealed ampule and weigh about 20 mg quickly and accurately. Transfer to volumetric flask, make to 200 mL with hexane, and mix. Carotene must dissolve with no residue. Dilute 10.0 mL to 100.0 mL with hexane. Makes a series of ≥ 5 dilutions to provide absorbances at a selected wavelength (440–460 nm) in the range of 0.07–0.7; results should plot essentially as a straight line. Alternately make a solution of carotene in hexane and determine concentration with spectrophotometer at 450 nm (see I.D.4.(a)3). Determine factor (concentration/A) to calculate carotene content.

D. Procedure

1. *Sampling.*   Samples should be representative of the bulk lot. Store in a freezer when received. Warm to room temperature just before the analysis. Prepare according to the following directions. Samples used are relatively large to obtain uniformity; size reduction is after alkaline digestion.

(a) Dry feed mixtures, premixes, concentrates, and fortified cereal products. Bulk sample should be 500–800 g. If necessary, grind to pass No. 30 sieve. Mix by rolling on paper or equivalent, guarding against loss of dust or fine particles. Breads and pastries may be dried in a freeze-dry apparatus (avoid light exposure) before grinding. Sticky, canned, or moist foods may be mixed in a blender or chopped, and representative small sections taken for the sample.

Weights for analytical samples: less than 5000 USP units/lb ($\sim$3000 μg/kg), weigh 40 g into 500 mL boiling flask; 5000–20,000 units/lb, weight 20–40 g into 250-mL or 500-mL flask; 20,000–80,000 units/lb, weigh 10–20 g into 250-mL flask; more than 80,000 units/lb, weigh 5–10 g into 125-mL or 250-mL flask.

(b) Fortified milk powders and dry mixes. Mix by rolling on paper or equivalent and use sample size as in Section I.D.1.(a).

(c) Butter and margarine. Use 1-lb bulk sample representative of the lot. Cut thin slices selected at random sites to make 10 g analytical samples. Do not warm and mix; water becomes separated from some samples and cannot be worked back in.

(d) Cheese and liver. Blend or use random selected thin slices, with sample size as in Section I.D.1.(a).

(e) Fats, oils, and liquid supplements. Warm to room temperature, mix thoroughly, and use sample size as in Section I.D.1.(a).

(f) Dry tablets. Select 10–20 representative of the lot. Grind to a fine powder and mix. Use only 1–2 g for assay, unless product is of low vitamin A content.

(g) Gelatin capsules. Select 5–10 representative of the lot. Warm to room temperature, cut capsules, express oil, and sample as in Section I.D.1.(a).

(h) Fluid milk and fortified fluid products. Mix or blend 500–1000-mL bulk sample; do not allow churning and separation of fat. Use 20–40-g sample.

2. *Alkaline Hydrolysis (Saponification, Digestion).*

(a) For all products except liquid samples containing molasses, or solid samples of high molasses or sugar contents. Add pyrogallol solution (mL) equal to 4 times sample weight (g). Place stirring bar in flask. Mix. As flask is swirled, add KOH solution (mL) equal to sample weight (g). Mix thoroughly. Reflux gently (approximately 2 drops/sec) for 30 min on a steam or boiling water bath. Agitate flask three to four times during refluxing to disperse any aggregates formed. Cool and add alcohol-H_2O (3 + 1 v/v) to about 20 mL below mark, and shake 1 min. Add 3 + 1 alcohol-H_2O to mark, mix well, and allow suspended matter to settle.

Note: Pyrogallol solution may not be required for antioxidant effect under all conditions; alcohol may be used instead.

(b) If sample is a viscous liquid or a powder containing high sugar or molasses contents, add equal volume H_2O and mix thoroughly. Add KOH and pyrogallol solution in reversed order, but follow other procedures as in Section I.D.2.(a).

Inspect diluted sample carefully. With some samples of high sugar content, two phases may separate. However, a small amount of sticky material adhering to flask after dilution does not affect results appreciably.

3. *Extraction.*

(a) For most products containing ≥ 1800 μg vitamin A/lb, little if any carotenoid pigment, nor high fat content. Transfer 5.0–10.0 mL of settled solution to the 50-mL or 60-mL centrifuge tube. Add 2 mL H_2O for each 5-mL solution. Add 20.0 mL hexane. Shake vigorously 1 min. Let phases separate; centrifuge briefly. (If vitamin A content is likely > 0.2 mg/mL, dilute portion 1+1−1+4 before extracting 5.0 mL). Draw lower layer from centrifuge tube with pipet and filler bulb and discard. Wash extract in tube once with 20 mL H_2O and centrifuge briefly. If hexane layer contains no more than traces of yellow pigment, transfer 1.0–10.0 mL (as required for colorimetry range) to colorimetric tube and proceed to colorimetry (Section I.D.5.).

(b) Diluted extracts forming two phases. Insert a 5.0-mL or 10.0-mL tilt dispenser into neck of boiling flask. Shake and remove measured amount before separation occurs. Small amount of solids will centrifuge out and cause no trouble. Proceed with extraction as in Section I.D.3.(a).

(c) For products with < 1800 μg vitamin A/lb, or containing carotenoid pigments requiring chromatography. Transfer 25.0–50.0 mL solution to a 125-mL or 250-mL separatory funnel. Add H_2O as in Section I.D.3.(a). Extract with 1–1.5 volumes of hexane for 1 min. When layers separate, drain lower layer to another separatory funnel and shake one or more times with an equal volume of hexane until essentially all carotenoid pigments are extracted. Combine extracts in first separatory funnel. Wash two or three times with equal volume of H_2O. If emulsions form, a little alcohol will help to break them. Drain H_2O. Swirl separatory funnel and again drain H_2O as completely as possible. Filter extract through paper containing about 5g anhydrous Na_2SO_4 into 100-mL volumetric flask (or smallest convenient volume). Rinse filter with small portions of hexane and make to volume. (Use a fume hood.)

(d) Margarine, butter, and high-fat samples giving low vitamin A recoveries. Transfer 10.0–20.0 mL of the diluted extract to a 125-mL separatory funnel. Add H_2O as in Section I.D.3.(a). Extract with hexane-ether $(1 + 2)$, following other procedures as in Section I.D.3.(c).

4. *Chromatography.* Required only if pigments need to be separated.

(a) Procedure.

(1) Evaporate aliquot of sample extract containing 30–100 μg vitamin A in hexane to about 10 mL, or evaporate vitamin A in hexane-ether solution just to dryness and add 10 mL hexane.

(2) Place small glass wool or cotton plug at constriction in chromatographic tube. Pack with alumina added in small portions to height of 6–7 cm, tamping firmly under vacuum. Add 0.5 cm Na_2SO_4, level, and

pack firmly. Do not continue drawing air through column; use immediately. Add 10–15 mL hexane to column, tap column several times, and adjust vacuum to a flow of 1–2 drops eluate/sec. Add solution to be chromatographed just as hexane disappears into top of column. Rinse container with 2–3 mL hexane and add to top of column just before it becomes dry. Elute carotene band with 4% acetone-in-hexane. Inspect column briefly with UV light. Retinol band should be within 1–2 cm of top of alumina (a light fluorescent band). Elute retinol with 15% acetone-in-hexane. Do not allow the column to become dry. Change receiver when retinol band is about two-thirds of the way down column (follow retinol band by brief inspection with UV light). Collect retinol fraction and make to convenient volume. A small amount of monohydroxy carotenoids (e.g., cryptoxanthin) may elute with retinol. Transfer 5.0–10.0 mL (as required for suitable color development) to colorimeter tube and evaporate (Section I.B.8.)

(3) Make carotene fraction to convenient volume with hexane. Read in photometer at selected wavelength (440–460 nm) with blank set with hexane. Calculate carotene content as follows:

$$\mu g \ carotene/g = C \times V/W$$

where C = concentration carotene in $\mu g/mL$ from curve or factor;
          V = final dilution volume (mL) of extract analyzed;
          W = sample weight (g).

5. *Colorimetry of Vitamin A.*

(a) Preparation of standard curve. Warm capsule of USP vitamin A reference standard to room temperature (be sure any solids have dissolved). Cut tip and express about 0.2 g oil into small tared beaker or watch glass. Weigh accurately. Transfer oil to volumetric flask and dilute with chloroform to 100 mL. Make ≥ 5 further dilutions so that aliquots to colorimeter tube treated as in Section I.D.5.(c) give A of 0.07–0.7. Plot A against μg vitamin A. Essentially a straight line should be obtained. Calculate factor (concentration/A_{620}) for determining vitamin A content of samples. Work in subdued light. Use solution as soon as possible; discard after 8 hr. Solution is not treated with KOH and extracted for making standard curve to avoid all possible sources of loss and error.

(b) Correction for carotenoids. A correction for all carotenoids based on carotene calibration is satisfactory at carotenoid levels where chromatography to remove them is unnecessary. Carotenoids form less than half as much blue color as equivalent amounts of vitamin A. The correction should not exceed 15% of the total vitamin A blue color readings.
Make series of ≥ 5 carotene solutions in hexane; read concentration at selected wavelength (440–460 nm). Evaporate 1 mL of each carotene solution, dissolve in 1 mL chloroform, and place in photometer, as in Section I.D.5.(c). Add

measured volume of colorimetric reagent, and determine blue color, as in Section I.D.5.(c). Using data relating A (absorbance) at 440 nm to A at 620 nm, determine the factor for correcting for the blue color caused by carotenoids based on the reading at 440 nm (or other selected wavelength). Subtract that correction from the total 620 nm reading in the determination of vitamin A.

(c) Determining vitamin A content. Use 620-nm filter or wavelength setting. Adjust galvanometer to 0 without radiation to photocell (dark current reading). Turn on colorimeter circuit and warm instrument to obtain stable readings. Evaporate solvent from colorimeter tube containing hexane extract of vitamin A (see Section I.B.8.). Immediately add 1 mL chloroform (or equivalent so ratio to colorimetric reagent is $\geq 1 + 6$) from pipette, washing down inside of tube. Place colorimeter tube containing 1 mL chloroform (blank) in instrument, add measured volume colorimetric reagent (Section I.C.7.), and adjust galvanometer to 0% A (100% T). This point must remain constant for series of determinations; repeat with blank only as necessary. Place tube containing sample solution in instrument, add measured volume colorimetric reagent, and read galvanometer at first transitory pause point in < 5 sec.

Color should begin to fade immediately and A decreases. For best results, A should be in the range 0.07–0.7. Examine contents in tube; the solution should be a clear blue without turbidity. On standing the blue color may be replaced by a red, lavender, or brown color.

(d) Recovery factor. Determine recovery of vitamin A periodically by adding known amount of vitamin A standard to sample (or food or feed blank, if available) and carry determination through entire procedure. Compare results with and without vitamin A addition and calculate recovery. If recoveries are < 95%, correct results for vitamin A by dividing by percentage recovery. Check procedures carefully for source if low recoveries are obtained.

6. *Calculation of Vitamin A Content.* Correction for carotenoids (C) is used only when carotenoids are present in extract containing vitamin A.

$$C = A_{440} \times f$$

where
A_{440} = reading of yellow color in extract in μg/mL
f = correction factor [Section I.D.5.(b)]
C = correction for carotenoids. (*Note*: If necessary, adjust 440 carotenoid and 620 vitamin A readings for respective dilution volumes.)

$$\mu\text{g vitamin A/g} = Ac_{620} \times S \times V/W$$

where
$Ac_{620} = A_{620} - C$;
S = slope of calibration curve (units vitamin A/A_{620} reading);
V = final dilution volume of vitamin A in colorimeter tube;
W = weight of sample in g.

Total vitamin A activity in RE (retinol equivalents = μg vitamin A + μg carotene/6. Total vitamin A activity in USP units = μg vitamin A × 3.33 + μg carotene × 1.67.

Note: If solids remain in boiling flask after alkaline digestion, results are increased slightly unless correction is made. Determining correction is difficult because some samples leave no residue. Maximum correction may be based on 10-g sample reducing volume in boiling flask by 3 mL.

II.   ULTRAVIOLET ABSORPTION METHOD

A.   Principle

The following references provide background information on this method (23,24,50,60,62,63,70,71). This method is based on measurement of absorption of a solution of retinol in isopropanol at 325 nm, where absorbance is maximum. The method is applicable to pharmaceutical preparations and vitamin A concentrates in which vitamin A content is relatively high and amounts of substances causing irrelevant absorption are relatively small and can be corrected for by taking additional readings at 310 nm and 334 nm (70,71). Care must be exercised in using the correction since it does not apply for some preparations (63,64,72). If tocopherol is present (absorption maximum, 298 nm), a correction is made employing a hydrogenation technique to destroy absorption due to retinol (73). Solutions with appreciable carotenoid contents are purified by chromatography (Section I.D.4.), but carotenoids are generally not a problem in samples to which this method is applied. Though somewhat simplified, the method is similar to the USP XX method (50).

B.   Equipment

1. *High-resolution Spectrophotometer with Quartz Optics.*   Narrow slit width adjustment is required. Use only matched quartz cuvettes, preferably of 1-cm i.d.; surfaces through which light beam passes must be clean and polished.

2. *Other Equipment Needed.*   See Section I.B.4–8 and Section I.B.13.

3. *Hydrogenation Assembly* (50,73,74).   Required only when tocopherol causes interference.

C.   Reagents

1. *See Sections I.C.1., I.C.2. and I.C.4–8.*

2. *Isopropanol.*   High-quality spectrophotometric grade, redistilled from all-glass apparatus.

3. *Palladium Catalyst (73,74).*   This may be obtained from some specialty chemical suppliers, or an equivalent catalyst as 5% palladium on an inert carrier.

4. *Source of Dry Hydrogen Gas Under Pressure.*

D. Procedure

1. *Sampling.* See Section I.D.1.(a) and Section I.D.1.(d–g) for applicable procedures.

2. *Alkaline Hydrolysis.* See Section I.D.2.

3. *Extraction.* See Section I.D.3. If recoveries are low, see Section I.D.3.(d). For some samples, amount of solution extracted must be increased to provide recommended concentrations of retinol in the solution analyzed.

4. *Spectrophotometry.* Use an aliquot of the extract which when made up to 100 mL will give an $A_{325 \text{ nm}}$ reading in the range of 0.3–0.8. Evaporate the aliquot to dryness under vacuum or nitrogen and quickly redissolve in isopropanol and dilute to 100.0 mL. Determine A with the spectrophotometer at 310, 325, and 334 nm, with isopropanol as the blank.

5. *Hydrogenation.* (Use only if interference from tocopherol.) Pipette 15 mL of isopropanol solution containing vitamin A (Section II.D.4.) into a 50-mL centrifuge tube, add about 0.2 g palladium catalyst, stir with glass rod, quickly attach the tube to the hydrogenator with microdispersion tube in place, and tighten connections securely. Adjust hydrogen gas pressure to 15 lb. Open the needle valve to obtain a smooth flow of hydrogen through the solution in the centrifuge tube and continue for 10 min. Bring the system slowly to atmospheric pressure (50,74). Check volume of solution in centrifuge tube and if not essentially the original volume, adjust with isopropanol. Add approximately 0.3 g chromatographic siliceous earth (Super-Cel), stir with glass rod, and centrifuge until solution is clear.

Test 1 mL of the solution for presence of vitamin A by evaporating solvent (Section I.B.8. is a convenient apparatus), dissolve in 1 mL chloroform, and add 6–10 mL color reagent (Section I.C.7.). If a detectable bluish color appears, hydrogenate for a longer time, or use a fresh, more active lot of catalyst.

Determine A of the untreated solution against the hydrogenated portion used as the blank at 310, 325, and 334 nm.

6. *Calculations.* Calculation of vitamin A content is based on $E^{1\%}_{1 \text{ cm}}$ of retinol in isopropanol = 1830.

Content of retinol in μg = $A_{325} \times 549/LC$

where L = internal diameter of the cuvette (1 cm is most convenient);
            C = concentration in grams, tablets, capsules, etc., of the original sample dissolved in the 100.00 mL of isopropanol;
            549 = factor converting $E^{1\%}_{1 \text{ cm}}$ to μg vitamin A.

If correction for irrelevant absorption is required, substitute A read at the three wavelengths into the following formula to obtain a corrected A.

$$A_{325 \text{ corr.}} = 6.815 A_{325} - 2.555 A_{310} - 4.260 A_{334.}$$

Then content of retinol in μg = $A_{325 \text{ corr.}} \times 549/LC$.

A correction is not used if substances causing irrelevant absorption are known to be absent. It also is not used if A_{325} is not less than $A_{325\ corr.}/1.03$, and not more than $A_{325\ corr.}/0.97$. The correction is used when $A_{325\ corr.}$ is less than $A_{325}/1.03$. To convert μg retinol to USP or IU vitamin A, multiply by 3.33.

III. FLUOROMETRIC METHOD

A. Principle

The following are background references for this method (23,60,75,76). This method depends on the fluorescence of retinol for measurement of vitamin A content. An extract of the sample is excited by radiation at 330 nm and fluorescent emission is measured at 480 nm. Quinine sulfate may be used as a secondary standard to calibrate the fluorometer for each series of determinations.

Fluorescent measurements are often more specific than absorbance measurements because many substances that absorb in the UV region do not fluoresce. However, in extracts of many types of samples, where fluorescent substances (e.g., phytofluene in blood) remain even after alkaline hydrolysis, extraction with hydrocarbon solvent and chromatography or a correction formula is required. In all fluorescent measurements, high concentrations of absorbing materials, including retinol, must be avoided because of self-absorption.

The method is useful for routine checking in quality control and in nutritional labeling of unfortified and fortified whole, skim, and dry milk products, since there are only small quantities of interfering substances in milk. The method is less accurate and specific for flavored milk drinks and infant formulas. It has been adapted for control purposes for dairy products (75). The part of the vitamin A activity due to provitamin A carotenoids is not measured by this method.

B. Equipment

1. *Spectrofluorometer or Filter Fluorometer.* Perkin-Elmer MPF series, or equivalent; Turner model 110 filter fluorometer, or equivalent. Use filters in the 330-nm excitation and 480-nm emission ranges and light source specified by the manufacturer.

2. *Water Bath.* Temperature controlled to 80°C, with openings in the cover to hold tubes with upper part of tubes exposed, or beaker partly filled with water immersed in steam bath so temperature can be controlled. (Must not allow alcohol to boil away.)

3. *Reaction Vessels.* Glass-stoppered centrifuge tubes (40 mL or 50 mL) or glass-stoppered Babcock 50% cream test bottles.

4. *Air Condenser.* For centrifuge tubes, use as purchased inner part of ℑ ground-glass joint to fit tube. For Babcock bottle, select short piece of glass tubing to just fit into neck of bottle and wrap with foil to hold in place.

5. *Automatic Shaker.*   180–260 cycles/min, or Vortex mixer (or shake by hand).

6. *Pipettes and Other Glassware.*   As required.

C.   Reagents

1. *Ethanol.*   USP or SD 3A. Check for low fluorescence. If necessary, purify by distilling from all-glass apparatus with approximately 25 g $AgNO_3$ crystals and 50 g KOH pellets/L ethanol. Discard first portions, collecting the distillate around 78°C. Store in all-glass container.

2. *Pyrogallol.*   (See Section I.C.4.).

3. *Potassium Hydroxide Solution.*   (See Section I.C.9.).

4. *0.1 N Sulfuric Acid.*   Slowly add, with stirring, 5.6 mL concentrated H_2SO_4 to H_2O to make to 2 L. Store in glass-stoppered bottle.

5. *0.1% Quinine Sulfate.*   Dissolve 1.0 g quinine sulfate hydrate in 1L of 0.1 N H_2SO_4. Store in tightly closed bottle in refrigerator. For standardization make further serial dilutions in 0.1 N H_2SO_4 as follows: 1 mL to 100 mL twice and then 2 mL to 50 mL. This solution contains 0.04 μg quinine sulfate/mL. Working standards are prepared by making a further series of dilutions 1–6 mL in 10 mL as required for working range of the fluorometer.

6. *Antifoaming Agent.*   Antifoam GF-10 or equivalent. Used when preparing powdered samples.

7. *USP Vitamin A Reference Solution.*   (*See Section E.*)

8. *Hexane.*   Commercial grade. Clear and free of nonhydrocarbon contaminants, boiling range 60–68°C.

9. *Isopropanol.*   Spectral grade.

D.   Procedure

With proper precautions, low-actinic glassware is not required. All glassware must be absolutely clean and free of fluorescent substances. Cuvettes must be clean, polished, and not touched with fingers; hold at top with clean tissue.

Note: Work in subdued light. Draw blinds; use Mylar film on windows, etc.

1. *Sampling.*

(a) Fluid milk and fluid formulas. Allow sample to attain room temp. If sample consists of more than one container, mix each without undue foaming and make a composite of at least 100 mL from each container, but not less than 10% from each. Stir thoroughly without causing foam production. Use 2 mL sample for analysis.

(b) Condensed milk. Dilute 20 mL of milk to 50 mL with H_2O and prepare as for fluid milk.

Note: If vitamin A content is to be expressed on a weight instead of volume basis, dilute 20 g to 50 mL.

(c) Powdered milk or dry milk products. If more than one container, mix each product by rolling on paper or equivalent. For the composite sample take 10 g or 10% from each container. Mix thoroughly by rolling on paper or equivalent. Transfer 20.0 g to 200-mL volumetric flask, add 1 g antifoaming agent, and dilute to approximately 180 mL with H_2O. Mix thoroughly and make to mark. Allow to stand 20–30 min and add H_2O to mark. Repeat until stable volume is attained.

2. *Alkaline Hydrolysis and Extraction.* Pipette 2 mL aliquot to reaction vessel. If fluorescent readings are too low, use 4 mL aliquot. Add 4 mL ethanolic pyrogallol, 1 mL KOH solution, and 1 mL H_2O. Mix thoroughly by swirling and shaking or use Vortex mixer.

Prepare a reagent blank with 4 mL ethanolic pyrogallol, 1 mL KOH solution, and 3 mL H_2O.

Attach air condenser. Reflux gently in water bath at $\geq 80°C$ for 30 min. Reject samples in any vessels with a substantial reduction in volume. Swirl sample two to three times during hydrolysis.

Cool samples to room temperature. Add 5 mL H_2O. Mix. Add 10.0 mL hexane. Insert glass stopper. Mix for 1 min on Vortex mixer, or by shaking vigorously, or 10 min on shaker apparatus. Centrifuge at about 1000 rpm to separate and clear hexane layer. Too-great a speed will break stoppered containers.

Remove upper layer with Pasteur pipette and filter bulb. Transfer to 25-mL volumetric flask. Add 10 mL hexane and repeat extraction. Transfer upper layer to volumetric flask and make to volume.

Note: A single extraction with 20 mL hexane without transfers is faster but may give lower recoveries.

3. *Preparation of Standard to Calibrate Fluorometer.* Warm capsule USP vitamin A reference standard (Section E) to room temperature. (Be sure any solids are dissolved.) Cut top and express approximately 0.2 g of oil into small tared beaker or watch glass. Weigh accurately. Transfer to 100-mL volumetric flask and dilute to mark with hexane. Mix thoroughly. Pipette 2.0 mL to 25-mL volumetric flask and dilute to mark with isopropanol. Make ≥ 4 solutions for standardization by diluting series of 1–5 mL to 10 mL with isopropanol. Change dilution range if necessary to obtain that suitable for fluorometer use. Use 2 mL of each solution for determination, as in Section III.D.2. Calculate concentrations of standards from data on bottle in which capsules were obtained.

4. *Calibration of Filter Fluorometer.* Insert filters in 330-nm and 480-nm ranges, such as Turner 7-60 primary and 75 secondary, or other filters recommended for model fluorometer used. Use excitation lamp suitable for filters selected.

Turn instrument on and allow to stabilize before taking readings (may require 20–30 min). Set range adjustment to 3X (Turner) or equivalent sensitivity with other instruments. Neutral filters and adjustable slit widths may be necessary to obtain desirable radiation intensity. Place opaque block in instrument and set control to zero. Remove block and take reading with hexane in the cuvette.

Read the series of hydrolyzed and extracted standard solutions (Section III.D.3) in duplicate (should agree closely).

Read each solution promptly so that irradiation does not destroy vitamin A and lower readings. Read quinine solutions in a similar fashion. Dilutions of vitamin A standards and quinine solutions should be selected to provide fluorescent readings in similar ranges with none above 80% full-scale deflection. The same conditions and instrument settings must be used for all subsequent analyses.

Plot retinol concentrations of standards against fluorescent readings corrected for hexane blank. Also plot quinine concentrations against corrected fluorescent readings. The plots should be essentially straight lines. Calculate the slope (units vitamin A/fluorescence) to obtain factor to calculate concentration of samples.

5. *Calibration of Spectrofluorometer.* Turn on instrument and allow to equilibrate before taking readings (may require 20–30 min). Set instrument at 330-nm excitation and 480-nm emission, with slit set initially at 8-nm band pass. Set dark current and zero controls to give zero reading with excitation shutter closed.

Slit widths may need to be adjusted by trial and error on instrument selected to obtain required sensitivity.

Intense excitation can cause destruction of vitamin A, resulting in erratic and decreasing readings on sample or standard solutions. Sample solutions should be read rapidly. The slit width of the excitation beam should be kept as narrow as practical and gain (sensitivity) set as high as possible for reasonably steady readings. Spectrofluorometers relying on intense excitation beams for sensitivity may not be suitable for this method.

Prepare standard solutions as in Section III.D.4. Place most concentrated standard solution (in 0.2–0.25 μg retinol/mL range) in cuvette, adjust slit widths and sensitivity as outlined in previous paragraph. Read each diluted standard solution prepared in duplicate. Read hexane blank in the cuvette. Without delay, read quinine solutions of concentrations to give readings in the same general range as vitamin A standards. Plot fluorescent readings of vitamin A standards, adjusted by subtracting the hexane blank, against concentrations of retinol in μg/mL. Plot fluorescent readings of quinine sulfate solutions, adjusted for hexane blank, against concentrations of quinine sulfate. The plots should be essentially straight lines; if not, the concentrations may be too high. Calculate the slope of the vitamin A plot to obtain a factor to determine vitamin A content of samples.

Once the standard and quinine solution have been read and found to be in the proper range, do not change sensitivity settings. Use those settings for all subsequent analyses, or reset as directed.

6. *Measurement of Sample Fluorescence.* Place hexane in cuvette as in Section III.D.4. or Section III.D.5., with settings as for calibrations, and read fluorescence blank. Similarly read sample extracts. Without delay, read one or more quinine working standard solutions. If readings of quinine solution(s) differ by more than ±2 from calibration value, calculate ratio to original reading to obtain factor by which to multiply vitamin A sample values to obtain corrected

value or reset sensitivity to give original reading on quinine solution. Recalibration is indicated if significant and consistent correction is required.

7. *Recovery Study.* Check recovery of vitamin A by adding standard in isopropanol at one to two multiples of amount in sample. Recoveries should be nearly quantitative.

8. *Calculation of Vitamin A Content.* Correct all fluorescence reading of samples by subtraction of reagent blank reading.

$$\mu\text{g vitamin A/g} = (C \times V/W^*) \times f$$

where C = concentration of vitamin A in μg/mL of solution read on fluorometer, from calibration curve or by multiplication of emission by slope of calibration curve;

V = final dilution volume of extract analyzed;

W^* = weight of sample in g (if sample was taken on volume basis, g and W are in volumetric units instead of g);

f = factor to correct for variable fluorescent response based on reading of quinine standard (not used if correction made by adjusting sensitivity).

USP units vitamin A/g $= (C \times 3.33 \times V/W) \times f$

IV. HIGH-PERFORMANCE LIQUID CHROMATOGRAPHY

A. Principle

The following references provide background information for this method (60,77–82). High-performance liquid chromatography (HPLC) is the newest method for vitamin A analysis dating from the early 1970s. Some advantages of the method are: relatively rapid and clean separations can be made; some costs and hazards are reduced because relatively small quantities of reagents are used; isomers can be separated more easily and precisely than by other methods; it can be modified to include other fat-soluable vitamins including provitamin A carotenoids; it has possibilities for full automation (see also Chapter 4).

The samples are prepared, hydrolyzed, and extracted by procedures similar to those outlined previously. A small aliquot of the extract containing vitamin A is injected into a relatively short, small-diameter column, packed with fine, uniform particles of absorbent. The vitamin A is rapidly eluted by a solvent mixture under pressure. As the components are eluted, they are monitored and measured continuously by a spectrophotometer, an integral part of the HPLC apparatus. Results are recorded graphically and components are identified by retention times of elution peaks as compared to known standards. Data from the graph are used to calculate concentration, or results are recorded by a computing integrator.

Although only small amounts of vitamin A are required for HPLC, large

(b) When carotene is determined as part of the analysis, carotene standards (Section IV.C.3.) also are carried through the procedure.

5. *Chromatography.* Operating conditions such as flow rate, sample size and injection, sensitivity, chart speed, and so on, must be determined on the system selected by trial and error in preliminary trials with vitamin A. Constant flow rates in the 1 to 1.5 mL/min range, sensitivities of 0.05 to 0.2 AUFS and chart speed of 0.5 cm/min have been used. Also see instructions supplied with components or systems chosen.

Before starting an analysis, pump column with the solvent system used for the separation for 20 min or longer if necessary to establish a stable base line. Following a determination, the column should be washed with 10 mL chloroform-methanol or methylene chloride-methanol (2 + 1), 10 mL methanol and 10 mL hexane mixture to remove polar contaminants. Use of a short disposable precolumn may extend life of HPLC columns and saves time.

The sample extract to be injected is evaporated to dryness under vacuum or nitrogen and dissolved in the solvent used for injection. The final dilution should provide a retinol concentration of about 0.5 μg/mL, or such that suitable readings will be obtained when 40–100 μL of the solution is injected. The retinol peak should be 100 times or more above "baseline noise."

6. *Detection and Quantitation of Vitamin A.* Set absorbance detector at 325 nm. Detectors set in the 310–340-nm region also may be found suitable.

Note: Fluorescence detection (325-nm excitation and 480-nm emission) may give increased specificity, but absorbance detection is less complicated.

(a) For silica single-phase column. Inject sample dissolved in hexane-cyclohexane (1 + 1) containing 1% isopropanol. The same solvent mixture is used for the separation. The most suitable solvent system may vary with column selected. Other solvent systems for single-phase separations of retinol are hexane containing 2–10% of ethyl ether, ethyl acetate, or dioxane.

(b) Reversed-phase column. Inject sample dissolved in methanol. Separation is with methanol containing 1–10% (typically 5%) H_2O. The most suitable solvent system may vary with column selected. Other solvent systems for reversed-phase separations of retinol are: Acetonitrile-H_2O (65 + 35), methanol-H_2O (80 + 20).

Depending on column used and operating conditions, all-*trans*-retinol should elute in 5–10 min. If present, 13-*cis*-retinol should elute 1–1.5 min earlier on a silica column. Traces of other isomers, such as the 9-*cis*-isomer, will elute between the 13-*cis* and all-*trans* forms.

The shape of the elution curves for retinol in standard and sample should be similar and the peaks should have the same retention times. The peaks should be sharp and the curves triangular-shaped without shoulders. Vitamin A contents may be calculated from peak heights relative to those of standards, or preferably from areas under the curves.

7. *Carotene.* In some materials such as butter, milk, margarine, and some mixed feeds, carotene must also be measured to obtain total vitamin A activity. On silica columns, carotene can be determined concurrently with retinol. With

(b) When carotene is determined as part of the analysis, carotene standards (Section IV.C.3.) also are carried through the procedure.

5. *Chromatography.* Operating conditions such as flow rate, sample size and injection, sensitivity, chart speed, and so on, must be determined on the system selected by trial and error in preliminary trials with vitamin A. Constant flow rates in the 1 to 1.5 mL/min range, sensitivities of 0.05 to 0.2 AUFS and chart speed of 0.5 cm/min have been used. Also see instructions supplied with components or systems chosen.

Before starting an analysis, pump column with the solvent system used for the separation for 20 min or longer if necessary to establish a stable base line. Following a determination, the column should be washed with 10 mL chloroform-methanol or methylene chloride-methanol (2 + 1), 10 mL methanol and 10 mL hexane mixture to remove polar contaminants. Use of a short disposable precolumn may extend life of HPLC columns and saves time.

The sample extract to be injected is evaporated to dryness under vacuum or nitrogen and dissolved in the solvent used for injection. The final dilution should provide a retinol concentration of about 0.5 μg/mL, or such that suitable readings will be obtained when 40–100 μL of the solution is injected. The retinol peak should be 100 times or more above "baseline noise."

6. *Detection and Quantitation of Vitamin A.* Set absorbance detector at 325 nm. Detectors set in the 310–340-nm region also may be found suitable.

Note: Fluorescence detection (325-nm excitation and 480-nm emission) may give increased specificity, but absorbance detection is less complicated.

(a) For silica single-phase column. Inject sample dissolved in hexane-cyclohexane (1 + 1) containing 1% isopropanol. The same solvent mixture is used for the separation. The most suitable solvent system may vary with column selected. Other solvent systems for single-phase separations of retinol are hexane containing 2–10% of ethyl ether, ethyl acetate, or dioxane.

(b) Reversed-phase column. Inject sample dissolved in methanol. Separation is with methanol containing 1–10% (typically 5%) H_2O. The most suitable solvent system may vary with column selected. Other solvent systems for reversed-phase separations of retinol are: Acetonitrile-H_2O (65 + 35), methanol-H_2O (80 + 20).

Depending on column used and operating conditions, all-*trans*-retinol should elute in 5–10 min. If present, 13-*cis*-retinol should elute 1–1.5 min earlier on a silica column. Traces of other isomers, such as the 9-*cis*-isomer, will elute between the 13-*cis* and all-*trans* forms.

The shape of the elution curves for retinol in standard and sample should be similar and the peaks should have the same retention times. The peaks should be sharp and the curves triangular-shaped without shoulders. Vitamin A contents may be calculated from peak heights relative to those of standards, or preferably from areas under the curves.

7. *Carotene.* In some materials such as butter, milk, margarine, and some mixed feeds, carotene must also be measured to obtain total vitamin A activity. On silica columns, carotene can be determined concurrently with retinol. With

the hexane-cyclohexane-isopropanol solvent system, carotene elutes in about 1 min. It is measured at 453 nm, using 2 in-line detectors for carotene and retinol, or determined in a separate procedure. Carotene also may be determined by simple column chromatography on alumina or magnesia.

8. *Identity and Validity.* The absorption curve of the material collected under the 325-nm peak can be scanned photometrically to establish the identity of all-*trans*-retinol (25). The material also is evaporated, dissolved in 0.2 mL chloroform and tested with 1–2 mL vitamin A colorimetric reagent (Section I.C.7.). A rapidly fading blue color is a positive test.

If a fraction believed to be 13-*cis*-retinol separates, it also will give a positive blue color test. Material from two or more eluates may need to be pooled to provide enough for the test. If the 13-*cis*-retinol fraction is examined spectrophotometrically, the 328-nm reading should exceed that at 325 nm.

If samples are spiked with the diluted standard solution at 50–100% the levels in samples and carried through the entire procedure, the retinol peak should be markedly enhanced and no significant new peak should appear. Results with unspiked and spiked samples may be used to calculate percentage recovery of vitamin A.

9. *Calculation.* If both all-*trans*-retinol and 13-*cis*-retinol are separated, calculate the content of each. The content of 13-*cis*-retinol can be calculated from data taken with the detector set at 328 nm, using the absorbance ratio, 1.08, of all-*trans*-retinol to 13-*cis*-retinol (25,78).

$$\text{Concentration in } \mu g/g^* = \frac{A \times B \times D}{B \times S}$$

where
- A = peak height (or area under the curve) of sample;
- B = peak height (or area under the curve) of standard;
- C = concentration of standard in $\mu g/mL$ at the same dilution volume as for sample solution;
- D = final dilution volume of sample;
- S = sample weight in g*;
- IU vitamin A/g* = $\mu g/g \times 3.33$.

If both all-*trans*- and 13-*cis*-retinol are calculated, then IU vitamin A = μg all-*trans*/.3 + μg 13-*cis*/.4 (25,78).

10. *Variations of HPLC Method.* If dry stabilized forms of vitamin A are absent from the sample and vitamin A esters are present in an easily extractable state, a determination without alkaline hydrolysis may be suitable (79,80,84,85). Simplification of the method by direct injection of a hydrolyzed extract without prior purification has been proposed (80,86). Vitamin A has been determined concurrently with other fat-soluble vitamins on the same column by several investigators (80–82,86–88).

*If sample is taken on volume basis, g and S are in volumetric units instead of g.

V. OTHER VITAMIN A METHODS

Other methods for vitamin A have been published that may be found advantageous in certain situations (23,24,60,64). Two of those methods are described briefly.

A. Anhydroretinol Method

This is a spectrophotometric method based on conversion of retinol to dehydroretinol by treatment with a dehydrating agent such as *p*-toluenesulfonic acid. Anhydroretinol has a distinctive absorption spectrum with a good peak at 399 nm. At that wavelength known contaminants do not interfere. Thus, it is claimed that the method can be used for samples containing impurities interfering in other methods without having to chromatograph the extract (63,89,90).

B. Maleic Anhydride Method for Vitamin A Isomers

The *cis-trans* isomers of retinol can be separated by HPLC (Section IV) and the vitamin A activity of the mixture of isomers can be calculated by taking account of the relative biopotencies of the components (35).

A chemical method for estimating the vitamin A activity of a mixture of

TABLE 7.2   Methods Suggested for Determining Vitamin A

Type of Material[a]	Colorimetric	Spectrophotometric	Fluorometric	HPLC
Pharmaceuticals	+	+		+
Vitamin A concentrates	+	+		+
Vitamin premixes	+			+
Fish oils	+	+		+
Mixed animal feeds	+			+
Fortified cereal foods	+			+
Butter and margarine	+			+
Livers, fish meals, etc.	+			+
Pet foods	+			+
Fluid and dry milk	+		+	+
Flavored milk drinks	+		+[b]	+
Infant and dietetic formulas	+		+[b]	+
Eggs	+			+
Snacks	+			
Prepared entrees	+			+

[a]Column chromatography may be required to remove certain interfering materials such as carotenoids from some samples.

[b]Limited application.

retinol isomers is based on differences in the reaction of various isomers with maleic anhydride under controlled conditions (21,24,51). Maleic anhydride reacts readily with all-*trans*- and 13-*cis*-retinols forming an additional product, which then prevents reaction with colorimetric reagents such as $SbCl_3$. Other principal isomers that might be present, the 9-*cis*, 9-13-di-cis, and 11-*cis* forms, react more slowly with maleic anhydride and blue colors are formed by reaction with $SbCl_3$. In the analysis, readings at 620 nm are obtained on solutions treated and untreated with maleic anhydride. From the difference in the two values, isomeric composition and biological potency of the sample are estimated by applying a special formula or using a table that relates maleic values to relative biopotencies (21).

VI. APPLICATION OF METHODS

More than one method may be suitable for determining vitamin A in a given product. Table 7.2 lists methods from this chapter used for vitamin A in various materials.

LITERATURE CITED

1. McCollum, E. V. and Davis, M. "The necessity of certain lipins in the diet during growth." *J. Biol. Chem.* **15**, 167 (1913).

2. McCollum, E. V. and Davis, M. "Observations on the isolation of the substance in butterfat which exerts a stimulating influence on growth." *J. Biol Chem.* **19**, 245 (1914).

3. Osborne, T. B. and Mendel, L. B. "The relation of growth to the chemical constituents of the diet." *J. Biol. Chem.* **15**, 311 (1913).

4. McCollum, E. V. and Kennedy, C. "The dietary factors operating in the production of polyneuritis." *J. Biol. Chem.* **24**, 491 (1916).

5. Rosenberg, H. R. *Chemistry and Physiology of the Vitamins*, revised reprint. Interscience Publishers, New York (1945).

6. Goodman, D. S. "Vitamin A transport and retinol-binding protein metabolism." In R. S. Harris, D. L. Munson, E. Diczfalusy, and J. Glover, Eds., *Vitamins and Hormones*, Vol. 32. Academic Press, New York, 167 (1974).

7. Thompson, J. N. "Fat-Soluble Vitamins." In M. Rechcigl, Jr., Ed., *Comparative Animal Nutrition*, Vol. 1. S. Krager, Basel, 99 (1976).

8. Moore, T. *Vitamin A.* Elsevier, New York (1957).

9. "Vitamin A and Carotene." In W. H. Sebrell, Jr. and R. S. Harris, Eds., *The Vitamins*, Vol. 1, 2nd ed. Academic Press, New York, 1 (1967).

10. Reti, L. "Sur l'état de combinaision de la vitamine A dans les huiles de foie." *Compt. Rend. Soc. Biol.* **120**, 577 (1935).

11. Neff, A. W., Parrish, D. B., Hughes, J. S., and Payne, L. F. "The state of vitamin A in eggs" *Arch. Biochem.* **21**, 315 (1949).

12. Moore, T. "The biochemistry of vitamin A in the general system." In R. A. Morton, Ed., *Fat-Soluble Vitamins.* Pergamon Press, New York, 223 (1970).

13. Goodwin, T. W. *Carotenoids.* Chemical Publishing Co., New York (1954).

14. Olson, J. A. "The metabolism of vitamin A." *Pharmacol. Rev.* **19**, 559 (1967).

15. Arens, J. F. and Van Dorp, D. A. "Synthesis of some compounds possessing vitamin A activity." *Nature* **157**, 190 (1946).

16. Isler, O., Huber, W., Ronco, A., and Kofler, M. "Synthese des vitamin A." *Helv. Chim. Acta* **30**, 1911 (1947).

17. Bauernfeind, J. C. and Cort, W. M. "Nutrification of foods with added vitamin A." *CRC Critical Rev. Food Tech.* **4**, 337 (1974).

18. Isler, O., Kläui, H., and Solms, U. "Vitamins A and carotene—3. Industrial preparation and production." In W. H. Sebrell, Jr. and R. S. Harris, Eds., *The Vitamins*, Vol. 1, 2nd ed. Academic Press, New York, 101 (1967).

19. "Nomenclature policy: generic descriptors and trivial names for vitamins and related compounds." *J. Nutr.* **112**, 7 (1982).

20. Aguilar, D. and Parrish, D. B. "Estimation of biopotency and isomerization of vitamin A in livers of four species." *Int. J. Vit. Nutr. Res.* **41**, 316 (1971).

21. Ames, S. R. and Lehman, R. W. "Estimation of the biopotency of vitamin A sources from their maleic values." *J. Assoc. Off. Agric. Chem.* **43**, 21 (1960).

22. Green, J. "Distribution of fat-soluble vitamins and their standardization and assay by biological methods." In R. A. Morton, Ed., *Fat-Soluble Vitamins.* Pergamon Press, New York, 71 (1970).

23. Olson J. A. "The determination of the fat-soluble vitamins: A, D, E, and K." In A. A. Albanese, Ed., *Newer Methods of Nutritional Biochemistry, Vol. 2. Academic Press, New York, 345 (1965).*

24. Roels, O. A. and Mahadevan, S. "Vitamin A." In P. György and W. N. Pearson, Eds., *The Vitamins*, Vol. 6. 2nd ed. Academic Press, New York, 139 (1967).

25. Schwieter, U. and Isler, O. "Vitamin A and carotene—2. Chemistry." In W. H. Sebrell, Jr. and R. S. Harris, Eds., *The Vitamins*, Vol. 1, 2nd ed. Academic Press, New York, 5 (1967).

26. Morton, R. A. "Chemical structure and physical properties." In R. A. Morton, Ed., *Fat-Soluble Vitamins.* Pergamon Press, New York, 27 (1970).

27. Baxter, J. G. and Robeson, C. D. "Crystalline aliphatic esters of vitamin A" and "Crystalline vitamin A." *J. Am. Chem. Soc.* **64**, 2407 and 2411 (1942).

28. Robeson, C. D. and Baxter, J. G. "Neovitamin A." *J. Am. Chem. Soc.* **69**, 136 (1947).

29. Robeson, C. D., Cawley, J. D., Weisler, L., Stern, M. H., Eddinger, C. C., and Chechak, A. J. "Chemistry of vitamin A—24. The synthesis of geometric isomers of vitamin A *via* methyl β-methylglutaconate." *J. Am. Chem. Soc.* **77**, 4111 (1955).

30. Robeson, C. D., Blum, W. P., Dieterle, J. M., Cawley, J. D., and Baxter, J. G. "Chemistry of vitamin A—25. Geometrical isomers of vitamin A aldehyde and an isomer of its α-ionone analog." *J. Am. Chem. Soc.* **77**, 4120 (1955).

31. Cama, H. R., Collins, F. D. and Morton, R. A. "Studies in Vitamin A—17. Spectroscopic properties of all-*trans* vitamin A and vitamin A acetate. Analysis of liver oils." *Biochem. J.* **50**, 48 (1951).

32. Shantz, E. M. "Isolation of pure vitamin A₂." *Science* **108**, 417 (1948).

33. Boldingh, J., Cama, H. R., Collins, F. D., Morton, R. A., Gridgeman, N. T., Isler, O., Kofler, M., Taylor, R. J., Welland, A. S. and Bradbury, T. "Pure all-*trans* vitamin A acetate and the assessment of vitamin A potency by spectrophotometry." *Nature* **168**, 598 (1951).

34. Kofler, M. and Rubin, S. M. "Physiochemical assay of vitamin A and related compounds." In R. S. Harris and D. J. Ingle, Eds., *Vitamins and Hormones*, Vol. 18. Academic Press, New York, 315 (1960).

35. Ames, S. K., Swanson, W. J., and Harris, P. L. "Biochemical studies on vitamin A—14. Biopotencies of geometric isomers of vitamin A acetate in the rat." 15. "Biopotencies of geometric isomers of vitamin A aldehyde in the rat." *J. Am. Chem. Soc.* **77**, 4134 and 4136 (1955).

36. Ganguly, J. and Murthy, S. K. "Vitamins A and carotene—4. Biogenesis of vitamin A and carotene." In W. H. Sebrell, Jr. and R. S. Harris, Eds., *The Vitamins,* Vol. 1, 2nd ed. Academic Press, New York, 125 (1967).

37. Smith, J. E. and Goodman, D. S. "Vitamin A metabolism and transport." In *Present Knowledge in Nutrition,* 4th ed. The Nutrition Foundation, New York, 65 (1976).

38. Wald, G. and Hubbard, R. "The chemistry of vision." In R. A. Morton, Ed., *Fat-Soluble Vitamins,* Pergamon Press, New York, 267 (1970).

39. Goodman, D. S. "Vitamin A metabolism." *Fed. Proc.* **39,** 2716 (1980).

40. Smith, J. E. and Goodman, D. S. "Retinol-binding protein and the regulation of vitamin A transport." *Fed. Proc.* **38,** 2504 (1979).

41. Peterson, P. A., Nilsson, S. F., Ostberg, L., Rask, L., and Vahlquist, A. "Aspects of the metabolism of retinol-binding protein and retinol." In R. S. Harris, P. L. Munson, E. Diczfalusy, and J. Glover, Eds., *Vitamins and Hormones,* Vol. 32. Academic Press, New York, 181 (1974).

42. DeLuca, H. F. "Retinoic acid metabolism." *Fed. Proc.* **38,** 2519 (1979).

43. Thompson, J. N., Howell, J. M., Pitt, G. A. J., and McLaughlin, C. I. "The biological activity of retinoic acid in the domestic fowl and the effects of vitamin A deficiency in the chick embryo." *Brit. J. Nutr.* **23,** 471 (1969).

44. Parrish, D. B. "Retinoic acid and reproduction of Japanese quail." *Nutr. Repts. International* **26,** 857 (1982).

45. Sporn, M. B. and Newton, D. L. "Chemoprevention of cancer with retinoids." *Fed. Proc.* **38,** 2528 (1979).

46. Rietz, P., Wiss, O., and Weber, F. "Metabolism of vitamin A and the determination of vitamin A status." In R. S. Harris, P. L. Munson, E. Diczfalusy, and J. Glover, Eds., *Vitamins and Hormones,* Vol. 32. Academic Press, New York, 237 (1974).

47. Glover, J., Jay, C. and White, G. H. "Distribution of retinol-binding protein in tissues." In R. S. Harris, P. L. Munson, E. Diczfalusy, and J. Glover, Eds., *Vitamins and Hormones,* Vol. 32, Academic Press, New York, 215 (1974).

48. Light, R. F., Alscher, R. P., and Frey, C. N. "Vitamin A toxicity and hypoprothrombinemia." *Science* **100,** 225 (1944).

49. Kläui, H. M., Hausheer, W., and Huschke, G. "Technological aspects of the use of fat-soluble vitamins and carotenoids and of the development of stabilized marketable forms." In R. A. Morton, Ed., *Fat-Soluble Vitamins,* Pergamon Press, New York, 113 (1970).

50. *The United States Pharmacopeia XX. The National Formulary XV.* The United States Pharmacopeial Convention, Rockville, Md. (1980).

51. Ames, S. R. "Methods for evaluating vitamin A isomers." *J. Assoc. Off. Anal. Chem.* **49,** 1071 (1966).

52. FAO/WHO. "Requirements of vitamin A, thiamine, riboflavine, and niacin." Rept. of a Joint FAO/WHO Expert Committee. FAO Nutrition Meeting Report Series No. 41; WHO Tech. Rept. Ser. No. 362, WHO, Geneva (1967).

53. Department of Health and Social Security. "Recommended intakes of nutrients for the United Kingdom." Repts. on Public Health and Medical Subjects No. 120, H. M. Stationary Office, London (1969).

54. National Research Council, Committee on Dietary Allowances. "Fat-soluble vitamins." In *Recommended Dietary Allowances,* 9th ed. National Academy of Sciences, Washington, D.C. (1980).

55. "Nutrition labeling," *Fed. Regist.* **38**(13), 2124; **38**(49), 6950 (1973).

56. Ames, S. R., Risley, H. A., and Harris, P. L. "Simplified procedure for extraction and determination of vitamin A in liver." *Anal. Chem.* **26,** 1378 (1954).

57. Kimble, M. S. "The photocolorimetric determination of vitamin A and carotene in human serum." *J. Lab. Chem. Med.* **24,** 1055 (1939).

58. Parrish, D. B. Unpublished. Kansas State University, Manhattan.

59. Dann, W. J. and Evelyn, K. A. "The determination of vitamin A with the photoelectric colorimeter." *Biochem. J.* **32**, 1008 (1938).

60. Parrish, D. B. "Determination of vitamin A in foods—a review." *CRC Crit. Rev. Food Sci. Nutr.* **9**, 375 (1977).

61. Callison, E. C., Hallman, L. F., Martin, W. F., and Orent-Keiles, E. "Comparison of chemical analysis and bioassays as measures of vitamin A value: yellow corn meal." *J. Nutr.* **50**, 85 (1953).

62. Association of Official Analytical Chemists. *Official Methods of Analysis,* 13th ed. Washington, D.C., Chapter 43 (1980).

63. Strohecker, R. and Henning, H. M. "Vitamin A." *Vitamin Assay-Tested Methods* (transl. by D. D. Libman). Verlag Chemie, Weinheim, Germany, 33 (1965).

64. Hashmi, M. Ul-H. "Vitamin A." *Assay of Vitamins in Pharmaceutic Preparations,* Wiley, New York, 19 (1973).

65. Carr, F. H. and Price, E. A. "Color reactions attributed to vitamin A." *Biochem. J.* **20**, 497 (1926).

66. Caldwell, M. J. and Parrish, D. B. "The effect of light on the stability of the Carr-Price color in the determination of vitamin A." *J. Biol. Chem.* **158**, 181 (1945).

67. Subramanyam, G. B. and Parrish, D. B. "Colorimetric reagents for determining vitamin A in feeds and foods." *J. Assoc. Off. Anal. Chem.* **59**, 1125 (1976).

68. Parrish, D. B. "Physico-chemical assay of vitamin A." In *Symp. Proc., the Biochemistry, Assay and Nutritional Value of Vitamin A.* Association of Vitamin Chemists, Chicago, Il. (1968).

69. Baskerville, C. and Hamor, W. A. "The chemistry of anaesthetics—1. Ethyl ether 4. Changes which occur in ethyl ether during storage." *Ind. Engr. Chem.* **3**, 387 (1911).

70. Morton, R. A. and Stubbs, A. L. "Symposium on spectroscopic analysis. Photoelectric spectrophotometry applied to the analysis of mixtures, and vitamin A oils." *Analyst* **71**, 348 (1946).

71. Morton, R. A. and Stubbs, A. L. "Studies in vitamin A. 4. Spectrophotometric determination of vitamin A in liver oils. Correction for irrelevant absorption." *Biochem. J.* **42**, 195 (1948).

72. Kobayashi, T. "Studies on the determination of vitamin A in the presence of contaminants having irrelevant absorption." *J. Vitaminol.* **12**, 256 (1966).

73. Quaife, M. L. and Biehler, H. "A simplified hydrogenation technique for the determination of blood plasma tocopherols." *J. Biol. Chem.* **159**, 663 (1945).

74. Freed, M. *Methods of Vitamin Assay,* 3rd ed. Interscience, New York, 363 (1966).

75. Thompson, J. N., Erdody, P., Maxwell, W. B., and Murray, T. K. "Fluorometric determination of vitamin A in dairy products." *J. Dairy Sci.* **55**, 1077 (1972).

76. Senyk, G. F., Gregory, J. F., and Shipe, W. F. "Modified fluorometric determination of vitamin A in milk." *J. Dairy Sci.* **58**, 558 (1975).

77. Thompson, J. N. "Analysis of vitamins in foods using high performance liquid chromatography." In *Symp. Proc., Application of High Pressure Liquid Chromatographic Methods for Determination of Fat Soluble Vitamins A, D, E, and K in Foods and Pharmaceuticals,* Association of Vitamin Chemists, Chicago, Il. (1978).

78. Egberg, D. C., Heroff, J. C., and Potter, R. H. "Determination of all-*trans* and 13-*cis* vitamin A in food products by high-pressure liquid chromatography." *J. Agric. Food Chem.* **25**, 1127 (1977).

79. Thompson, J. N., Hatina, G., and Maxwell, W. B. "High performance liquid chromatographic determination of vitamin A in margarine, milk, partially skimmed milk, and skimmed milk." *J. Assoc. Off. Anal. Chem.* **63**, 894 (1980).

80. Widicus, W. A. and Kirk, J. R. "High pressure liquid chromatographic determination of vitamins A and E in cereal products." *J. Assoc. Off. Anal. Chem.* **62**, 637 (1979).

81. Thompson, J. N. "Trace analysis of vitamins by liquid chromatography." In J. F. Lawrence, Ed., *Trace Analysis,* Vol. 2. Academic Press, New York, 1 (1982).

82. Parrish, D. B. "Recent developments in chromatography of vitamins in foods and feeds." In J. F. Lawrence, Ed., *Food Constituents and Food Residues: Their Chromatographic Determination,* Marcel Dekker, New York (Chapter 3, 1984).

83. Lehman, R. W. "A statistical procedure for estimating vitamin A assay variations caused by particulate distribution of dry vitamin A in feed samples." *J. Assoc. Off. Anal. Chem.* **43**, 15 (1960).

84. Aitzetmüller, K., Pilz, J., and Tosche, R. "Fast determination of vitamin A palmitate in margarine by HPLC." *Fette:Seifen:Anstrichm.* **81**, 40 (1979).

85. Landen, W. O., Jr., and Eitenmiller, R. R. "Application of gel permeation chromatography and nonaqueous reverse phase chromatography to high pressure liquid chromatographic determination of retinyl plamitate and β-carotene in oil and margarine." *J. Assoc. Off. Anal. Chem.* **62**, 283 (1979).

86. DeVries, J. W., Egberg, D. C., and Heroff, J. C. "Concurrent analysis of vitamin A and vitamin E by reversed phase high performance liquid chromatography." In G. Charalambous, Ed., *Liquid Chromatographic Analysis of Food and Beverages,* Vol. 2. Academic Press, New York, 477 (1979).

87. Rose, W. P. "Simultaneous determination of vitamins A, D, and E in fortified food products by HPLC." In *Symp. Proc., Application of High Pressure Liquid Chromatographic Methods for Determination of Fat Soluble Vitamins A, D, E, and K in Foods and Pharmaceuticals,* "Association of Vitamin Chemists, Chicago, Il. (1978).

88. Williams, R. C., Schmit, J. A., and Henry, R. A. "Quantitative analysis of the fat-soluble vitamins by high-speed liquid chromatography." *J. Chromatogr. Sci.* **10**, 494 (1972).

89. Budowski, P. and Bondi, A. "Determination of vitamin A by conversion to anhydrovitamin A." *Analyst* **82**, 751 (1957).

90. Müller, V., v. Lengerken, J., Kirmas, D., and Wetterau, H. "Beiträge zur Vitamin-A-Bestimmung in industriell hergestellten Futtermitteln—2. Mitt. Die Bestimmung von Vitamin A in Mischfuttermitteln." *Nahrung* **20**, 47 (1976).

8 Carotenes

Kenneth L. Simpson, Samson C. S. Tsou, and C. O. Chichester

GENERAL CONSIDERATIONS

Carotenoids are pigments found in yellow, orange, red, and green plants as well as in many animals. Some are split into retinals or vitamin A compounds and are thus precursors to retinoids. The carotenoids are polyenes and classified into two groups: [1] carotenes, hydrocarbons such as α-, β-, and γ-carotenes, and [2] xanthophylls, oxygenated hydrocarbons such as cryptoxanthin lutein and their esters. Epidemiologic evidence suggests a physiologic role for intact β-carotene in cancer prevention (1).

A. Physicochemical Properties

About 500 carotenoids have now been identified. Their structures are generally characterized by eight repeating isoprenoid units with attached methyl groups, symmetry around the center of the molecule, and a system of conjugated double bonds, which is responsible for the yellow to deep red color. But, these carotenoids differ in degree of saturation, cyclization, oxidation, and/or carbon addition or subtraction from the basic (carbon) skeleton. According to the nomenclature established by the International Union of Pure and Applied Chemistry Commission, the stem name "carotene" is used with specific designations for end groups (2). Thus, β-carotene [I] is β,β-carotene; α-carotene [II] is β,ϵ-carotene; γ-carotene [III] is β,ψ-carotene; lycopene [IV] is ψ,ψ-carotene; β-cryptoxanthin [V] is β,β-carotene-3-1; echinenone [VI] is β,β-carotene-4-one;

185

and β-zeacarotene [VII] is 7',8'-dihydro-β-ψ-carotene (Figure 8.1). The more common of these carotenoids have trivial names and these will be used in this chapter.

The provitamin carotenoids, which exhibit vitamin A activity, contain a β-ionone (cyclohexenyl) ring at either one or both ends of the polyene chain (Figure 8.1). This ring and the terminal groups of the chain (retinyl structure) determine the retinoid activity. Lycopene is devoid of provitamin A activity, but the other six carotenoids in Figure 8.1 are vitamin A-active and represent some of the more commonly found types. Based on structure, about 50 carotenoids would be expected to exhibit provitamin A activity (3). Bauernfeind (4)

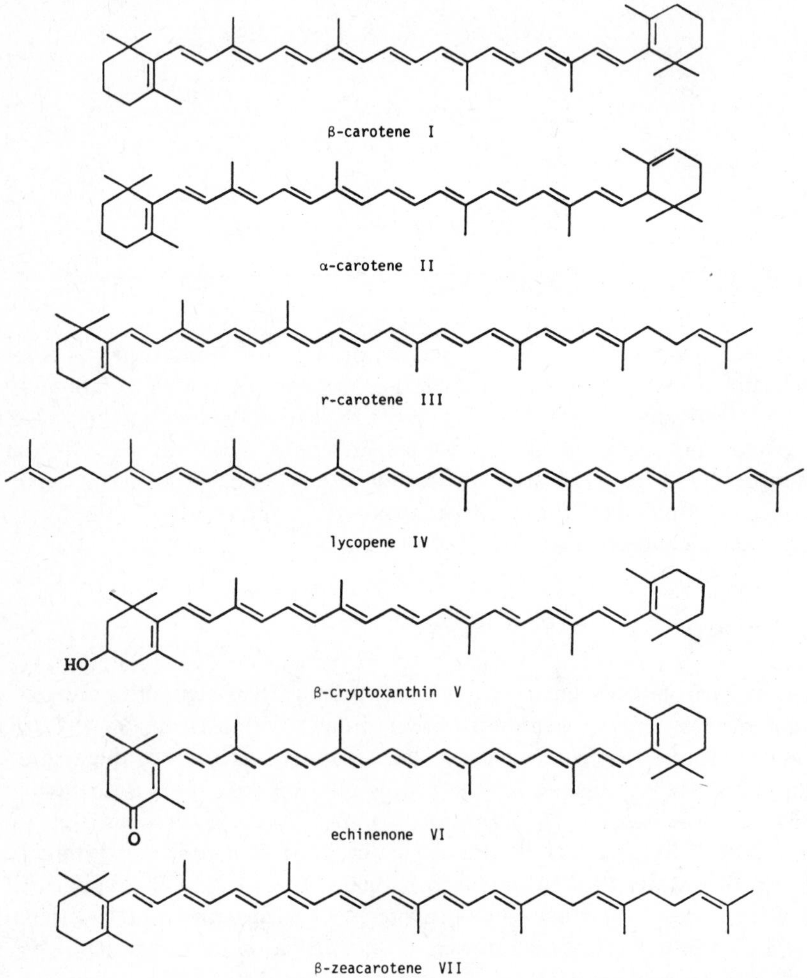

FIGURE 8.1 Structure of some common carotenoids.

lists 32 provitamin carotenoids and apocarotenols with significant sources for each (Table 8.1).

The ability to synthesize the basic terpenoid structure is thought to be limited to plants (Protista and higher plants). Animals are capable of making a number of alterations in the basic structure, including the cleavage of some carotenoids, leading to the formation of apocarotenals and retinal. Animals can biosynthesize acetyl coenzyme A (CoA) into farnesyl pyrophosphate (FPP) leading to squalene and the steroids, but are unable to convert FPP into geranylgeranyl pyrophosphate (GGPP) and then to phytoene and the carotenoids (Figure 8.2).

Carotenoids with vitamin A activity are fat soluble and readily dissolve in benzene, petroleum ether, chloroform, and carbon disulfide but dissolve only slightly in ethanol. Carotenoids are sensitive to light and oxidation and stable to heat in an oxygen-free atmosphere, except for some stereoisomeric changes. In general, carotenoids are all *trans*-isomers; some natural mono-*cis* and poly-*cis* forms do exist.

Carotenoids exhibit characteristic absorption spectra. The major absorption maxima of some common carotenoids in different solvents are listed in Table 8.2. Solvents interact with carotenoids and alter the spectral qualities. The first harmonic of the electronic spectrum approaches the visual spectrum with seven double bonds in conjugation. With increased desaturation, the absorption spectra shift to longer (red) wavelengths.

TABLE 8.1 Representative Types of Carotenoids and Apocarotenoids with Provitamin A Activity[a]

Carotenoids	Activity (%)
β-Carotene	100
α-Carotene	50–54
3,4-Dehydro-β-carotene	75
3,4,3′,4′-Bisdehydro-β-carotene	38
γ-Carotene	42–50
7,8′-Dihydro-γ-carotene	20–40
β-Carotene 5′,6′diepoxide	21
α-Carotene 5,6-epoxide	25
β-Carotene 5,6,5′,6′diepoxide	Active
3-Keto-β-carotene	52
3-Hydroxy-β-carotene	50–60
4-Hydroxy-β-carotene	48
β-Apo-2′-carotenal	Active
β-Apo-8′-carotenal	72
β-Apo-10′-carotenal	Active
β-Apo-12′-carotenal	120
Lycopene	Inactive
Lutein	Inactive

[a]From Bauernfeind (4).

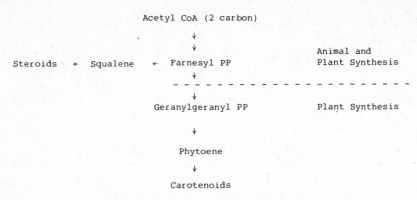

```
                    Acetyl CoA (2 carbon)
                              ↓
                              ↓                    Animal and
   Steroids   ←   Squalene   ←   Farnesyl PP       Plant Synthesis
                              ↓
       - - - - - - - - - - - - - - - - - - - - - - - -
                              ↓
                    Geranylgeranyl PP              Plant Synthesis

                              ↓

                         Phytoene

                              ↓

                       Carotenoids
```

FIGURE 8.2   Animal and plant terpene synthesis.

A hydroxyl group does not affect the chromophore, whereas a conjugated carbonyl group may affect the spectrum. Acyclic carotenoids exhibit a sharp, three-fingered spectrum, although some of this sharpness is lost with the addition of each ring. The addition of a carbonyl in conjunction results in the loss of most, if not all, fine structure. The effects of substituents and solvents on the absorption maxima are listed in Table 8.3.

Compounds such as magnesium oxide, alumina, microcel C, and silica gel used in chromatographic procedures may shift the absorption spectra of carotenoids and xanthophylls. β-Carotene suffers the least shift from magnesium oxide, while silica gel shifts the spectrum considerably (Figure 8.3). This light absorption property of the carotenoids is universally used for quantitative determinations. The molar extinction coefficient (ϵ) is used when the carotenoid's molecular weight is known. However, the specific extinction coefficient ($E_{1\,cm}^{1\%}$) is most commonly used and is the extinction of a 1% solution in a 1-cm path at a given wavelength. The $E_{1\,cm}^{1\%}$ values for selected carotenoids are listed in Table 8.4.

The relationship between ϵ and $E_{1\,cm}^{1\%}$ is: $\epsilon = E_{1\,cm}^{1\%} \times \dfrac{\text{mol. wt.}}{10}$ A useful relationship between absorption and quantity is as follows:

$$\text{mg} = \frac{A \times \text{dil} \times \text{mL} \times 10}{E_{1\,cm}^{1\%}}$$

where A = absorbance;
          dil = dilution factor;
        mL = total mL of sample.

In a sample analysis, the total number of milligrams in a sample is determined by measuring the absorbance (A) in a 1-cm cuvette, taking into account the total size of the sample (mL) and any dilutions (dil) that had to be made to bring it on scale (0–1.0 A).

TABLE 8.2 Main Absorption Maxima of Some Common Carotenoids[a,b]

Carotenoid	Hexane	Ethanol	Acetone	Chloroform	Benzene	Petroleum Ether
Astaxanthin	468	478	480	485	478	468
Canthaxanthin	467	474		482	480	463
α-Carotene	420 442 472	423 444 473	424 448 476	433 457 484		422 444 473
β-Carotene	(425) 450 477	(427) 449 475	(429) 452 478	435 461 485	(435) 462 487	(425) 448 475
β-Carotene 5,6 epoxide	423 444 473			459 492	460 492	447 478
β-Carotene 5,6,5',6' epoxide	417 440 468	418 442 471		424 448 477	426 451 481	443 471
γ-Carotene	437 462 492	(440) 460 489	(439) 461 491	446 475 509	447 477 510	437 462 494
ζ-Carotene	380 400 425			384 405 430		378 400 425
β-Cryptoxanthin	(425) 446 475	(428) 449 473		(435) 459 485		425 449 476
Echinenone	(423) 459 (483)	461	460	471	470 (490)	456 (482)
Lutein	420 445 475	422 445 474		435 458 485	433 458 487	421 445 474
Lycopene	448 473 504	446 472 503	448 474 505	458 484 518	455 487 522	446 472 505
Neurosporene	416 440 470	416 441 470		424 451 480		414 439 467
Phytoene	276 286 297	277 287 298		280 291 303		276 286 298
Phytofluene	331 347 366			337 354 374		331 347 367
β-Zeaxanthin	407 427 454	(405) 428 455		(414) 439 465		406 428 454
Zeaxanthin	(426) 450 480	(428) 450 478	452 479	(434) 459 488	(440) 463 491	424 449 476

[a]Adapted from Davies (5).

[b]Figures in parentheses represent the shoulder.

TABLE 8.3   Effects of Substituents and Solvents on the Main Absorption Maxima of Carotenoids[a]

Substituents		
Change	Position	Effect
Double bond	Chain	+7 to +35 nm
Double bond	Ring	+5 to +9 nm
First carbonyl	Chain	+28 nm
Second carbonyl	Chain	+1 to +7 nm
First carbonyl	Ring	+7 nm
Second carbonyl	Ring	+5 to +9 nm
First and second epoxide	5,6	−8 nm
First and second epoxide	5,8	−20 nm
Trans → cis		−4 nm
Solvents		
Type		Effect
Ethanol, hexane, light petroleum		Small effect
Benzene, chloroform		+15
Carbon disulfide		+35

[a]Adapted from Vetter et al. (6).

Vitamin A or retinol activity of carotenoids has been assayed by: [1] feeding the carotenoid to a test animal under prescribed conditions; [2] measuring the activity of the cleavage enzyme on the test carotenoid to yield retinal; and [3] examining its structure, one-half of which at least, resembles retinol. The precise retinol equivalent of each provitamin carotenoid is not definitely known, since the carotenoid utilization by the animal in question depends upon the carotenoid source, the species of the animal, and the nutritional status of the animal at the time of feeding. It is also possible that the digestion process alters some carotenoids into their active forms.

United States Pharmacopeia arbitrarily assigned that 0.6 μg of β-carotene or 1.2 μg of other provitamins is equivalent to 1 USP unit or 1 International Unit (IU) of vitamin A or 0.1 μg of retinol. The IU is commonly used in nutrition data books and nutrition labels.

Since the utilization of the provitamin A compounds are considerably less than that of retinol, the unit is now expressed as retinol equivalents (8):

$$
\begin{aligned}
1 \text{ retinol equivalent (RE)} &= 1 \text{ μg retinol} \\
&= 6 \text{ μg } \beta\text{-carotene} \\
&= 12 \text{ μg other provitamin A compounds} \\
&= 3.33 \text{ IU activity from retinol} \\
&= 10 \text{ IU vitamin A activity from } \beta\text{-carotene.}
\end{aligned}
$$

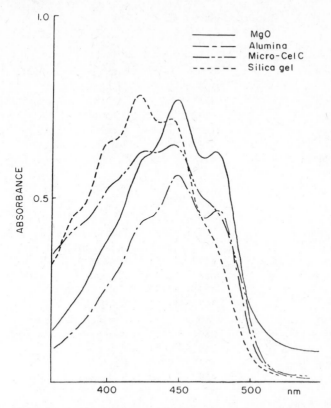

FIGURE 8.3 Absorption spectra of β-carotene after chromatography on magnesium oxide, alumina, microcel C, and silica gel columns (7).

For products containing β-carotenes and other provitamin A carotenoids,

$$\text{Total retinol equivalent} = \frac{\mu g\ \beta\text{-carotene}}{6} + \frac{\mu g\ \text{other provitamins A}}{12}$$

B. Occurrence and Stability of the Carotenoids

It has been estimated that 10^8 tons of carotenoids are produced each year (9) by the earth's biomass. The major carotenoids are not provitamin A precursors, although β-carotene and related provitamin A-active pigments do occur widely. The carotenoids are found in all photosynthetic tissues; in some nonphotosynthetic tissues, such as roots, flowers, seeds, fruits, vegetables; and in the Protista (yeast, fungi, and bacteria). The yellow, orange, and red pigments are present in skin, organs, and flesh of birds, insects, salmon, and in the exoskeleton of shellfish. Animal products such as eggs, milk, butter, and cheese contain carotenoids in addition to retinols.

The carotenoids are altered or partially destroyed by acids, bases (in some instances), lipoxygenases, and light, especially in the presence of oxygen or some

TABLE 8.4 $E_{1\,cm}^{1\%}$ **Values for Selected Carotenoids**[a]

Carotenoid	(nm)	$E_{1\,cm}^{1\%}$	Solvent
Canthaxanthin	466	2200	Light petroleum petroleum ether
α-Carotene	444	2800	Light petroleum
β-Carotene	453	2592	Light petroleum and hexane
β-Carotene	453	2620	Ethanol
β-Carotene	465	2396	Chloroform
β-Carotene	484	2008	Carbon disulfide
β-Carotene 5,6,5',6'di- epoxide	451	2394	Benzene
γ-Carotene	462	2760	Hexane
γ-Carotene	462	3100	Light petroleum
ζ-Carotene	400	2555	Hexane
β-Cryptoxanthin	452	2386	Light petroleum
Echinenone	458	2158	Light petroleum
Lutein	445	2550	Ethanol
Lutein	458	2236	Benzene
Lycopene	472	3450	Light petroleum
Lycopene	487	3370	Benzene
Neurosporene	440	2918	Hexane
Phytoene (15-*cis*)	286	757	Hexane
Phytofluene	347	1577	Hexane
β-Zeacarotene	427	1940	Hexane
Zeaxanthin	452	2340	Light petroleum

[a]Selected from Davies (5).

metals. The degradation steps result in the formation of *cis-trans* isomers, epoxides, and chain cleavage, leading to discoloration, and loss of vitamin A activity.

The degradation of the plant carotenoids has been reviewed Simpson et al. (10). When exposed to light, especially in the presence of acid and/or iodine, all the *trans* isomers change into *cis-trans* isomers. This results in a shift in the absorption maxima to shorter wavelengths, loss of extinction, formation of "*cis*" peak and partial loss of biological activity. The effect of isomerization on the loss of biological activity is listed in Table 8.5. Zechmeister (11) and Davies (5) have reviewed the carotenoid *cis*-isomers.

Lipoxygenases are known to act on carotenoids where these carotenes act as secondary substrates for the fat oxidizing system. The activity of a heat-labile lipoxygenase-like enzyme is implicated in the discoloration of red fish (12). Carotenoid losses occur during food processing, cooking, dehydration (13), accelerated storage, and extrusion cooking (14,15). Microcel-C degrades β-carotene into 4-hydroxy and 4-keto derivatives (16).

In-chain epoxides of carotenoids have been shown to split into apocarotenals when chromatographed on magnesium oxide (17). Epoxides are formed during fluorescent light-induced autoxidation of β-carotene in fatty acid solvents (18).

TABLE 8.5 Provitamin A Activity of *Cis-trans* Isomers

Cis-isomer	Relative Biological Potency[a]
All-*trans*-β-carotene	100
Neo-β-carotene U	38
Neo-β-carotene B	53
All-*trans*-α-carotene	53
Neo-α-carotene U	13
Neo-α-carotene B	16
All-*trans*-γ-carotene	27–42
Neo-γ-carotene P	19
All-*trans*-cryptoxanthin	57
Neo-cryptoxanthin U	27
Neo-cryptoxanthin A	42

[a]Zechmeister (11).

Epoxide formation is shown to occur in overripe tomatoes (19). The initial step in the breakdown of carotenes is the postulated formation of an epoxide at the 5,6 double bond.

During extraction and chromatography, carotenoid samples should be protected from exposure to sunlight, mercury lamps, and fluorescent lights; the *cis*-isomer of β-carotene was identified as α-carotene in a tomato extract, in spite of these precautions (personal observation). Although some losses and artifact production are unavoidable, normal precautions such as the following can minimize these losses: [1] preventing prolonged exposure to light, oxygen, heat, acid, and lipoxy type enzymes; [2] storing at low temperature ($< -20°C$) under nitrogen; [3] avoiding acetone as storage solvent; and [4] using antioxidants and sulfites to protect the carotenes.

C. Existence of Bound Forms and Their Release

There is a precursor relationship between carotenes and the retinoids. In a sense, carotene is a bound form of vitamin A, until it is split into retinal. The carotenoids of vegetables, fruit, animal, or animal product origin are usually found associated with lipid fractions, complexed with protein or esterified.

During the digestion process, the pigments are released by digestive enzymes, solubilized by bile salts, and oxidatively cleaved within the mucosal cell forming retinal and several apocarotenals. The retinal is reduced to retinol, which is then esterified and transported to the liver. The metabolism of α-carotene results in the formation and subsequent storage of vitamin A and α-vitamin A in the liver (20).

Some carotenoids are absorbed directly from the digestive tract into the blood, then deposited in various parts of the body, such as the fat depot, adrenal cortex, atheromatous plaques, skin, shell, and in milk or eggs (14).

D. Sample Preservation

A sample for analysis should represent the material from which it is taken; the portion of the tissue, which the data represents should be specified. Freezing and storage at $-20°C$ in the dark under nitrogen is recommended (21). Tissues that contain lipoxygenase should be blanched and treated with an antioxidant prior to freezing. Since some leaching losses occur with steam or hot water blanching, weighing before and after blanching is recommended. Hot-air drying, especially in the sun, is not recommended since serious degradation may occur. Vacuum drying of blanched samples has been reported to result in negligible losses (22). However, analysis of fresh tissue is always preferred.

   The carotenoid solutions may be stored in the refrigerator in petroleum ether and related solvents or benzene; acetone or unprotected chloroform should not be used.

METHODS AVAILABLE

Bioassay, solvent partitioning, and chromatographic techniques can be used to determine the carotenoid or provitamin A content.

A. Biological Method

Bioassay determines the actual retinol activity of foods or feeds. Vitamin A-depleted rats are fed several levels of the sample and the weight gains with these are compared with those fed known quantities of β-carotene. Differences in the bioavailability of carotenoids from different sources are taken into account. The method is tedious, expensive, time-consuming, subject to errors and variations, and cannot measure the individual isomers. In general, these bioassays have been replaced by physicochemical methods.

B. Physicochemical Methods

These methods measure the amount of various carotenoids without indicating the actual biological potency in terms of vitamin A. All these procedures use some method of extraction, usually followed by saponification and physical methods of separating the pigments. Quantification is based on their light-absorbing properties at 450 nm.

   1. *Phase Separation and Countercurrent Distribution.*   Separations based on polarity are often used as a preparatory step to chromatographic procedures. The hydrocarbons are soluble in petroleum ether and xanthophylls are distributed between a nonpolar petroleum ether and an alcohol-H_2O mixture, depending on the number of oxygen substitutions. The Craig countercurrent distribution method based on this principle is now seldom used due to cost, space required,

time needed for separations, possible epoxide formation, and the need for further chromatography of fractions (5).

2. *Gas-Liquid Chromatography (GLC).* GLC analysis is not possible because of the high melting point (MP) of the carotenoids and their thermal instability. But, the hydrogenated derivatives can be separated by GLC. When the parent carotenoid is hydrogenated, identical derivatives will result from a number of different carotenoids. Thus, α-carotene, β-carotene, and ε-carotene would form the same hydrogenated compound and would be indistinguishable from each other. The method is good for size (GLC-Mass Spectrometer) and xanthophyll separations. The main drawback is the need to chromatograph hydrogenated derivatives (23).

3. *Thin-Layer Chromatography (TLC).* TLC techniques are excellent for identification and preliminary purification of carotenoids. The adsorption plate is streaked with an extract and developed in a nitrogen atmosphere. The spots may be identified by their color or made visible by reaction with antimony trichloride (24) or iodine vapor. R_f values are calculated. The spot may be scraped from the plate, extracted from the adsorbent, and its quantity determined by spectrophotometry. Quantitative (97%) recoveries of standards were reported by Targan et al. (25), but the recovery is not routinely that high (26). Table 8.6 lists some important provitamin A compounds and retinoids with adsorbent and solvent systems (5,22,24–29). Due to differences in the polarity of carotenoids, a single adsorbent-solvent system will not resolve all the carotenoids. The adsorbed compounds should be protected from light and oxidation during analysis.

TABLE 8.6 Selected Relative R_f Values of Carotenoids and Related Compounds on TLC Systems[a]

Compounds	A	B	C	D	E
α-Carotene	0.96	0.96	0.80		
β-Carotene	0.92	0.97	0.74	1.00	0.90–1.00
γ-Carotene		0.20	0.41		
Cryptoxanthin	0.73	0.44			
Lycopene		0.84	0.13		
Lutein	0.65	0.21			
Zeaxanthin	0.39	0.19			
Retinyl esters					0.90–1.00
Retinal				0.65	0.69
Retinoic acid				0.08	0.08
Retinol					0.33
β-Apo-8′-carotenal				0.67	
β-Apo-10′-carotenal				0.71	

[a]Systems: A, CaCO$_3$-MgO-Ca(OH)$_2$ 30+6+4; PE-Acetone-CHCl$_3$-MeOH 50+50+40+1 (27); B, silica gel, 3% MeOH in C$_6$H$_6$ (28); C, MgO, benzene-PE 90+10 (29); D, silica gel-acetone:PE 10+90 (24); and E, silica gel G, benzene-ethyl ether 90+10 (25).

TLC of carotenoids is useful for quantitative purposes such as detecting impurities from other techniques and determining the purity of standards. Paper chromatography is also useful in carotenoid separations (5,30).

4. *Column Chromatography.* Open-column chromatography is widely used to isolate and individually separate carotenoid pigments. Structural differences between the carotenoids and their varying affinities toward adsorbents lead to the formation of distinct adsorption bands or fractions. The pigment in each fraction is eluted or cut from the column and quantitated by spectral analysis. Several adsorbents, solvents, and elution patterns are used. The AOAC procedure is based on the above and is widely used due to its low-cost operations and visual monitoring of the separations (31).

The AOAC method is a crude method which gives a good estimate for tissues that contain β-carotene as the only carotene, such as green leaves. The method tends to overestimate where a complex mixture exists (e.g., β-carotene, α-carotene, lycopene, etc.) or carotenoid esters are present as in fruit (Table 8.7). Some simple modifications are suggested that reflect the correct extinction coefficient λ_{max} and need for saponification of some fruit samples.

5. *High-Performance Liquid Chromatography (HPLC).* HPLC is a rapid, reproducible, sensitive, and quantitative method for carotenoid analysis. The lower detection limits for lycopene, α-carotene, and β-carotene are 3.95, 37.2, and 38.5 pmoles, respectively, with a SF 770 Spectroflo monitor variable wavelength detector set (Kratos Inc.) at 470 nm (32). Several column-solvent systems are used to separate the carotene pigments (Table 8.8). Pigments are identified by retention times and quantified by peak area or peak height. Within the 20–2,000 pmole range, there is a linear relationship between the amount of pigment injected and the peak area, with a linear correction coefficient of 0.991–0.998 (36).

With microparticle column packing, flexibility of normal, reverse-phase, and gradient solvent-adsorbent systems and the use of on-line UV/Vis detectors and integrators, HPLC is the method of choice for carotenoid separations. However,

TABLE 8.7   Provitamin A Activity of Selected Fruits and Vegetables[a]

Commodity	HPLC Method (mg β-carotene/100 g)	AOAC Method (mg β-carotene/100 g)
Carrot	7.06	9.87[b]
Pumpkin	5.09	10.03
Orange	0.73	2.68
Papaya	0.44	0.99
Persimmon	0.63	2.88
Spinach	3.35	2.62 (3.55)[c]

[a]C. S. Tsou (unpublished data).

[b]Combination of HPLC and AOAC.

[c]Measurement at 436 nm, $E^{1\%}_{1cm}$ 1960.

TABLE 8.8 Selected HPLC Columns and Solvent Systems of Carotenoid Separation

System	Column	Solvents	Remarks
1	Basic alumina	Benzene-hexane (1 + 5) plus 0.01% BHT	For carotene only
2	Spherisorb	THF-hexane (1 + 5) plus 0.01% BHT	For cryptoxanthin only
3	Magnesia	Acetone-hexane gradient system	Good resolutions of α-carotene, β-carotene, ξ-carotene, α-cryptoxanthin, β-cryptoxanthin Low temperature control 16°C Need 30 min for each sample
4	Spherisorb	0–40% of acetone in hexane containing 0.1% methanol	No separation of α-carotene and β-carotene Separate *cis-trans* isomers of lutein and bacterioruberin
5	Partisil-5/ODS 5 μm	8% chloroform in acetonitrile (2 mL/min)	Resolve α-carotene, β-carotene, and lycopene
6	Merck RP18 10 μm	Linear gradient of methanol/ acetonitrile (25 + 75) - H_2O (1.5 mL/min)	Separate xanthophylls and carotenes in single run. Resolve *cis-trans* isomers of β-carotene and other carotenoids. Methanol/acetonitrile (25 + 75) may be used isocratically to separate carotenes
7	RCM C18 cartridge 5 μm	Solvent gradient of 3% H_2O in methanol-10% THF in methanol (2.0 mL/min)	Separate xanthophylls and carotenes in single-run THF-methanol (10 + 90). May be used isocratically for carotene separation Relatively short time for re-equilibration

(Continued)

TABLE 8.8 Selected HPLC Columns and Solvent Systems of Carotenoid Separation (*Continued*)

System	Column	Solvents	Remarks
8	Zorbax ODS 7 μm 25 × 0.46 cm	Acetonitrile-dichloromethane-methanol (70 + 20 + 10) (1.0 mL/min)	Resolve lutein, zeaxanthin, canthaxanthin, β-cryptoxanthin, echinenone, lycopene, torulene, α-carotene, β-carotene
9	Merck RP18 10 μm	Acetone-methanol-acetonitrile (20 + 40 + 40) (0.7 mL/min)	Resolve β-cryptoxanthin, lycopene, α-carotene, β-carotene

Sources: 1, Reeder and Park (33); 2, *Ibid.*; 3, Stewart (34); 4, Fiksdahl et al. (35); 5, Zakaria et al. (32); 6, Braumann and Grimme (36); 7, Tsou and Simpson (37); 8, Nelis and DeLeenheer (38); 9, Tsou, unpublished data.

it is premature to recommend any specific system that can be used for a variety of samples. HPLC results are more precise than those obtained by AOAC column chromatography procedures (Table 8.9).

ANALYTICAL METHODOLOGY

I. OPEN-COLUMN CHROMATOGRAPHY

A. Principle

Carotenoid pigments are extracted by a suitable process and purified if necessary by saponification; the purified carotenoids are separated by chromatography on a MgO-Hyflo Super Cel column. Quantification is by measuring light absorption at a suitable wavelength.

B. Equipment

1. *Homogenizers.* (Braun homogenizer, electric blenders with Teflon gasket, Polytron from Brinkmann Instruments using a combination of sonic oscillation and mechanical blades.)

2. *Fritted Glass Funnels.* Coarse porosity.

3. *Filter Flasks.*

4. *Refrigerated Centrifuge.*

5. *Separatory Funnels.* With Teflon stopcock.

6. *Steam Bath.*

7. *Rotary Vacuum Evaporator.*

TABLE 8.9 Comparison of Provitamin A Analyses (μg/mL) in Valencia Orange Juice

	AOAC		HPLC				
Sample	Total Carotene[a]	Retinol Equivalent[b]	α-Carotene	β-Carotene	Cryptoxanthin	Total Carotene	Retinol Equivalent[b]
A	1.86	0.31	0.15	0.23	1.22	1.60	0.15
B	2.14	0.36	0.13	0.20	1.08	1.41	0.16
C	1.60	0.27	0.11	0.14	1.08	1.31	0.14

Source: Reeder and Park (33).

[a]AOAC (39.014). (31)

[b]Our calculation.

8. *Vacuum Desiccator.*

9. *Chromatography Tubes.*   Pyrex glass 22 × 175 mm or 18 × 160 mm with constricting end.

10. *Recording Spectrophotometer.*

C.   Reagents

1. *Methanol.*   USP grade.

2. *Acetone.*   Dry alcohol-free.

3. *Petroleum Ether.*   B.P. 40–60°C.

4. *Ethyl Ether.*   Peroxide-free.

5. *Hexane.*   B.P. 60–70°C, distilled over KOH.

6. *Anhydrous Sodium Sulfate.*

7. *Magnesium Oxide.*   Sea Sorb 43.

8. *Diatomaceous Earth, Hyflo Super Cel.*   Adsorbent: Mix intimately equal quantities by weight of MgO and Hyflo Super Cel in a large bottle. Make a large batch and test before use for recovery of carotene.

9. *Carotene Standard.*

(a) 90% β- and 10% α-carotene mixture.   Dissolve 50 mg of this in hexane and dilute to 500 mL with hexane. Use fresh solutions and dilute as needed for calibration curves.

(b) Use pure 100% β-carotene for specific purposes.

D.   Procedure

Sample Preparation for Analysis

1. *Extraction.*   A universal method does not exist to extract these fat-soluble pigments from different food and biological materials. Hydrocarbons, provitamin A compounds, and single-oxygen xanthophylls are among the more easily extracted carotenoids. For total extraction, several solvents might be tried to compensate for the polarity variation among the carotenoids and for sample matrix. Acetone, methanol, and ethanol are often used either singly or in combination because of their dual solubility. Mechanical disruption accelerates the extraction. The sample should be extracted until it becomes colorless or the extracting solvent used remains colorless.

(a) Weigh 2–25 g of representative sample, estimated to contain 10–500 μg of carotenes.

(1) Homogenize all moist materials such as fresh, frozen, and canned fruits and vegetables to puree consistency; add a known weight of H_2O, if necessary. Blanch fresh and frozen foods to inactivate enzymes prior to blending. Wash fruits canned in thick syrup two or three times with H_2O before blending. Sun-dried fruits such as apricots, prunes, peaches, and

so on, should be ground in a food chopper and a representative sample rehydrated first with a known amount of H_2O and then blended with more H_2O to puree consistency.

(2) Pulverize all dry samples to fine powder and rehydrate a weighed sample by covering with enough quantity of hot H_2O for 5–10 min.

(3) Materials such as butter, lard, and margarine, with high lipid content, are directly saponified omitting this extraction step.

(b) Homogenize with 30 mL acetone in a blender with the motor mounted above the blades to minimize leakage.

(c) Transfer the homogenate to a large fritted glass funnel, rinsing with 20 mL acetone. Stir well and draw off the acetone extract into a filter flask under reduced pressure. Add successively 10-mL portions of acetone to complete the extraction.

(1) Alternatively, the homogenized sample can be transferred to a 250-mL centrifuge flask, treated with required amounts of acetone, and centrifuged.

(2) Fluid milk samples coagulate on treatment with acetone or other extractant, resulting in a clear upper layer; the carotenoid pigments are in this layer, which can be easily removed.

(3) Fruits and vegetables are also extracted with methanol (methanol-slurry, 1 + 1), followed by sequential extractions with acetone or acetone-hexane, 1 + 1 mixture (22).

(4) Addition of dry ice during homogenization reduces any possible artifacts.

(d) Transfer the extract quantitatively to a large separatory funnel with Teflon stopcock, with two 10-mL portions of H_2O and three 15-mL portions of hexane. Shake the contents gently for 30–60 sec and allow the layers to separate.

(1) If there is a slight yellow color in the lower acetone-H_2O layer, add either acetone or 5% Na_2SO_4 (aq) solution gradually down the sides of funnel to transfer the pigments into the hexane layer and to prevent emulsions.

(2) Sometimes there could be a single layer or phase; if so, proceed to step I.D.1(f).

(e) Draw the water-acetone layer into a second separatory funnel and re-extract with 25-mL portions of hexane two or three times and transfer the hexane extract to the first separatory funnel.

(f) Pour 100 mL H_2O through the combined hexane extracts. Allow layers to separate and discard the lower aqueous phase. Repeat the washings one or two times.

(1) As the polar solvent (acetone) is being removed, break up any emulsion that is likely to happen by adding NaCl. All traces of acetone

of acetone must be removed prior to saponification to prevent aldol condensation artifacts (5).

(g) Wash the dried hexane extract over anhydrous Na_2SO_4; collect the dried extract quantitatively and concentrate it under nitrogen or rotatory vacuum evaporator to a known volume of 10–25 mL.

At this point, the extract may be chromatographed and spectrally analyzed or further purified by saponification.

2. *Saponification.*

(a) Mix equal volumes of the hexane extract and 5–10% KOH in methanol. Heat the mixture on a steam table for 5–15 min, preferably in the dark under nitrogen or keep in the dark at 5–20°C under nitrogen for 12–16 hr. Remove hexane from the mixture either by heat or a stream of nitrogen. Saponification is complete if only one phase remains.

(1) Choice of hot or cold procedure depends upon the time available, heat sensitivity of the pigments analyzed, or presence of carotenoid esters, which are not satisfactorily split in the cold procedure (5). Antioxidants can be added but this is not necessary where nonoxidizing conditions are maintained; little loss of most carotenes occurs during the actual saponification in both procedures. The pH should remain high during saponification. Samples with a high fat content require more KOH. Milk and animal tissues can be saponified directly with 5% KOH in absolute ethanol (milk-KOH, 1 + 4, tissue-KOH, 1 + 8) at 75°C for 25 min (39).

(b) Cool the alkaline mixture and transfer successive portions to a separatory funnel containing an equal volume of hexane. Add H_2O slowly without shaking and discard the aqueous phase. Repeat the process until all KOH is removed.

(1) Add acetone to facilitate the washing out of methanolic KOH from saponified samples that do not contain carotenals. Loss of pigments, partitioned between the two phases on washing out the alkali, can be avoided by adding acetone to the methanolic KOH and by using small aliquots of sample extract. NaCl can be added to break up any emulsions formed during saponification.

(c) Dry the washed hexane extract over anhydrous Na_2SO_4 and concentrate as in Section I.D.1(g). The residue is dissolved in a known volume of either hexane or petroleum ether. Saponification removes chlorophylls that cochromatograph with certain xanthophylls. Saponified xanthophyll esters are readily separated from the carotenes on the basis of polarity; this results in good chromatographic resolution of carotene and common provitamin A xanthophylls such as β-cryptoxanthin. However, saponification should be avoided when the carotenoid ester is to be assayed, carbonyl carotenoids are present, or the carotenoid is likely to be altered by saponification.

3. *Chromatography Separation.*

(a) Total carotenes from unsaponified sample extracts.

(1) Column preparation.

(i) Attach the adsorption tube (22 × 175 mm) to a filter flask and pack a plug of glasswool into the constriction. Apply vacuum and add enough adsorbent to make a column about 2 cm in length. Press down the adsorbent firmly twice with a suitable plunger and loosen the adsorbent surface around the edges with a thin spatula. Add more adsorbent and continue stepwise to a column length of 10 cm.

(ii) Add a 1-cm layer of anhydrous Na_2SO_4 on top of the adsorbent. Wet the column by washing with 25–50 mL hexane. While the last 2–5 mL hexane is still above the Na_2SO_4, turn off the vacuum and transfer the adsorption column to another clean filtration flask.

(2) Adsorption and elution.

(i) Pour the extract onto the column and apply suction. Rinse the container with 5–10-mL portions of hexane, pouring each rinsing onto the column. Keep the washings small so that the extract may be adsorbed in a narrow band in the upper portion of the column.

(ii) Elute the adsorbed band with 50 mL of 10% acetone in hexane by pouring small successive volumes of this elutant onto the column.

(iii) Collect the "carotene" fraction in a clean flask and concentrate it to dryness in a rotary vacuum apparatus. Dissolve the residue in a suitable final volume of hexane to a carotene concentration of 1–4 µg/mL. Quantitate spectrophotometrically.

Comment: The above AOAC method (31) is widely used; values for carotene and vitamin A in the food composition tables are from this method. The method chromatographically separates the carotenes from the oxygenated compounds, but does not separate individual carotenes. Figure 8.4 shows the type of column separation that was obtained from peach puree using the AOAC method modified for use with a 1 + 3 column (MgO-Hyflo Super Cel) (40).

A simple introduction of a solvent schedule (Figure 8.5, 40) separates α-carotene and β-cryptoxanthin from the xanthophyll and carotene bands of the peach. A visual comparison of Figures 8.4 and 8.5 shows the oversimplification of measuring the "carotene" band and calling it β-carotene.

Table 8.6 lists several fruits and vegetables in which the HPLC method (to be described later) and the AOAC method are compared. Three examples are illustrated:

1. Spinach. The AOAC method excludes the more polar compounds such as xanthophylls and chlorophylls and only measures β-carotene, since the other carotene levels are negligible. We have found a consistent loss in the AOAC method due to losses on the column. On the other hand, the use of AOAC recommended values (436 nm and $E\,{}^{1\%}_{1\,cm}$ 1960) results in an overestimation.

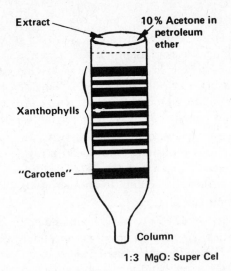

FIGURE 8.4 Separation of the carotenoids from cling stone peaches on a 1 + 3 magnesium oxide-Hyflo Super Cel column (40).

2. Carrot, pumpkin, orange, papaya. These fruits and vegetables represent complex mixtures of provitamin A compounds and inactive carotenoids. These are mainly included as β-carotene resulting in an overestimation.

3. Fruits containing esters. Persimmon contains esterified cryptoxanthin

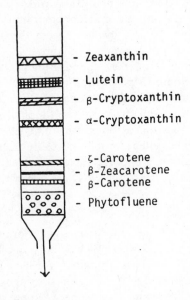

FIGURE 8.5 Separation of peach carotenoids without saponification (40).

which would have the same visual spectrum as β-carotene and chromatograph with it. On saponification, cryptoxanthin could be excluded as a xanthophyll in the AOAC method.

There are many modifications of the AOAC method. In the present chapter, it is suggested that the type of carotenoid content be considered and that the acetone-hexane mixture be evaporated to dryness and a pure solvent be used to measure the absorbances using recognized extinction coefficients. Since lycopene has no provitamin A activity, it is often eliminated by stopping the chromatograph before the red pigment is eluted. In the literature examples, lycopene was excluded from tomato analysis of carotenes (41) or not mentioned as being included or excluded in tomato analysis (42).

(b) Individual carotenes from saponified extract samples.

(1) Column preparation. Proceed as in Section I.D.3(a)(1) but use a 18 × 160-mm absorption tube.

(2) Adsorption, resolution, and elution.

(i) Pour an appropriate aliquot of the extract in petroleum ether onto the column followed by 5–10-mL portions of petroleum ether to form a narrow band in the upper portion of the column.

(ii) Add petroleum ether until the phytofluene band separates from β-carotene. The separation can be monitored since phytofluene fluoresces under black light. When the two bands are separated, add 1% ethyl ether in petroleum ether followed by 2% ethyl ether. When γ-carotene separates from lycopene, increase to 5% ethyl ether. Develop further with 2% acetone in petroleum ether until β-zeacarotene separates from γ-carotene. Increase to 5% acetone to further resolve bands.

(iii) Stop developing the chromatograph after phytofluene is eluted.

(iv) Run the column dry and extrude the column carefully under pressure. Cut the different bands from the column and elute the individual pigments from the adsorbent with acetone.

(v) Evaporate the different pigment fractions to dryness under reduced pressure and dissolve the residue in a suitable final volume to a carotene concentration of 1–4 μg/mL. Xanthophylls in the column can be further resolved with larger proportions of acetone (20%) in petroleum ether. Representative column separations are shown for corn (Figure 8.6) and tomato (Figure 8.7) using 1% acetone in petroleum ether as the developing solvent. Figure 8.8 shows the complexity of band separation and identification of pigments where *cis*-isomers abound, as in a tangerine or tomato or as artifacts.

Some fractions require further purification. The β-zeacarotene obtained from the column is often contaminated with its own *cis*-isomer or γ-carotene and can be rechromatographed on basic alumina III (activity grade). Develop the column with 1% diethyl ether in petroleum ether. γ-Carotene can be rechromatographed

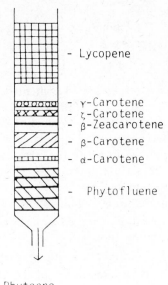

Phytoene

FIGURE 8.6 Chromatographic separation of carotenoids from corn on 1 + 2 magnesium oxide-Hyflo Super Cel (43).

on alumina III with petroleum ether. β-Carotene can be rechromatographed on MgO-Hyflo Super Cel, 1 + 2.

(c) Quantification of individual carotenoid fractions. Set the spectrophotometer to the appropriate wavelength (λ_{max} from Table 3), dissolve the fraction in the listed solvent, make up to a known volume, and make any necessary dilutions. Calculate milligrams by the expression:

$$mg = \frac{A \times \text{dilution} \times \text{total mL} \times 10}{E_{1\ cm}^{1\%}}$$

Comment: This method separates provitamin A and non-provitamin A precursors from the extract. Each individual band or fraction can be assigned a microgram value that can be converted to retinol equivalents by use of appropriate factors. The method is slow and requires practice at column packing and pigment identification and rechromatography. Often the solvent schedule that works in purifying pigments from one tissue does not work for another because of interfering substances. Separations, while qualitatively correct, lend themselves to pigment degradation due to the long chromatographic procedure and subsequent purification steps.

4. *Spectrophotometry.* Determination of concentration. A recording spectrophotometer is preferred over the fixed wavelength or filter spectrophotometer.

(a) Wait 30 min after turning the power on and set instrument to read at the λ_{max} for the specific pigment in the pure solvent.

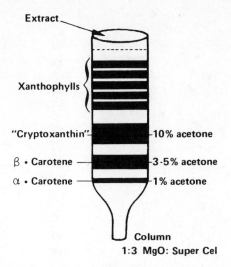

FIGURE 8.7 Chromatographic separation of carotenes from tomato fruits on 1 + 2 magnesium oxide-Hyflo Super Cel (43).

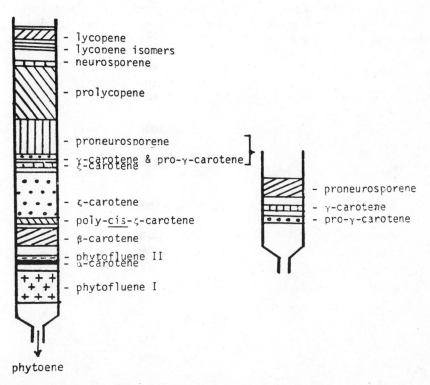

FIGURE 8.8 Chromatographic separation of carotenes from the tangerine tomato fruit on 1 + 2 magnesium oxide-Hyflo Super Cel (44).

(b) Prepare a standard calibration curve plotting absorption against concentration of a series of freshly prepared standard solutions (0.2–2.6 μg/mL). Measure the absorbancy of final sample solutions from Section I.D.3(a)(2)(iii) and Section I.D.3(b)(2)(v). Determine the concentration by reference to the standard curve.

5. *Calculation.* Calculate the carotene content of the original sample using:

$$\mu g\,\text{carotene}/g = \text{concentration}\,(\mu g/mL) \times \frac{\text{final volume}}{\text{sample, g wt.}} \times \text{dilution}$$

where concentration is from Section I.D.4(b); final vol. (mL) is from Section I.D.3(a)(2)(iii); sample wt. (g) is from Section I.D.1(a); and dilution (mL) is from Section I.D.1(g).

II. ALUMINA COLUMN CHROMATOGRAPHY FOR BLOOD/ PLASMA (45)

A. Principle

Following denaturation with 95% ethanol, the pigments are extracted with petroleum ether and separated on an alumina column. Absorbancy at 463 nm is the basis of quantification.

B. Equipment

1. *Chromatography Tubes.* Pyrex 22 × 175 mm with constricted ends.
2. *Refrigerated Centrifuge.*
3. *Rotary Vacuum Evaporator.*
4. *Spectrophotometer.*
5. *Separatory Funnels With Teflon Stopcocks.*

C. Reagents

1. *Petroleum Ether.* B.P. 30–60°C.
2. *95% Ethanol.*
3. *Acetone.*
4. *Alumina for Chromatography.* To alumina in a bottle add 6% H_2O, stopper, shake, and equilibrate for 1 hr.

D. Procedure

1. *Extraction.*

(a) Denature serum or plasma by the slow addition of an equal volume of 95% ethanol in a large centrifuge tube.

(b) Centrifuge and transfer the clear alcohol extract to a small separatory funnel. Add two volumes of petroleum ether, shake vigorously, and let stand until two layers separate.

(c) Discard the lower layer and concentrate the top petroleum ether layer to a small known volume with a stream of nitrogen or in a rotary vacuum evaporator.

2. *Chromatography Separation.*

(a) Column preparation. Proceed as in Section I.D.3(a)(1), but use deactivated alumina as the adsorbent. Wet the column by washing with petroleum ether.

(b) Adsorption and elution.

(1) Transfer pigments in a minimal volume of petroleum ether to top of column, as in Section I.D.3(a)(2)(i).

(2) Elute first the fraction containing β-carotene, α-carotene, less polar precursors such as phytofluene, and carotenoid esters with petroleum ether.

(3) Elute next lycopene and compounds with similar polarities with petroleum ether-acetone, 96 + 4 mixture.

(4) Elute finally lutein, zeaxanthin, and vitamin A alcohol with petroleum ether-acetone, 60 + 40 mixture.

(5) Collect the eluted fractions in different tubes and evaporate the fractions to dryness under vacuum; dissolve each fraction in a known volume of petroleum ether.

3. *Spectrophotometry.* Determination of concentration. Quantify by measuring absorbancy of the various eluted fractions as in Section I.D.4(a),(b),(c).

Comment: Since other carotenes are eluted with β-carotene, the estimate of provitamin A would be high, depending on the nature of the polyenes present. The method has been made into a micromethod by using capillary glass tubes (39).

III. THIN-LAYER CHROMATOGRAPHY (TLC)

A. Principle

TLC has mainly been used as a qualitative tool in the identification of carotenoids and in the detection of impurities. Samples are spotted or streaked on a suitable adsorbent supported by glass, plastic, or metal. Identification is based on the distance that the spot or band has moved. Quantification is made by the use of a densitometer or by removing the spot from the plate, extracting the compound, and quantifying based on light absorption properties.

B. Equipment and Reagents

    1. *Glass TLC Chamber.*

    2. *TLC Plates.*   Obtained commercially or spread with suitable adsorbent and binder (Table 8.6).

    3. *Reagent-Grade Solvents (Table 8.6).*

C. Procedure

A line is drawn on the plate about 1.5 cm from the bottom edge. Solvents (usually distilled or reagent grade) are selected appropriate to the separation scheme. The plate is spotted or streaked by use of a capillary pipette containing the saponified extract. The plate is dried under a stream of nitrogen and placed in the TLC chamber containing the developing solvent. The plate is removed from the chamber when the solvent front has advanced 10–15 cm up the plate. The spots may be identified directly if they are colored or made visible by reaction with antimony trichloride (24) or iodine vapor. R_f values are calculated as the distance from the center of the spot to the origin divided by the distance traveled by the solvent front. The spot may be scraped from the plate, extracted from the adsorbent, and its quantity determined in a spectrophotometer.

    Comment: Thin-layer chromatography has proven to be an indispensible tool in the qualitative aspects of carotene analysis. It has often been used as a preparative procedure. The method has been reported to be used for quantitative determination of carotenes. Targan et al. (25) report a 97% recovery of β-carotene standards using TLC, although the recovery is not routinely that high. Because of the difference in polarity of carotenoids, no single plate or solvent system will resolve all the carotenoids. A gradient is not practical, although solvent changes have been used. The basic advantages of the method are that it is simple and quick. It can be used for detecting impurities in fractions from other techniques, as well as determining the purity of standards.

    Table 8.6 lists the important provitamin A compounds and retinoids with the plate and solvent systems. The individual references should be consulted for details. The R_f values in Table 8.6 are relative values. Important references include Stahl (26), Davies (5), DeRitter and Purcell (22), and Hagar and Stransky (27).

    Paper chromatography (not covered here) has also found application in carotenoid separations, although TLC is probably more widely used because of its versatility (5). An excellent review of paper chromatography has been completed recently by Sestak (30).

VI.   HIGH-PERFORMANCE LIQUID CHROMATOGRAPHY (HPLC)

A. Principle

Following extraction and filtration the carotenoid pigments are separated, identified, and estimated at the same time by HPLC. Identification and quantification are based on retention time and peak area or peak height of individual pigments.

B. Equipment

Basic HPLC system:

1. *Solvent Delivery System.* Constant-rate pump with capacity of more than 3 mL/min and 2000 psi.

2. *Detector.* Either visible or UV detector. Variable wavelength detector with stop-scan capacity is preferable.

3. *Injection System.* Injector with sample valve or equivalent to precisely deliver 1–10 μL sample.

4. *Syringe.* Hamilton 710 or equivalent.

5. *Recorder with Integrator.*

6. *Column.* Various types of columns may be used (Table 8.8). A matched guard column is recommended.

7. *Solvent Programming System.* Programmer or equivalent to deliver gradient solvent system.

8. *Sample Clarification and Preparation System.*

    (a) Sampler Filter and Filter Holder. Sample clarification kit (Waters Associates or equivalent).

    (b) Sep-Pak C18 Cartridge (optional, but recommended), (Waters Associates).

C. Reagents

All reagents are HPLC grade. Filter solvents through 0.5 μm filter and degas under low pressure before use.

1. *Benzene.*
2. *Hexane.*
3. *Acetone.*
4. *Methanol.*
5. *Acetonitrile.*
6. *Chloroform.*
7. *Tetrahydrofuran.*
8. *Basic Alumina.*
9. *Spherisorb.*
10. *Magnesia.*
11. *HPLC Column.*
12. *α-Carotene-Type V.*
13. *β-Carotene-Type IV.*

Recrystallize these standards and use freshly prepared standard solutions. α- and β-carotene can be obtained from carrots or commercially. Solvents and columns used under different conditions are summarized in Table 8.8.

D. Procedure

1. *Preparation of Samples for Analysis.*

(a) Extract and saponify, if necessary, as described under Section I.D.1 and 2.

(1) Concentration of samples and elimination of some impurities contribute to sensitive and precise assays (46).

(b) Dissolve the samples in a solvent that has a polarity similar or close to that of the initial eluting solvent.

(1) Carotenoids dissolved in a more polar solvent can be absorbed in a reversed-phase Sep-Pak C18 and eluted by a less polar solvent. Filter the samples through a 0.5-μm membrane prior to injection.

(c) Store samples under refrigeration and nitrogen in the dark on a routine basis.

2. *Separation Methods.*   Available HPLC methods for carotenoid analysis are classified into four groups based upon the adsorbent-solvent system. General comments on these may help in selecting appropriate conditions that are suitable for the sample and the available facilities. Column techniques are not discussed here, however information is available in reference (47).

(a) Isocratic solvent system on normal-phase adsorbent.   It is difficult to develop a complete carotenoid profile with a single system of this nature. Systems 1 and 2 listed in Table 8.8 were developed to separate α-carotene, β-carotene, and cryptoxanthin by using two columns and two isocratic solvent combinations. Reeder and Park (33) have demonstrated an important advantage of the HPLC method by this system. Table 8.9 lists the carotenoids of orange juice determined by HPLC compared to the AOAC method. The AOAC method not only overestimates the quality of provitamin A by including carotenoids beside the three listed in the table, but overestimates the provitamin A activity since it cannot separate α-carotene and cryptoxanthin from β-carotene.

(b) Normal phase with gradient solvent system.   There are several systems reported that use a normal phase with a solvent gradient to separate mixtures of carotenes and xanthophylls (34,35,48,49,50). The long reequilibration period required at the initial stage for subsequent analysis is a disadvantage of this type of system. Figure 8.9 shows a successful resolution of α-carotene, β-carotene, ζ-carotene, α-cryptoxanthin, and β-cryptoxanthin on magnesium oxide by a gradient elution by an acetone-hexane mixture (34). Analytical HPLC on silica for the separation of carotenoids was investigated by Fiksdahl and co-workers (35). No separation of the double-bond positional isomers, α-carotene, and β-carotene was achieved on the silica column. This system is thus less desirable for provitamin A analysis.

(c) Reverse-phase isocratic solvent system.   This system uses column materials, such as octadecylsilane-bonded silica. The retention mechanism of reverse-phase chromatography relies on the hydrophobic interaction between

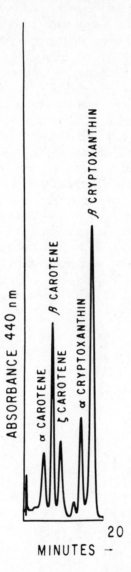

FIGURE 8.9 HPLC chromatogram of the principal carotenes and cryptoxanthin in citrus juice separated on magnesium oxide eluted with an acetone-η-hexane gradient solvent system (34).

the nonpolar hydrocarbon layer, solute, and relatively polar mobile phase. Under this system, only weak hydrophobic forces comparable to the partitioning between immiscible solvents are operative. These weak forces are far less destructive than ionic and polar forces in conventional chromatography, as demonstrated by Braumann and Grimme (36) in the rechromatography of the xanthophyll fraction of spinach, which had been separated on a low-pressure silica gel column. There is no system so far reported to separate all pigments by a single-step system with isocratic solvents. By careful selection of column and solvent, however, it is possible to resolve major carotenoids with provitamin A activity in a single-step isocratic system. Zakaria et al. (32) demonstrated that lycopene, α-carotene, and β-carotene can be separated by a Partisil-5/ODS column, eluted by 8% chloroform in acetonitrile. This system may not be able to resolve more polar xanthophylls, but is good for provitamin A carotenoids.

More recently Nelis and DeLeenheer (38) reported the separation of α-carotene, β-carotene, echinenone, and β-cryptoxanthin from the non-provitamin A compounds—lutein, zeaxanthin, canthaxanthin, lycopene, and torulene. This 32-min separation was on Zorbax ODS column (Dupont) with acetonitrile-dichloromethane-methanol as the mobile phase (Table 8.8 and Figure 8.10). Tsou (unpublished data) was able to separate some common carotenoids (β-cryptoxanthin, α,β-carotene, lycopene) on a Merck RP 18 column using acetone-methanol-acetonitrile (Table 8.8). Broich et al. (53) reported a good recovery of lycopene, α- and β-carotene, and retinyl esters on a Supelcosil LC-18 ODS-C18-5-μm packed column (Supleco). The 100-μL plasma sample was rapidly extracted and chromatographed with a solvent system of methanol-acetonitrile-

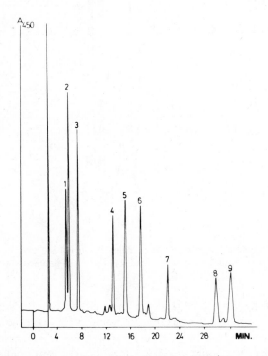

FIGURE 8.10 Separation of carotenoid standards on Zorbax ODS (25 cm × 0.46 cm). The mobile phase consisted of acetonitrile-dichloromethane-methanol (70 + 20 + 10, v/v). Flow rate was 1 mL/min and detection was at 450 nm. Peak identification: 1, lutein; 2, zeaxanthin; 3, canthaxanthin; 4, β-cryptoxanthin; 5, echinenone; 6, lycopene; 7, torulene; 8, α-carotene; 9, β-carotene (38).

chloroform (47 + 47 + 6). Two detection wavelengths were used for the carotenoids (466 nm) and retinyl esters (325 nm).

Peng et al. (54) also reported a β-carotene separation from plasma. These
authors used 500 μL plasma, a rather harsh perchloric acid extraction step, and
a complicated HPLC solvent system.

(d) Reverse-phase column with gradient solvent system. Both stepwise
gradient and single-step gradient elutions on reverse-phase chromatography
demonstrate successful separations of photosynthetic pigments (36,38,51).
Braumann and Grimme (36) reported that a column packed with Sil-60 RP-
18 10 μm (Riedel-de Hann, Hannover, FRG) and eluted with a linear gradient
of methanol-acetonitrile (25 + 75)-H$_2$O solvent system can resolve all the
chloroplastic pigments isolated from spinach and *Chlorella fusca*. This system
is able to separate *cis*-isomers and oxidation products from their parent
compounds (Figure 8.11). Isocratic runs on a 10-μm RP-18 column with
methanol-acetonitrile (25 + 75) give a complete resolution of chlorophyll b,
chlorophyll a, and β-carotene.

One drawback of the reverse-phase column with gradient solvent system is
the long re-equilibration period required with the initial solvent. The application
of a radial compressed cartridge does reduce the necessary back-washing time.
The radial compression module applies hydraulic pressure to compress a flexible
wall cartridge radially, thus producing a highly efficient column bed that is free
of voids and channels. Separations and re-equilibration are carried out while the
cartridge is under compression. RCM C18 cartridge 5 μm (Waters Associates)
eluted with a gradient solvent system of 3% water in methanol to 10% tetrahydrofuran (THF) in methanol resolved most carotenoids within 30 min. Re-
equilibration with the initial solvent for 10 min gave reproducible results (Table
8.10). An isocratic solvent of 10% THF in acetonitrile was found to resolve
cryptoxanthin, lycopene, α-carotene, and β-carotene within 25 min. With refinement, the RCM C18 method demonstrates potential as a routine method
for provitamin A analysis.

3. *Determination.* A suitable amount of standard carotene solution is injected into the chosen column-solvent system; retention time and the peak area
for the standard carotene sample are recorded in the resulting HPLC chromatogram. A suitable aliquot of the purified test material is then injected into the
column and the chromatogram developed under identical conditions. The pigment peaks (fractions) from the sample are identified on the basis of retention
time and quantified by the peak area.

CONCLUSION

Our interest in carotenoids stems from the fact that many foods are brightly
colored with these pigments. They are also germain to this chapter since 50–
60 of the approximately 500 carotenoids now known possess provitamin A

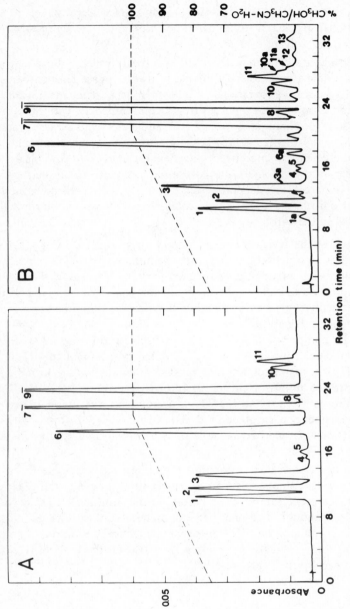

FIGURE 8.11 Chromatogram of a total pigment extract from *C. fusca*. (A) Extract immediately injected after preparation. (B) Extract aged for 3 hr and injected. Column, 10 μm RP-18; eluent; linear gradient of methanol-acetonitrile (25 + 75 v/v) - water as indicated by the dotted line; flow rate; 1.5 mL/min; sample volume, 5 μL. The peaks are: 1, neoxanthin; *cis*-neoxanthin; 2, trihydroxy-α-carotene; 3, violaxanthin; 3a, *cis*-violaxanthin; 4, lutein; 5, antheraxanthin; 6, lutein; 6a, *cis*-lutein; 7, chlorophyll b; 8, chlorophyll a isomer; 9, chlorophyll a; 10, α-carotene; 10a, *cis*-α-carotene; 11, β-carotene; 11a, *cis*-β-carotene; 12, chlorophyll a; 10, α-carotene; 10a, *cis*-α-carotene; 11, β-carotene; 11a, *cis*-β-carotene (36).

TABLE 8.10 Retention Times of Selected Carotenoids Separated by RCM C18 Cartridge with Gradient Elution

Injection	Neoxanthin	Violaxanthin (time in minutes)	Lutein	β-Carotene
1	3.45	4.24	7.42	26.5
2	3.46	4.26	7.47	26.7
3	3.48	4.27	7.49	26.9
4	3.46	4.25	7.46	26.6
5	3.48	4.28	7.51	26.7
Mean	3.47	4.26	7.46	26.7
SD	0.01	0.02	0.04	0.1

Source: Simpson (52).
Solvent gradient: A, H_2O-MeOH (3 + 97); B, THF-MeOH (10 + 90); 0–100% B 10-min curve 8; 10 min re-equilibration with solvent A between runs.

activity. The task of the vitamin A analyst is to separate and quantitate the provitamin A compounds from the inactive carotenoids. Further, the activity varies between β-carotene and the other carotenoids.

The methods detailed in this book range from the rather crude chromatographic procedure of the AOAC method to the sophisticated HPLC method. The HPLC method is clearly the method of choice, however, it may not be available. It is hoped that the caution and modifications mentioned in this chapter will allow a good estimation of the provitamin A content of plant and animal products.

ACKNOWLEDGMENT

This publication contains data that was obtained as a direct result of a USAID grant (DAN-1406G-35-1061-00) "Provitamin A Content in Foods in Southeast Asia," from the Office of Nutrition, Bureau for Science and Technology, U.S. Agency for International Development.

Rhode Island Agricultural Experiment Station Contribution No. 2108.

LITERATURE CITED

1. Peto, R., Doll, R., Buckley, J. D., and Sporn, M. B. "Can dietary β-carotene materially reduce human cancer rates?" *Nature* **290**, 201 (1981).

2. Isler, O. (Ed.) *Carotenoids.* Birkhauser Verlag, Basel, 851–864 (1971).

3. Straub, O. "List of natural carotenoids." In O. Isler, Ed., *Carotenoids.* Birkhauser Verlag, Basel, 771–850 (1971).

4. Bauernfeind, J. C. "Carotenoid vitamin A precursors and analogs in foods and feeds." *J. Agric. Food Chem.* **20**, 456 (1972).

5. Davies, B. H. "Analytical methods—carotenoids." In T. W. Goodwin, Ed., *Chemistry and Biochemistry of Plant Pigments*, Pt. 4. Academic Press, London, 38–165 (1976).

6. Vetter, W., Englert, G., Rigassi, N., and Schwieter, U. "Spectroscopic methods." In O. Isler, Ed., *Carotenoids*. Birkhauser Verlag, Basel, 189–266 (1971).

7. Tanaka, Y., Katayama, T., Simpson, K. L., and Chichester, C. O. "Stability of carotenoids on silica gel and other adsorbents." *Bull. Jap. Soc. Sci. Fish.* **46**, 799 (1981).

8. National Research Council, Food and Nutrition Board. *Recommended Dietary Allowances*, 9th ed. National Academy of Sciences, Washington, D.C. (1980).

9. Weedon, B. L. C. "Occurrence." In O. Isler, Ed., *Carotenoids*. Birkhauser Verlag, Basel, 29–60 (1971).

10. Simpson, K. L., Lee, T-C., Rodriguez, D. B., and Chichester, C. O. "Metabolism in senescent and stored tissues." In T. W. Goodwin, Ed., *Chemistry and Biochemistry of Plant Pigments*, Pt. 4. Academic Press, London, 780–842 (1976).

11. Zechmeister, L. *Cis-trans Isomeric Carotenoids, Vitamins A and Arylpolyenes*. Springer-Verlag, Vienna (1962).

12. Tsukuda, N. "Studies on the discoloration of red fishes—6. Partial purification and specificity of the enzyme responsible for carotenoid discoloration in red fish skin." *Bull. Jap. Soc. Sci. Fish.* **36**, 725 (1970).

13. Maeda, E. E. and Salunkhe, D. K. "Retention of ascorbic acid and total carotene in solar dried vegetables." *J. Food Sci.* **46**, 1288 (1981).

14. Simpson, K. L. and Chichester, C. O. "Nutritional significance of carotenoids." *Ann. Rev. Nutr.* **1**, 351–374 (1981).

15. Lee, T-C., Chen, T., Alid, G., and Chichester, C. O. "Stability of vitamin A and provitamin A (carotenoids) in extrusion cooking processing." *AICHE Symp Ser.* **74**, 192 (1978).

16. Rodriguez, D. B., Tanaka, Y., Katayama, T., Simpson, K. L., Lee, T-C., and Chichester, C. O."Hydroxylation of β-carotene on microcel-C." *J. Agric. Food Chem.* **24**, 819 (1976).

17. Cyronak, M. J., Osianu, D., Britton G., and Simpson, K. L. "Transformation of 13,14 and 11,13-monoepoxy-canthaxanthin on magnesia." *J. Agric. Food Chem.* **26**, 712 (1978).

18. Carnevale, J., Cole, E. R., and Crank, G. "Fluorescent light catalyzed autoxidation of β-carotene." *J. Agric. Food Chem.* **27**, 462 (1979).

19. Ben-Aziz, A., Britton, G., and Goodwin, T. W. "Carotene epoxides of *Lycopersicon esculentum*." *Phytochem.* **12**, 2759 (1973).

20. McAnally, J. S. and Szymanski, C. D. "Metabolism of alpha-carotene." *Nature* **210**, 1366 (1966).

21. Seely, G. R. and Meyer, T. H. "The photosensitized oxidation of β-carotene." *Phytochem. Photobiol.* **13**, 27 (1971).

22. DeRitter, E. and Purcell, A. E. "Carotenoid analytical methods." In J. C. Bauernfeind, Ed., *Carotenoids as Colorants and Vitamin A Precursors: Technological and Nutritional Applications*. Academic Press, New York (1981).

23. Taylor, R. F. and Ikawa, M. "Gas chromatography, mass spectroscopy, and high-pressure liquid chromatography of carotenoids and retinoids." *Methods in Enzymol.* **67** (1980).

24. Singh, H., John, J., and Cama, H. R. "Separation of beta-apocarotenals and related compounds by reverse phase paper and TLC." *J. Chromatogr.* **75**, 146 (1973).

25. Targan, S. R., Merrill, S., and Schwabe, A. D. "Fractionation and quantification of β-carotene and vitamin A derivatives in human serum." *Clin. Chem.* **15**, 479 (1969).

26. Stahl, E. *Thin Layer Chromqtography*. Springer Verlag, New York (1969).

27. Hager, A. and Stransky, H. "The carotenoid pattern and the occurrence of the light induced xanthophyll cycle in various classes of algae." *Arch. Microbiol.* **71**, 132 (1970).

28. Rodriguez, D. B., Raymundo, L. C., Lee, T-C., Simpson, K. L., and Chichester, C. O. "Carotenoid pigment changes in ripening *Momordica charantia* fruits." *Ann. Bot.* **40**, 615 (1976).

29. Schwieter, F., Bollinger, H. R., Chopard-dit-Jean, L. H., Englert, G., Koffer, M., Konig, A., Van-planta, C., Ruegg, R., Vetter, W., and Isler, O. "Synthesen in der Carotenoid-Reike 19 Mitteilung: Physikalische eigenschaften der carotine." *Chimia. Switz.* **19**, 294 (1965).

30. Sestak, Z. "Paper chromatography of chloroplast pigments (chlorophylls and carotenoids)—Pt. 3." *Photosynthetica* **14**, 239 (1980).

31. Association of Official Analytical Chemists. *Official Methods of Analysis,* 13th ed. Washington, D.C. (1980).

32. Zakaria, M., Simpson, K. L., Brown, P. R., and Krstulovic, A. "Use of reversed phase HPLC analysis for the determination of provitamin A carotenes in tomatoes." *J. Chromatogr.* **176**, 109 (1979).

33. Reeder, S. K. and Park, G. Y. "A specific method for the determination of provitamin A carotenoids in orange juice." *J. Assoc. Off. Anal. Chem.* **58**, 595 (1975).

34. Stewart, I. "High performance liquid chromatographic determination of provitamin A carotenoids in orange juice." *J. Assoc. Off. Anal. Chem.* **60**, 132 (1977).

35. Fiksalh, A., Mortensen, J. T., and Liaaen-Jensen, S. "High pressure liquid chromatography of carotenoids." *J. Chromatogr.* **157**, 111 (1978).

36. Braumann, T. and Grimme, L. H. "Reversed-phase high-performance liquid chromatography of chlorophylls and carotenoids." *Biochim Biophys. Acta* **637**, 8 (1981).

37. Tsou, S. C. and Simpson, K. L. Unpublished.

38. Nelis, H. J. C. F. and DeLeenheer, A. P. "Isocratic nonaqueous reversed-phase liquid chromatography of carotenoids." *Anal. Chem.* **55**, 270 (1983).

39. McLaren, D. S., Read, W. W. C., Awdeh, Z. L., and Tchalian, M. "Micro-determination of vitamin A and carotenoids in blood and tissue." In D. Glick, Ed., *Methods of Biochemical Analysis,* Vol. 15. Wiley, New York (1967).

40. Gebhardt, S. E., Elkins, E. R., and Humphrey, J. "Comparison of two methods for determining the vitamin A value of Clingstone peaches." *J. Agric. Food Chem.* **25**, 629 (1977).

41. Watada, A. E., Aulenbach, B. B., and Worthington, J. T. "Vitamin A and C in ripe tomatoes as affected by stage of ripeness at harvest and supplementary ethylene." *J. Food Sci.* **41**, 856 (1976).

42. Mathews, R. F., Crill, P., and Lagascia, S. J. "β-carotene and ascorbic acid contents of tomato as affected by maturity." *Proc. Fla. State Hort. Soc.* **87**, 214 (1974).

43. Chang, Yu-Huey. "Studies on the carotenoids of tomato and corn." M.S. Thesis, University of Rhode Island, Kingston (1977).

44. Glass, R. G. "Carotenoids in plants." Ph.D. Thesis, University of Rhode Island, Kingston (1975).

45. Krinsky, N. I., Cornwall, D. G., and Oncley, J. L. "The transport of vitamin A and carotenes in human plasma." *Arch. Biochem. Biophys.* **73**, 223 (1958).

46. Waters Association Technical Sheets Nos. 4438 and 4439.

47. Simpson, C. F. "Appendix II: Column packing techniques." In C. F. Simpson, Ed., *Practical High Performance Liquid Chromatography.* Heyden and Son, London (1976).

48. Stewart, I. "Provitamin A and carotenoid content of citrus juice." *J. Agric. Food Chem.* **25**, 1132 (1977).

49. Stewart, I. and Wheaton, T. A. "Continuous flow separation of carotenoids by liquid chromatography." *J. Chromatogr.* **55**, 325 (1971).

50. Iriyama, K., Yoshiura, M., and Shiraki, M. "Micro-method for the qualitative and quantitative analysis of photosynthetic pigments using high performance liquid chromatography." *J. Chromatogr.* **154**, 302 (1978).

51. Eskins, K., Scholfield, C. R., and Dutton, H. J. "High-performance liquid chromatography of plant pigments." *J. Chromatogr.* **135**, 217 (1977).

52. Simpson, K. L. "Relative value of carotenoids as precursors of vitamin A." *Proc. Nutr. Soc.* **42**, 7 (1983).

53. Broich, C. R., Gerber, L. E., and Erdman, Jr., J. W. "Determination of lycopene, α- and β-carotene and retinyl esters in human serum by reversed-phase HPLC." *Lipids.* **18**, 253–258 (1983).

54. Peng, Y-M., Beaudry, J., Alberts, D. S., and Davis, T. P. "HPLC of the provitamin A β-carotene in plasma." *J. Chromatogr.* **273**, 410–414 (1983).

9 Vitamin D

Laxman Singh

GENERAL CONSIDERATIONS

The name vitamin D was given in the early 1920s to the active component present in cod liver oil, which could cure or prevent rickets, the disease characterized by defective ossification, disturbance of calcium uptake, and a resulting weakness and deformation of the bones (1).

A. Vitamin Forms, Isomers, Nomenclature

The most important forms of vitamin D are vitamin D_2 (ergocalciferol or calciferol) and vitamin D_3 (cholecalciferol). Ergocalciferol is formed by ultraviolet irradiation of the provitamin ergosterol, which is synthesized only by plants, mainly yeasts and fungi. Cholecalciferol is formed by the ultraviolet irradiation of provitamin 7-dehydrocholesterol, which in turn is synthesized from cholesterol found in animal tissues (2). Vitamin D_1 was an earlier preparation consisting of a 1 + 1 complex of the active compound with lumisterol, an inactive isomer (3).

The structural formulas of vitamins D_2 and D_3 are shown in Figure 9.1 and various physical and chemical properties are summarized in Table 9.1. Chemical structure of the vitamins differs only in the side chain attached to C-17. Ergocalciferol has an additional double bond at C-22 and methyl group instead of hydrogen at C-24.

Following the IUPAC rules for steroid nomenclature (3), the full notation for ergocalciferol is 9,10-seco-(5Z,7E)-5,7,10(19),22-ergostatetraen-3-β-ol. An understanding of chemical configuration is helpful in the development of analytical methods for vitamins D. Due to the close structural relationships of the two vitamins, most of their chemical properties are similar and, therefore, their

221

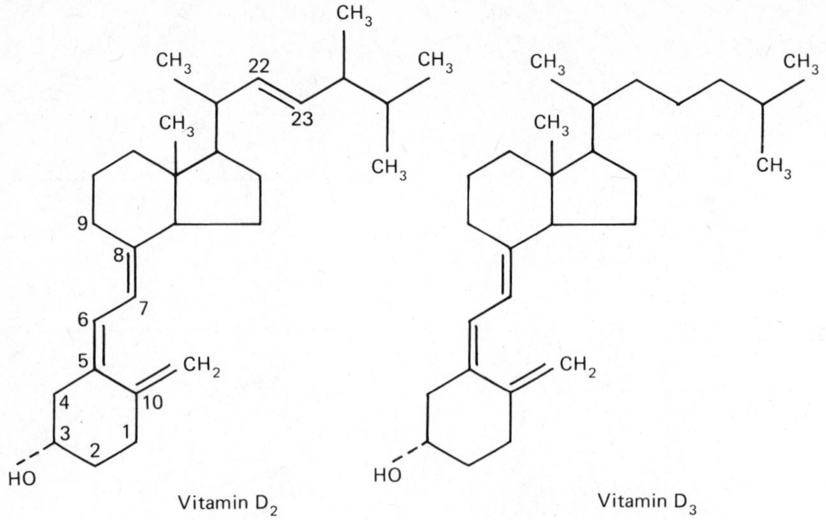

FIGURE 9.1   Structure of vitamin D$_2$ and vitamin D$_3$.

analytical methods are also identical. The main difference, however, between the two vitamins is that D$_2$ is not biologically active for birds.

Irradiation of provitamin D (ergosterol or 7-dehydrocholesterol) with ultraviolet light generates a mixture of diene and triene isomers (1). According to generally accepted reaction sequence, provitamin converts to previtamin (D$_2$ or D$_3$), which in turn may convert to tachysterol and/or lumisterol. Conversion of previtamin to vitamin D is strictly a thermal transformation. All these isomerization reactions are known to be reversible in nature. Vitamin D also undergoes *cis/trans*-isomerization. Being a complex polycyclic ring molecule, 64 different isomers are possible in theory. In practice, the triene isomers are of significance from a chemical analysis point of view, since they also react similar to vitamin D. Isotachysterol, tachysterol, and 5,6-*trans* calciferol are the main triene isomers in that respect.

TABLE 9.1   Physical and Chemical Properties of Vitamins D (2,4,5)

	D$_2$	D$_3$
Empirical formula	C$_{28}$H$_{44}$O	C$_{27}$H$_{44}$O
Molecular weight	396.6	384.6
Melting point (°C)	115–118	84–88
Absorption maximum (nm)	265	265
Specific absorption (E$_{1\text{cm}}^{1\%}$)	459	473
Optical rotation [α] in alcohol	+103°–+106°	+105°–+112°
Potency (IU/g)	40 Million	40 Million
Biological activity	Mammals	Mammals and birds

Vitamin D is considered both a vitamin and hormone. This essential micronutrient is ingested along with food. Some individuals can get adequate vitamin D through sunlight activation of 7-dehydrocholesterol in their skin and do not need vitamin D supplementation. Vitamin D is converted in the kidney to the most active metabolite 1,25-dihydroxyvitamin D_3 [1α,25,$(OH)_2$,D_3] and functions in the intestine and bones. This metabolite carries out all the known functions of vitamin D and is considered to be a hormone; thus, vitamin D is a prohormone. There are also other vitamin D metabolites.

Vitamin D is involved in normal mineralization of bone and endochondral calcification and prevents rickets in the young and osteomalacia and osteoporosis in the adult. Parathyroid hormone and vitamin D prevent hypocalcemic tetany. Despite adequate vitamin D intake, some bone diseases occur due to defective vitamin D metabolism and lack of circulating vitamin D metabolites.

Prolonged intake of excessive doses of vitamin D leads to hypercalcemia or hypercalciuria (abnormal calcium levels) in blood serum. Prolonged hypercalcemia causes irreversible renal, heart, and aortic damage.

B. Occurrence and Stability

Vitamin D is present in nature in very low amounts and only in few food materials, for example, fish liver oil and eggs. Nonfortified milk, butter, cheese, and ice cream, and animal liver contain only traces of vitamin D (6). Dairy products sold often are fortified with vitamin D. Generally, vitamin D as such is fairly stable. However, the presence of minerals and other constituents in samples affects its stability. Vitamin D is sensitive to heat. It is also sensitive to air. Therefore, antioxidants are used during the assay. Saponification and other heat treatments cause thermal isomerization of vitamin D to previtamin D and therefore proper care should be taken during analysis to prevent this from occurring. Greenbaum (7) has reviewed vitamin D forms and their stabilities, availabilities, and actions.

Vitamin D is found in the animal body or animal product in both free and esterified forms. Most of the bound vitamin D in animals is esterified at the C-3 position with fatty acids or other acids. However, in most analytical systems such as those listed in Table 9.2, vitamin D is present in its free, unesterified form. Small quantities of diene and triene isomers may also be present. Saponification and extraction are frequently necessary to release vitamin D from the sample matrix and to remove fat from the unsaponifiable phase. In some cases, when stabilized powders and beadlets are used as a source, it becomes necessary to hydrolyze the sample before vitamin D can be extracted.

In addition to isomers, another consideration for vitamin D assay is the presence of other fat-soluble vitamins, such as A, E, and carotenoids. In most samples, these vitamins are present many times (50–100) the amount of vitamin D. These compounds interfere in analyses and must be removed before an accurate determination of vitamin D can be made.

One International Unit (IU) of vitamin D is the activity of 0.025 μg of

TABLE 9.2   Types of Vitamin D Samples

Preparation	IU/g
1. Crystalline vitamin D	40,000,000
2. Vitamin D concentrates	
a. Resins	≥ 20,000,000
b. Oily solutions	≥ 100,000
c. Powders, capsules, tablets, and aqueous dispersions	≥ 25,000
3. Multivitamin preparations	
a. Oily solutions	500–100,000
b. Powders, capsules, tablets, and aqueous dispersions	200–25,000
4. Mixed feeds, premixes, pet foods	2–200
5. Milk, margarine, foods	≤ 2

crystalline cholecalciferol. The United States Pharmacopeia (USP) Unit and the International Chick Unit (IC) are identical to IU. Due to 3% difference in the molecular weights of vitamin D_2 and D_3, the IU for D_2 is equivalent to 0.0258 μg (8). The United States Recommended Daily Allowance (USRDA) for vitamin D is 400 IU.

METHODS AVAILABLE

Several review publications have emerged over the past few years that cover recent developments in vitamin D analysis (2,9–13). Recently, Parrish (6) published a thorough review on determination of vitamin D in foods. The choice of method depends on the type of samples, saponification, and solvent extraction procedures. Several methods are available and categorized as physicochemical, chromatographic, and biological methods.

A.   Physicochemical Methods

Spectrophotometry

Ultraviolet spectrophotometry is one of the earliest methods used to determine vitamin D in fairly concentrated and pure forms. The absorbance of vitamin D solution in ethanol is determined at 265 nm and vitamin D content is calculated from the appropriate specific extinction and absorption values. Other solvents such as hexane and cyclohexane can also be used. This method is applicable only for vitamin D in highly purified forms because the isomers of vitamin D, other vitamins, and impurities interfere. Vitamin D tablets and dry dispersions have been analyzed after appropriate extraction and purification (9). The spectrophotometric method, however, has very limited use.

Infrared spectrophotometry of vitamin D dissolved in carbon disulfide between 10 nm and 11 nm and nuclear magnetic resonance (NMR) spectroscopy of vitamin D in deuterochloroform are used to differentiate between pure vitamin D_2 and D_3 (9).

Colorimetric assay using antimonytrichloride reagent ($SbCl_3$ dissolved in $CHCl_3$) is the basis of several tested, generally accepted, and official procedures to estimate vitamin D in the final purified extract (9,10,16,17). Vitamin D gives an orange-yellow color with $SbCl_3$ and the absorbance is measured at 500 nm. The earlier procedure had been improved over the years to the present form. Addition of acetyl chloride to $SbCl_3$ reagent increased the stability of the color, speed of color development, and sensitivity (14,15). The $SbCl_3$ reagent, with ethylene dichloride as the solvent, is stable for at least 10 weeks and reacts with vitamin D to give a salmon-pink color (16,17).

Vitamins A, E, and other interfering compounds are removed from the final sample extract by adsorption or partition chromatography, since vitamin A also reacts with $SbCl_3$ to form a deep blue color. Acetic anhydride, which inhibits the $SbCl_3$–vitamin D reaction, is utilized to correct any nonspecific absorbance (i.e., $SbCl_3$ reading for nonvitamin D color) due mainly to any residual traces of vitamin A or its oxidation products.

Vitamin D triene *trans*-isomers, especially tachysterol and isotachysterol, also react with $SbCl_3$ reagent. Treatment with maleic anhydride inactivates tachysterol. Absorbancy values before and after maleic anhydride treatment are used to correct for isotachysterol, when its presence is established by a confirmatory test (18).

All these improvements are utilized in the recent AOAC procedure (17). Reproducible results are claimed for vitamin D concentrates and pharmaceutical preparations. The results are less satisfactory for samples with low vitamin D content.

Other reagents used in developing color complexes with vitamin D include trifluoroacetic acid, trichloroacetic acid, glycerol dichlorohydrin, and iodine-ethylene dichloride (6). The dichlorohydrin reaction with vitamin D compounds in the presence of acetyl chloride, differentiates vitamins D_2 and D_3 from ergosterol and 7-dehydrocholesterol; and ergosterol from 7-dehydrocholesterol.

Absorption and partition chromatography are most common for reducing or eliminating vitamins A, E, and their decomposition products. Phosphate-treated deactivated alumina chromatography eliminates tocopherols and vitamin A decomposition products, partition chromatography with polyethylene glycol 600 and celite separate vitamin D from vitamin A alcohol, and absorption chromatography on Florex removes vitamin A decomposition products and any traces of polyethylene glycol (19). Chromosorb W is preferred over Celite as a stationary phase for partition chromatography (20). Panalaks (21) used several chromatographic steps to determine vitamin D in the range of 0.2–0.4 IU/g present in fortified whole milk and skim milk. These include: removal of cholesterol on digitonin-impregnated Celite, removal of vitamin A alcohol by partition chromatography on Celite-polyethylene glycol, removal of carotenoids and decomposition products of vitamin A on the basic alumina column, and finally purification on a silicic acid microcolumn to eliminate subsequent colorimetric interfering substances.

Vitamin D in pharmaceuticals is determined by the USP chemical method (16). After saponification of the sample in alcoholic KOH in the presence of butylated hydroxytoluene (BHT), the vitamin is extracted with ethyl ether and the ether extract is dried and evaporated. Hexane solution of the residue is chromatographed on a siliceous earth-polyethylene glycol 600 partition column, prepared in isooctane. Hexane elution separates vitamin D from A, which remains on the column. The concentrated eluate is layered next on a Fullers earth absorption column. Elution with benzene removes vitamin D from the column. This final eluate is concentrated and treated with $SbCl_3$-acetyl chloride reagent in ethylene dichloride. A second aliquot is treated with acetic anhydride followed by $SbCl_3$ reagent. Absorbances are measured initially at 500 nm and at 550 nm, 45 sec after the initial reading, to correct for any nonspecific color development.

The AOAC method is based on the USP method and includes an additional treatment with maleic anhydride to inactive vitamin D *trans* isomers. This is significant for samples where resins are the source of vitamin D supplements. Three column chromatographic purifications are used depending on the samples. Methods were developed for concentrates and for multivitamin preparations (17,22–26).

Thin-Layer Chromatography (TLC)

This is an easy and rapid method for identification of vitamin D, adapted for quantitative assays. Vitamin A, E, and isomers of vitamin D are separated on appropriate absorbent and solvent systems. TLC methods have been used to study vitamin decomposition during alkaline hydrolysis and thermal isomerization to previtamins, and to detect and assay vitamin D in crude irradiation mixture (9). USP identification tests for ergocalciferol and cholecalciferol employ TLC (4). Silica gel plates are more widely used than alumina plates (27). The preferred solvent system for silica gel plates is cyclohexane and ether (1 + 1). Other solvent systems include chloroform, 9 + 1 hexane-ethyl acetate, 6 + 4 cyclohexane-chloroform, and 98 + 2 benzene-methanol (28). Detection is usually done by spraying with antimony trichloride-acetyl chloride reagent. For quantitative analysis, a sample extract is streaked on silica gel plate and the chromatogram is developed in suitable solvent. Vitamin D (and previtamin D) bands are scraped and eluted in chloroform and concentration of vitamin D measured colorimetrically using antimony trichloride reagent (9).

Gas-Liquid Chromatography (GLC)

These methods have been developed to determine vitamin D in low concentrations. Several reviews have recently appeared on this technique (29,30,31). Kobayashi et al. used GLC for vitamin D determination in multivitamin preparation (32), preparation containing excess amounts of vitamin E (33), and in tuna liver and resin oils (34). Extensive purification of the samples is required before injecting onto the GLC column. These pretreatments include TLC, column chromatography on phosphate-treated alumina, and digitonin-celite chromatography. TMS ether derivative formation was found necessary in most cases. GLC has been used to monitor synthesis of vitamin D, to assay vitamin D in pharmaceutical preparation, tissues, fortified dried milk, and other products with low vitamin D content (29,35,36,37).

GLC methods for vitamin D are not widely used despite the claim for high sensitivity. Calciferols are converted to pyrocalciferols in the column operating at high temperatures. Separation of different isomers is not very efficient. Furthermore, extensive sample cleanup is required. Thus, this technique does not lend itself for routine analyses.

High-Performance Liquid Chromatography (HPLC)

This is the latest new technique for vitamin D analysis. It offers greater speed, sensitivity, and specificity to individual vitamins and their isomers. Furthermore, it lends itself to the simultaneous determination of vitamins A, D, and E (61). Burns et al. (38) presented a rationalization of the chromatographic behavior of vitamin D_2, D_3, and related compounds in adsorption HPLC.

The choice of the system for vitamin D depends on [1] the presence of vitamin D isomers, [2] the presence of the other fat-soluble vitamins, and [3] the concentration of vitamin D in samples. Since previtamin and vitamin D are separated, each with a different retention time, it is essential that both these are measured for the total "potential vitamin D." HPLC methods are suitable for the groups of samples mentioned in Table 9.2.

USP XX (16) assay methods for pure cholecalciferol and pure ergocalciferol utilize HPLC technique, with 70 + 30 + 1 chloroform-n-hexane-tetrahydrofuran as mobile phase (4,5).

Hofsass et al. (39) published a detailed procedure for determination of vitamin D_3 in resins, oils, and dry concentrates with and without vitamin A. Normal-phase silica column and 1.6% ethanol in isooctane as mobile phase were used. Retention times for previtamin and vitamin D_3 were 7.4 min and 10.5 min, respectively. The method worked well in most concentrates. However, the limitations were the lack of separation of previtamin D and 5-6-*trans*-vitamin D and the use of fixed previtamin/vitamin conversion factor. Meanwhile, DeVries et al. (40) used 0.35% amyl alcohol in n-hexane as mobile phase. A previtamin conversion factor was determined for each system. These two methods were collaboratively studied for concentrates (41).

The official AOAC method for resins is based on the method of DeVries et al. (40,42). The extraction procedure was improved using ether and pentane to resolve the discrepancies in values between chemical and HPLC methods for resin-containing powders (43). DeVries et al. (44) developed a two-column method to separate vitamin D from A and E in multivitamin samples. The first, a reverse-phase Lichrosorb RP 8 (10 μm) cleanup column using 50 + 50 + 2 acetonitrile-methanol-water solvent, separates vitamin D from A, E, and other interferences. The second, a normal-phase silica column (10 μm Partisil) using 0.35% amyl alcohol in n-hexane as the mobile phase separates vitamin D from its isomers. Few recommendations for improvement of this method were made on the basis of collaborative studies (45). Another HPLC method for multivitamin preparation of oil, dry concentrate, and gelatin capsule did not involve any saponification (46).

Premixes, mixed feeds, and pet foods containing 2–200 IU vitamin D/g are analyzed by AOAC method (47). After extraction and before cleanup reverse-phase HPLC, alumina column chromatography is performed to remove tocopherols. Final determination is still made on a normal-phase silica analytical column. For livestock feed supplements, normal-phase Porasil column for cleanup and reverse-phase C18 column for final analyses were used (48). Lein et al. analyzed animal feed premixes on a Lichrosorb NH_2 column preceded by silica precolumn for cleanup (49).

Fortified milk and milk powders have been analyzed for vitamin D by HPLC by several workers. Thompson et al. (50) developed a method for fortified milk, which involved saponification, ether extraction, chromatography on HAPS, and HPLC on 5-μm Lichrosorb Si 60 and 0.6% isopropanol in hexane as mobile phase. This procedure was recently improved for fortified milk, margarine, and infant formulas (51). Milk was saponified overnight at room temperature with 1% ethanolic pyrogallol and KOH. Hexane extract of the digest was first chromatographed on 5-μm silica column and vitamin D fraction was rechromatographed on reverse phase (Spherisorb 10 ODS) using 1 + 9 methanol-acetonitrile solvent system. Recovery of vitamin D was reported to be 96–99% with coefficient of variation of 3%. Another method for instant nonfat dried milk involved Sep-Pak and Partisil column cleanup and final HPLC on Lichrosorb NH_2 (52). AOAC method (53,54) utilizes the same cleanup and analytical (silica) column as for multivitamin preparations. Detection up to 15 IU/quart and separation of D_2 and D_3 in milk were reported (55). A method for margarine requires dual chromatographic cleanup before final analysis on reverse-phase analytical column (56).

Animal feeds containing low levels of vitamin D_3 (0.5–4 IU/g) were analyzed by Cohen et al. (57). Steps in this procedure are: sample extraction with dichloromethane, sequential cleanup on a Sep-Pak silica cartridge followed by Sephadex LH-20, and on a HPLC silica column followed by analysis on a phenyl column.

HPLC method separates D_2 and D_3 while determining both in the same sample (55,58,59). This is used for the analysis of vitamin D metabolites and analogs including 25-OH-cholecalciferol and 1,25-$(OH)_2$-cholecalciferol (60). An automated HPLC system for simultaneous determination of vitamin A, D, and E has been described (61). An interlaboratory evaluation of 12 vitamin D assay methods, which included chemical, GLC, and HPLC procedures, showed that HPLC is the most promising (62).

B. Biological Methods

The most used biological methods for determination of vitamin D are the "line test" with rats and bone ash with chicks (4,63). In the rat curative test, weanling rats are placed on a rachitogenic diet for a 16–25-day vitamin D depletion period. Daily supplements of test material and reference standards are then supplied in the diet. After 7–12 days, animals are sacrificed and the proximal end of a tibia or distal end of a radius or ulna is split and stained with silver nitrate. A line is formed and degree of calcification of rachitic metaphysis is recorded. Length and width of this line are the basis of estimation of potency.

Standard bioassay of vitamin D products intended for poultry is a prophylactic test based on determination of percentage of bone ash. Newly hatched chicks are fed graded levels of test preparation and reference standard of vitamin D_3 for a period of 21 days. The birds are then killed and bone ash percentage of dry, fat-free tibia is determined as a measure of vitamin D_3 International Chick Units. Toe ash measurements can also be used as a response to vitamin D.

Biological methods are time consuming, expensive, and lack precision, but are specific and sensitive. In a comparative study of vitamin D_3 methods, the coefficient of variation (c.v.) in chick bioassay was found to be 15%, with a single determination variation of $\pm 30\%$. Chemical assay on resins on oil, on the other hand, showed less than 2% c.v. (64). Bioassays, however, will continue to be required to verify validity of new assays and to establish the antirachitic activity of new compounds and isomers. Using the chick assay, for example, the antirachitic activity of 5,6-*trans*-vitamin D_3 was found to be less than 5% of cholecalciferol (65).

ANALYTICAL METHODOLOGY

I.   COLORIMETRIC METHOD

A.   Principle

This method is based upon the measurement of the salmon-pink color that develops when D vitamins interact with $SbCl_3$ in ethylene dichloride. The absorbance of the pink solution at 500 nm is proportional to the concentration of vitamin D. Prior to color development, and depending on the sample matrix to be analyzed, vitamin D needs to be purified from interfering substances according to the summary outline presented in Table 9.3. The purpose of the chromatographic treatment is to separate vitamin D from vitamins A, E, and carotenes, as well as BHT. Treatment of the extracts with maleic anhydride removes the *trans*-isomer tachysterol. Lumisterol, provitamins, suprasterols, and polymers do not interfere in the colorimetry. Acetic anhydride, which completely and selectively inhibits the vitamin D–$SbCl_3$ reaction, is used in some instances to correct for the presence of any decomposition products of vitamin A that may not have been removed during sample purification.

The method is based on the procedure developed by AOAC, and is applicable to single and multiple vitamin preparations as well as to fortified food and food matrices, generally containing 200 IU/g vitamin D or more. Acceptable results, however, have also been obtained with systems containing smaller concentrations of this vitamin.

TABLE 9.3 Scheme for Chemical Analysis of Vitamin D Preparations

Preparation	D Content IU/g	Saponification	Alumina Chromatography	PEG-Florex Chromatography	Maleic Anhydride Treatment	Spectrophotometry 500 + 550nm	500 nm only
Resins	≥20,000,000				X		X
Vitamin D Concentrates							
a. oils	≥100,000	X			X		X
b. powders, etc.	≥25,000	X			X		X
Samples containing vitamins A & E	≥200	X	X	X		X	
Samples without other vitamins	≥200	X	X		X		X

The assay must be completed promptly, and sample exposure to air and light must be minimized through the use of antioxidants, inert gases, and low-actinic glassware.

B. Equipment

1. *Flasks.* With ground joints, suitable for the saponification of the sample to be assayed.

2. *Condensers.* Water or air-cooled, with suitable ground joints.

3. *Water Bath.* Thermostatically controlled for supplying heat for saponification and solvent removal. Thermoregulated hot plates and steam baths may also be used.

4. *Flash Evaporator or Rotary Evaporator.* For solvent removal.

5. *Vacuum Pump.* Or other system suitable for solvent removal and chromatography.

6. *Ultraviolet Lamp.* The lamp should provide weak ultraviolet radiation in the longer (360 nm) region. Suitable commercial models are available.

7. *Spectrophotometer.* Any model suitable to read at 500-nm and 550-nm wavelength using 2-cm tubes or 1-cm cuvets.

8. *Chromatography Tubes.*

(a) For columns I and III (steps D.1 and D.3) 20-mm × 150-mm (i.d.) glass tube with a 250-mL bulb at the top and a coarse fritted glass disc about 30 mm from the bottom, which is constricted to 8 mm below the disc and fitted with a Teflon stopcock.

(b) For column II (step D.2) same as above but 300 mm long and without reservoir.

C. Reagents

All reagents should meet ACS specifications or be of reagent grade unless otherwise specified.

1. *Solvents.*

(a) Acetic anhydride, 95%.

(b) Acetyl chloride, colorless; distill if necessary.

(c) 95% ethanol, SD3A denatured alcohol.

(d) Benzene

(e) Ethyl ether, peroxide and acid free.

(f) Ethylene dichloride (1,2-dichloroethane), nanograde or redistilled reagent grade.

(g) Isooctane (2,2,4-trimethylpentane), acid free.

(h) Petroleum ether (pet ether) reflux over KOH pellets for 1 hr and collect fraction distilling between 40°C and 65°C.

(i) Polyethylene glycol 600, peroxide and acid free.

(j) Toluene, acid free.

(k) Solvent hexane.

2. *Ethyl Ether–Petroleum Ether Eluants.*   8% and 30% ether in petroleum ether.

3. *Sodium Ascorbate Solution.*   Dissolve 3.5 g ascorbic acid in 20 mL 1 N NaOH. Prepare fresh daily.

4. *Potassium Hydroxide Solutions.*   3% (w/v), 6% (w/v), and 50% (w/w) in H_2O.

5. *20% Pyrogallol Solution.*   Dissolve 20 g pyrogallol in alcohol and dilute to 100 mL.

6. *10% Sodium Sulfide Solution.*   Dissolve 120 g $Na_2S\cdot9H_2O$ in 20 mL H_2O and dilute to 100 mL with 87% glycerol.

7. *0.01% β-Carotene Solution In Isooctane.*

8. *0.1% BHT Solution In Toluene.*

9. *Ethoxyquin Solution.*   0.05 mg/mL in pet ether.

10. *Sodium Sulfate.*   Anhydrous, granular.

11. *Color-Inhibiting Solution.*   Isooctane-toluene-acetic anhydride, 1 + 1 + 1.

12. *Maleic Anhydride Solutions.*

(a) 10% Stock solution. Dissolve 10 g maleic anhydride (distilled, b.p. 196°C) in 100 mL toluene (clear solution, stable for 1 month).

(b) 1% Working solution. Just before use dilute aliquot with toluene to obtain 1% solution.

13. *Column Chromatographic Material.*

(a) Alumina, Type 1076 (E. Merck).

(b) Disodium hydrogen phosphate, $Na_2HPO_4\cdot2H_2O$.

(c) Diatomaceous earth, acid washed Chromosorb W, 80–100 mesh (150–180 μm) or Celite 545 (Johns-Manville), 90% > 125 μm.

(d) Granular fullers earth, Florex - XXS (Floridin Co). Sieve and retain 80–100 mesh portion.

14. *Color Reagent.*   Prepare two stock solutions: *Solution A*: Dissolve about 100 g $SbCl_3$ (dry, crystalline, and if necessary, distilled) in 400 mL ethylene dichloride. Add 2 g anhydrous alumina, mix, and filter through paper into 500-mL volumetric flask. Dilute to volume with ethylene dichloride and mix. Absorbance of solution, determined in 2-cm cell at 500 nm with spectrophotometer against ethylene dichloride should be <0.070. (*Caution*: $SbCl_3$ is toxic and corrosive. Avoid contact with skin and eyes and breathing vapor.) *Solution B*: Mix under hood 100 mL colorless, distilled acetyl chloride and 400 mL ethylene dichloride and store in cool place. Mix 90 mL Solution A and 10 mL Solution B. Store in brown glass bottle and use within 7 days; discard if any color develops.

15. *Vitamin Standards.* USP Reference Standard Ergocalciferol (vitamin D_2) or cholecalciferol (vitamin D or D_3). Dissolve about 25 mg calciferol reference standard, accurately weighed, in 100 mL of 20% toluene in isooctane solution containing 0.5 mg BHT/mL. Solution is stable for 1 month, if kept in dark room at room temperature. On day of assay, pipette 2 mL concentrated standard solution into 100-mL volumetric flask and dilute to volume with 20% toluene in isooctane. This solution contains about 200 IU/mL.

D. Chromatographic Column Preparation

1. *Column I, Alumina.* For samples with low vitamin D content containing other fat-soluble vitamins:

(a) Preparation and deactivation of phosphate-treated alumina. Sieve alumina and collect 50–150 μm (30–80 mesh) fraction. Heat 250 g sieved alumina with 1.6 L H_2O and 20 g $Na_2HPO_4 \cdot 2H_2O$ in 2-L Erlenmeyer flask 30 min on steam bath, swirling occasionally. Cool, swirl gently, and decant upper layer, which may contain suspension of fine particles. Filter residue by suction on paper using a Buchner funnel. Transfer alumina to 22-cm-diameter porcelain disk. Dry in 150°C oven for 3 hr, mixing occasionally to prevent lumping. Cool disk in a vacuum desiccator. Store activated alumina in airtight (rubber-stoppered) container.

Weigh 30 g dried alumina into 100-mL Erlenmeyer flask, add 1.5 mL H_2O by pipette, and close flask with rubber stopper. Heat 5 min on steam bath. Vigorously shake warm flask until powder is free flowing. Cool and let stand 15 min. Check activity of this batch of deactivated phosphate-treated alumina (5% water) by column performance test (see below). If column performance is < 97%, repeat deactivation, using a different amount of H_2O.

(b) Preparation of column. Add 40 mL pet ether to deactivated alumina, swirl, and transfer to tube, using petroleum ether. Let packing settle, maintain head of ≥ 0.5 cm liquid on column throughout assay, and use nitrogen gas to regulate flow rate at 4–5 mL/min. (Phosphate-treated alumina column can be used for only one assay.)

2. Column II, Diatomaceous Earth. For samples containing other fat-soluble vitamins:

(a) Preparation of polyethylene glycol 600. Diatomaceous earth mixture. Magnetically stir 125 mL isooctane and 25 g Celite 545 in screw-cap, wide mouth bottle to obtain slurry. Add, dropwise, and with magnetic stirring, 10 mL polyethylene glycol 600 and stir 2 min.

Chromosorb W can also be used in place of Celite; its larger particle size offers better packaging properties than Celite (25).

(b) Preparation of column. Fill the tube halfway with isooctane. Pour about half of slurry in portions into tube and let settle by gravity. Then apply gentle suction and add remainder of slurry in small portions, packing each portion with 20-mm disk plunger. When solid surface has formed, remove vacuum, and add about 2 mL isooctane. Space under fritted glass disk must be empty. Check packing of column with 1 mL β-carotene solution, which should pass through column as horizontal band. Otherwise, repeat packing. Check recovery by column performance test (see below) together with Florex column. Use 1000 IU vitamin A alcohol as detector.

3. *Column III, Florex.* For use along with Column II.

(a) Preparation and deactivation of Florex. Eliminate small particles as follows: Suspend 200 g Florex in 500 mL ethanol and boil few min in 1 L round-bottomed flask. Decant upper layer containing colloidal suspension. Shake with 250 mL ethanol and decant upper layer. Repeat washing with two 250-mL portions of ether. (*Caution*: Perform ether washing and evaporation under hood.) Dry suspension on steam bath at 100°C, using aspirator, and store in air-tight container. Weigh 10 g dried Florex into 50-mL Erlenmeyer. Add 1.6 mL H_2O by pipette, stopper flask, and heat 5 min on steam bath. Gently swirl warm flask to obtain free-flowing powder. Cool, and let stand 15 min. Check activity of deactivated Florex (16% H_2O) by column performance test. If performance is < 97%, repeat deactivation, using different volume of water.

(b) Preparation of column. Add 20 mL pet ether to flask, swirl, and transfer Florex with pet ether to tube; let packing settle. Regulate flow rate at 2 mL/min with stopcock. Elute with 50 mL isooctane and discard eluate. Maintain head of 1 cm liquid on column throughout assay.

4. *Column Performance Test.* Pipette 10 mL solution containing 5 μg crystalline cholecalciferol (or ergocalciferol)/mL pet ether onto column I, and elute with pet ether, collecting eluate in 250 mL flask. Evaporate to dryness under vacuum in 40°C water bath. Evaporate 10.0 mL untreated calciferol solution in same way. Cool and restore atmospheric pressure with nitrogen without delay. Separately dissolve each residue in 10.0 mL 20% toluene in isooctane. Pipette 2 mL into a 2-cm cell, add 5 mL color reagent from rapid delivery pipette and mix. Measure absorbance at 500 nm against blank consisting of 2 mL 20% toluene in isooctane and 5 mL color reagent.

% Performance $= 100\,(A/A_0)$, where A and A_0 refer to absorbances of solutions with and without chromatography respectively.

This column performance test can also be used to check the three columns together. Result of performance tests should be between 97% and 103%; if not, repeat deactivation of column materials with different volumes of water and recheck by performance test.

E. Procedure

1. *Sample Preparation and Saponification.*

(a) Vitamin D resins in cans. For resins containing about 25,000,000 IU vitamin D/g, scatter sample by sharp blows on outside of container. Into 100-mL flask, accurately weigh 0.8 g (estimated to contain 20,000,000 IU vitamin D) of largest lumps from lower part of container. Avoid powdering the sample to prevent any surface oxidation. Dissolve sample in toluene and dilute to volume. Dilute aliquot to about 400 IU vitamin D/mL with pet ether (dilution: 5 mL to 100 and 2 mL to 50). Pipette 5 mL, containing about 50 μg (2000 IU) into round-bottomed boiling flask. Evaporate to dryness on flash evaporator, under vacuum at < 40°C. Cool, restore atmosphere with nitrogen, and continue immediately with maleic anhydride treatment, without saponification or chromatography.

(b) Oil solutions.   Weigh accurately about 1 g sample estimated to contain about 4000 or more IU of vitamin D/g and less than 75 mg α-tocopherol acetate into saponification flask. For each g of sample, add 10 mL 20% pyrogallol solution, 1 mL 20% sodium ascorbate solution, 25 mL ethanol, and 4 mL 50% aq KOH solution, and then reflux 30 min on a steam bath.

(c) Capsules or tablets.   Weigh, preferably more than 10 capsules or tablets estimated to contain about 4000 or more IU vitamin D into a sapon-ification flask. For each 5 g sample, add 10 mL 20% sodium ascorbate solution and warm on steam bath for about 10 min, swirling occasionally. Crush remaining solid with blunt glass rod, warm 5 min longer, and add three drops of sodium sulfide solution. Add dropwise, with gentle swirling, 20 mL 20% pyrogallol solution and then, all at once, 10 mL 50% aqeous KOH solution, followed by dropwise addition, with gentle swirling, 25 mL ethanol, mix, and then reflux 30 min on a steam bath.

(d) Dry preparation and aqueous dispersions.   Weigh accurately 1–5 g, estimated to contain 4000 IU or more vitamin D and less than 75 mg α-tocopherol acetate, into saponification flask. For each 5-g sample, add in small quantities and with gentle swirling, 25 mL ethanol, 10 mL 20% sodium ascorbate solution, 20 mL pyrogallol solution, and 10 mL 50% aqueous KOH solution, mix, and reflux 30 min on a steam bath.

2. *Extraction.*   Extract the unsaponifiable matter from steps E1.(b), (c), and (d) by one of the following two methods.

(a) Benzene extraction.   To the hot saponified mixture, add 5 mL 20% pyrogallol solution and then cool. Add without delay 100 mL benzene, mix, and transfer to separation funnel without rinsing. Add 40 mL 6% aqueous KOH solution, shake vigorously 10 sec, let layers separate (2–3 min), and discard still turbid aqueous layer. Wash benzene layer with 40-mL portions of H_2O, until neutral to phenolphthalein (usually 4–5 washings). Drain last few drops of H_2O, add two sheets of 9-cm filter paper (in strips) to funnel, and shake until benzene layer is clear. Store this solution in stoppered flask and use appropriate aliquots for further analysis. During washing, the turbid aqueous layer contains droplets of benzene. As droplets have same vitamin D concentration as benzene layer, determination of concentration of vitamin D in benzene layer is not influenced by loss of these droplets.

(b) Ether-hexane extraction.   Cool the saponified mixture rapidly under running H_2O and transfer to a conical separator, rinsing the saponification flask with two 15-mL portions of H_2O, 10 mL of ethanol, and two 50-mL portions of ether. Shake the combined saponified mixture and rinsings vigorously for 30 sec and allow to stand until both layers are clear. Transfer the aqueous phase to a second conical separator, add a mixture of 10 mL of ethanol and 50 mL of solvent hexane, and shake vigorously. Petroleum ether or pentane can also be used instead of hexane. Allow to separate, transfer the aqueous phase to a third conical separator, rinsing the second separator with two 10-mL portions of solvent hexane, adding the rinsings to the first separator. Shake the aqueous phase in the third separator with 50 mL of solvent hexane, and add the hexane phase to the first separator. Wash the combined ether-hexane extracts by shaking vigorously with three 50-mL portions 6% KOH solution, and finally wash with 50-mL portions H_2O vigorously until last washing is neutral to pheolphthalein. Drain any remaining drops of H_2O from the combined ether-hexane extracts, add two sheets of 9-cm filter paper, in strips, to the separator, and shake. Transfer the washed ether-hexane extracts to a round-bottomed flask, rinsing the separator and paper with solvent hexane. Combine the hexane rinsings with the ether-hexane extracts concentrate to 100 mL. Make appropriate dilution, if necessary, for further analysis.

3. *Solvent Removal.*

(a) Multivitamin samples.   Pipette an aliquot, estimated to contain 3000 IU of vitamin D, of either benzene or ether-hexane extract, into boiling flask. Add 1 mL ethoxyquin solution and evaporate to dryness under vacuum in a water bath at about 40°C. Cool, restore atmospheric pressure with nitrogen, and continue with the three-column chromatography separation without delay.

(b) Samples without other fat-soluble vitamins.   Pipette an aliquot, estimated to contain 2000 IU of vitamin D, from either benzene or ether-hexane extract, into a boiling flask. Evaporate to dryness under vacuum in a water bath at about 40°C. Cool and restore atmospheric pressure with nitrogen.

For vitamin D concentrates such as resins ($\geq$ 100,000 IU/g) proceed with maleic anhydride treatment.

For lower-potency samples, continue with one-column alumina chromatography separation.

4. *Chromatography.*

(a) Alumina (column I).   Dissolve residue from solvent removal step in 5 mL pet ether. Transfer to column I with aid of 10 mL pet ether, let liquid drain, and wash with 10 mL pet ether. Elute column, in 10-mL portions, with 200 mL 8% ether–pet ether, and discard eluate. Elute column with 150 mL 30% ether–pet ether, collecting eluate in boiling flask. Add 1 mL ethoxyquin solution. Evaporate eluate to dryness under vacuum at < 40°C. Cool, restore atmospheric pressure with nitrogen, and continue without delay as in 3.(b). (For samples containing no vitamin A, continue with maleic anhydride treatment.)

(b) Polyethylene glycol 600 diatomaceous earth (Column II) and Florex (Column III). Dissolve the residue from Section E.4(a) in 3 mL isooctane. Start draining the isooctane solvent from column II; as the solvent passes into the column, pipette 2-mL aliquot of sample solution on the column. As the last of the aliquot passes into the column, rinse down the sides with three 1-mL portions of isooctane. Then add isooctane to the column from a dropping funnel or reservoir, maintaining the flow rate to about 2 mL/min and drain the isooctane eluate into the Florex (column III). Always maintain about 1 cm of this eluate on top of column III by adjusting the stopcock of this column. Monitor the fluorescent vitamin A band (or ethoxyquin) in column II with a portable UV lamp (at 360 nm) at frequent time intervals. Stop the addition of isooctane when the front of the vitamin A band reaches 3 cm from the bottom of column II. All the vitamin D will now be in column III while vitamin A is retained on column II. Detach column II and elute vitamin A with isooctane and this column is ready for the next sample.

Discard the isooctane eluate from column III and elute the vitamin D from this column with 150 mL benzene. Collect the eluate in a boiling flask, and evaporate to dryness under vacuum at 40°C. Cool, restore atmospheric pressure with nitrogen, and proceed without delay to maleic anhydride treatment.

5. *Tachysterol Inactivation by Maleic Anhydride.* Dissolve residue, estimated to contain about 2000 IU vitamin D, from steps E1(a), 3(b), 4(a), or 4(b) in 2 mL 1% maleic anhydride solution in round-bottomed flask; stopper the flask and swirl. Let stand 30 min in the dark at room temp. Pipette 8 mL isooctane into the flask and mix. This final solution is ready for colorimetry.

6. *Color Development and Spectrophotometry.*

(a) Multivitamin samples. Set the spectrophotometer to read the absorbancy at 500 nm. Use a set of four matched cuvets or tubes.

Pipette 2 mL of 20% toluene in isooctane into the first tube which is the reagent blank. Pipette 2 mL freshly diluted standard vitamin D solution into tube 2, 2 mL purified sample to tube 3, and 1 mL of purified sample and 1 mL color inhibitor to tube 4. Add 5 mL color reagent from an automatic pipette to the reagent blank tube, mix, and use this blank to set for zero absorbancy at 500 nm. Add 5 mL each of the color reagent to the other tubes and mix. Determine the absorbance of these solutions (first reading) exactly 45 sec after the addition of the color reagent.

Immediately adjust the spectrophotometer to zero absorbancy at 550 nm with the reagent blank and measure the absorbance of the other tubes 45 sec after the first reading.

For some batches of $SbCl_3$ reagent, 45 sec may not be sufficient for maximum color development; determine the exact time for each batch of the reagent with standard vitamin solution. Use this time for the reading at 500 nm and measure 45 sec later at 550 nm.

(b) Samples without other fat-soluble vitamins. Absorbance correction step is omitted for these samples. Pipette 2 mL each of 20% toluene in isooctane, freshly diluted standard vitamin D solution, and sample solution (from maleic anhydride treatment step) to three different cuvets. Add 5 mL color reagent quickly to each cuvet and mix. Measure the absorbance of the standard and sample at 500 nm, after setting the instrument to zero absorbance with the reagent blank.

7. *Calculations.*

(a) **Multivitamin samples.** Designate absorbance as follows:

$A_{1(500)}$ = sample absorbance at 500 nm

$A_{2(500)}$ = standard absorbance at 500 nm

$A_{3(500)}$ = sample and inhibitor absorbance at 500 nm

$A_{1(550)}$ = sample absorbance at 550 nm

$A_{2(550)}$ = standard absorbance at 550 nm

$A_{3(550)}$ = sample and inhibitor absorbance at 550 nm

Calculate the vitamin D (μg or IU) content of the sample:

$$\text{Vitamin D}/\text{g sample} = \frac{C}{W} \times \frac{A_D}{A_{2(500)}}$$

where C = μg or IU cholecalciferol or ergocalciferol in 2 mL Standard (1 μg = 40 IU);

W = weight of original sample (μg) in each 2 mL of final sample solution used in color development;

A_D = corrected sample absorbance.

Calculate the corrected sample absorbance A_D as follows:

$$A_D = \frac{q}{q - p} \times A_{1(500)} - \frac{1}{q - p} \times A_{1(550)}$$

where $p = A_{2(550)}/A_{2(500)}$ and $q = A_{3(550)}/A_{3(500)}$.

In spectrophotometer with ≤ 10-nm band pass, absorbance of standard solution at 550 nm will be negligible. Then p is <0.01 and for this spectrophotometer,

$$A_D = A_{1(500)} - \frac{A_{1(550)}}{q}$$

If q is <1, it should be taken as 1, to avoid systematic errors.

(b) **Samples without other vitamins.** Calculate μg or IU of vitamin D/g sample using the equation:

$$\text{Vitamin D}/\text{g sample} = \frac{C}{W} \times \frac{A_{1(500)}}{A_{2(500)}}$$

where $C =$ μg or IU of vitamin D in 2 mL standard solution;

$W =$ weight of original sample in each 2 mL of final sample

$=$ solution used in color development;

$A_{1(500)} =$ absorbance of sample at 500 nm;

$A_{2(500)} =$ absorbance of standard at 500 nm.

8. *Confirmation of Identity for Isotachysterol.* This test is designed to confirm the absence of isotachysterol in samples of resins and concentrates.

Prepare sample residues (steps 3, 4, and 5) containing about 2.5 mg vitamin D (100,000 IU) and dissolve in 10.00 mL 0.1% BHT solution. Pipette 4 mL of this solution into each of two 10-mL volumetric flasks. To one flask, add 2 mL 10% maleic anhydride solution. Place plastic tube over neck of flask. Fill flask with nitrogen and close tube with pinch cock. Heat 3 hr in dark in 100°C water bath and cool. Dilute the solutions (treated with maleic anhydride and untreated) to volume with 0.1% BHT solution. Quantitatively transfer untreated solution to 200-mL volume flask and dilute to volume with 0.1% BHT solution. Determine the absorbance of treated and diluted-untreated solutions after mixing with color reagent as described in color development step (6b)

$$\text{Residual color value (\%)} = 5 \times (A/A_u)$$

where A and A_u are the absorbance values of treated and diluted untreated solutions, respectively. Residual color values $\leq 5\%$ are considered negative for isotachysterol. Isotachysterol can also be determined quantitatively (18).

II. HIGH-PERFORMANCE LIQUID CHROMATOGRAPHY

A. Principle

In HPLC, vitamin D and its isomers are separated from interfering substances at ambient temperatures on a reverse-phase HPLC cleanup column. An analytical silica-type column separates vitamin D and previtamin D from other isomers and impurities. Vitamin D is the sum of vitamin D and previtamin D.

The method is applicable to a variety of samples including foods, mixed feeds, premixes, pet foods, dairy products, and other foods as well as to multivitamin preparations and vitamin D concentrates. Methods of saponification and sample preparation vary depending on the type of sample to be analyzed and are summarized in Table 9.4.

Use of a blanket of inert gas and low actinic glasswares are recommended to protect the vitamin D-containing solutions during assay.

B. Equipment

1. *Liquid Chromatograph.* Hewlett-Packard 1010A, or equivalent, with 254 nm (or variable wavelength) UV detector with two columns: cleanup and ana-

TABLE 9.4 Scheme for HPLC Analysis of Vitamin D Preparations

Preparation	D Content IU/g	Saponification	Alumina Chromatography	HPLC Cleanup	HPLC Analytical External Standard	HPLC Analytical Internal Standard
Resins	> 20,000,000				X	
Vitamin D Concentrates						
a. oils	> 100,000	X			X	
b. powders, etc.	> 25,000	X			X	
Multivitamin samples	> 200	X		X		X
Mixed feeds, premixes, and pet foods	2–200	X	X	X	X	
Milk and milk powder	> 0.5	X		X	X	

lytical. Peak height or area (integration counts) can be used to quantitate vitamin D.

2. *Cleanup Columns.*

(a) For multivitamin samples. Stainless steel, 300 $\times$ 0.6 (i.d.) mm, packed with 10-μm particle size Lichrosorb RP-8 (E. Merck), passing the system suitability test. Typical operating conditions: flow rate 1.4 mL/min (ca. 750 psi); detector sensitivity, 0.32 AUFS; temperature, ambient; injection volume, 500 μL; solvent system, acetonitrile-methanol-H_2O (50 + 50 + 2).

(b) For mixed feeds, foods, etc. Stainless steel, 250 $\times$ 4.6 (i.d.) mm, packed with 10-μm particle size Lichrosorb RP-18 (E. Merck, Applied Science Labs). Typical operating conditions: flow rate, 1.4 mL/min; detector sensitivity 0.08 AUFS; temperature, ambient; injection volume, 500 μL; solvent system, acetonitrile-methanol-H_2O (50 + 50 + 5).

(c) For milk and milk powder. Stainless steel 250 $\times$ 4.6 (i.d.) mm, packed with 10-μm particle size Sil-60D-10CN (Perkin-Elmer). Typical operating conditions: flow rate, 1 mL/min; detector sensitivity, 0.128 AUFS; temperature, ambient; injection volume, 500 μL; mobile phase, hexane containing 0.35% *n*-amyl alcohol.

3. *Analytical Column.* Stainless steel, 250 $\times$ 4.6 (i.d.) mm, packed with 5-μm particle size Partisil-5 (Whatman), passing the system suitability test. Typical operating conditions: flow rate, 2.6 mL/min; detector sensitivity, 0.016 AUFS; temperature, ambient; injection volume, 200 μL; solvent system, hexane containing 0.35% (v/v) *n*-amyl alcohol.

4. *Alumina Column* (For Mixed Feeds, Foods, etc.). Alumina columns can be used for one assay only.

(a) Chromatography tube. 150 $\times$ 20 mm (i.d.) with a 250-mL bulb at the top and a coarse fritted glass disc 30 mm from the bottom, which is constricted to 8 mm below the disc and fritted with a Teflon stopcock.

(b) Column preparation. Heat 250 g alumina overnight at 750°C. Cool and store in vacuum desiccator. Weight 30 g dried alumina into 100-mL Erlenmeyer. Pipette 2.7 mL H_2O into flask, and stopper. Heat 5 min on steam bath. Vigorously shake the warm flask until powder is free-flowing. Cool and let stand 30 min.

Add 40 mL pet ether to the deactivated alumina, swirl, and transfer to tube, using petroleum ether. Let packing settle. Maintain head of >0.5 cm liquid on column throughout assay.

C. Reagents

1. *Solvents.*

(a) Methanol, HPLC grade.

(b) *n*-Amyl alcohol, reagent grade.

(c) Acetonitrile, HPLC grade.

(d) Ethanol, reagent.

(e) Toluene, reagent or nanograde.

(f) Ether, peroxide, and acid-free ethyl ether.

(g) Pentane.

(h) Hexane (spectro-grade). Dry n-hexane by passing through column 60 $\times$ 8 cm i.d. containing 500 g 50–250 μm silica dried 4 hr at 150°C.

2. *Sodium Ascorbate Solution.* Dissolve 3.5 g ascorbic acid in 20 mL 1N NaOH. Prepare fresh daily.

3. *Sodium Sulfide Solution.* Dissolve 12 g $Na_2S \cdot 9H_2O$ in 20 mL H_2O and dilute to 100 mL with 87% glycerol.

4. *Antioxidant Solution.* BHT in hexane:

(a) 10 mg/mL.

(b) 1 mg/mL.

5. *Petroleum Ether.* Reflux over KOH pellets and collect fraction distilling between 40°C and 60°C.

6. *Potassium Hydroxide Solutions.*

(a) 50% (w/w), dissolve 50 g KOH in 50 mL H_2O and cool. Prepare fresh.

(b) 3% in alcohol. Dissolve 3 g KOH in H_2O, add 10 mL ethanol, and dilute to 100 mL with H_2O. Prepare fresh.

7. *Ether-Hexane Eluants.* 8% and 40% ether in hexane.

8. *Alumina.* Neutral, Type 1097 (E. Merck).

9. *Mobile Phase A (For Cleanup Column).*

(a) Acetonitrile-methanol-H_2O, 50 + 50 + 2, for multivitamin samples.

(b) Acetonitrile-methanol-H_2O, 50 + 50 + 5, for mixed feeds.

(c) Hexane containing 0.35% n-amyl alcohol for milk samples.

10. *Mobile Phase B (For Analytical Column).* Hexane containing 0.35% (v/v) n-amyl alcohol.

11. *Internal Standard Solution (For Multivitamin Preparations).* Accurately weigh 15 mg USP $\Delta4,6$ cholestadienol into 200-mL volumetric flask and dilute to volume with toluene-mobile phase B, 10 + 190.

12. *System Suitability Standard Solution.* Use USP Vitamin D Assay System Suitability Reference Standard or prepare solution containing 2 mg vitamin D_3 and 0.2 mg *trans*-vitamin D_3/g in vegetable oil. Peaks of *trans*-vitamin D_3 and previtamin D_3 must have about the same peak heights. If necessary, increase previtamin D_3 content by warming oil solution for about 45 min at 90°C. Store solution at 5°C.

13. *Vitamin D Standard Solutions.* USP Reference Standard ergocalciferol (vitamin D_2) or cholecalciferol (vitamin D or D_3). Prepare different concentrations as follows:

(a) 1 mg/mL. Accurately weigh 50 mg vitamin D standard in a 50-mL amber volumetric flask. Dissolve without heat in toluene, and dilute to volume with toluene (Solution A).

(b) 50 μg/mL.   Dilute 5 mL solution A to 100 mL with toluene. Prepare fresh.

(c) 1.25 μg/mL.   Dilute solution A with 5 + 95 toluene-mobile phase B.

(d) 1.5 μg/mL.   Dilute solution A with mobile phase A (Reagent 9b).

D.   System Suitability Test

1. *Cleanup Column (For Multivitamin Samples).*   Pipette 5 mL vitamin D standard solution (50 μg/mL) into an amber volumetric flask, add two to three crystals BHT, replace air with nitrogen, and heat under reflux, in 90°C water bath, for 45 min to form previtamin D. Cool, add 10.0 mL internal standard solution (Reagent 11), and evaporate to dryness under vacuum by swirling in water bath at 40°C. Cool under running H_2O and restore atmospheric pressure with nitrogen. Dissolve residue immediately in 10 mL 1 + 1 acetoitrile-methanol and chromatograph 500 μL. In the chromatogram, vitamin D, previtamin D, and internal standard should appear as a single peak with a retention time of about 7 min.

2. *Analytical Column.*   Dissolve 0.1 g system suitability standard solution (Reagent 12) in 100 mL toluene-mobile phase B (5 + 95) and inject 200 μL. Determine peak resolution between previtamin D and *trans*-vitamin D as:

$$R = \frac{2D}{B + C}$$

where D = distance between peak maxima of previtamin and *trans*-vitamin D;

B = peak width of previtamin D;

C = peak width of *trans*-vitamin D.

Performance is satisfactory if R is ≥ 1.0.
(*Note*: Relative retention times are approximately 0.4 min for previtamin, 0.5 min for *trans*-vitamin, and 1.0 min for vitamin D.)

E.   Calibration of HPLC Columns

1. *For Samples with Vitamin D Levels Below 200 IU/g.*   Inject 500 μL vitamin D standard (2.5 μg/mL) diluted in appropriate mobile phase A (Reagent 9b or 9c) on to the cleanup column through sample valve and 200 μL vitamin D standard (1.25 μg/mL/Reagent 13c) on to analytical column. Adjust operating conditions or detector for largest possible on-scale peak of vitamin D.

Determine retention time of vitamin D on both columns and peak height of vitamin D on analytical column. Retention time on RP-18 column should be between 15 min and 25 min and on Sil-60D-10 CN between 10 min and 20 min.

2. *For Multivitamin Samples.*

(a) Vitamin D response factor.   Pipette 4 mL vitamin D standard solution (50 μg/mL) and 10 mL internal standard solution (Reagent 11) into 100-

mL amber volumetric flask and dilute to volume and mobile phase B (Reagent 10). Store this working solution at 0°C. Inject 200 μL onto analytical column. Detect peak heights of vitamin D_3 and internal standard and calculate response factor of vitamin D:

$$F_D = \frac{(P_{ir} \times W_r \times V_{ir})}{(P_r \times W_{ir} \times V_r)}$$

where F_D = response factor of vitamin D;
$\quad P_{ir}$ = peak height of internal standard in working standard solution;
$\quad P_r$ = peak height of vitamin D in working standard solution;
$\quad W_{ir}$ = mg internal standard weighed;
$\quad W_r$ = mg vitamin D standard weighed;
$\quad V_{ir}$ = final dilution of internal standard in working standard (2000 mL);
$\quad V_r$ = final dilution of vitamin D standard in working standard (25,000 mL).

b. Previtamin D response factor.   Pipette 5 mL vitamin D standard solution into 100-mL amber volumetric flask, add two to three crystals of BHT, replace air with nitrogen, and heat and 45 min in subdued light in 90°C water bath and under nitrogen reflux atmosphere. Cool, add 10 mL internal standard solution (Reagent 11), and dilute to volume with mobile phase B. Inject 200 μL of this heated working standard solution onto analytical column. Determine peak heights of vitamin D, previtamin D, and internal standard.

Calculate vitamin D as percent of amount in unheated solution:

$$q\% = \frac{(F_D \times P_D \times V_r \times W_{ir} \times 100)}{(P_{ir} \times V_{ir} \times W_r)}$$

where F_D = response factor for vitamin D;
$\quad P_D$ = peak height of vitamin D in heated solution;
$\quad V_r$ = final dilution of vitamin D in heated solution (20,000 mL);
$\quad V_{ir}$ = final dilution of internal standard in heated solution (2000 mL);
$\quad W_r$ = mg vitamin D standard weighed;
$\quad W_{ir}$ = mg internal standard weighed;
$\quad P_{ir}$ = peak height of internal standard in heated solution.

Previtamin D content = $p\%$ = $100 - q\%$

Response factor for previtamin D:

$$F_{pre} = \frac{(p\% \times P_{ir} \times V_{ir} \times W_r)}{(100 \times P_{pre} \times V_{pre} \times W_{ir})}$$

where q = vitamin D (%);

$\quad F_{pre}$ = response factor of previtamin D;

$\quad W_r$ = mg vitamin D standard weighed;

$\quad W_{ir}$ = mg internal standard weighed;

$\quad P_{pre}$ = peak height of previtamin D in heated solution;

$\quad V_{pre}$ = final dilution of previtamin D in heated solution (20,000 mL);

$\quad P_{ir}$ = peak height of internal standard in heated solution;

$\quad V_{ir}$ = final dilution of internal standard in heated solution (2000 mL);

$\quad p\%$ = previtamin D content.

(c) Conversion factor (C_F)—previtamin to vitamin D. Calculate C_F from two determinations performed on different days: $C_F = F_{pre}/F_D$.

3. *For Resins and Vitamin Concentrates.* C_F—previtamin to vitamin D. Pipette 4 mL vitamin D standard solution (1 mg/mL) into 25-mL volumetric flask. Add 1 mL toluene and dilute to volume with mobile phase B (Reagent 10). Store in ice bath. Inject 20 μL onto analytical column through sampling valve and adjust operating conditions of detector to obtain maximum on scale peak heights. Repeat injection and average peak height.

Pipette 5 mL vitamin D standard solution (1 mg/mL) into 25-mL volume flask, add a few crystals of BHT, displace air with nitrogen, and attach reflux condenser. Heat in a 90°C water bath in dark under nitrogen for 45 min and cool. Dilute to volume with mobile phase B. Inject 20 μL onto column under the same conditions as above. Detect the peak height of heated vitamin D and of previtamin D formed. Calculate calibration factor:

$$F = \frac{\dfrac{5K}{4} - L}{M}$$

where F = calibration factor;

$\quad K$ = peak height of unheated vitamin D;

$\quad L$ = peak height of heated vitamin D;

$\quad M$ = peak height of previtamin D formed.

F. Procedure

1. *Sample Preparation.*

(a) Food, premixes, mixed feeds and pet foods.

(1) Isolation of unsaponifiable matter from powder. Accurately weigh about 25 g powdered sample (preferably particle size <1 mm) into saponification flask. Add 80 mL ethanol, 2 mL sodium ascorbate solution, a pinch of Na_2EDTA, and 10 mL 50% aqueous KOH solution. Reflux 30 min on steam bath under nitrogen with stirring. Cool and extract with five 60-mL portions of ether in saponification flask; decant each time and

transfer ether layer to a 1-L separator containing 100 mL H_2O. Shake ether layer in separator (A), let separate and transfer aqueous phase to 500-mL separator (B). Extract aqueous phase with 60 mL ether and transfer ether layer to separator (A). Wash combined ether extracts with 100 mL 0.5 N KOH solution and then 100-mL portions of H_2O until last washing is neutral to phenolphthalein. Add 150 mL pet ether, wait ½ hr to separate from last drop of H_2O, and add two sheets of 9-cm filter paper in strips to separator. Shake, add 1 mg BHT, and transfer to boiling flask, rinsing separator and paper with pet ether. Evaporate solution by swirling (Rotavapor) under nitrogen stream in 40°C water bath. Dissolve residue immediately in 5 mL hexane and continue with alumina column chromatography.

(2) Alumina column chromatography.

Transfer sample solution to column with aid of three 10-mL portions of hexane. Discard eluate (contains carotenoids). Elute column with seven 10-mL portions of 8 + 92 ether-hexane mixture and discard eluate (contains tocopherols). Elute the column next with seven 10-mL portions of 40 + 60 ether-hexane. Monitor the column for fluorescent vitamin A band under UV light (360 nm) with a portable UV lamp. Discard first 20–25 mL of eluate and then collect the eluate in a boiling flask until the vitamin A band reaches 3 cm above the disc.

(3) Solvent removal and extract preparation for HPLC.

Evaporate solution by swirling (Rotavapor) under nitrogen stream in 40°C water bath. Transfer to centrifuge tube, rinsing flask with 2–3 mL ether, evaporate ether, and dissolve in 1 mL methanol with warming. Add 1 mL acetonitrile and cool. Centrifuge and use clear supernate for injection onto cleanup column.

(b) Milk and milk powder.

(1) Saponification of fluid milk.

Pipette 200 mL milk into 1-L saponification flask. Add 200 mL ethanol, 5 g sodium ascorbate, and 50 mL 50% aqueous KOH solution. Reflux 45 min on steam bath. Cool rapidly under running water.

(2) Saponification of milk powder.

Accurately weigh about 50 g milk powder into saponification flask. Add 100 mL alcohol, 25 mL 25% aqueous sodium ascorbate solution, and 25 mL 50% (w/w) aqeous KOH solution. Reflux 45 min on steam bath. Cool rapidly under running water.

(3) Extraction.

Extract the saponified mixture Section F.1.b(1) or (2) as follows. Transfer the mixture to separator with two 30-mL portions H_2O and two 100-mL portions ether. Shake vigorously 30 sec and let stand for the layers to clear. Transfer the aqueous lower phase to second separator. Shake with 20 mL ethanol and 100 mL pentane and let stand for separation.

Transfer the lower aqueous phase to third separator and the upper pentane phase to first separator.

Wash second separator with two 20-mL portions of pentane and transfer the washings to first separator. Shake the aqueous phase in third separator with 100 mL pentane, discard the aqueous layer, and transfer pentane phase to first separator. Wash combined pentane extracts with three 100-mL portions of freshly prepared 3% KOH solution in dilute ethanol (Reagent 6b), shaking vigorously. Then wash with 100-mL portions of H_2O until the washing is neutral to phenolphthalein. Drain the last few drops of H_2O, add two sheets 9-cm filter paper in strips to separator and shake.

Transfer the pentane extract to boiling flask, rinsing separator and paper with pentane.

Hexane can be substituted for pentane (16).

(4) Solvent removal and extract preparation for HPLC.

To the dried ether-pentane extract in boiling flask add 1 mL BHT solution (Reagent 4b). Evaporate to dryness under vacuum by swirling with water and restore atmospheric pressure with nitrogen. Dissolve residue immediately in 2–3 mL 5 + 95 toluene-mobile phase B (Reagent 10).

Transfer the solution to 10-mL boiling flask, rinse 500-mL boiling flask with pentane, and collect the rinsings in the 10 mL flask. Evaporate under nitrogen stream at room temperature. Dissolve residue immediately in 2.0 ml 5 + 95 toluene-mobile phase A (Reagent 9c). This extract is ready for the HPLC cleanup column.

(c) Multivitamin Samples.   These samples could be dry material, aqueous dispersions, or solution in oils.

(1) Saponification.

(i) Dry materials and aqueous dispersions.

Weigh accurately into a saponification flask an amount of sample (≥ 0.5 g) estimated to contain 5000 IU vitamin D. With gentle swirling, add slowly 25 mL ethanol, 5 mL 20% (w/v) sodium ascorbate solution, and 3 mL freshly prepared 50% (w/w) aqueous KOH solution. Reflux 30 min on water bath at 90°C. Cool rapidly under running H_2O.

(ii) Formulation in oil.

Weigh accurately into a saponification flask an amount of sample (≥ 0.5 g) estimated to contain about 5000 IU vitamin D. Add 1 mL of 20% aqueous sodium ascorbate, 25 mL ethanol, and 2 mL 50% aqueous KOH. Reflux 30 min on a water bath at 90°C. Cool rapidly.

(2) Extraction.

Extract saponified mixture with ether and pentane as described under F.1.(b)(3) but use only one-half the volume of reagents.

(3) Solvent removal and extract preparation for HPLC.

Add 5 mL internal standard (Reagent 11) and 100 µL BHT (Reagent

4a) to the washed pentane extract in boiling flask and evaporate to dryness under vacuum by swirling in water bath at 40°C. Cool under running water and restore atmospheric pressure with nitrogen. Dissolve residue immediately in 5 mL acetonitrile-methanol (1 + 1). This extract is ready for use on the cleanup column.

(d) Vitamin D concentrates without other vitamins—dry material and aqueous dispersions.

(1) Saponification.

Weigh accurately into a saponification flask a quantity sample estimated to contain about 100,000 IU. With gentle swirling, add slowly 2 mL aqueous sodium ascorbate, 25 mL ethanol, and 5 mL aqueous KOH and reflux 30 min on a water bath at 90°C. Cool rapidly.

(2) Extraction.

Extract saponified mixture with ether and pentane as described in F.I.b(3) but use only one-half the volume of reagents.

(3) Solvent removal and extract preparation for HPLC.

Evaporate the washed pentane extract to dryness under vacuum by swirling in water bath at about 40°C. Cool rapidly and restore atmospheric pressure with nitrogen. Dissolve residue immediately in 2 mL toluene and transfer to 10-mL amber volumetric flask, rinsing with 1-mL portions of mobile phase B (Reagent 10). Dilute to volume with mobile phase B. Proceed with the assay on analytical column without any cleanup.

(e) Vitamin D concentrate in oil.   Accurately weigh amount of oil containing 500,000 IU into 50-mL volumetric flask. Dissolve in 10 mL toluene, and dilute to volume with mobile phase B (Reagent 10). Proceed to assay on analytical column without any cleanup.

(f) Resins.   Shatter sample by sharp blows on outside of container. Into 100-mL flask, accurately weigh about 0.8 g (estimated to contain about 20,000,000 IU vitamin D) of largest lumps from lower part of container. (Avoid powdering the resin sample to prevent any surface oxidation.) Dissolve in toluene and dilute to volume with toluene. Pipette 5 mL into 100-mL volumetric flask, add 15 mL toluene, and dilute to volume with mobile phase B (Reagent 10). (Concentration = 10,000 IU or 0.25 mg vitamin D/mL). Proceed to assay on analytical column without any cleanup.

2. *Determination.*

(a) Foods, feeds and milk samples. Vitamin levels below 200 IU/g.

(1) Cleanup.

Inject 500-μL sample solution onto cleanup column through sampling valve and adjust operating conditions of detector to give largest possible on-scale peaks for vitamin D. Collect fraction between 3 min before and 3 min after vitamin D peak, in 10-mL volumetric flask. Add 1 mL antioxidant solution and evaporate to dryness under nitrogen. Dissolve residue immediately in 2 mL 5 + 95 toluene-mobile phase B (Reagent 10). Use this solution for injection onto analytical column.

(2) Assay.

Inject 200 μL solution (a) onto analytical column through sampling valve, and adjust operating conditions of detector to give largest possible on-scale peaks of vitamin D. Measure peak height of vitamin D. Use same operating conditions and inject standard solution [(1.25 μg/mL (Reagent 13c)]. Measure peak height of vitamin .

(3) Calculation.

Vitamin D in IU/g sample =

$$CF \times \frac{P}{P'} \times \frac{W'}{W} \times \frac{V}{V'} \times 40{,}000$$

where P = peak height of vitamin D in sample solution;
$\quad$ CF = correction factor of 1.25 for previtamin D formed during refluxing for saponification;
$\quad$ P' = peak height of vitamin D in reference solution;
$\quad$ W = g sample;
$\quad$ W' = mg reference standard;
$\quad$ V = final dilution of sample (mL);
$\quad$ V' = final dilution of reference standard solution (mL)
(USP Reference Standard: 40,000 IU vitamin D/mg).

(b) Multivitamin Samples.

(1) Cleanup.

Inject 500 μL working sample solution onto cleaning column through sampling valve and adjust operating conditions of detector to give largest possible on-scale peaks for vitamin D_3. Collect fraction with retention times of 5–9 min corresponding to vitamin D_3 peak, in 10-mL volumetric flask. Add 50 μL antioxidant solution and evaporate to dryness under vacuum by swirling in water bath at <40°C. Cool under running water and restore atmospheric pressure with nitrogen. Dissolve residue immediately in 5 mL 5 + 95 toluene-mobile phase B. Use this solution for injection onto analytical column.

(2) Assay.

Inject 200 μL solution (1), onto analytical column through sampling valve, and adjust operating conditions of detector to give largest possible on-scale peaks of vitamin D_3. Measure peak heights of vitamin D_3, previtamin D_3, and internal standard.

(3) Calculation.

Vitamin D in IU/g sample =

$$F_D \times \frac{P_D + (P_{pre} \times CF)}{P_{ir}} \times \frac{W_{ir}}{W_s} \times \times \frac{V_s}{V_{ir}} \times 40,000$$

where F_D = response factor of vitamin D;
P_{ir} = peak height of internal standard in sample solution;
P_D = peak height vitamin D peak in sample solution;
P_{pre} = peak height previtamin D peak in sample solution;
CF = conversion factor;
W_{ir} = weight of internal standard in mg;
W_s = weight of sample in g;
V_s = final dilution of sample solution (50 mL);
V_{ir} = final dilution of internal standard solution (2000 mL)
(USP Reference Standard: 40,000 IU vitamin D/mg).

(c) Resins and concentrates without other vitamins.
   (1) Assay.

Inject 20 μL vitamin D standard solution and prepared sample solution onto column through sampling valve with detector adjusted to obtain maximum on scale peak height. Measure peak heights of vitamin D and previtamin D. Repeat injections and reinject standard solution after every four sample injections to verify that response remains constant.

   (2) Calculation.

Average peak heights obtained for standard replicates and sample duplicates and use in calculating:
IU vitamin D/g sample=

$$\frac{P_D + (P_p \times CF)}{P_R} \times \frac{W'}{W} \times \frac{V}{V'} \times 40,000$$

where P_D = peak height of vitamin D in sample;
P_p = peak height of previtamin D in sample;
P_R = peak height of vitamin D in standard;
CF = calibration factor, previtamin D/vitamin D;
W' = weight of vitamin D standard in mg;
W = weight of sample in g;
V = final dilution of sample solution;
V' = final dilution of vitamin D standard solution
(USP Reference Standard: 40,000 IU vitamin D/mg).

LITERATURE CITED

1. Havinga, E. "Vitamin D, example and challenge." *Experentia* **29**, 1181 (1973).

2. Harris, R. S. "Vitamin D group." In W. H. Sebrell, Jr. and R. S. Harris, Eds., *The Vitamins*, Vol. 3. Academic Press, New York, 155 (1971).

3. Bell, P. A. "The chemistry of vitamins D." In D. E. M. Lawson, Ed., *Vitamin D*. Academic Press, New York, 1 (1978).

4. "Cholecalciferol." *In The United States Pharmacopeia*, 20th ed. Mack Printing, Easton, Penn., 147 (1980).

5. "Ergocalciferol." *In The United States Pharmacopeia*, 20th ed. Mack Printing, Easton, Penn., 282 (1980).

6. Parrish, D. B. "Determination of vitamin D in foods: A review." *CRC Crit. Rev. Food, Sci. Nutr.*, **12**, 29 (1979).

7. Greenbaum, S. B. "Vitamin D: A review of its forms, stability, availability, and action." *Feedstuffs*, **45**, 30 (1973).

8. Norman, A. W. "Problems relating to the definition of an International Unit for vitamin D and its metabolites." *J. Nutr.*, **102**, 1243 (1972).

9. Strohecker, R. and Henning, H. M. "Vitamin D." In *Vitamin Assay-Tested Methods*, Verlag Chemie, Gmbh., 254, (1965).

10. Freed, M. *Methods of Vitamin Assay*, 3rd ed. Interscience, New York, 345–362 (1966).

11. DeLuca, H. F. and Blunt, J. W. "Vitamin D." In *Methods in Enzymol.*, **18**, 709 (1971).

12. Norman, A. W. (Ed.) *Vitamin D, Molecular Biology and Clinical Nutrition.* Marcel Dekker, New York (1980).

13. Lawson, D. E. M. (Ed.) *Vitamin D.* Academic Press, New York (1978).

14. Nield, C. H., Russell, W. C. and Zimmerli, A. "A spectrophotometric determination of vitamins D2 and D3." *J. Biol. Chem.*, **136**, 73 (1940).

15. Zimmerli, A., Nield, C. H., and Russell, W. C. "A modified antimony trichloride reagent for the determination of certain sterols and vitamins D2 and D3." *J. Biol. Chem.*, **148**, 245 (1943).

16. "Vitamin D assay." In The United States Pharmacopiea, 20th ed. Mack Printing, Easton, Penn., 934 (1980).

17. Association of Official Analytical Chemists. *Official Methods of Analysis*, 13th ed. Washington, D.C., 747–750 (1980).

18. DeVries, E. J., Mulder, F. J., and Borsje, B. "Analysis of fat-soluble vitamins—15. Confirmation of isotachysterol in vitamin D concentrates." *J. Assoc. Off. Anal. Chem.* **60**, 989 (1977).

19. Osadca, M. and DeRitter, E. "Modification of USP vitamin D assay to remove interference of vitamin E." *J. Pharm. Sci.* **57**, 309 (1963).

20. Mulder, F. J., DeVries, E. J., and Borsje, B. "Analysis of fat-soluble vitamins. XIV Collaborative study of the determination of vitamin D in multivitamin preparations." *J. Assoc. Off. Anal. Chem.* **60**, 151 (1977).

21. Panalaks, T. "Colorimetric method of the determination of vitamin D in fortified whole and partially skim fluid milk." *J. Off. Anal. Chem.* **54**, 1299 (1971).

22. Mulder, F. J., DeVries, E. J., and Borsje, B. "Chemical analysis of vitamin D in concentrates and its problems—12. Analysis of fat-soluble vitamins." *J. Assoc. Off. Anal. Chem.* **54**, 1168 (1971).

23. Mulder, F. J. and DeVries, E. J. "Analysis of fat-soluble vitamins—13. Chemical vitamin D assay in vitamin D and multi-vitamin preparations." *J. Assoc. Off. Anal. Chem.* **57**, 1349 (1974).

24. Quackenbush, F. W., Banes, D., and Derse, P. H. "Report of Ad Hoc Committee on vitamin D methodology, AOAC." *J. Assoc. Off. Anal. Chem.* **58**, 330 (1975).

25. Mulder, F. J., DeVries, E. J., and Borsje, B. "Analysis of fat-soluble vitamins—14. Collaborative study of the determination of vitamin D in multivitamin preparations." *J. Assoc. Off. Anal. Chem.* **60**, 151 (1977).

26. Mulder, F. J., Borsje, B., Van Strik, R., and DeVries, E. J. "Analysis of fat-soluble vitamins—19. Collaborative studies on the chemical assay for vitamin D concentrates." *J. Assoc. Off. Anal. Chem.* **61**, 261 (1978).

27. Ponchon, G. and Fellers, F. X. "Thin-layer chromatography of vitamin D and related sterols." *J. Chromatogr.* **35**, 53 (1968).

28. Bollinger, H. R. and Konig, A. "Vitamins, including carotenoids, chlorophylls and biologically active quinones—2. TLC of fat-soluble vitamins, carotenoids, chlorophylls and quinones." In E. Stahl, Ed., *Thin-Layer Chromatography*, 2nd ed. Springer-Verlag, New York, 264–291 (1969).

29. Sheppard, A. J., Prosser, A. R., and Hubbard, W. D. "Gas chromatography of fat-soluble vitamins: A review." *J. Amer. Oil Chem. Soc.* **49**, 619 (1972).

30. Kobayashi, T. "Gas-liquid chromatographic determination of vitamin D." *Methods Enzymol.* **67**, 347 (1980).

31. DeLeenheer, A. P. "Gas-liquid chromatography of vitamin D and analogs." *Methods Enzymol.* **67**, 335 (1980).

32. Kobayashi, T. and Adachi, A. "Gas-liquid chromatographic determination of vitamin D in multivitamin preparation." *J. Nutr. Sci. Vitaminol.* **22**, 41 (1976).

33. Kobayashi, T. and Adachi, A. "Gas-liquid chromatographic determination of vitamin D in multivitamin preparations containing excess amounts of vitamin E." *J. Nutr. Sci. Vitaminol.* **22**, 209 (1976).

34. Kobayashi, T., Adachi, A., and Furuta, K. " Gas-liquid chromatographic determination of vitamin D_3 in tuna liver and vitamin D_3 resin oils." *J. Nutr. Sci. Vitaminol.* **22**, 215 (1976).

35. Murray, T. K., Erdody, P., and Panalaks, T. "Determination of vitamin D2 and D3 in pharmaceuticals by gas-liquid chromatography." *J. Assoc. Off. Anal. Chem.* **51**, 839 (1968).

36. Wilson, P. W., Lawson, D. E. M., and Kodicek, E. "Gas-liquid chromatography of ergocalciferol and cholecalciferol in nanogram quantities." *J. Chromatogr.* **39**, 75 (1969).

37. Edlund, D. O., Fillippini, F. A., and Datson, J. K. "Gas-liquid chromatographic determination of vitamin D2 in multiple vitamin tablets containing minerals and vitamin E acetate." *J. Assoc. Off. Anal. Chem.* **57**, 1089 (1974).

38. Burns, D. T., Mackay, C., and Tillman, J. "Rationalization of the chromatographic behavior of vitamin D2/D3 and related compounds in adsorption HPLC." *J. Chromatogr.,* **190**, 140 (1980).

39. Hofsass, H., Grant, A., Alicino, N. J., and Greenbaum, S. B. "High-pressure liquid chromatographic determination of vitamin D3 in resins, oils, dry concentrates, and dry concentrates containing vitamin A." *J. Assoc. Off. Anal. Chem.* **59**, 251 (1976).

40. DeVries, E. J., Zeeman, J., Esser, R. J., Borsje, B., and Mulder, F. J. "Analysis of fat-soluble vitamins—21. High pressure liquid chromatographic assay methods for vitamin D in Vitamin D concentrates." *J. Assoc. Off. Anal. Chem.* **62**, 129 (1979).

41. Mulder, F. J., DeVries, E. J., and Borsje, B. "Analysis of fat-soluble vitamins—23. High performance liquid chromatographic determination of vitamin D in concentrates. Collaborative study." *J. Assoc. Off. Anal. Chem.* **62**, 1031 (1979).

42. Association of Official Analytical Chemists. *Official Methods of Analysis*, 13th ed. Washington, D.C., 751–752 (1980).

43. Mulder, F. J., DeVries, E. J., and Borsje, B. "Analysis of fat-soluble vitamins—24. High performance liquid chromatographic determination of vitamin D in vitamin D resin containing powders: collaborative study." *J. Assoc. Off. Anal. Chem.* **64**, 58 (1981).

44. DeVries, E. J., Zeeman, J., Esser, R. J., Borsje, B., and Mulder, F. J. "Analysis of fat-soluble vitamins—23. High performance liquid chromatographic assay for vitamin D in vitamin D3 and multi-vitamin preparations." *J. Assoc. Off. Anal. Chem.* **62**, 1285 (1979).

45. DeVries, E. J., Mulder, F. J., and Borje, B. "Analysis of fat-soluble vitamins—25. High performance liquid chromatographic determination of vitamin D in multivitamin preparations: Collaborative study." *J. Assoc. Off. Anal. Chem.* **64**, 61 (1981).

46. Lofty, P. A., Jordi, H. D., and Bruno, J. V. "Determination of vitamin D in multivitamin preparation by high performance liquid chromatography." *J. Liq. Chromatog.* **4**, 155 (1981).

47. Changes in Methods. "Vitamin D in mixed feeds, premixes, and pet foods. Liquid chromatographic method-official first action." *J. Assoc. Off. Anal. Chem.* **65**, 494 (1982).

48. Ray, A. C., Dwyer, J. N., and Reagor, J. C. "High pressure liquid chromatographic determination of vitamin D3 in livestock feed supplements." *J. Assoc. Off. Anal. Chem.* **60**, 1296 (1977).

49. Lein, D. G., Campbell, H. M., and Cohen, H. "High pressure liquid chromatographic determination of vitamin D3 in mineral feed premixes." *J. Assoc. Off. Anal. Chem.* **63** 1149 (1980).

50. Thompson, J. N., Maxwell, W. B., and L'Abbe, M. "High performance liquid chromatographic determination of vitamin D in fortified milk." *J. Assoc. Off. Anal. Chem.* **60**, 998 (1977).

51. Thompson, J. N., Hatina, G., Maxwell, W. B., and Duval, S. "High performance liquid chromatographic determination of vitamin D in fortified milk, margarine, and infant formulas." *J. Assoc. Off. Anal. Chem.* **65**, 624 (1982).

52. Cohen, H. and Wakefield, B. "High-pressure liquid chromatographic determination of vitamin D3 in mineral feed premixes." *J. Assoc. Off. Anal. Chem.* **63**, 1149 (1980).

53. Changes in Methods. "Vitamin D in fortified milk and milk powder. High performance (pressure) liquid chromatographic method—official first action." *J. Assoc. Off. Anal. Chem.* **64**, 524 (1981).

54. DeVries, E. J. and Borsje, B. "Analysis of fat-soluble vitamins—27. High-performance liquid chromatography and gas-liquid chromatographic determination of vitamin D in fortified milk and milk powder. Collaborative study." *J. Assoc. Off. Anal. Chem.* **65**, 1228, 1982.

55. Muniz, J. F., Wehr, C. T., and Wehr, H. M. "Reverse phase liquid chromatographic determination of vitamins D_2 and D_3 in milk." *J. Assoc. Off. Anal. Chem.* **65**, 791 (1982).

56. Van Niekerk, P. J. and Smit, S. C. "The determination of vitamin D in margarine by high pressure liquid chromatography." *J. Am. Oil Chem. Soc.* **57**, 417 (1980).

57. Cohen, H. and Lapointe, M. "Determination of low levels of vitamin D3 in animal feeds, using Sephadex LH-20 and normal phase high-pressure liquid chromatography." *J. Assoc. Off. Anal. Chem.* **63**, 1158 (1980).

58. Wiggins, R. A. "Separation of vitamin D_2 and vitamin D_3 by high-pressure liquid chromatography." *Chem. and Ind.* **841** (1977).

59. Osadca, M. and Araujo, M. "High pressure liquid chromatographic separation and identification of vitamin D_2 and D_3 in the presence of fat-soluble vitamins in dosage forms." *J. Assoc. Off. Anal. Chem.* **60**, 993 (1977).

60. Tanaka, Y., DeLuca, H. F., and Ikekawa, N. "High pressure liquid chromatography of vitamin D metabolites and analogs." *Methods Enzymol.* **67**, 370 (1980).

61. Abdou, H. M., Russo-Alesi, F. M., and Fernandez, V., "An automated high pressure liquid chromatographic system for simultaneous determination of A, D, and E." *Pharm. Technol.* **5**, 40 (1981).

62. Borsje, B., Craenen, H. A. H., Esser, R. J. E., Mulder, F. J., and DeVries, E. J. "Analysis of fat-soluble vitamins—18. Inter-laboratory comparison of vitamin D assay methods." *J. Assoc. Off. Anal. Chem.* **61**, 122 (1978).

63. Association of Official Analytical Chemists. *Official Methods of Analysis*, 13th ed. 770–774 (1980).

64. Mulder, F. J. and Van Strik, R. "Analysis of fat-soluble vitamins—17. Comparison of chemical and biological assays of vitamin D." *J. Assoc. Off. Anal. Chem.* **61**, 117 (1978).

65. Borsje, B., Heyting, A., Roborgh, J. R., Ross, D. B., and Shillam, K. W. G. "Analysis of fat-soluble vitamins—16. Antirachitic activity of 5,6-trans-vitamin D_3 alone and in the presence of 5,6-cis-vitamin D_3 resin using chick bioassay." *J. Assoc. Off. Anal. Chem.* **60**, 1003 (1977).

10 Vitamin E

Indrajit D. Desai and Lawrence J. Machlin

GENERAL CONSIDERATIONS

Vitamin E was initially discovered as an antisterility factor in rats, but it has now been generally recognized as essential for all animals including man. It occurs predominantly in plant foods such as vegetable oils and their products, whole-grain cereals, and green leafy vegetables, whereas animal products such as meats, milk, and eggs contain small amounts of this vitamin. Vitamin E is a naturally occurring antioxidant, which specifically inhibits the oxidation of unsaturated fatty acids.

A. Nomenclature and Structure

The term vitamin E refers to a group of four naturally occurring tocols and four tocotrienols having a common molecular structure made up of a chromanol and an isoprenoid side chain, each one exhibiting different stereochemistry and biological activity (1). Vitamin E activity in plant foods derives from α-, β-, γ-, and δ-tocopherols and corresponding tocotrienols. In animal tissues α-tocopherol is the predominant form. The nutritionally important isomers of α-tocopherol are the naturally occurring *d*-α-tocopherol and chemically synthesized *dl*-α-tocopherol and their acetates or succinate esters, which are used as food additives and in pharmaceutical preparations. α-Tocopherol is 2,5,7,8-tetramethyl-2-(4′,8′,12′-trimethyl tridecyl)-6-chromanol.

Naturally occuring *d*-α-tocopherol is 2R,4′R,8′R-α-tocopherol, with structure (Figure 10.1) and is designated as RRR-α-tocopherol. The epimer of *d*-α-to-

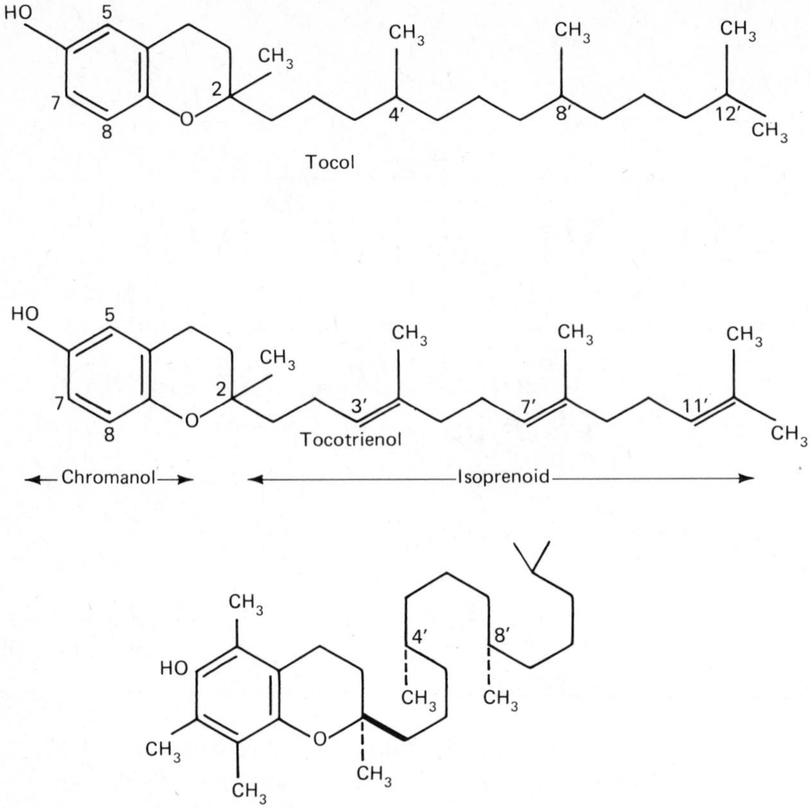

RRR-α-tocopherol (formerly *d*-α-tocopherol)

FIGURE 10.1 Basic structure of tocol and tocotrienol compounds.

copherol, *l*-α-tocopherol or 2S,4′R,8′R is designated as 2-epi-α-tocopherol. Totally synthetic *dl*-α-tocopherol obtained by synthesis using synthetic phytol, is a mixture of four racemates or pairs of enantiomers in unspecified proportions; this is now termed as all-rac-α-tocopherol; the international standard now used is the all-rac-α-topheryl acetate (2). The partially synthetic racemic tocopherol, obtained by synthesis using natural phytol is a mixture of approximately equimolar amounts of RRR-α-tocopherol and 2-epi-α-tocopherol and is termed as 2-ambo-α-tocopherol; this racemic-α-tocopheryl acetate was the former international standard.

The term vitamin E is now used as a generic descriptor for tocol and tocotrienol derivatives, which exhibit the biological activity of α-tocopherol; tocopherols serve as generic descriptors for all methyl tocols. The term tocopherol is not now considered synonymous with the term vitamin E. The nomenclature of tocopherol compounds in this chapter is summarized in Tables 10.1 and 10.2.

TABLE 10.1 Nomenclature and Physical Properties of Tocol and Tocotrienol Compounds

Trivial Name	Structure Designation	Empirical Formula	Molecular Weight	Absorption Max. (nm)	$E_{cm}^{1\%}$ In Alcohol
Tocol					
α-Tocopherol	5,7,8-Trimethyltocol	$C_{29}H_{50}O_2$	430	292	70–73.7
β-Tocopherol	5,8-Dimethyltocol	$C_{28}H_{48}O_2$	416	297	86–87
γ-Tocopherol	7,8-Dimethyltocol	$C_{28}H_{48}O_2$	416	298	90–93
δ-Tocopherol	8-Methyltocol	$C_{27}H_{46}O_2$	402	298	91.2
Tocotrienol					
α-Tocotrienol	5,7,8-Trimethyltocotrienol	$C_{29}H_{44}O_2$	424		
β-Tocotrienol	5,8-Dimethyltocotrienol	$C_{28}H_{42}O_2$	410		
γ-Tocotrienol	7,8-Dimethyltocotrienol	$C_{28}H_{42}O_2$	410		
δ-Tocotrienol	8-Methyltocotrienol	$C_{27}H_{40}O_2$	396		

TABLE 10.2 Nomenclature of α-Tocopherols

	Trivial Name	Revised Designations
1	d-α-tocopherol	2R,4'R,8'R-α-tocopherol or RRR-α-tocopherol
2	l-α-tocopherol	2S,4'R,8'R-α-tocopherol or 2-epi-α-tocopherol
3	dl-α-tocopherol (fully synthetic)	all-rac-α-tocopherol
4	dl-α-tocopherol (partially synthetic mixture of 1 and 2)	2-ambo-α-tocopherol

B. Physical and Chemical Properties

Tocopherols are pale yellow, viscous oils. Some tocopherols can be crystallized, and they are freely soluble in oils, fats, acetone, ethanol, $CHCl_3$, ethyl ether, and other fat solvents. They are stable to visual light but are destroyed by ultraviolet light and darken gradually on continued exposure to light.

Tocopherols fluoresce maximally by excitation at 295 nm; they are stable to heat and alkali in the absence of oxygen and stable to acid. They are slowly oxidized by atmospheric air, rapidly by alkali in the presence of air, and more rapidly by ferric, auric, ceric, silver, and nitrate ions. Tocopherols are effective antioxidants due to the free phenolic hydroxyl group; δ-tocopherol is the most effective antioxidant.

Tocopheryl acetates are less readily soluble in ethanol and practically unaffected by the oxidizing influences of air, visual light, and ultraviolet light.

Vitamin E deficiency is manifested by a variety of symptoms that are highly variable from species to species. Some of these are: testicular degeneration, fetus resorption, deposition of ceroid pigments in the musculature of small intestine and uterus, increased fragility of erythrocytes, increased urinary excretion of creatine, etc. Current information on certain biochemical, hematological, and clinical aspects is available (3). Compared with vitamins A and D, vitamin E is relatively nontoxic.

C. Occurrence

Tocopherols occur in high concentrations (0.1–0.3%) in wheat germ, corn, sunflower seed, rape seed, and soybean oils and in alfalfa and lettuce. The α-form is the major component along with the β-, γ-, and δ-forms. The δ-form constitutes 30% of the mixed tocopherols in soybeam oil. In plant material, tocopherols occur free and esterified. During the processing of vegetable oils into margarine and shortenings, vitamin activity is lost. In dehydrated foods and foods where there is extensive autooxidation, vitamin level is considerably decreased. The decomposition products of tocopherols include dimers, trimers, dihydroxy compounds, quinones, etc. In animal tissues, α-tocopherol occurs free or esterified in the nonsaponifiable lipid portions; in blood, it is associated with lipoproteins.

All-rac-α-tocopherol acetate or succinate is the major constituent in pharmaceuticals and concentrates. When used in feed premixes and in food fortification, the tocopherols are "protected" against oxidation by a coating of wax, fat, gelatin, vegetable gum, or a combination of these. Fortified oils contain both the natural RRR-α-tocopherol and the added synthetic forms in addition to the β-, γ-, and δ-forms.

D. Reference Standard and Biological Activity of Vitamin E Compounds

Vitamin E activity is commonly measured in international units (IU). One IU of vitamin E is considered equivalent to 1 mg of synthetic dl-α-tocopheryl acetate (all-rac-α-tocopheryl acetate) with which the biopotencies of all other forms of tocopherols and tocotrienols are compared. The average biopotencies of various natural and commercially available forms of vitamin E compounds, obtained by various bioassays such as rat fetal resorption test, erythrocyte hemolysis test, etc., are presented in Table 10.3. The activity of naturally occurring RRR-α-tocopherol is higher than synthetic all-rac-α-tocopherol, because 2-epi-α-tocopherol, produced in the racemic mixture during synthetic manufacture, is only about 20–25% as active as RRR-α-tocopherol (4,5). The lower biological activity of the l-form is mainly because of its poor retention in the body (6,7). α-Tocotrienol and β-tocopherol occurring mainly in cereal grains are about 40% as active as α-tocopherol (8), whereas γ-tocopherol present mainly in vegetable

TABLE 10.3 Relative Biological Activity of Vitamin E Compounds

Vitamin E Compound	Relative Biological Activity (IU per mg)	References
2-ambo-α-tocopheryl acetate or dl-α-tocopheryl acetate (former International Std.)	1.00	2
all-rac-α-tocopheryl acetate (current International Std.)	1.00	2
all-rac-α-tocopherol	1.10	2
RRR-α-tocopheryl acetate or d-α-tocopheryl acetate	1.36	2
RRR-α-tocopherol or d-δ-tocopherol	1.49	2
2-epi-α-tocopherol or l-α-tocopherol	0.21–0.24	4,5
β-Tocopherol	0.50	10
γ-Tocopherol	0.10	10
α-Tocotrienol	0.30	10

oils such as soybean oil has only about 10% activity of that of α-tocopherol (9). One practical approach to expressing vitamin E activity of various forms of tocopherols in mixed human diets is to multiply α-tocopherol values by a factor of 1.2 (10).

E.   Sample Preparation, Preservation, and General Precautions

Fresh plant and animal tissues, unsupplemented food and feed, and oils will contain natural α-tocopherol associated with many other reducing substances. Premixes and supplemented food/feed will contain, in addition, synthetic α-tocopheryl acetate coated with protectants. Sample materials require preparatory treatment.

Fresh plant and animal tissues require homogenization in a Waring Blender or an Omni-mixer. The loss of tocopherols due to heat generated during homogenization is prevented by immersing a blending cup in a bucket containing mixture of ice and H_2O. The homogenates can either be freeze-dried or converted into acetone powder. Dried foods and feeds should be ground into fine powder prior to extraction.

Premixes containing wax- or fat-coated tocopherols and food and feed fortified with these premixes are extracted with hot hexane; gelatin or vegetable gum-coated materials are boiled with dilute H_2SO_4 before extraction with ethanol.

Biological fluids such as plasma and serum do not require preparatory and purification steps and are stored in frozen condition. Oils and fats also do not require this step.

Among the pharmaceuticals and concentrates, tablets are powdered and agitated with warm H_2O to dissolve H_2O-soluble components; capsules are agitated with warm H_2O to break the capsule and dissolve the capsule; liquid materials are used as such without any pretreatment.

All samples and solutions of tocopherols are stored in the dark at $-20°C$, if the analysis is not completed in 1 day. Analysis should be done preferably in subdued light. Evaporate tocopherol solutions with nitrogen or under vacuum. A thin film of dry tocopherol will oxidize very rapidly.

Trace amounts of nonspecific reducing substances and metal ion contaminations can interfere with the vitamin E analyses. Only all-glass apparatus and glass-stoppered tubes and reagent bottles should be used. Silicone stopcock grease, rubber, polyethylene, crayon-type marking pencil, and so on, must never be used. However, cork stoppers, if well protected with aluminum foil can be used.

All glassware should be soaked overnight in sulfochromic acid or 8 N nitric acid or dilute hydrochloric acid (1 + 2) prior to thorough washing with plenty of tap water. Several rinsings with distilled water followed by an additional rinsing with glass-distilled water must be routinely carried out. Final rinsing should be carried out with redistilled ethanol or purified acetone prior to heat drying in an oven. Clean glassware should be stored in dustproof cabinets until use.

Purity of chemicals and solvents is a critical factor in the analysis of vitamin E. Only certified analytical grade pure chemicals should be used.

METHODS AVAILABLE

Following initial extraction and saponification, the unsaponifiable fraction from the test sample is purified to isolate tocopherol-containing fractions. The tocopherol content of these fractions can be estimated by several methods; these are categorized under biological, physical, and chemical methods.

A. Biological Methods

The methods most commonly used for the bioassay of vitamin E are based on fetal resorption in female rats, erythrocyte-hemolysis with dialuric acid or hydrogen peroxide, muscular dystrophy, and liver storage.

1. *Fetal Resorption Bioassay.*   This classical method for testing the biological activity of vitamin E compounds measures the reproductive performance in successfully mated female rats in producing viable offspring (11–13). The general procedure for a typical fetal resorption bioassay of vitamin E follows:

(a) Female rats weighing between 40–50 g are placed on a vitamin E-free basal diet.

(b) After 30–40 days on the vitamin E-free diet, female rats weighing about 150 g are mated with colony males of proven fertility.

(c) The females are observed daily for ascertaining fertilization by examining vaginal smears for spermatozoa.

(d) The pregnant rats are divided into groups of 10 rats in each group and different levels of standard (*dl*-α-tocopheryl acetate contining 1.0 IU of vitamin E/mg) and unknown test sample are fed in food or olive oil over 5 successive days beginning on the day 5 of pregnancy.

(e) On day 20 of pregnancy, each rat is sacrificed and the uterus examined for viable fetuses and implantation sites. Only animals that have at least four implantation sites are evaluated. At least one viable fetus indicates a positive response, whereas no living fetus indicates a negative test.

(f) Vitamin E activity is determined by calculating the percentage of rats in each group having positive response (percent litter efficiency) and by converting these to probits or similar units by referring to statistical tables and plotting against dose (in mg) or log of dose to give the median fertility dose (dose of vitamin E required for 50% litter efficiency). A ratio of the median fertility values for the standard dose and the test dose is the relative biopotency of the sample in international units.

The classical fetal resorption-rat bioassay is laborious and time consuming, but has the advantage of being more specific than indirect bioassays such as erythrocyte-hemolysis and liver storage tests. Female rats, if maintained on a vitamin E-deficient diet for a prolonged period of time, may fail to conceive in spite of repeated matings (14). This irreversible sterility is associated with ceroid pigment formation in the uterus (15).

2. *Erythrocyte-Hemolysis Test.*

(a) Hemolysis with dialuric acid.   A modified version (16) of the original test (17) is based on the degree of susceptibility of erythrocytes from vitamin E-deficient and -supplemented rats to in vitro hemolysis by dialuric acid. Procedure:

(1) Male or female rats weighing about 100 g are depleted of vitamin E by feeding a vitamin E-deficient diet until the erythrocytes show 90–99% hemolysis. This may require a period of 3–4 weeks.

(2) An appropriate amount of test dose dissolved in small amount (0.2 mL) of olive oil is administered orally by stomach tube.

(3) After 40–44 hr of the test dose, erythrocytes are collected and tested for in vitro hemolysis by dialuric acid, and percentage hemolysis is calculated.

(4) The biopotency of the test substance containing vitamin E is determined from the reduction in the in vitro erythrocyte hemolysis of the test rats' as compared with vitamin E-deficient rats.

The hemolysis test in general compares well with fetal-resorption and liver-storage bioassays but proper precautions are needed in eliminating interference by contaminants from unclean glassware and synthetic antioxidants to obtain reliable results. More details about this test can be obtained from the original publications (16,17).

(b) Hemolysis with hydrogen peroxide.   This is a test for the assessment of vitamin E status in humans wherein hydrogen peroxide instead of dialuric acid is used for in vitro hemolysis of erythrocytes (18–20).

3. *Muscular Dystrophy Bioassay.*   Muscular dystrophy is a common manifestation of vitamin E deficiency in many species of animals and has been used as an index for testing the biopotency of vitamin E compounds in rabbits (21,22), chicks (5,7,23), and ducklings (24). A typical test using rats or rabbits may involve raising animals on vitamin E-deficient diet and determining the relative biopotency of a test sample against vitamin E standard using muscular dystrophy lesions on thighs and/or creatinuria as indices of bioassay. The chick bioassay is carried out by raising 1-day-old chicks on a basal vitamin E-deficient diet with and without supplements of vitamin E standard and test samples. After a period of 4–6 weeks, lesions of muscular dystrophy on breast muscle are scored on a scale ranging from 0 for absence of dystrophy to 4 for maximal dystrophy (5,7,23). Other indices such as thiobarbituric acid index and hydrolytic activity of lysosomal enzymes (23) and serum enzyme activities of aspartate aminotranferase and lactic dehydrogenase (24) have also been used in conjunction with nutritional muscular dystrophy in animals.

4. *Liver Storage Bioassay.*   Bioassay based on storage of tocopherols in tissue such as liver have been developed on the assumption that vitamin E stores in

the liver of rats (25,26) and chicks (27–29) show a linear response to the level of vitamin E in the diet. In a typical liver storage bioassay, groups of 1-day-old chicks are placed on a vitamin E-deficient diet and then given supplements of standard tocopherol or test material for a period of 3 days (short assay) or 13 days (long assay). The chicks are sacrificed at the end of a test period and liver vitamin E content determined as described under physicochemical methods.

B. Chemical and Physical Methods of Vitamin E Analysis

1. *Colorimetry.*   This widely used method is based on Emmerie and Engel's reaction (30) in which tocopherols reduce ferric ions to ferrous ions; ferrous ions form a red-colored complex with α,α'-dipyridine which can be measured at 520 nm. The reaction is unstable and requires that all samples be read at 30 sec after starting the reaction. Many nonspecific reducing substances such as carotenoids, vitamin A, and sterols interfere with this colorimetric measurement of tocopherols, and, hence, this method is more suitable for purified extracts or eluate fractions from thin-layer, paper, or column chromatography. A modified Emmerie-Engel procedure (31) uses bathophenanthroline (4,7-diphenyl-1,10-phenanthroline) instead of α,α'-dipyridine, whereby a more sensitive and stable chromophore is developed that eliminates the need for timing each reaction. The background absorbancy of this new reaction employing orthophosphoric acid as stabilizing agent is low and many samples can be simultaneously handled with great accuracy.

2. *Spectrophotometry.*   The physical properties and absorption characteristics of various tocopherols as shown in Tables 10.1 and 10.2 can be used to directly measure spectra of these compounds at specific wavelengths in natural products (32) and pharmaceutical preparations. However, this method is useful only when the samples to be examined are in pure and concentrated form, since tocopherols have low intensity of absorption in ultraviolet light and impurities can interfere with the absorbance measurements.

3. *Spectrofluorometry.*   Spectrofluorometric assay of tocopherols involves measurement of fluorescence at 295-nm and 340-nm wavelengths at which maximum excitation and emission, respectively, are obtained. An extract of the sample is prepared in an appropriate solvent such as ethanol or hexane and the fluorescence is measured and compared against a standard of known concentration of tocopherols in the same solvent. Selection of a proper solvent is very important since different solvents can alter fluorescence measurements. Fluorescence spectrometry is very useful for measuring free and esterified tocopherols, since only free tocopherols exhibit fluorescence whereas esterified tocopherols require hydrolysis by ethereal lithium aluminum hydride to form free fluorescing tocopherols (33). Tocopherols in extracts of tissues, foods, and pharmaceuticals are measured spectrofluorometrically after hydroxyalkoxypropyl-Sephadex chromatography to remove the impurities (34).

4. *Chromatographic Methods.*
    (a) Paper chromatography.   Separation and identification by the method

involves two-dimensional chromotography on zinc carbonate-impregnated paper with a solvent mixture of benzene in cyclohexane (30% v/v) for the first dimension and 75% ethanol in H_2O for the second. Tocopherol spots are identified under ultraviolet light, after spraying the paper with 0.7% sodium fluorescein in H_2O. The method is cumbersome, time consuming, and not very accurate for individual tocopherols (35).

(b) Thin-layer chromatography (TLC).   A two-dimensional TLC on silica gel G, alumina, or magnesium phosphate is efficient in the separation and estimation of individual tocopherols (36–44). Different solvent systems such as benzene-ethanol, hexane-ethanol, benzene-ethyl ether, cylohexane-benzene, and petroleum ether-isopropyl ether have been used. Adsorbant coating contains sodium fluorescein for the visualization of tocopherol spots under UV light.

The chromatogram in Figure 10.2 shows the separation of all tocopherols

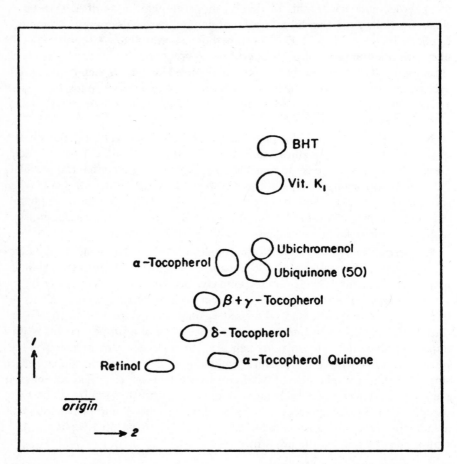

FIGURE 10.2   Thin-layer chromatography of tocopherols, tocotrienols, and other lipid components on silica gel G (37).

and the corresponding tocotrienols from overlapping components such as retinol, tocopherol quinone, ubiquinone, and ubichromanol. Tocopherol esters, if present, can be estimated by conversion to the free forms by lithium aluminum hydride (33).

Individual spots are quantitatively removed with ethanol and the tocopherol content is measured by colorimetry or spectrofluorometry procedures.

A detailed TLC procedure based on AOAC method will be described later (45).

(c) Column chromatography. Column chromatography is effective in separating nonspecific interfering lipid materials associated with tocopherols prior to final analysis. Adsorbents such as Florex (28,35), Decalso (46), and Celite 545-digitonin have been used; Florex treated with HCl and $SnCl_2$ (47) is recommended for satisfactory removal of carotenoids, vitamin A, and sterols.

Complete separation of individual tocopherols and tocotrienols by column chromatography has not been achieved. Adsorbents such as deactivated alumina (36), zinc carbonate (48), secondary magnesium phosphate (49,50), florisil, and silicic acid (51) have been used with limited success.

(d) High-performance liquid chromatography (HPLC). HPLC systems are being used for continuous monitoring of the separation and estimation of vitamin E compounds. Corosil II column eluted under pressure either with 5% diisopropyl ether in hexane (45) or with 0.5% tetrahydrofuran in η-hexane (52) at a flow rate of 1–1.5 mL/min has been successful in separating all forms of tocopherols and tocotrienols. Another column (Jascopack WC-03-500) was developed for high-pressure/high-speed liquid chromatography of vitamin E compounds in vegetable oils using 2% diisopropyl ether in hexane as a mobile phase applied at a flow rate of 0.8 mL/min (53). HPLC is the method of choice for routine analysis and quality control analysis in government and industrial laboratories. Survey of methodology and the detailed HPLC method for simultaneous assay of vitamins A and E are in the chromatography procedures chapter.

(e) Gas-liquid chromatography (GLC). GLC has been used successfully for routine analysis of tocopherols, tocopheryl esters, and other tocopherol derivatives such as trimethyl silyl ethers.

Instrumental set-up of gas-liquid chromatography is a standard gas chromatographic unit equipped with hydrogen flame or β-argon ionization detector and a suitable Pyrex glass or stainless steel column containing silanized inert support made up of Gaschrom, Chromsorb, or Celite. The column is filled with a stationary liquid phase of choice in concentration ranging from 1–10% of the column weight. A variety of silicone-type liquid phases such as SE-30 (54-61), SE-52 (62), QF-1 (56), XE-60 (63), Apiezon N or L (54,59,60), and OV-17 or 1 (60,64) have been used, but SE-30 has been commonly used by most for routine analysis of tocopherols. A mixture of SE-52 and XE-60 liquid phases has also been used for the separation of tocopherols and their trimethylsilyl ethers (65–67).

The relative retention times of unknown tocopherols are determined by injecting internal standards such as cholestane, octacosane, or squalene and known reference standards of tocopherol compounds or their derivatives (55–61,65–67).

GLC procedure (AOAC) for tocopheryl acetate analysis of pharmaceuticals will be described in detail (45,68).

ANALYTICAL METHODOLOGY

I. COLORIMETRIC PROCEDURE FOR BIOLOGICAL FLUIDS

A. Principle

The method is based on the oxidation of xylene-extracted tocopherols of the blood sample by ferric chloride and the pink complex of ferrous ions with bathophenanthroline is measured colorimetrically at 536 nm. This is a modification of Emmerie and Engel's method (25,26,68) and is useful for blood serum and plasma and other fluids.

B. Equipment

   1. *Spectrophotometer.*
   2. *Centrifuge.*
   3. *Vortex Mixer.*
   4. *Centrifuge Tubes.*

C. Reagents

   1. *Absolute Ethanol (Redistilled).*
   2. *Xylene (Redistilled).*
   3. *4,7-Diphenyl-1,10-Phenanthroline (Bathophenanthroline) Reagent.* Dissolve 400 mg in purified absolute ethanol and make up to 100 mL with the same solvent.
   4. *Ferric Chloride Reagent.* Dissolve 60 mg of $FeCl_3 \cdot 6H_2O$ in purified absolute ethanol and make up to 100 mL with the same solvent. Store in amber bottle for no more than 1 week in a refrigerator or use fresh solution every time.
   5. *Orthophosphoric Acid, 85% Analytical Reagent Grade.* Dilute solution of 0.5 mL/100 mL purified absolute ethanol is used.
   6. *Vitamin E Stock Solution.* Dissolve 100 mg of *dl*-α-tocopherol in purified absolute ethanol and make up to 100 mL with the same solvent. Put it in an amber bottle and store in a refrigerator where it is stable for several weeks.
   7. *Vitamin E Standard Solution.* Dilute 2 mL of stock solution to 100 mL with purified absolute ethanol. Stable for several days in amber bottle placed in a refrigerator.

D. Procedure

1. Pipette 0.6 mL of serum or plasma, 0.6 mL of vitamin E standard, and 0.6 mL of glass-distilled H_2O in three 15-mL glass-stoppered centrifuge tubes marked "test," "standard," and "blank," respectively.

2. Add 0.6 mL of purified absolute ethanol to tubes marked "test" and "blank" and 0.6 mL of glass-distilled H_2O to tube marked "standard," stopper, and mix with a Vortex mixer.

3. Add 0.6 mL of purified xylene to all tubes. Stopper and mix on a Vortex mixer for 2 min.

4. Centrifuge all tubes for 5 min at 3000 rpm.

5. Exactly 0.4 mL of serum or plasma-xylene extract from each centrifuge tube is carefully pipetted into fresh, appropriately labeled, glass-stoppered test tubes containing 0.2 mL of bathophenanthroline reagent and mixed.

6. Add 0.2 mL of ferric chloride reagent followed by 0.2 mL of ortho-phosphoric acid solution. The contents of the tube are mixed thoroughly on a Vortex mixer after every addition of reagents. The order of reagent addition is critical. Orthophosphoric acid as a chelating agent of residual ferric ions, reduces carotene interference, and stabilizes the color.

7. Read the absorbance of the "test" and "standard" at 536 nm using 1.2 mL semimicrocuvettes and a suitable spectrophotometer set to zero with the "blank" cuvette.

E. Calculation

Concentration of vitamin E or tocopherols in mg per 100 mL of serum or plasma can be calculated as follows:

$$\frac{\text{Absorbance of "test"}}{\text{Absorbance of "standard"}} \times \text{concentration of "standard" in mg/100 mL}$$

The method is simple and sensitive and does not require timing of the color reaction and use of correction factors to compensate for the carotene effect. A standard curve and recovery test should occasionally be run to check the accuracy of the method under variable analytical conditions.

II. COLORIMETRIC PROCEDURE—THIN-LAYER AND OXIDATIVE CHROMATOGRAPHY

A. Principle

Tocopherols reduce ferric ions to ferrous ions, which readily react with batho-phenanthroline to form a stable red chromophore, in the presence of phosphoric acid. The background absorbancy of this reaction is low and the absorbance of this chromophore is measured at 536 nm. This modified Emmerie-Engel procedure is used to measure tocopherols isolated from foods and feeds.

Extensive purification procedures remove interfering compounds such as chlorophylls, xanthophylls, carotenoids, sterols, and other lipid components. Two-dimensional TLC separates tocopherol components for final colorimetry. Rapid and reliable estimates are obtained for the different vitamin E analogs in foods (69,70), vegetable oils (40,41,43,71), edible plant leaves (72,73), and algae (74,75).

Procedural steps for naturally occurring α-tocopherol:

1. Hot ethanol extraction of sample.
2. Saponification of lipid extract with alcoholic KOH.
3. Separation of tocopherols by two-dimensional TLC on alumina.
4. Colorimetry of individual tocopherol analogs or total tocopherols.

Procedural steps for fortified synthetic α-tocopheryl acetate:

1. Extraction.
2. Oxidative chromatography to isolate α-tocopheryl acetate.
3. Saponification of the acetate.
4. Colorimetry of α-tocopherol from the acetate ester.

B. Equipment

1. *Spectrophotometer.*   Beckman Model DU or equivalent with matched cells (1-cm light path; 1.6 mL).

2. *Spectrophotometric Colorimeter.*   Bausch & Lomb Spec. 20 or equivalent.

3. *Soxhlet Extractor.*   Goldfisch or equivalent.

4. *Chromatogram Sheet.*   Alumina adsorbent without fluorescent indicator, for vitamin E assay. Type X6062. Heat for 30 min at 105°C in air oven for activation, if necessary.

5. *Pipettes.*   Ultramicro, 50 μL capacity.

6. *Developing Chamber.*   Pyrex, Corning Glassworks 69664.

7. *Sprayer.*   Aerosol propellent.

8. *Vials.*
   (a) Glass with screw caps, 1.8 mL capacity.
   (b) Glass with polyethylene stoppers, 25 mL capacity.

9. *Chromatography Tubes.*   Pyrex 18 (i.d.) × 270 mm with constricted end.

10. *Ultraviolet Lamps.*   366-nm or 254-nm wavelength.

C. Reagents

1. *Petroleum Ether.*
   (a) Purified, boiling range 35–60°C. Redistill from KOH pellets and Zn granules or dust, discarding first and last 5%.

(b) High boiling 60–71°C.

2. *Ethanol, Absolute.* Redistill from Al granules and KOH pellets.

3. *Anhydrous Ethyl Ether.* Redistill from Al granules or dust and KOH pellets, discarding first and last 5%.

4. *Isopropyl Ether.*

5. *Cyclohexane.*

6. *Petroleum Ether–Absolute Ethanol Mixture.* Dilute 600 mL of pet ether (l.b.) to 1 L with absolute ethanol.

7. *Anhydrous Sodium Sulfate.* Granular and powdered.

8. *Ascorbic Acid.*

9. *Benzene.*

10. *0.172 M Orthophosphoric Acid.* Dilute 1.1 mL 86% H_3PO_4 to 100 mL with absolute ethanol.

11. *0.002 M Ferric Chloride Solution.* Dissolve 55 mg $FeCl_3 \cdot 6H_2O$ in 100 ml of absolute ethanol and store in amber glass bottle at 5°C.

12. *0.003 M Bathophenanthroline Solution.* Dissolve 100 mg 4,7-diphenyl-1,10-phenanthroline in 100 mL absolute ethanol. Store in amber glass bottle at 5°C. Prepare fresh solution every 3 weeks.

13. *1% Phenolphthalein in Absolute Ethanol.*

14. *2',7'-Dichlorofluorescein Solution.* Dissolve 3 mg dye in 100 mL absolute ethanol.

15. *Diatomaceous Earth.* Celite 501 or equivalent inert filter aid.

16. *Fuller's Earth.* Florex AA-RVM grade, 60–100 mesh.

17. *Ceric Sulfate-Treated Fuller's Earth.* Add a mix of 0.5 mL H_2SO_4 and 5 mL H_2O to 4.8 g $Ce(HSO_4)_4$ and stir. Dilute to 100 mL with H_2O. Warm in hot H_2O bath and shake until all $Ce(HSO_4)_4$ is dissolved. Cool to 35–40°C. Distribute this solution immediately onto 200 g of Fuller's earth. Spread out in a large glazed porcelain dish. Stir gently but thoroughly and dry 48 hr in 60°C oven. Store in tightly capped bottle.

18. *Standard α-Tocopherol.* Dissolve 100 mg RRR-α-tocopherol in 100 mL absolute ethanol and store at 5°C.

19. *Potassium Hydroxide Solution.* Dissolve 80 g KOH pellets in 50 mL H_2O.

D. Procedure

1. *Sample Extraction.* Sample size varies from a minimal 1 g to 40 g; with an estimated α-tocopherol content of 0.1–0.2 mg, use 10 g for most foods and feeds. For foods supplemented at low levels using high-potency premixes, use about 40 g.

(a) Oils and fats. Liquify the fat if necessary, mix thoroughly and weigh an aliquot containing approximately about 0.2 mg of α-tocopherol, into a 125-mL round-bottom flask.

(b) Dairy products. Transfer to a separatory funnel 60 mL of milk or condensed milk product or reconstituted milk powder and add an equal volume of absolute ethanol and shake. Add 150 mL ethyl ether, shake 30 sec, add 150 mL pet ether, and shake 30 sec. Allow layers to separate and remove ether layer. Repeat the extraction twice with 25 mL ethanol, 100 mL ethyl ether, and 100 mL pet ether. Combine ether layers and evaporate to 50 mL. Evaporate a 10-mL aliquot and weigh lipid. Evaporate the remaining 40-mL extract or an aliquot containing approximately 1 g lipid and approximately 0.15 mg of α-tocopherol, in 125-mL round-bottom flask under nitrogen on a steam bath. Proceed immediately to saponification.

(c) Dry foods, feeds, feed concentrates, and premixes containing α-tocopheryl acetate added directly or in a dry carrier.   Grind the sample, if coarse, to a fine powder. Weigh a suitable amount into Soxhlet thimble. Add 100 mL absolute ethanol and boiling chip to the flask and mark the liquid level. Assemble the extraction apparatus with condenser and extract on a steam bath for 16 hr (or overnight).

Extract 4 hr with a Goldfisch extractor, stopper the flask, cool to room temperature and add ethanol to restore to the original volume.

Transfer the extract to a separatory funnel; rinse the flask with 100 mL H_2O followed by 50 mL pet ether and add the rinses to the funnel. Add approximately 0.5 g anhydrous Na_2SO_4 and shake for 10 min. Allow layers to separate, drain, and discard the H_2O layer. Dilute the pet ether extract to 50 mL. Evaporate a 10-mL aliquot and weigh the lipid. Proceed with the 40 mL extract as in Section II.D.1(b).

(d) Products in (c) above, supplemented with α-tocopheryl acetate in gelatin, vegetable gum, or dextrin matrix. Proceed as in Section II.D.1(c) starting with a suitable amount of sample. Retain the pet ether extract after discarding the H_2O layer. Transfer quantitatively the contents of Soxhlet thimble to a round-bottom flask with a total of 50 mL 2.5 N H_2SO_4. Reflux 30 min on a hot plate. Cool to room temperature and transfer the contents to a separating funnel and rinsing the flask with 50 mL absolute ethanol. Extract with two 75-mL and one 50-mL portions of pet ether. Combine this pet ether extract with the pet ether extract from hot alcohol extraction. Evaporate these combined extracts under nitrogen to less than 50 mL and dilute to 50 mL.

Evaporate a 10-mL aliquot and weigh the lipid. Proceed with the 40-mL extract as in Section II.D.1(b).

This extract is not suitable to determine the supplemental α-tocopheryl acetate by oxidative chromatography.

Wet samples such as plant and animal tissues, and so on. Grind thoroughly in a large mortar, a weighed sample with two to three times its weight of anhydrous powdered Na_2SO_4, to a dry mixture. Transfer quantitatively the mixture to one or two Soxhlet thimbles, using absolute ethanol as rinse liquid. Proceed as in Section II.D.1(c).

2. *Saponification-Reextraction.*   Add 4 mL absolute ethanol and 0.3 g ascorbic acid for each gram (or fraction of gram) of lipid residue in the 125-mL

round-bottom flask. Heat to boiling under reflux in a boiling H_2O bath. Add 1 mL of KOH solution for each gram of lipid residue and reflux 15 min.

Exclusion of air or addition of ascorbic acid is essential to restrict the oxidation of tocopherols under alkaline conditions.

Stopper the flask and cool the contents rapidly in running water. Transfer the solution to a separating funnel with 20 mL H_2O. Rinse the flask with 25 mL ethyl ether and extract with two 25-mL portions ethyl ether, the nonsaponified material.

Add NaCl to break up any emulsion.

Combine ethyl ether extracts and wash with equal volumes H_2O until neutral to phenolphthalein.

Prior to H_2O wash, the ethyl ether extract should be washed twice with equal volumes H_2SO_4 (1 + 1), if the original samples contain BHA or ethoxyquin. If ether becomes visible in the H_2SO_4 (1 + 1) wash, wash this acid layer once with ethyl ether and add this ethyl ether to the unsaponafiable ether extract.

Filter the washed ethyl ether extract through granular anhydrous Na_2SO_4 into a small flask and rinse with ethyl ether; concentrate the dry extract under nitrogen by gentle warming and dilute to 10 mL with ethyl ether. Suitable aliquots are used in TLC and in colorimetry.

3. *Thin-Layer Chromatography (TLC).*   TLC of α-tocopherol should be performed in subdued light or in darkness; TLC is sensitive to ambient humidity. Recovery factor for alumina TLC under the most suitable solvent systems should be determined first with standard tocopherol before the samples are analyzed.

(a) Recovery factor.   Depending on ambient relative humidity, choose a suitable solvent system from Table 10.4, to get an R_f value of 0.5–0.7 for α-tocopherol. The alumina sheet must be activated before use at > 60% humidity.

Transfer quantitatively 10 μL standard tocopherol solution (contains 10 μg) to a spot about 2 cm from the lower and left edges of alumina sheet. Rinse pipette with ether and add to the spot. Dry spot with nitrogen jet everytime.

Place the alumina sheet immediately in TLC chamber and develop in the

TABLE 10.4   TLC of α-Tocopherol—Humidity Conditions

	Solvent Systems	
Relative Humidity (%)	1st Dimension Benzene-Ether	2nd Dimension Pet Ether-Isopropyl Ether
< 20	60 + 40 + 1% H_2O	50 + 50 + 1% H_2O
20	60 + 40	50 + 50
40	90 + 10	80 + 20
60	100 + 0	90 + 10
	Cyclohexane-Benzene	
> 60	20 + 80	100 + 0

first-dimension solvent system, until the solvent front moves about 15–16 cm from bottom of sheet. Remove sheet from chamber and dry with nitrogen. Place the sheet immediately in the second chamber, after turning the sheet 90° counterclockwise and develop in the second-dimension solvent system until the solvent front moves about 15–16 cm from the bottom of sheet. Remove the sheet from second chamber and dry with nitrogen gas.

Spray sheet lightly with dichlorofluorescein solution and allow sheet to dry completely for 5 min. Locate tocopherol spot under UV light and circle this spot and spot of comparable size from unused but sprayed portion of sheet for blank.

Avoid excessive use of UV light and allow a safety margin of about 5 mm while circling tocopherol and blank spots.

Cut out both spots and transfer to two separate 25-mL vials, containing 1.4 mL bathophenanthroline solution; elute after replacing cap, swirling, and standing for 15 min. Determine the tocopherol content colorimetrically.

$$\text{Recovery factor} = \frac{\mu\text{g of } \alpha\text{-tocopherol recovered from sheet}}{\mu\text{g of standard } \alpha\text{-tocopherol applied to spot}}$$

The value may range from 75–85% but should be constant within the same laboratory.

(b) Separation of α-tocopherol.   Pipette a suitable aliquot (from Section II.D.2) containing about 10–20 μg α-tocopherol into 1.8-mL vial and reduce the volume to 0.1–0.2 μL by evaporating ethyl ether under nitrogen. With a micropipet, transfer slowly the entire vial contents to form a small spot about 2 cm from lower and left edges of alumina sheet. Rinse the vial with a few drops of ethyl ether and transfer the rinse to the spot. Dry spot with nitrogen jet.

Spot standard α-tocopherol about 2 cm from lower and right edges of the same alumina sheet and dry the spot. Place the sheet immediately in the first chamber and develop as in Section II.D.3(a).

Identify α-tocopherol spot of sample by comparison with standard tocopherol spot. Elute the sample tocopherol as described in Section II.D.3(a). Any bright blue fluorescent spot about 1 cm above α-tocopherol spot is due to any residual ethoxyquin.

(c) Colorimetry.   Set up the Beckman spectrophotometer to measure at 536 nm.

Transfer 1.0 mL of bathophenanthroline solution from each vial [Section II.D.3(b)] to a 15-mL centrifuge tube, add 0.3 mL $FeCl_3$ solution dropwise, and swirl. Add 0.3 mL H_3PO_4 solution exactly 15 sec after the addition of the last drop of $FeCl_3$ and swirl. The color, formed after 3 min, is stable for 90 min.

Centrifuge, if necessary, to settle adsorbent particles. Transfer supernate to separate cells and measure the absorbance of test spot against that of blank spot.

Prepare a calibration curve by measuring the absorbance of a series of standard solutions of α-tocopherol. Determine the amount of α-tocopherol in the sample using the calibration curve and the recovery factor.

This colorimetry procedure is applicable to samples low in lipid and the use of spectrophotometer.

4. *Colorimetry for α-Tocopherol Equivalents or Total Reducing Substances.* Ethyl ether extract of nonsaponifiable material from step II.D.2 is used in colorimetry. Matched 13-mm colorimeter tubes should be used with Spec 20 colorimeter, set to measure at 536 nm. Subdued lighting conditions are essential.

(a) Calibration curve.   Prepare a series of standard solutions containing 5–50 μg of α-tocopherol in pet ether–absolute ethanol mixture.

Transfer exactly 4 mL pet ether–absolute ethanol solvent mixture (reagent blank) and 4 mL of standard tocopherol (5 μg) solution to separate 25-mL vials. To the standard tocopherol solution, add 1.0 mL bathophenanthroline solution and swirl; add exactly 0.5 mL $FeCl_3$ solution dropwise and swirl. Exactly 15 sec after the addition of last drop of $FeCl_3$, add 0.5 mL H_3PO_4 solution and swirl. The color formed after 3 min is stable for 90 min. Repeat the steps for the reagent blank.

Transfer solutions to matched colorimeter tubes and measure A at 536 nm. Repeat using the series of standard α-tocopherol solution. Plot A against μg of tocopherol and draw the best fitting smooth curve through 6 points and origin.

New calibration curve must be prepared for new reagent solutions and also checked daily.

(b) Colorimetry of samples.   Transfer accurately aliquot of ethyl ether extract from Section II.D.2., estimated to contain 20 μg of α-tocopherol or equivalent reducing substances to 25-mL vial. Evaporate to dryness under nitrogen and add immediately 4 mL of pet ether–absolute ethanol solvent mixture. Swirl and dissolve the sample. Add exactly 1.0 mL bathophenanthroline solution and continue as in Section II.D.4(a) to measure A at 536 nm.

If the color formed is too dark for accurate A measurement, dilute the solution with reagent blank and read A again. For extract samples containing more than 100 mg of lipid or unsaponifiable matter, the final colored solution must be centrifuged at 2500 rpm for 10 min, before colorimetry.

Determine the α-tocopherol or total equivalent of reducing substances in μg/6 mL from the standard calibration curve.

5. *Calculations.*

(a) α-Tocopherol from TLC separation.

$$\text{mg } \alpha\text{-tocopherol}/\text{g composited sample} =$$
$$\mu\text{g } \alpha\text{-tocopherol measured} \times \frac{1.4}{1.0} \times \frac{x}{y} \times \frac{v}{w} \times \frac{1}{1000} \times \frac{1}{W}$$

where x = total mL of extract before saponification;
       y = mL of x used for saponification;
       v = total mL of unsaponifiable extract;
       w = mL of unsaponifiable extract used for spotting on TLC;
       $^1/_{1000}$ = factor to convert μg to mg;
       1.4   = mL of bathophenanthroline solution used for elution;
       1.0   = mL of eluate used;
       W = weight in grams of composited assay sample.

(b) α-Tocopherol or equivalent total reducing material from colorimetry.

$$\text{mg } \alpha\text{-tocopherol equivalent/g composited sample} =$$
$$\mu\text{g } \alpha\text{-tocopherol measured} \times \frac{x}{y} \times \frac{a}{b} \times \frac{1}{1000} \times \frac{1}{W}$$

Where x = total mL of extract before saponification;
       y = mL of x used for saponification;
       a = total mL of unsaponifiable extract;
       b = mL of a used in colorimetry measurement;
       W = weight in grams of composited assay sample.

6. *Oxidative Chromatography for Added α-Tocopherol Acetate.*

(a) Sample extraction.   Grind thoroughly a weighed amount of wet sample with two to three times its weight of powdered anhydrous Na_2SO_4 in a large motar until dry.

Samples are extracted with 50 mL purified ethyl ether in a glass-stoppered flask by shaking for 15 min and allowing the solids to settle. Use 10-mL aliquot of the extract to determine the lipid content by evaporating the solvent slowly. Transfer a suitable aliquot containing about 1 g lipid and 0.1 mg of supplemental tocopherol compounds to a 125-mL round-bottom flask and evaporate under nitrogen just to dryness. Redissolve the residue in 4 mL pet ether.

Extracted samples of dairy products [Section (II.D.1(b)] are evaporated just to dryness under nitrogen and the residue is dissolved in pet ether. Fat or oil sample is dissolved in pet ether. Extracted samples of dry food and feed [Section II.D.1.(c)] in pet ether are used as such.

(b) Oxidative chromatography.

(1) Column preparation.

Place a small wool plug at the constricted end of the chromatography tube. Layer uniformly on top of this plug in the following order: 3 g Fuller's earth, 3 g $Ce(HSO_4)_4$-treated Fuller's earth, 3-mm layer Fuller's earth, 3 g $Ce(HSO_4)_4$-treated Fuller's earth, 4 g Fuller's earth, and 5-mm layer of diatomeceous earth. Ensure uniform packing of each adsorbent. Wash the column with 200 mL pet ether by using suction. Always keep a layer of solvent above the top of the adsorbent column.

A new column should be used for each assay.

(2) Separation of α-tocopheryl acetate.

Transfer quantitatively 4 mL pet ether extract estimated to contain about 0.1 mg α-tocopherol acetate to top of the column. If this extract contains less than 0.5 g of lipid, add olive oil to increase the lipid level to this minimal level.

Rinse with five 1.0-mL portions of pet ether for quantitative transfer. During transfer, keep the column covered with minimal solvent by avoiding suction. Elute the column with 100 mL benzene. Collect the eluate and evaporate to about 4 mL on steam bath under nitrogen gas; evaporate just to dryness under nitrogen with reduced heat. Dissolve the residue in pet ether–absolute ethanol solvent and dilute to 10 mL. Use about 4 mL for saponification and a suitable aliquot for colorimetry.

(c) Saponification. Transfer accurately a suitable aliquot from Section II.D.6(a) (about 4 mL) estimated to contain about 20 μg tocopherol to a 125-mL round-bottom flask and evaporate to dryness under nitrogen. Saponify as described under Section II.D.2. Concentrate the dry ethyl ether extract to a small volume in 25-mL vial.

(d) Colorimetry

(1) Assay the concentrated ethyl ether extract from the saponification step Section II.D.6(c) for α-tocopherol as described under Section II.D.4.

(2) Assay about 5 mL of the pet ether–absolute ethanol extract of the eluate from Section II.D.6(b)(2) for α-tocopherol equivalent of extraneous reducing substances still present (not removed by oxidative chromatography) by colorimetry procedure as described under Section II.D.4.

(e) Calculations

(1) mg of reducing substances before saponification/g sample =

$$\mu\text{g of substances determined} \times \frac{x}{y} \times \frac{10}{w} \times \frac{1}{1000} \times \frac{1}{W}$$

where x = total mL extract from Section II.D.1. or first sample extract;

y = mL extract used in oxidative chromatography;

w = mL taken for colorimetry;

W = weight in grams of composited assay sample;

10 = mL solution from chromatography.

(2) mg of α-tocopherol after saponification/1 g sample =

$$\mu\text{g of α-tocopherol measured} \times \frac{x}{y} \times \frac{10}{v} \times \frac{1}{1000} \times \frac{1}{W}$$

where $v =$ mL taken for saponification and the rest are as in Section
         II.D.6(e)(1).

(3) mg of α-tocopherol/1 g sample $=$

mg of tocopherol after saponification
                  $-$ mg of reducing substances before saponification

(4) mg of α-tocopheryl acetate/1 g sample $=$

mg of α-tocopherol $\times$ 1.098.

When excessive amounts of other isomers of α-tocopheryl acetate are
present in the feed or food sample ($> 15\%$), TLC on the ethyl ether extract
from the oxidative chromatography and saponification steps, should be
done to correct for these non-α-tocopheryl acetate in the final calculation
[Section II.D.6(e)(3)].

7. *Identification and Determination of RRR- or All-Rac-α-Tocopherol.* Estimation of the above analogs is necessary to express the total vitamin E activity
of a sample in IU. Following initial extraction and saponification, extraneous
color is removed by chromatography on ceric sulfate-treated Fuller's earth. The
extract is purified by Mg silicate column to isolate α-tocopherol, which is then
oxidized by ferricyanide. Optical rotation of ferricyanide oxidation product of
all-rac-α-tocopherol is negligible; RRR- form shows positive optical rotation
and is estimated on this basis. Details of this method are available in the AOAC
procedures.

III. GAS LIQUID CHROMATOGRAPHY—PHARMACEUTICAL
      PREPARATIONS

A. Principle

From pure pharmaceutical preparations devoid of interfering material, tocopherols are extracted with hexane and injected into chromatography columns.
Tocopherol peaks are identified on the basis of retention times and estimated
by measuring peak areas. RRR- and all-rac-α-tocopherols and acetate and hydrogen succinate esters can be separated and estimated using either the internal
or external standard method. This procedure is based on the AOAC method
(45,68).

B. Equipment

1. *Gas Chromatograph.*   With glass-lined sample introduction system, on-
column injection and either hydrogen flame detector or β-Ar ionization detector.
Operating conditions: temperature of column 270–285°C, injection system 295°C,
detector 295°C, chart speed 0.33″/min; β-Ar detector 900 V dc; adjust nitrogen

or argon carrier flow for α-tocopherol peak appearance 23–27 min after sample injection.

2. *Filtering Assembly.*   Millipore filter holder, microfiber glass filter disc, and filtrator.

3. *Glass Column.*   Pyrex glass 2.4 m × 4 mm i.d. uniform bore.

4. *Hamilton Micro-Syringes.*

C. Reagents

1. *Hexane.*

2. *Column Material.*   5% SE-30 on Gas Chrom Q 100–120 mesh.

3. *RRR- or All-Rac-α-Tocopherol.*

4. *RRR- or All-Rac-α-Tocopheryl Acetate.*

5. *RRR- or All-Rac-α-Tocopheryl Hydrogen Succinate.*

6. *Standard Solutions.*   Dissolve 100 mg of each vitamin E analog or reference standard in a 100-mL flask either in hexane (for external standard) or in internal standard solution. Store under nitrogen in amber flasks in refrigerator.

7. *Internal Standard Solution.*

(a) Dissolve 500 mg hexadecyl palmitate in hexane in a 500-mL flask and dilute to volume (cetyl palmitate, primary internal standard Analabs no. LMS-067 or equivalent), or

(b) Dissolve 500 mg dotriacontane (Eastman Kodak no. 3555) in 500 mL hexane.

D. Procedure

1. *Sample Preparation.*

(a) Grind tablets to a powder. Extract a known weight of the powdered sample with four 25-mL portions of hexane. Filter through the filter assembly into a receiver.

(1) Dilute with hexane to a final concentration of 1 mg vitamin E/mL (use the label claim as basis) for external standard method.

(2) Evaporate hexane under nitrogen stream and dilute with internal standard solution to a final concentration of 1 mg vitamin E/mL.

(b) Dissolve sealed capsules in hexane under nitrogen gas, warming if necessary. Open slip-capsules and dissolve both contents and capsule parts in hexane. If capsule material does not disintegrate, cut open the capsule and remove the contents with hexane and dissolve. Dilute to a final concentration of 1 mg vitamin E/mL as in Section III.D.1(a).

(c) If the same is not directly extractable with hexane, disperse the sample in H_2O and extract by any suitable procedure described under Section II.D.1(a–d). Evaporate the solvent under nitrogen and dissolve in hexane. Dilute as in Section III.C.1(a).

(d) Dilute liquid and injectible samples with either hexane or internal standard solution to a final concentration of 1 mg vitamin E/mL. Inject directly μL aliquots of product onto GLC column, if the product is immiscible with hexane. Follow the procedure for external standard method.

2. *Injection Technique.* External standard method. Draw 1 μL air into the barrel of 10 μL Hamilton microsyringe, insert needle into sample, and draw desired volume into barrel; remove needle from sample solution and draw 1 μL air into barrel. To ensure uniformity in volume, check sample volume between the same microliter range on the calibration scale each time the sample is drawn. The injection technique is not critical for internal standard method.

3. *Column Preparation.*

(a) Packing. Fill the glass tube with 5% SE-30 on Gas-chrom Q to within 10 cm of injection point and 2–5 cm of column exit. Pack uniformly by vibrating the column during filling. Place glasswool plugs, one extending from the top of adsorbent to top of carrier gas inlet arm at column injection end and the second filling the space between packing and septum at exit.

(b) Conditioning. Condition column 24 hr at 285°C and 80 mL/min carrier gas flow. Cool column with gas flowing and then connect column outlet to the detector. Raise the temperature of the chromatograph to operating temperature and carrier gas flow rate. Check instrument stability by recording base line. Base-line drift should be less than 1% in 30 min.

Following a direct sample injection, the column is sometimes rendered unusable for 1–4 hr. Under this condition, increase column temperature for short time to expel sample contaminants or wait for base-line stabilization at column operating temp.

4. *Column Performance Check and Calibration.*

(a) Check column performance by observing separation of α-tocopheryl and α-tocopheryl acetate peaks and expressing as peak resolution.

$$\text{Peak resolution} = 2D/(B + C)$$

where D is the distance between the analog peak maxima; B is the base width of α-tocopheryl acetate peak; and C is the base width of α-tocopherol peak. Peak resolution values are determined with equal weights of α-tocopherol and α-tocopheryl acetate; use a sample size that will peak at about 50% full scale. If peak resolution is about less than 1.0, column and instrument are performing satisfactorily.

There will be gradual loss in peak resolution; install new column when the value becomes more than 1.0.

(b) Internal and external standard methods.

(1) Internal standard method:

Inject 2–5 μL of standard solutions to produce peaks for tocopherol analog and internal standard, that are about 50% full scale. Measure the area of the peaks with integrator or by peak height times width at half peak height, recording sensitivity and retention times. Calculate RF (relative response factor) for standard solution.

$$RF = Q_s/Q_d$$

where Q_s = peak area for tocopherol analog and Q_d = peak area for internal standard. Repeat this calibration until RF is constant or within 2% for three consecutive injections and for each tocopherol analog.

(2) External standard method.

Inject standard solutions of tocopherol (2–5 μg range) and measure peak areas. Plot response in area against μg injected; use about three points in duplicate. Prepare standard curve for each tocopherol analog, daily.

5. *Identification of Analog Peaks.* Compare retention times of sample peaks and standard tocopherols and identify the components on the basis of relative retention times in Table 10.5.

α-Tocopherol and its hydrogen succinate analog have similar retention times. To distinguish between the two in a sample, proceed as follows: Perform GLC analysis on sample extract. To another aliquot of extract, add 1 mL of acetic anhydride–pyridine (2 + 1) mixture and shake 10 min. Evaporate solution under nitrogen gas, dilute to original volume with η-hexane, and perform GLC analysis. If sample peak shifts to the α-tocopheryl acetate position, it contains α-tocopherol; if it does not, the sample contains α-tocopherol hydrogen succinate.

6. *Determination.*

(a) Internal standard method. Inject a suitable aliquot of sample solution to produce response comparable with that of standard solution as described in Section III.D.4(b)(1). Measure the peak areas of sample component analogs and internal standard.

$$\text{mg of tocopherol analog/g sample} = Q_s/Q_d \times \frac{\text{declared potency}}{RF}$$

TABLE 10.5 Relative Retention Times

Tocopherol Analogs	External Standard	Internal Standard	
		Hexadecyl Palmitate	Dotriacontane
α-Tocopherol	0.9	0.53	0.75
α-Tocopheryl acetate	1.0	0.62	0.86
α-Tocopheryl hydrogen succinate	0.9	0.54	0.76

where $\quad Q_s \quad = \quad$ Peak area for tocopherol analog;

$\qquad Q_d \quad = \quad$ peak area for internal standard;

$\qquad$ RF $\quad = \quad$ relative response factor as determined in Section III.D.4(b)(1).

(b) External standard method.   Inject 2 μL sample extract from Section III.D.1(a)(1). Measure each peak area from the sample component analogs. Convert the peak area to amount of tocopherol analog using the calibration plot prepared in Section III.D.4(b)(2).

$$\text{mg of tocopherol analog/g sample} = \frac{x}{y} \times \frac{v}{W}$$

where $\quad x \quad = \quad$ μg read from calibration curve;

$\qquad y \quad = \quad$ volume injected;

$\qquad v \quad = \quad$ volume of total extract;

$\qquad W \quad = \quad$ weight of composited assay sample.

(c) To convert these mg weights to IU, multiply by the conversion factors in Table 10.3.

ACKNOWLEDGMENT

Financial support from the Natural Sciences and Engineering Research Council of Canada and the University of British Columbia is gratefully acknowledged.

LITERATURE CITED

1. IUPAC-IUB Commission on Biochemical Nomenclature. "Nomenclature of tocopherols and related compounds." *Eur. J. Biochem.* **46**, 217 (1974).

2. American Pharmaceutical Association. *National Formulary,* 14th ed. Washington, D.C. (1975).

3. Lubin, B. and Machlin, L. J., Eds., "Vitamin E—biochemical, hematological and clinical aspects." *Ann. N.Y. Acad. Sci.* **393** (1982).

4. Ames, S. R. "Isomers of alpha-tocopheryl acetate and their biological activity." *Lipids* **6**, 281 (1971).

5. Scott, M. L. and Desai, I. D. "The relative anti-muscular dystrophy activity of the d-and l-epimers of α-tocopherol and of other tocopherols in the chick." *J. Nutr.* **83**, 39 (1964).

6. Desai, I. D., Parekh, C. K., and Scott, M. L. "Absorption of d- and l-alpha tocopheryl acetates in normal and dystrophic chicks." *Biochim. Biophys. Acta* **100**, 280 (1965).

7. Desai, I. D. and Scott, M. L. "Mode of action of selenium in relation to biological activity of tocopherols." *Arch. Biochem.* **110**, 309 (1965).

8. Slover, H. T. "Tocopherols in foods and fats." *Lipids* **6**, 291 (1971).

9. Bieri, J. G. and Poukka Evarts, R. "Vitamin E activity of α-tocopherol in the rat, chick and hamster." *J. Nutr.* **104**, 850 (1974).

10. Food and Nutrition Board, National Research Council. *Recommended Dietary Allowances.* National Academy of Sciences, Washington, D.C. (1980).

11. Joffe, M. and Harris, P. L. "The biological potency of natural tocopherols and certain derivatives." *J. Am. Chem. Soc.* **65**, 925 (1943).

12. Harris, P. L. and Ludwig, M. I. "Relative vitamin E potency of natural and synthetic α-tocopherol." *J. Biol. Chem.* **179**, 1111 (1949).

13. Ames, S. R., Ludwig, M. I., Nelan, D. R., and Robeson, C. D. "Biological activity of an l-epimer of d-α-tocopheryl acetate." *Biochem.* **2**, 188 (1963).

14. Raychaudhuri, C. and Desai, I. D. "Ceroid pigment formation and irreversible sterility in vitamin E deficiency." *Science* **173**, 1028 (1971).

15. Desai, I. D., Fletcher, B. L., and Tappel, A. L. "Fluorescent pigments from uterus of vitamin E-deficient rats." *Lipids* **10**, 307 (1975).

16. Friedman, L., Weiss, W., Wherry, F., and Kline, O. L. "Bioassay of vitamin E by the dialuric acid hemolysis method." *J. Nutr.* **65**, 143 (1958).

17. Rose, C. S. and Gyorgy, P. "Specificity of hemolytic reaction in vitamin E-deficient erythrocytes." *Am. J. Physiol.* **168**, 414 (1952).

18. Gyorgy, P., Cogan, G., and Rose, C. S. "Availability of vitamin E in the newborn infant." *Proc. Soc. Exptl. Biol. Med.* **81**, 536 (1952).

19. Nitowsky, H. M., Cornblath, M., and Gordon, H. H. "Studies of tocopherol deficiency in infants and children—2. Plasma tocopherol and erythrocyte hemolysis in hydrogen perioxide." *Am. J. Dis. Child.* **92**, 164 (1956).

20. Horwitt, M. K. "Vitamin E and lipid metabolism in man." *Am. J. Clin. Nutr.* **8**, 451 (1960).

21. Hove, E. L. and Harris, P. L. "Relative activity of the tocopherols in curing muscular dystrophy in rabbits." *J. Nutr.* **33**, 95 (1947).

22. Fitch, C. D. and Diehl, J. F. "Metabolism of l-alpha-tocopherol by the vitamin E-deficient rabbit." *Proc. Soc. Exptl. Biol. Med.* **119**, 553 (1965).

23. Desai, I. D. and Scott, M. L. "Bioassays for orally administered and injected tocopherols: A relationship with tissue peroxidizability and lysosomal enzymes." *Proc. 7th Int. Cong. Nutr.* **5**, Hamburg, 643 (1966).

24. Jager, F. C. and Verbeek-Raad, J. A. "Methods for determining the vitamin E requirement in ducklings—2. Myopathy, serum enzymes and serum proteins." *Int. J. Vit. Res.* **40**, 597 (1970).

25. Bolliger, H. R. and Bolliger-Quaife, M. L. "Analytical methods and their use in evaluation of vitamin E." *Vitamin E, Atti 3rd Cong. Int.,* 30 (Venice 1955) Valdonega Verona (1956).

26. Mason, K. E. "Distribution of vitamin E in tissues of the rat." *J. Nutr.* **23**, 71 (1942).

27. Bunnell, R. H. "The vitamin E potency of alfalfa as measured by the tocopherol content of the liver of the chick." *Poultry Sci.* **36**, 413 (1957).

28. Pudelkiwicz, W. J., Matterson, L. D., Potter, L. M., Webster, L., and Singsen, E. P. "Chick tissue-storage bioassay of alpha-tocopherol: Chemical analytical techniques and relative biopotency of natural and synthetic alpha-tocopherol." *J. Nutr.* **71**, 115 (1960).

29. Dicks, M. W. and Matterson, L. D. "Chick liver storage bioassay of alpha-tocopherol: Methods." *J. Nutr.* **75**, 165 (1961).

30. Emmerie, A. and Engel, C. "Colorimetric determination of α-tocopherol (vitamin E)." *Rec. Trav. Chim.* **57**, 1351 (1938).

31. Tsen, C. C. "An improved spectrophotometric method for the determination of tocopherols using 4,7-diphenyl-1,10-phenanthroline." *Anal. Chem.* **33**, 849 (1961).

32. Lambertsen, G. and Braekkan, O. R. "The spectrophotometric determination of α-tocopherol." *Analyst* **84**, 706 (1959).

33. Duggan, D. E. "Spectrofluorometric determination of tocopherols." *Arch. Biochem. Biophys.* **84**, 116 (1959).

34. Thompson, J. N., Erdody, P., and Maxwell, W. B. "Chromatographic separation and spectrophotofluorometric determination of tocopherols using hydroxyalkoxypropyl Sephadex." *Anal. Biochem.* **50**, 267 (1972).

35. Analytical Methods Committee, Society for Analytical Chemists. "The determination of tocopherols in oils, foods and feeding stuffs." *Analyst* (London) **84**, 356 (1959).

36. Bunnell, R. H. "Vitamin E assay by chemical means." In P. Gyorgy and W. N. Pearson, Eds., *Vitamins*, Vol. 6. Academic Press, New York, 261 (1967).

37. Bieri, J. G. "Chromatography of tocopherols." In G. V. Marinett, Ed., *Chromatographic Analysis*, Vol. 2. Marcel Dekker, New York, 459 (1969).

38. Bunnell, R. H. "Modern procedures for the analysis of tocopherols." *Lipids* **6**, 245 (1970).

39. Stowe, H. D. "Separation of β- and α-tocopherol." *Arch. Biochem. Biophys.* **103**, 42 (1963).

40. Rao, M. K. G., Rao, S. V., and Acharya, K. T. "Separation and estimation of tocopherols in vegetable oils by thin-layer chromatography." *J. Sci. Food Agric.* **16**, 121 (1965).

41. Lovelady, H. G. "Separation of β- and α-tocopherols in the presence of α- and δ-tocopherols and vitamin A acetate." *J. Chromatogr.* **78**, 449 (1973).

42. Pennock, J. F., Hemming, F. W., and Kerr, J. D. "A reassessment of tocopherol chemistry." *Biochem. Biophys. Res. Commun.* **17**, 542 (1964).

43. Whittle, K. J. and Pennock, J. F. "The examination of tocopherols by thin-layer chromatography and subsequent colorimetric determination." *Analyst* **92**, 423 (1967).

44. Chow, C. K., Draper, H. H., and Csallany, A. S. "Method for the assay of free and esterified tocopherols." *Anal. Biochem.* **32**, 81 (1969).

45. Association of Official Analytical Chemists. *Official Methods of Analysis*, 13th Ed. 752 (1980).

46. Diplock, A. T., Green, J., Edwin, E. E., and Bunyan, J. "Studies on vitamin E— 4. The simultaneous determination of tocopherols, ubiquinones and ubichromanols in animal tissues: A reconsideration of the Keilin-Hartree heart preparation." *Biochem. J.* **76**, 563 (1960).

47. Pudelkiewicz, W. J. and Matterson, L. D. "Effect of coenzyme Q_{10} on the determination of tocopherol in animal tissue." *J. Biol. Chem.* **235**, 496 (1960).

48. Bieri, J. G., Pollard, C. J., Prang, I., and Dam, H. "The determination of α-tocopherol in animal tissues by column chromatography." *Acta Chem. Scand.* **15**, 783 (1961).

49. Bro-Rasmussen, F. and Hjarde, W. "Determination of α-tocopherol by chromatography on secondary magnesium phosphate." *Acta Chem. Scand.* **11**, 34 (1957).

50. Bro-Rasmussen, F. and Hjarde, W. "Quantitative determination of the individual tocopherols by chromatography on secondary magnesium phosphate." *Acta Chem. Scand.* **11**, 44 (1957).

51. Dick-Bushnell, M. W. "Column chromatography in the determination of tocopherol: Florisil, silicic acid and secondary magnesium phosphate." *J. Chromatogr.* **27**, 96 (1967).

52. Cavins, J. F. and Inglett, G. E. "High-resolution liquid chromatography of vitamin E isomers." *Cereal. Chem.* **51**, 605 (1974).

53. Abe, K., Yaguchi, Y., and Katsui, G. "Quantitative determination of tocopherols by high-speed liquid chromatography." *J. Nutr. Sci. Vitaminol.* **21**, 183 (1975).

54. Kofler, M., Sommer, P. F., Bollinger, H. R., Schmidli, B., and Vecchi, M. "Physiochemical properties and assay of the tocopherols." *Vitamins Hormones* **20**, 407 (1962).

55. Nicolaides, N. "The use of silicone rubber gums or grease in low concentration as stationary phase for the high temperature gas chromatographic separation of lipids." *J. Chromatogr.* **4**, 496 (1960).

56. Wilson, P. W., Kodicek, E., and Booth, V. H. "Separation of tocopherols by gas-liquid chromatography." *Biochem. J.* **84**, 524 (1962).

57. Bieri, J. G. and Andrews, E. L. "The determination of α-tocopherol in animal tissues by gas-liquid chromatography." *Iowa State J. Sci.* **38**, 3 (1963).

58. Carroll, K. K. and Herting, D. C. "Gas-liquid chromatography of fat-soluble vitamins." *J. Am. Oil Chem. Soc.* **41**, 473 (1964).

59. Slover, H. T., Shelley, L. M., and Burks, T. L. "Identification and estimation of tocopherols by gas-liquid chromatography." *J. Am. Oil Chem. Soc.* **44**, 161 (1967).

60. Slover, H. T., Lehmann, J., and Valis, R. J. "Vitamin E in foods: Determination of tocols and tocotrienols." *J. Am. Oil Chem. Soc.* **46**, 417 (1969).

61. Rudy, B. C., Mahn, F. P., Senkowski, B. Z., Sheppard, A. J., and Hubbard, W. D. "Collaborative study of the gas-liquid chromatographic assay for vitamin E." *J. Assoc. Off. Anal. Chem.* **55**, 1211 (1972).

62. Nair, P. P. and Turner, D. A. "The application of gas-liquid chromatography to the determination of vitamin E and K." *J. Am. Oil Chem. Soc.* **40**, 353 (1963).

63. Libby, D. A. and Sheppard, A. J. "Gas-liquid chromatographic method for the determination of fat-soluble vitamins—1. Application to vitamin E." *J. Assoc. Off. Agr. Chem.* **47**, 371 (1964).

64. Lovelady, H. G. "Separation of individual tocopherols from human plasma and red blood cells by thin-layer and gas-liquid chromatography." *J. Chromatogr.* **85**, 81 (1973).

65. Nair, P. P., Sarlos, I., and Machiz, J. "Microquantitative separation of isomeric dimethyltocols by gas-liquid chromatography." *Arch. Biochem. Biophys.* **114**, 448 (1966).

66. Nair, P. P. and Machiz, J. "Gas-liquid chromatography of isomeric methyltocols and their derivatives." *Biochim. Biophys. Acta* **144**, 446 (1967).

67. Nair, P. P. and Luna, Z. "Identification of α-tocopherol from tissues by combined gas-liquid chromatography, mass spectrometry and infrared spectroscopy." *Arch. Biochem. Biophys.* **127**, 413 (1968).

68. Sheppard, A. J. and Hubbard, W. D. "Collaborative study of GLC method for vitamin E." *J. Pharm. Sci.* **68** (1), 115 (1979).

69. Ames, S. R. "Determination of vitamin E in foods and feeds: A collaborative study." *J. Assoc. Off. Anal. Chem.* **54**, 1 (1971).

70. Desai, I. D., O'Leary, L. P., and Schwartz, N. "Vitamin E status of proprietary infant formulas available in Canada." *Nutr. Rep. Int.* **6**, 83 (1972).

71. Herting, D. C. and Drury, E. E. "Vitamin E content of vegetable oils and fats." *J. Nutr.* **81**, 335 (1963).

72. Roughan, P. G. "A simple and rapid method for the quantitative determination of α-tocopherol (vitamin E) in leaves." *Anal. Biochem.* **19**, 461 (1967).

73. Burcke, C. "The distribution and stability of α-tocopherol in subcellular fractions of broad bean leaves." *Phytochem.* **7**, 693 (1968).

74. Antia, N. J., Desai, I. D., and Romilly, M. J. "Tocopherol, vitamin K and related isoprenoid quinone composition of a unicellular red algae (Porphyridium Cruentum)." *J. Phycol.* **6**, 305 (1970).

75. Dasilva, E. J. and Jensen, A. "Content of α-tocopherol in some blue-green algae." *Biochim. Biophys. Acta* **239**, 345 (1971).

11 Vitamin K

Raymond Berruti

GENERAL CONSIDERATIONS

Vitamin K activity was established as a distinct dietary factor in 1935 and is now an officially recognized vitamin entity that is required by all warm-blooded animals to insure proper prothrombin levels in the blood. Without adequate amounts of vitamin K, a specific lowering of the prothrombin occurs and the blood will not coagulate properly. In the absence of this vitamin factor, warm-blooded animals will bleed to death, because almost any injury that causes a rupture of the blood vessel walls will hemorrhage spontaneously (1–3).

The term "vitamin K" is a generic one that can be applied to many different chemical compounds, all having vitamin K activity. The degree of vitamin K activity and the biological effectiveness possessed by each of these compounds varies with its structure and its functional group nature, as well as with its own distinct chemical and physical properties. Stability, a quality absolutely essential if the compound is to be used in animal feeds, also varies greatly from one compound to the other (4–6).

Vitamin K activity is shared by a large group of very closely related naphthoquinones. The most widely known occurring naturally are phylloquinone and farnoquinone, and the numerous synthetics such as menadione, acetomenaphthone, menadione sodium diphosphate, menadione sodium bisulfite, menadione sodium bisulfite complex, and menadione dimethylpyrimidinol bisulfite (3,7). Obsolete designations include K_3, prothrombin factor, "koagulations," vitamin and antihemorrhagic vitamin.

A. Structures and Properties

1. Phylloquinone (K₁)

Phylloquinone (K_1) is the naturally occurring vitamin K_1, which is of vegetable origin. It is heat stable, but is unstable to light, and thus is easily destroyed. It is a difficult and costly compound to synthesize and its occurrence as a viscous oil makes it difficult, if not impossible, to incorporate in microquantities uniformly dispersed into finished feeds. Although often used in research and in products for human consumption, vitamin K_1 was never accepted as a practical source of vitamin K for fortification of animal feeds because of these drawbacks.

The structure of phylloquinone (K_1) has been established as 2-methyl-3-phytyl-1,4-naphthoquinone (Figure 11.1). The empirical formula is $C_{31}H_{46}O_2$ and the molecular weight is 450.68. The quinone moiety was established on the basis of oxidation-reduction reactions. Because of the yellow color of K_1, it was readily apparent that the quinone was the 1,4-rather than the red-colored 1,2-quinone; also, the oxidation-reduction potential of the compound was similar to that of many other known 1,4-quinones. The nature of the side chain was established by oxidation and by hydrogenation experiments. Hydrogenation established that the side chain contains one carbon-to-carbon double bond, since the compound consumed 1 mole of hydrogen in excess of that required for the reduction of the naphthoquinone moiety. On the basis of the oxidation products, phylloquinone was formulated as 2-methyl-3-phytyl-1,4-naphthoquinone and the structure was finally confirmed by synthesis (8).

The best sources of vitamin K_1 are alfalfa, spinach, cabbage, kale, cauliflower, and other leafy vegetables. Vitamin K_1 activity is also present in tomatoes and soybean oil, but, in general, fruits and cereals are very poor sources of the vitamin.

2. Farnoquinone (K₂)

Farnoquinone or vitamin K_2 is found in many microorganisms, especially bacteria, but molds, yeasts, and fungi contain very little vitamin K activity. From the practical standpoint of nutrition, it is important that the microorganisms in

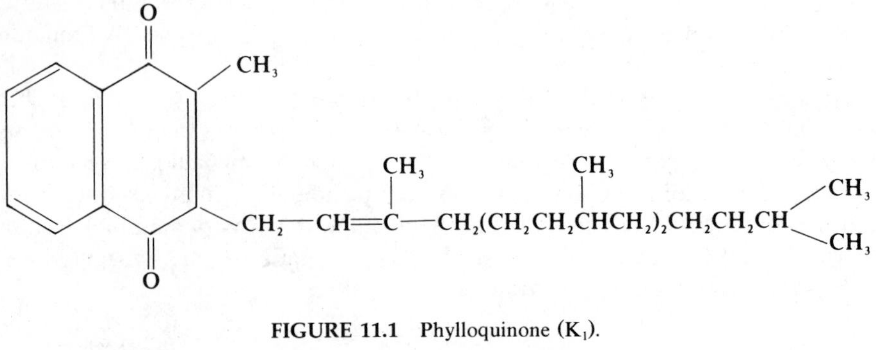

FIGURE 11.1   Phylloquinone (K_1).

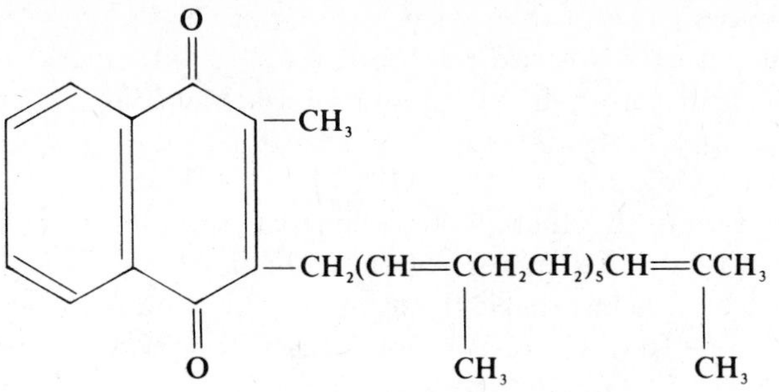

FIGURE 11.2   Vitamin K$_2$.

the intestinal tract produce abundant quantities of the vitamin (9). Most putrefied animal and plant materials also contain high amounts due to bacterial growth. Animal tissues contain very little vitamin K$_2$, although milk and eggs contain small amounts. Hog liver is the richest animal source known (9).

The structure of K$_2$ has been established as 2-methyl-3-farnesyl-farnesyl-1,4-naphthoquinone (Figure 11.2). The empirical formula is C$_{41}$H$_{56}$O$_2$ and the molecular weight is 580.86. The methods used for establishing the structure of vitamin K$_1$ and the knowledge gained from the proof of the structure of this vitamin were useful for the elucidation of structure of vitamin K$_2$. The nature of the quinone moiety of vitamin K$_2$ was established exactly as described for the determination of the structure of vitamin K$_1$. The side chain was assumed to contain 6 double bonds, since hydrogenation of vitamin K$_2$ appeared to require 6 moles of hydrogen in addition to that consumed by the naphthoquinoid ring system. However, recent studies have indicated that two forms of vitamin K$_2$ may actually exist, one being the structure in Figure 11.2 and the other being 2-methyl-3-all-*trans*-farnesylgeranyl geranyl-1,4-naphthoquinone (Figure 11.3), sometimes designated as K$_{2\,(35)}$ (8).

B. Important Synthetic Vitamin K Activity Sources

1. Menadione

As work continued in this field, it became obvious that the activity of the naturally occurring vitamin K active compounds resulted from the naphthoquinone nucleus, although the degree of activity was definitely modified by the

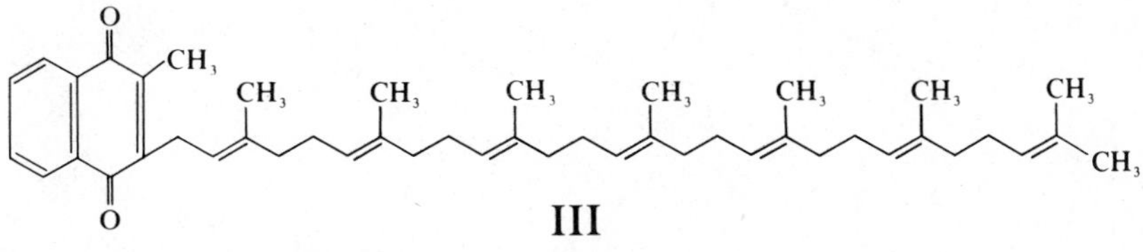

III

FIGURE 11.3   Vitamin K$_{2(35)}$

rest of the molecule. Thus, the search was started for simple naphthoquinones, and attention was soon focused on 2-methyl-1,4-naphthoquinone (menadione), commonly and correctly referred to as K_3 (10). Menadione (Figure 11.4) was found to have three times the biological activity of K_1. Its empirical formula is $C_{11}H_8O_2$, and its molecular weight is 172.17.

Despite its vitamin K efficacy, menadione has several serious disadvantages. It is unstable to light, it requires normal amounts of bile to be effective as an aid in the control of hemorrhagic disease, it is toxic, and is irritating to the skin and also to the respiratory tract; it combines with the protein of feeds, which inactivates it (11–13). For these reasons, menadione is not a preferred source of K activity and is no longer used in the fortification of animal diets.

2. Menadione Sodium Bisulfite (MSB)

Early in the 1940s, a water-soluble menadione derivative was introduced in the pharmaceutical industry that seemingly overcame most of the disadvantages of menadione. Its water solubility increases the rate of absorption of the vitamin into the bloodstream, even in the absence of adequate amounts of bile, and this water-soluble compound does not have the irritating properties of menadione itself (2,14). Menadione sodium bisulfite (Figure 11.5) is the bisulfite addition product of menadione with sodium bisulfite in exactly 1:1 molar proportions. It is a white crystalline solid and its empirical formula is $C_{11}H_8O_2 \cdot NaHSO_3 \cdot 3H_2O$ and its molecular weight is 330.29.

Despite its decided improvement over menadione as a practical source of vitamin K activity, MSB has certain characteristics that render its use difficult in many applications. MSB is sensitive to light and air and its water solutions soon deteriorate. Observations showed that even the purest MSB products decompose when stored in their own containers and rapidly turn into amorphous, pink–red-colored masses. When allowed to stand in air, they undergo changes, predominantly on the surface, due to the action of moisture and aerial oxygen. This external change is evident first by the appearance of a yellow and subsequently a pinkish color. Accordingly, a definite increase is also observed in the toxicity. These phenomena are apparently connected with the onset of isomerization into hydroquinone sulfonate and its subsequent oxidation by air to the corresponding quinone of greater toxicity (3). Carmak and co-workers (15)

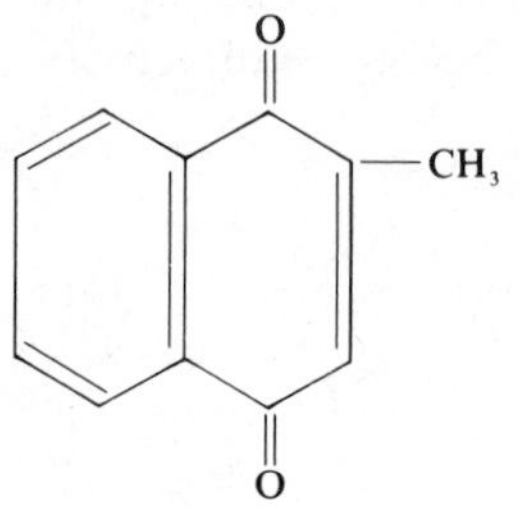

FIGURE 11.4 Menadione.

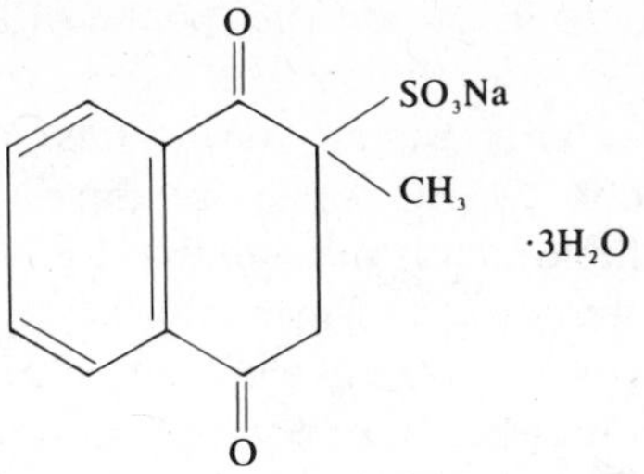

FIGURE 11.5 Menadione sodium bisulfite (MSB).

definitely established that at least two isomeric forms of MSB are formed; their relative proportions depend on the reaction conditions (Figure 11.6). Compound B exhibits very marked antihemorrhagic activity comparable to the parent quinone, whereas compound A exhibits only a small portion of the activity. More recently, Charles (16) has theorized that as many as nine isomers may be present in MSB, each with a different vitamin K activity dependent upon its molecular structure.

3. Menadione Sodium Bisulfite Complex (MSBC)

To overcome the undesirable effects that complicate the practical use of an MSB preparation, Moore and Kirchmeyer (17) found that several times the amount of bisulfite must be used during the manufacturing process and that this excess bisulfite must be allowed to coprecipitate with the MSB to form the crystalline sodium bisulfite complex of menadione. The double complex thus formed is MSBC. The U.S. Pharmacopeia XX (11) describes menadione sodium bisulfite complex as containing not less than 63% and not more than 75% of menadione sodium bisulfite trihydrate ($C_{11}H_8O_2 \cdot NaHSO_3 \cdot 3H_2O$) and not less than 30.0% and not more than 38.0% of sodium bisulfite ($NaHSO_3$).

MSBC has all the necessary requirements of safety and effectiveness in the absence of bile. Griminger (18) reported that supplementation of a diet deficient

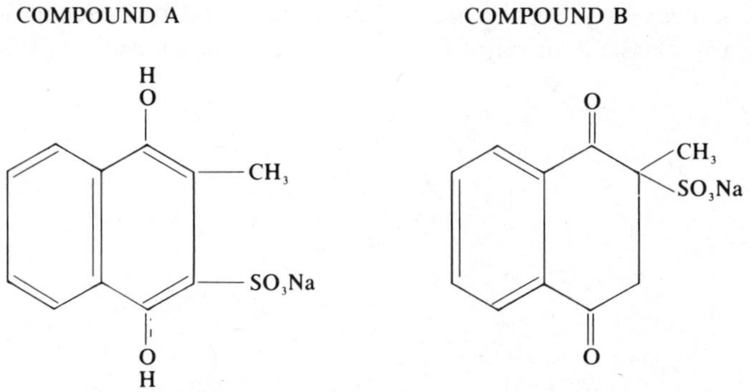

COMPOUND A   COMPOUND B

FIGURE 11.6 Isomeric forms MSB.

in vitamin K with 0.8 mg of menadione per pound of feed, or an equal amount of MSBC, containing 33% menadione, was necessary to reduce the plasma prothrombin times of poults to normal during their first weeks. Thus, it was shown that a water-soluble MSBC was three times as effective, per mole of menadione, as was fat-soluble menadione and that 1 g MSBC of 0.33 g menadione content can adequately replace 1 g of menadione.

In its pure form, MSBC is extremely water soluble and is stable to light, air, but not heat. The compound has marked, well-substantiated, and well-defined biological activity (14). The compound is often called "Stabilized Menadione Sodium Bisulfite" in contrast to the ordinary MSB. However, this stability designation does not refer to its stability in modern feeds and feed manufacturing operations, but merely to its ability to retain its potency when stored for long periods of time in closed containers.

When used in the form of a premix for feeds, however, MSBC exhibits instability, losing its original potency rapidly and changing in appearance and composition. This undesirable incompatibility characteristic was found to be the result of the action of the minerals, moderate heat, and moisture encountered in feed manufacturing operations (19). The pelleting operation, which subjects feed ingredients to extremes of moisture, heat, and pressure, is even more destructive to all sensitive vitamins and especially to vitamin K active substances (20).

4. Menadione Dimethylpyrimidinol Bisulfite (MPB)

A new vitamin K active molecule which exhibits enhanced antihemorrhagic activity and superior stability was introduced in 1966 (21). For the sake of relating MBP (Figure 11.7) to the vitamin K-active compounds ordinarily used in feeds, it may be considered to be an MSB in which the sodium has been replaced by the weakly basic substance, dimethylpyrimidinol. MPB is a well-defined compound having a definite molecular structure free of isomeric substances. Its empirical formula is $C_{17}H_{18}O_6N_2S$ and its molecular weight is 378.39.

C. Metabolic Role

Vitamin K is necessary for the maintenance of normal blood coagulation. According to the classical theory (9), two different phases are involved and are

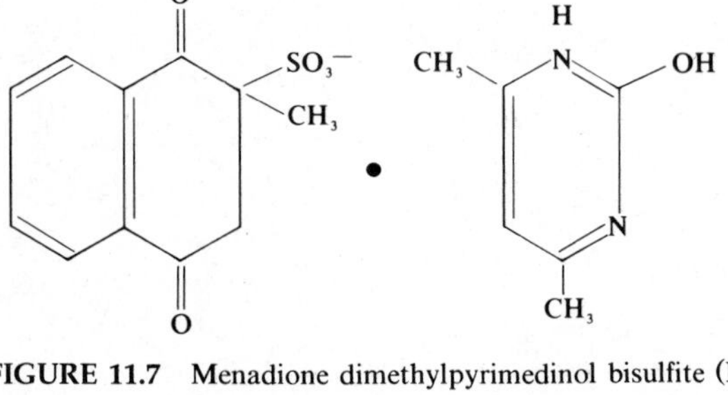

FIGURE 11.7   Menadione dimethylpyrimedinol bisulfite (MPB).

represented schematically by the following reactions:

$$\text{PROTHROMBIN} \xrightarrow[\text{Thromboplastin}]{\text{Calcium}} \text{THROMBIN}$$

$$\text{FIBRINOGEN} \xrightarrow{\text{Thrombin}} \text{FIBRIN}$$

The end result, which constitutes the second step of the process, is the transformation of fibrinogen, a soluble blood plasma protein, into fibrin, a solid and insoluble protein. This reaction is carried out by an enzyme, the thrombin. Thrombin does not occur in the blood, since otherwise the blood would not be fluid, but the precursor of thrombin, namely, prothrombin, is present in plasma. The first phase of blood coagulation, therefore, is the conversion of prothrombin into thrombin. This process involves the action of another enzyme, thromboplastin (thrombokinase) in the presence of calcium ions. While the latter are present in blood plasma, thromboplastin is a normal cell constituent, but not a blood constituent.

During vitamin K deficiency, the prothrombin concentration is lowered. Yet vitamin K should not be considered a part of the prothrombin molecule, but rather an activator of a prothrombin precursor in the liver where both the precursor and prothrombin are formed (22). Most speculation on vitamin action has centered on the possibility that the vitamin is in some manner utilized to stabilize the hydrogen on the α-position of the glutamyl acid residue of α-carboxyglutamic acid. Since vitamin K influences the prothrombin concentration, it is assumed that vitamin K is involved in the prothrombin formation (8). This synthesis is apparently accomplished in the liver, because partial destruction of the liver greatly reduces the prothrombin level in blood and because symptoms of a vitamin K deficiency, even in the presence of normally adequate amounts of this vitamin, have been observed frequently in cases of liver damage such as cirrhosis and hepatitis. In all these cases, the prothrombin concentration could not be influenced by vitamin K when given orally or injected intravenously or intramuscularly. That a special mechanism for the formation of prothrombin actually exists is furthermore suggested by the fact that excessive feeding of vitamin K will not cause the prothrombin to rise above a certain level (9).

Vitamin K dietary deficiency in humans is practically unknown, and only in a few pathological or emergency conditions is administration of the vitamin indicated (23). In fact, in complete contrast to most other vitamins, the vitamin K group is not permitted by law in any over-the-counter preparations for human use, and the use of vitamin K activity is strictly governed on a prescription basis only. Synthesis of the vitamin by microorganisms in the intestinal tract is usually sufficient to supply the needs of most animals, with the notable exception of poultry and swine (6). Thus, it can be seen that the commercial need for vitamin K activity supplementation exists primarily in the area of animal feeds and feeding.

METHODS AVAILABLE

A. Microbiological and Biological Methods

Generally speaking, most of the vitamins can be determined in one form or another by physical, chemical, microbiological, and biological estimation. Because of the nature of the various chemical compounds constituting the vitamin K group, microbiological methods have not proven satisfactory. Similarly, the biological assay methods for vitamin K activity must be viewed somewhat differently from the biological methods applied to certain other vitamins.

Since chemical methods of analysis are not sufficiently sensitive, one cannot distinguish between biologically active and inactive isomers of the same vitamin K compound (24). The establishment of the total vitamin K activity in complete animal feeds can only be accomplished by biological means.

The earliest quantitative biological estimation of vitamin K attempted was the measurement of simple clotting time of whole blood in chicks (9). If a very large number of chicks are used, the average blood clotting time has a fairly close relation to the activity of the vitamin K active substances. However, since clotting time is measured in minutes, there is great variation between the clotting time of individuals. Greater precision is attained with absolute specificity when the whole blood prothrombin time method of Quick (25) is adopted to the chick assay. This method is now the only generally accepted means of accurately estimating the vitamin K activity content of feeds and feed ingredients.

Thus, vitamin K activity can be measured biologically by determination of the degree of lowering of elevated prothrombin times in vitamin K-depleted chickens under standard conditions (26). However, this testing procedure is costly, tedious and requires the development of great skill in handling the chicks, the performance of the prothrombin determinations, and preparation of reagents, diets, environment, etc. Many factors influence the results and the effects of each of these must be isolated and controlled. It has been found that some experts in carrying out such tests have had to spend several years to perfect their technique. Because of this, it is quite understandable that few feed manufacturers are able to test the vitamin K they purchase for its biological activity in such a manner but instead rely on chemical determinations of liberated menadione content. For detailed discussions on the biological determination of vitamin K activity by prothrombin time determinations, it is suggested that the papers of Quick and Stefanini (27) and McCormick and Kopp (28) be consulted.

B. Spectroscopic Assay

The vitamins K_1, K_2, and 2-methyl-1,4-naphthoquinone (menadione) can be estimated by means of their absorption spectra, provided the compounds are essentially free from other absorbing materials and are not present in the reduced hydroquinone form. For a description of such methods, the appropriate editions of the U.S. Pharmacopeia and the National Formulary should be consulted (11,29).

C. Chemical Assays

These methods are dependent on specific properties of the vitamin K forms present in a given material. In many cases, they are specific for pure forms of the vitamin. The reduction-oxidation method, for example, is suitable for pure menadione; however, it is nonspecific, since any quinone will give the same reaction.

Water-soluble derivatives of menadione can be determined by the ethylcyanoacetate method. This is most suitable for use with vitamin premixes in animal feeds. This method is based on the reaction between ethylcyanoacetate and menadione in the presence of ammonia as described by Pinder and Singer (30). The drawback of this method is that it does not have sufficient sensitivity for determining the low levels of vitamin K activity normally present in finished feeds (1–10 ppm). A more sensitive method for determination of microgram quantities is the measurement of the hydrazone formed by the reaction between menadione and 2,4-dinitrophenylhydrazine (31).

D. Chromatographic Methods

Various chromatographic techniques for the determination of menadione have been described. The gas-liquid chromatographic technique for the detection of menadione is very sensitive and has been applied to pharmaceutical products (32). However, water-soluble derivatives of menadione must be converted to menadione before they can be chromatographed. As a result, sensitivity is lost and when applied to the determination of microgram quantities in feedstuffs, the technique has not yet proved to be of value.

ANALYTICAL METHODOLOGY

I. REDUCTION-OXIDATION METHOD

A. Principle

This method involves the reduction of the quinone moiety of vitamin K to the hydroquinone form, and reoxidation to the quinone form with ceric sulfate. Water-soluble derivatives may be converted to the oil-soluble menadione form for measurement. This procedure is most suitable for pure menadione or derivatives (33).

B. Procedure

1. *Menadione Determination.*
   (a) Weigh accurately about 150 mg menadione and transfer to a 150-mL flask. Add 15 mL glacial acetic acid and 15 mL 3 N HCl, and swirl the flask

until the menadione is dissolved. Then add about 3 g zinc dust and close the flask with a stopper bearing a Bunsen valve. Shake well and allow to stand in the dark for 1 hr, with frequent shaking.

(1) A Bunsen valve is a simple device, easily assembled in the laboratory, which permits gas to escape from a flask but which prevents atmospheric gases from entering.

(b) Rapidly decant the solution through a pledget of cotton into another flask. Immediately wash the reduction flask with three 10-mL portions of freshly boiled and cooled H_2O.Combine filtrate and washings. Add 0.1 mL *ortho*-phenanthroline and immediately titrate the combined filtrate and washings with 0.1 N ceric sulfate. Perform a blank determination as well, and correct final titration value for blank.

2. *Conversion of Water-Soluble Derivatives to Menadione.*   Dissolve about 300 mg (accurately weighed) water-soluble derivatives in 20 mL H_2O in a separatory funnel. Add 5 mL in NaOH, and extract the precipitated menadione with three 20-mL portions of chloroform. Wash the combined chloroform extracts with 10 mL H_2O, filter chloroform extracts through filter paper moistened with chloroform, and wash filter paper with 5 mL chloroform. Evaporate the combined chloroform solutions in a 150-mL flask to dryness with the aid of a current of air and proceed as described in Section B.1(a), beginning with the addition of glacial acetic acid.

3. *Calculation of Results.*   Each mL of exactly 0.1 N ceric sulfate used in the titration is equivalent to 8.609 mg of menadione (33,34). The amount of menadione in the original sample can be calculated on the basis of the initial sample weight.

(a) Ceric sulfate is standardized as per USP XVII (33) using arsenic trioxide as the primary standard. One mL of exactly 0.1 N ceric sulfate contains 33.22 mg. Then 2 M ceric sulfate (mol. wt. 332.24) is equivalent to 1 M menadione (mol. wt. 172.17), and thus each mL 0.1 N ceric sulfate is equivalent to 8.60 mg menadione or 16.51 mg menadione bisulfite trihydrate (mol wt. 330.29), and so on.

(b) For known forms of the water-soluble derivatives, the following conversions are useful:

Menadione $\times$ 1.919 = menadione sodium bisulfite trihydrate
Menadione $\times$ 3.030 = menadione sodium bisulfite complex
Menadione $\times$ 2.197 = menadione dimethylpyrimidinol bisulfite
Menadione $\times$ 4.074 = menadione sodium diphosphate anhydrous

(c) A typical calculation would be:

$$\frac{\text{mL 0.1 N ceric sulfate} \times 8.609 \times 100}{\text{weight of sample}} = \% \text{ menadione}$$

II. ETHYLCYANOACETATE METHOD FOR WATER-SOLUBLE MENADIONE DERIVATIVES

A. Principle

This method is based on the formation of a colored complex between ethylcyanoacetate and menadione in the presence of ammonia, as previously described by Pinder and Singer (30). However, in this procedure the violet-blue color formed by the direct reaction of menadione, ethylcyanoacetate, and alcoholic ammonia is measured at 575 nm, rather than the yellow color produced when the initial complex between menadione and ethylcyanoacetate is treated with sodium hydroxide. This technique is used for the determination of water-soluble menadione derivatives in vitamin premixes for animal feeds.

B. Reagents

1. *0.1 N Iodine Solution.*   Weigh out 25 g KI and dissolve in 20 mL H_2O in a 150-mL beaker. Weigh out 9.8 g reagent grade iodine and add to the KI solution. Stir until iodine is completely dissolved. After solution is complete, transfer to a glass-stoppered liter bottle and dilute to approximately 750 mL with H_2O. Mix thoroughly, store in dark, and let stand 24 hr before using to insure solution of iodine.

2. *0.1 N Sodium Thiosulfate.*   Prepare a 0.1 N solution by dissolving 25 g $Na_2S_2O_3 \cdot 5H_2O$ in 500 mL freshly boiled and cooled H_2O containing 0.1 g Na_2CO_3. Dilute to 1000 mL with boiled, cooled H_2O.

3. *Starch Indicator.*   Prepare a 1% starch solution by dispersing 2 g "water-soluble" starch in 10 mL H_2O, and adding slowly to 200 mL boiling H_2O; boil 2 min.

4. *Ammonium Hydroxide–Isopropanol Solution.*   Prepare by mixing equal volumes of isopropyl alcohol (99%) and concentrated NH_4OH.

5. *Ethylcyanoacetate Solution.*   Prepare by dissolving 3 g ethylcyanoacetate (Eastman Kodak) in isopropyl alcohol (99%) to make a solution containing approximately 30 mg/mL.

6. *Menadione Standard.*   Weigh approximately 100 mg menadione USP Reference Standard (USP) accurately. Transfer to a 100-mL amber volumetric flask using isopropyl alcohol (99%). Make certain all menadione is dissolved before bringing to final volume with isopropyl alcohol.

(a) Amber glassware prevents destruction of menadione by light.

C. Procedure

1. Weigh approximately 15 g vitamin premix (sample) accurately and transfer to 150 mL beaker. Add exactly 100 mL H_2O by means of a pipette. Stir well for at least 10 min to insure complete extraction and solution of the menadione

complex. Filter through Whatman No. 12 filter paper. If solution is cloudy, refilter through the same filter paper until a clear solution is obtained.

2. Pipette 40 mL clear filtrate into a 100-mL clear glass volumetric flask. Add 1 to 2 drops starch solution (Reagent 3) and titrate with 0.1 N iodine (Reagent 1) until the first permanent blue color appears. Dispel the blue color with 1 drop 0.1 N $Na_2S_2O_3$ (Reagent 2). Bring to volume with H_2O and mix well.

(a) The use of iodine is important because it oxidizes the easily removed sodium bisulfite from the menadione sodium bisulfite complex, which tends to bleach the color formed in the procedure.

3. Prepare six amber 100-mL volumetric flasks: three for the menadione standard solution and three for the sample. Into each of the three standard flasks, pipette exactly 2 mL menadione standard solution (Reagent 6). Add H_2O to approximately 90 mL.

4. Into each of the sample flasks, pipette 10 mL of the iodine-treated sample solution. Add H_2O to approximately 90 mL.

5. Set one standard and one sample flask aside for use as blanks. Add 3 mL isopropyl alcohol to the sample blank and 1 mL isopropyl alcohol to the standard blank.

6. Into the four remaining flasks (two standards and two samples) carefully add exactly 1 mL of ethylcyanoacetate solution (Reagent 5) by means of a buret. Then add exactly 2 mL isopropyl alcohol to the sample flasks only.

(a) All flasks (blanks, standards, and samples) will contain the equivalent of 3 mL isopropyl alcohol. The blanks do not contain ethylcyanoacetate.

7. Into each of the six flasks, add exactly 1 mL of NH_4OH isopropanol solution (Reagent 4). Make the addition from a buret. Immediately upon addition of the alcoholic ammonia, stopper the flask and shake vigorously. Work as rapidly as possible, and when all six flasks have been treated in this manner, bring to volume with H_2O, shake and set aside for 10 min. Read at 575 nm in a suitable colorimeter.

(a) The amounts of ethylcyanoacetate and alcoholic ammonia solutions should be carefully controlled since varying amounts will change the amount of color produced.

(b) The violet-blue color is not completely stable and will fade on standing. When the reactants are mixed together under the conditions described, peak color is produced very rapidly and is stable for 20–25 min, which is ample time to conduct each series of two determinations, one set of samples and one standard.

D. Calculation

The menadione content is calculated from the absorbance of the test and sample solutions by the following formula:

$$\frac{\text{Absorbance of sample solution-absorbance of sample blank}}{\text{Absorbance of standard solution-absorbance of standard blank}} \times$$

$$\frac{\text{weight of standard in 2-mL aliquot}}{\text{weight of sample in 10-mL aliquot}} \times 100 = \% \text{ menadione}$$

III. 2,4-DINITROPHENYLHYDRAZINE METHOD FOR MENADIONE

A. Principle

Menadione is released from the combined forms present in feedstuffs, concentrates, and premixes by extraction with ethanol and treatment with sodium carbonate. It is extracted with 1,2-dichloroethane. The extracted menadione is reacted with 2,4-dinitrophenylhydrazine (DNPH) to form a blue-green hydrazone complex; the optical density is then measured at 635 nm (31,35). The lower limit of detection by this method is 1 ppm menadione.

B. Reagents

1. *96% (v/v) Ethanol.* Dilute absolute ethanol with H_2O.

2. *40% Ethanol.* Dilute Reagent 1 with H_2O to bring to 40%.

3. *10% Tannin Solution.* Weigh 10 g tannin and bring to 100 mL with H_2O.

4. *10% Sodium Carbonate Solution.* Prepare by weighing out 10 g Na_2CO_3 and dissolving in H_2O. Bring final volume to 100 mL.

5. *DNPH.* Dissolve 40 mg DNPH in about 40 mL boiling absolute ethanol, allow to cool, and transfer to a 50-mL volumetric flask. Add 1 mL concentrated HCl ($d = 1.19$) and make up to volume with absolute ethanol. Prepare immediately before use.

6. *Ammoniacal Ethanol.* Mix one volume of absolute ethanol with one volume of concentrated NH_4OH ($d = 0.91$).

7. *Menadione Standard.* Dissolve 20 mg menadione in 1,2-dichloroethane and dilute to 200 mL with the same solvent. Dilute aliquots of this stock solution with 1,2-dichloroethane to obtain a series of solutions with menadione concentrations between 2 and 10 $\mu g/mL$. These solutions must be prepared immediately before use.

C. Procedure

All operations must be carried out away from direct light, using apparatus of amber glass where necessary.

1. *Test Sample.* From the finely divided sample, take a test sample according to the presumed menadione conent, for example, 0.1–5.0 g for concentrates and

premixes, 20–30 g for feedstuffs. Transfer the sample to a 250-mL flask with ground glass stopper without delay.

2. *Extraction.* Add to the test sample exactly 96 mL 40% ethanol (Reagent 2) and shake mechanically for 15 min at room temperature. Then add 4.0 mL tannin solution (Reagent 3), mix, transfer the extract into a centrifuge tube, centrifuge at 3000–5000 rpm and decant.

Place 20–40 mL, accurately measured, of the extract in a 250-mL separatory funnel, add 50 mL 1,2-dichloroethane, mix, and add by pipette 20 mL Na_2CO_3 solution (Reagent 4). Shake vigorously for 30 sec, collect the dichloroethane phase in a 100-mL separatory funnel. Add 20 mL H_2O, shake again for 15 sec, collect the dichloroethane phase and remove traces of water with strips of filter paper.

For concentrates and premixes, take an aliquot of the extract and dilute with 1,2-dichloroethane to obtain a menadione concentration of 2–10 μg/mL. For feedstuffs, evaporate an aliquot of the extract to dryness under reduced pressure in a rotary vacuum evaporator under nitrogen on a water bath at 40°C. Rapidly treat residue with 1,2-dichloroethane to obtain a solution containing 2–10 μg/ mL.

3. *Hydrazone Formation.* Transfer 2.0 mL of the extract obtained in Section C.2 to a 10-mL volumetric flask and add 3.0 mL DNPH (Reagent 5), securely stopper the flask with a cork or Teflon stopper to prevent evaporation, and heat for 2 hr at 70°C on a water bath. Allow to cool, add 3.0 mL ammoniacal ethanol (Reagent 6), mix, make up to volume with absolute ethanol, and mix again.

4. *Measurement of the Optical Density.* Measure the optical density of the blue-green colored complex with spectrophotometer at 635 nm, using a reagent blank obtained by treating 2.0 mL 1,2-dichloroethane as indicated in Section C.3. Determine the quantity of menadione by reference to a calibration curve established for each series of analyses.

5. *Calibration Curve.* Treat 2.0 mL of menadione standard solutions (Reagent 7) as described in Section C.3. Measure the optical density as indicated in Section C.4. Plot the calibration curve with the optical density values as ordinates and the corresponding quantities of menadione (in μg) as abscissae.

6. *Calculation of Results.* Calculate the menadione content of the sample by taking account of the weight of the test sample and of the dilutions carried out in the course of the analysis.

$$\frac{\text{μg Menadione from standard curve} \times 100}{\text{μg of Sample represented in final dilution}} = \% \text{ Menadione}$$

Menadione values obtained can be converted to other forms using the same conversion factors given in Method I.

7. *Reproducibility.* The difference between the results of two parallel determinations carried out on the same sample must not exceed:

20%, in relative value, for menadione contents less than 10 ppm;

2 ppm, in absolute value, for content between 10 and 14 ppm;

15% in relative value, for contents between 14 and 100 ppm;

15 ppm, in absolute value, for contents between 100 and 150 ppm;

10%, in relative value, for contents greater than 150 ppm.

IV. MODIFIED 2,4-DINITROPHENYLHYDRAZINE METHOD FOR COMBINED FORMS OF MENADIONE

A. Principle

This modification allows the determination of combined menadione in feedstuffs, concentrates, and premixes when the relative concentration of foreign substances is such to cause a distortion of the absorption curve for the color obtained with the formation of the hydrazone (36). As a criterion for the need for chromatography, the ratio of absorption of the sample at 635 nm to that at 550 nm is measured; if this ratio is less than 2.0 or 2.5, chromatography to remove the interfering substances is needed. If, even after chromatographic separation, the ratio is still less than 2.0, chromatography should be repeated with a longer column.

In this modification, the dichloroethane solution obtained is evaporated and the residue take up in cyclohexane. The cyclohexane solution is chromatographed on a column of purified Fuller's earth; an aliquot of the eluate is evaporated to dryness, dissolved in dichloroethane, and determined by the usual colorimetric method with DNPH.

B. Reagents

All reagents (1–7) listed under Method III are required.

8. *Purified Fuller's Earth.*   A suitable brand of Fuller's earth (Floridin XS°) is purified by boiling with concentrated HCl, decanting, and then washing with H_2O until the reaction is neutral. The earth is then dried at 37°C overnight; the water content is determined and brought to about 40%. Before use, it is tested with menadione in cyclohexane; the vitamin should pass completely through the column under the conditions described below in C.

(a) The solution is used in a test to ensure that the purified Fuller's earth used in column is not absorbing any menadione but is allowing it to pass completely through the column. A solution of approximately 20 μg menadione/mL is used. Prepare a suitable amount of solution, dissolving the menadione in cyclohexane. The UV absorption at 250 nm of the solution leaving the column should be the same as the UV absorption of the solution entering the column.

C. Procedure

1. *Preparation of the Solution for Chromatography.*   An aliquot of the dichloroethane solution containing an expected amount of 5–50 μg menadione is evaporated to dryness at low temperature (about 40°C) under nitrogen as described in Section III.C.2. The residue is dissolved in about 1 mL of cyclohexane.

2. *Chromatography.*   About 2 g of purified Fuller's earth are poured into a chromatographic column, about 5 mm (i.d.) × 15 cm, provided with a plug of cotton-wool or other suitable device, and washed with 3–4 mL cyclohexane. The solution of menadione obtained in Section C.1 is transferred quantitatively to the column, and the effluent is collected in a graduated cylinder fitted with a glass or Teflon stopper. Cyclohexane is added to the column and the effluent is collected to 10 mL. The solution is mixed by inversion, and an aliquot is taken corresponding to about 15 μg of menadione and evaporated under a stream of nitrogen at about 40°C. The residue is dissolved in 2 mL of dichloroethane and the solution is analyzed by the DNPH method described previously (Method III).

V.   METHOD FOR WHOLE BLOOD PROTHROMBIN CLOTTING TIME

Each 2-mL vial of chick embryo extract is diluted with 10 mL of 0.025 M $CaCl_2$ in 0.85% NaCl. This thromboplastin–$CaCl_2$ solution is held in the water bath at 37°C. Blood is obtained by heart puncture whereby 0.1 mL of 1.34% sodium oxalate in the syringe is simultaneously mixed with 0.9 mL of blood. The oxalated blood (0.2 mL) is immediately incubated at 37°C for 1 min, after which 0.14 mL of thromboplastin–$CaCl_2$ mixture is added. The time required for this mixture to clot on gently tilting the tube is accurately observed.

A curve of blood prothrombin concentration against prothrombin clotting time in seconds can be drawn for each species. Prothrombin clotting time is normal in the range of 12–20 sec for most species and increasingly abnormal above 30 sec. A commercial lypholized chick embryo extract (Difco) is a suitable source of thromboplastin for avian studies.Rabbit brain thromboplastin serves well for studies in humans and other animals.

VI.   METHOD FOR WHOLE BLOOD CLOTTING TIME

About 1 mL of free-flowing blood is caught in 2 × 15 test tubes. The tubes are suspended in a water bath at 38°C and agitated mechanically until the blood is seen to form a gelatinous clot. This requires 3–4 min for normal blood. In acute vitamin K deficiency, blood may not clot even in 30 min.

Sufficient free-flowing blood for this test can be obtained from chickens by piercing the exposed wing vein. Admixture with tissue juice must be avoided, so that in most species blood is collected by heart or vein puncture using a 5- or 10-mL silicone-coated syringe.

LITERATURE CITED

1. Goodhart, R. S. and Shils, M. E. Eds. *Modern Nutrition in Health and Disease*, 6th ed. Lea and Febiger, Philadelphia, 170 (1980).

2. Scott, M. L., Nesheim, M. C., and Young, R. J. *Nutrition of the Chicken*. M. L. Scott & Associates, Ithaca, New York, 160 (1969).

3. Berruti, R. "Vitamin K for animal feed use." *World Feeds and Protein News* 7, 13 (1972).

4. Vogel, H. and Knobloch, H. *Chemie und Technik der Vitamine*, 3rd ed. Ferdinand Enke Verlag, Stuttgart, Germany, 308 (1950).

5. Griminger, P. "Vitamin K activity in chickens: Phylloquinone and menadione in presence of stress agents." *J. Nutr.* 87, 337 (1965).

6. Scott, M. L. "Vitamin K: New information on metabolism, stability and requirements." *Feedstuffs* 44 (30), 32 (1972).

7. Ewing, W. R. *Poultry Nutrition*, 5th ed. The Ray Ewing Co., Pasadena, Calif., 995 (1963).

8. Wagner, A. F. and Folkers, K.. *Vitamin and Coenzymes*, Vol. 12. Interscience, New York, 428 (1966).

9. Rosenberg, H. R. *Chemistry and Physiology of the Vitamins*. Interscience, New York 481 (1945).

10. Almquist, H. J. "The early history of vitamin K." *Am. J. Clin. Nutr.* 28, 656 (1975).

11. *The United States Pharmacopeia*, 20th ed. Mack Printing, Easton, Penn., 472 (1980).

12. *Federal Register*, 3051 (1963).

13. Quick, A. J., Hussey, C. V., and Callentine, G. E. "Vitamin K requirements of adult dogs and the influence of bile on its absorption from the intestine." *Am. J. Physiol.* 176, 239 (1954).

14. Frost, D. V. and Spruth, H. C. "Control of hemorrhagic condition in chickens with menadione sodium bisulfite." *Poultry Sci.* 34, 56 (1955).

15. Carmack, M., Moore, M. B., and Balis, M. E. "The structure of the antihemorrhagic sodium bisulfite addition product of 2-methyl-1,4-naphthoquinone (menadione)." *J. Am. Chem. Soc.* 72, 844 (1950).

16. Charles, O. W. "A review of the isomeric structures and properties of menadione bisulfites." *Feedstuffs* 44 (11), 35 (1972).

17. Moore, M. B. and Kirchmeyer, F. J. U.S. Patent No. 2,367,302 (1945).

18. Griminger, P. "On the vitamin K requirement of turkey poults." *Poultry Sci.* 36, 1227 (1957).

19. Day, E. J. "Evaluation of a new vitamin K compound." Proceedings of the Texas Nutrition Conference, 32 (1967).

20. Charles, O. W. and Huston, T. M. "The biological activity of vitamin K materials following storage and pelleting." *Poultry Sci.* 51, 1421 (1972).

21. Food Additive Regulation 121.286. *Federal Register* 40FR30108, July 17 (1975).

22. Suttie, J. W. "Current understanding of vitamin K function." Proceedings of the 39th Semiannual American Feed Manufacturers Association, 39 (1980).

23. Frick, P. G., Riedler, G., and Brogli, H. "Dose response and minimal daily requirement for vitamin K in man." *J. Appl. Physiol.* 23(3), 387 (1967).

24. Charles, O. W. "The relationship of chemical and physical properties to biological activity of various vitamin K active substances." *Proc. Sixth Eur. Poult. Conf. World Poult. Sci. Assoc.*, 3 (1980).

25. Quick, A. J. *Hemorrhagic Diseases*, Lea and Febiger, Philadelphia (1957).

26. Griminger, P. "Relative vitamin K potency of two water-soluble menadione analogues." *Poultry Sci.* 44, 210 (1965).

27. Quick, A. J. and Stefannini, M. "Experimentally induced changes in the prothrombin level of the blood IV." *J. Biol. Chem.* 175, 945 (1948).

28. McCormick, J. B. and Kopp, J. B. "Semimicro prothrombin time test chamber." *Am. J. Clin. Pathol.* **48**, 511 (1967).

29. *The United States Pharmacopeia,* 17th ed. Mack Printing, Easton Penn., 468 (1965).

30. Pinder, J. L. and Singer, J. H. "Examination and determination of 2-methyl-1:4-naphthoquinone." *Analyst* **65**, 7 (1940).

31. Zijl, H.J.M. van, and Geerling, H. "Vitamine-K_3 en vitamine-K_3-bisulfiet." *Chemisch Weekblad* **55**, 597 (1959).

32. Libby, D. A. and Sheppard, A. J. "Gas liquid chromatographic method for the determination of fat soluble vitamins 2 Application to menadione." *J. Assoc. Off. Anal. Chem.* **48**, 973 (1965).

33. *The United States Pharmacopeia,* 17th ed. Mack Printing, Easton, Penn., 1082 (1965).

34. *The United States Pharmacopeia,* 14th ed. Mack Printing, Easton, Penn., 948 (1950).

35. "Determination of menadione (Vitamin K_3)." *Off. J. Eur. Communities* No. L 108/23, 22.4.74.

36. Gaudiano, A., Bellmonte, G., Sanzini, E., Gilardi, G., and Civalleri, S. "La vitamina K negli integratori per mangimi." *Rivista della Societa Italiana di Scienza dell' Alimentazione* **6** (3), 193 (1977).

12 Vitamin C (L-Ascorbic and Dehydro-L-Ascorbic Acids)

Omer Pelletier

GENERAL CONSIDERATIONS

Although L-ascorbic acid is widely distributed in the animal and plant kingdoms, enzymes for its biosynthesis from D-glucose or D-galactose in man, monkey, guinea pig, Indiana fruit bat, and several species of passeriformes birds are lacking due to genetic defects (1).

L-ascorbic acid is essential for the prevention and cure of scurvy, a disease that has been known since ancient times. In the first part of the sixteenth century, Jacques Cartier, during his exploration of Canada, found that the natives prevented and cured scurvy by drinking extracts from the bark and needles of pine trees, which we know provided L-ascorbic acid. In the eighteenth century, scurvy was traced to a lack of fresh fruits and vegetables in the diet. Some of the characteristics of scurvy are loosening of teeth, swollen joints, petechial hemorrhages from venules, and subcutaneous and intestinal hemorrhages, which can be attributed to defects in collagen synthesis (2). During the process of collagen synthesis, ascorbic acid participates in the hydroxylation of particular prolyl and lysyl residues previously incorporated into peptides linkages (3).

The name "ascorbic acid" was suggested in 1933 by Szent-Gyorgy and Haworth, whereas the name "vitamin C" was adopted following Drummond's publication in 1920 of the "nomenclature of the so-called accessory food factors (vitamin C)" (4).

L-ascorbic acid has the empirical formula $C_6H_8O_6$ which accounts for a molecular weight of 176. It forms colorless crystals (M.P. 192°C) freely soluble in water; slightly soluble in acetone, methanol and ethanol; and insoluble in ether, benzene, chloroform, fats, and fat solvents. L-ascorbic acid contains a dienol group that not only contributes reducing action but also confers acidic behavior to the molecule. Solutions of L-ascorbic acid greater than $1.2 \times 10^{-4}M$ show an intense absorption maximum at 245 nm which moves to 265 nm following dilution to $0.6 \times 10^{-4}M$ owing to increased dissociation of the acid (5). The oxidation-reduction potential E_0^1 is 0.166 V at pH 4.0 and 35°C. On oxidation with moderate oxidants, L-ascorbid acid yields dehydroascorbic acid, which may slowly undergo irreversible conversion to diketogulonic acid:

$$
\begin{array}{ccc}
\text{O=C} & \text{O=C} & \text{CO}_2\text{H} \\
\text{HO-C} & \text{O=C} & \text{O=C} \\
\text{HO-C O} & \text{O=C O} & \text{O=C} \\
\text{H-C} & \text{H-C} & \text{H-C-OH} \\
\text{HO-C-H} & \text{HO-C-H} & \text{HO-C-H} \\
\text{CH}_2\text{OH} & \text{CH}_2\text{OH} & \text{CH}_2\text{OH} \\
\text{L-Ascorbic Acid} & \text{Dehydro-L-ascorbic acid} & \text{2,3-Diketogulonic acid}
\end{array}
$$

Oxidation of L-ascorbic acid in solution in presence of oxygen is facilitated by such factors as alkaline pH and particularly by ferric and cupric ions. All these effects are accelerated by increases in temperature (6). L-ascorbic acid is quite stable to air oxidation in aqueous metaphosphoric acid solution (7). The presence of oxygen will promote oxidation of L-ascorbic acid by ascorbic acid oxidase, which is naturally present in certain foods (e.g., cucumber).

Dehydroascorbic acid is neutral in solution and, on treatment with reducing agents such as hydrogen sulfide and homocysteine, is reduced to ascorbic acid. Dehydroascorbic acid may be quantitatively oxidized with an equimolar amount of sodium hypoiodite to oxalic acid and L-threonic acid. Dehydroascorbic acid in solution has maximum stability at approximately pH 2–3 at 25°C, and its stability decreases at both higher and lower pH (8). Dehydroascorbic acid is transparent in the region 230–280 nm and shows a weak absorption band at 300 nm (5). Dehydroascorbic acid is readily reduced to ascorbic acid in the animal body and is utilized by humans in a manner comparable to ascorbic acid (9). Above pH 7 dehydroascorbic acid rapidly saponifies to diketogulonic acid.

Diketogulonic acid has no antiscorbutic activity. Diketogulonic acid displays a maximum absorption at 290 nm (10). In alkaline medium diketogulonic acid will be decomposed to threonic, xylonic and oxalic acids.

D-isoascorbic acid, also named D-araboascorbic acid and erythorbic acid, is a stereoisomer (mirror image according to Fischer convention) of L-ascorbic acid. According to certain food regulations (e.g., the Food and Drug Act and Regulations, Canada), D-isoascorbic acid or L-ascorbic acid may be used as preservatives for certain foods such as frozen fruits, preserved fish, preserved meats, meat by-products, and pickles. It has been demonstrated experimentally that D-isoascorbic acid can cure scurvy in guinea pigs previously deprived of vitamin C but that intakes 20 times larger than L-ascorbic acid were not quite as effective as the latter (11). Thus, to determine accurately the vitamin C content of foods to which D-isoascorbic acid has been added as a preservative, it is necessary to differentiate L-ascorbic acid from D-isoascorbic acid.

METHODS AVAILABLE

A. Bioassays

A reasonably satisfactory bioassay based upon the determination of the minimum quantity of product required to protect a guinea pig from scurvy was described by Sherman et al. (12) in 1922. More recently, bioassays have been utilized only for research purposes to determine if certain compounds have a certain activity as compared with L-ascorbic acid. The activity of compounds such as D-ascorbic acid and D-isoascorbic acid cannot be readily converted into L-ascorbic acid equivalents. D-ascorbic acid was found to be rapidly metabolized and excreted by guinea pigs, but given in sufficient amounts could maintain the weight and survival of the animals; although the teeth of these animals showed a normal dentin, hemorrhages of the joints were not prevented (13). D-isoascorbic acid had less than one-twentieth the activity of L-ascorbic acid for curing scurvy (11), but upon discontinuation of intakes, its rate of disappearance from guinea pigs' organs was about four times more rapid (14).

B. 2,6-Dichloroindophenol Reduction

2,6-Dichloroindophenol is a dye that has been often referred to as Tillman's reagent by the name of the person who introduced this reagent for measuring the antiscorbutic activity of lemon juice (15). When an aqueous solution of this blue dye is added to an acidic solution of ascorbic acid, it is reduced by ascorbic acid, which is oxidized to dehydroascorbic acid; the reduced dye is colorless, but dye added after all the ascorbic acid has been oxidized, gives a pink color to the acidic solution. (Figure 12.1)

Measurement of L-ascorbic acid by direct titration with 2,6-dichloroindophenol has been and still is about the most popular method because it is simple and rapid, and in many cases not less specific than several of the other methods based on oxido-reduction. Direct titration yields valid vitamin C measurements in cases where the sample composition is known not to have more than negligible

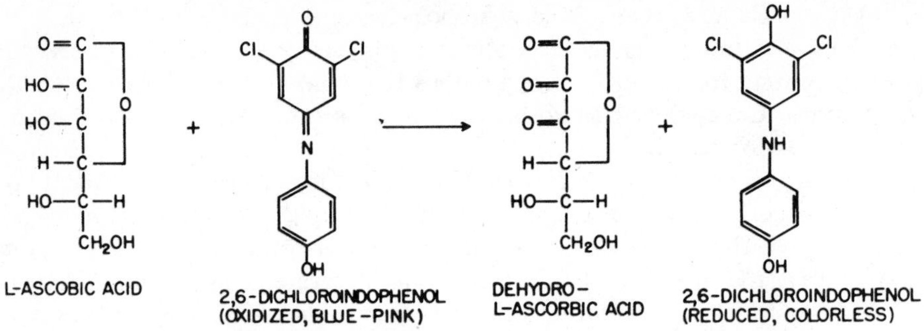

Figure 12.1　Reaction of 2,6-dichloroindophenol.

amounts of interfering substances and when the concentration of dehydroascorbic acid is negligible or irrelevant. Thus, the method is unquestionably applicable to certain types of samples such as fresh citrus fruit juice and multivitamin tablets that do not contain minerals. However, it has been demonstrated that dehydroascorbic acid, which has vitamin C activity (9), can be present in significant amounts in fruit drinks (16,17) and in a variety of cooked and processed food (18–22). In other cases, the presence of dehydroascorbic acid may arise from the preparation of samples for analysis due to the presence of ascorbic acid oxidase, or ferric or cupric ions. Numerous substances capable of reducing the dye may result from the preparation and processing of food and include reductones and reductic acid (7,23,24), ferrous and stannous ions (7,25,26), sulfite, thiosulfate (7), and D-isoascorbic acid. Other substances naturally present in foods or biological materials that may be oxidized by the dye, comprises tannins, betanin (27,28), and sulfhydryl compounds such as cysteine and glutathione. In other cases, the materials to be analyzed may contain natural or added colors that render the end point difficult to judge visually. Because of the numerous shortcomings of 2,6-dichloroindophenol for measuring vitamin C, it is not surprising that many ways have been proposed to circumvent or eliminate these sources of inaccuracy and imprecision.

　　The formation of dehydroascorbic acid during the preparation of plant samples for analysis can be minimized by stabilizing the samples with cold trichloroacetic acid solution in presence of ethylenediaminetetraacetic acid (EDTA) (29). This compound will effectively chelate copper and other metals that are associated with the loss of ascorbic acid while the trichloroacetic acid will precipitate enzymes and prevent ascorbic acid oxidation (29).

　　Various reagents have been proposed for reducing dehydroascorbic acid prior to titration. Reduction with H_2S followed by removal of excess H_2S by bubbling nitrogen has been described as being satisfactory by King (30). Besides being open to question with regard to specificity for dehydroascorbic acid (31,32), the use of H_2S presents risks of flammability and toxicity and it is a rather unpleasant and time-consuming procedure.

　　Hughes (32) demonstrated that at pH values greater than 6.8, homocysteine rapidly reduced dehydroascorbic acid to ascorbic acid. Measurements were made photoelectrically within 30 sec after addition of a known amount of dye in excess of the total ascorbic acid content, which according to Hughes (32) avoided interference by homocysteine. Because other substances such as alloxan, dehydroreductic acid, and dehydroreductones were also reduced by homocysteine, Hughes (32) utilized blanks where boric acid was used to destroy dehydroascorbic acid before the homocysteine treatment. The only disadvantage found with this procedure by personal experience was the difficulty in judging the end point because of the unstability of the dye even in the absence of vitamin C. Subsequently, Hughes (33) selected to use a cation-exchange resin to remove color material and interfering reducing substances from urine. Howard and Constable (34) applied homocysteine reduction and used boric acid blanks to determine total vitamin C in urine following oxidation of ascorbic acid and removal of interfering pigments with charcoal.

Gero and Candido (35) used 2,6-dimercaptopropanol in slight excess to reduce dehydroascorbic to ascorbic acid at pH 6.8; excess 2,6-dimercaptopropanol was removed by precipitation with cadmium chloride before titration with 2,6-dichloroindophenol. Precipitation of other thiols by cadmium chloride improved the specificity of the method, but there was no comment about possible interference from alloxan, dehydroreductic acid, and dehydroreductones (35), which have been shown to be reduced by homocysteine in presence or absence of boric acid (32).

Various other means besides cation exchange resins (33) and charcoal (34) have been proposed to eliminate interference of colors with the titration of ascorbic acid with 2,6-dichloroindophenol. Bhattacharya and Ganguly (36) used an anion-exchanger to separate ascorbic acid from edible dyes in extracts from pharmaceutical preparations. Various solvents have also been tried to extract selectively and measure the excess of a known quantity of 2,6-dichloroindophenol following the oxidation of ascorbic acid. The method of Robinson and Stotz (37) utilized xylene extraction followed by photometric measurement. Gero (38) found isoamyl alcohol a suitable replacement for xylene because it increased sensitivity about three times. Nadkarni (39) investigated the use of various solvents for the purpose of extracting the dye for visual detection after addition of only a basic excess; ethyl ether proved to be very effective and was utilized for determining the ascorbic acid content of several fruits and a few vegetables. The only apparent drawbacks of utilizing ether are its flammability and toxicity, which require special precautions.

A very simple means of detecting the end point of titration with 2,6-dichloroindophenol, has been used by Pelletier and Morrison (40) for determining ascorbic acid in colored fruit drinks. This modification consists of determining the end point by observing a slight reversal of the decrease in absorbance at the moment that excess dye is added.

The reduced ions of iron, copper, and stannum may reduce 2,6-dichloroindophenol and thus can produce falsely elevated ascorbic acid values. Chapman et al. (41) made a thorough study of various procedures that has been proposed for eliminating or reducing the ferrous iron interference in ascorbic acid assays and concluded that in presence of ferrous iron, a sodium acetate–hydrochloric acid buffer at pH 0.65 (25) gave reliable results for titration in the presence of ferrous iron but only in the absence of copper salts; the use of 2.5% sulfuric acid gave results comparable with those obtained with the sodium acetate–hydrochloric acid buffer, but was not recommended because of the unstability of ascorbic acid in sulfuric acid (41). Methods using H_2O_2 to oxidize ferrous iron gave unsatisfactory recoveries of ascorbic acid (41). Pelletier and Morrison (26) found the sodium acetate–hydrochloric acid buffer inefficient in presence of stannous chloride or in presence of ferrous sulfate with traces of oxalic acid as might occur in certain foods. Lugg (7) suggested that in presence of ferrous sulfate, advantage could be taken of the more rapid rate of aerial oxidation of ferrous salts as compared with ascorbic acid, but this appeared unsatisfactory (26) because ferric and traces of cupric ions could cause oxidation of ascorbic acid. Pelletier and Morrison (26) conducted aerial oxidation in presence of EDTA to chelate effectively the oxidized metal ions and prevent the oxidation of ascorbic acid.

The effect of pH on the condensation of formaldehyde with ascorbic acid and several reducing substances has been thoroughly studied by Lugg (7) for the purpose of improving the estimation of ascorbic acid with 2,6-dichloroindophenol. Lugg (7) carried condensations at pH 1.5 and 3.5; ascorbic acid was found to condense readily at pH 3.5 but very slowly at pH 1.5, whereas sulfites, thiosulfates, cysteine, and H_2S-treated pyruvic acid readily condensed at both pH levels to form nonreducing or feebly reducing substances; on the other hand, reductones, thiourea, and ferrous salts did not condense appreciatively at either pH. Consequently titration after condensation at pH 1.5 minus titration at pH 3.5 represents ascorbic acid. These principles have been subsequently utilized with modifications by Mapson (23) and Robinson and Stotz (37). Kuusi (24) compared the latter two methods for the assay of ascorbic acid in presence of reductones and concluded that the method of Robinson and Stotz (37) appeared to give the most reliable results; the xylene-extraction step of the latter method possibly contributed additional specificity. Pelletier (42) reported that extraction of ascorbic acid from enriched evaporated or condensed milk with an acetic acid–metaphosphoric acid solution removed heat-generated reducing substances believed to be protein derivatives and that it was only necessary to do condensation with formaldehyde at pH 3.5 to provide blanks representing the amount of 2,6-dichloroindophenol reduced by reductones types of compounds.

Owen and Iggo (43) recommended the use of p-chloromercuribenzoic acid to precipitate and remove the sulfhydryl type of reducing compounds with the exception of sulfites. They reported that p-chloromercuribenzoic acid only removed part of the interfering reducing substances from urine and that formaldehyde condensation was preferable in that case (43).

Continuous-flow systems can be used to monitor the decrease in absorbance of 2,6-dichloroindophenol produced after mixing with an ascorbic acid solution. In 1967, Nesset et al. (44) and Beyer (45) presented diagrams of very simple manifolds of flowthrough systems applicable to solutions containing only a few mg ascorbic acid per mL. A somewhat more complex system including on-flow dialysis was utilized by Gary et al. (46) for the determination of ascorbic acid directly from plasma. The Technicon Instrument Corporation (Tarrytown, New York) has proposed a simple manifold (Industrial method no. 252-73A) with on-line dialysis applicable to ascorbic acid concentrations ranging from 20 mg/ mL to 100 mg/mL with a 15-mm flow cell. The time delay between mixing of sample and dye was specified only with the technique of Nesset et al. (44); those authors pointed out that the 50-sec period required for mixing and reading might need to be adjusted to a shorter period for materials containing considerable amounts of reduced sulfhydryl compounds in the filtrate. Saindelle et al. (47) proposed a more complex but possibly more accurate automated method: the sample is mixed with formol at pH 1.1 to condense with sulfhydryl compounds, then, 2,6-dichloroindophenol is added simultaneously with a buffer that adjusts pH to 3.7; rapidly thereafter, excess dye is extracted with isoamyl alcohol and its absorbance measured at 500 nm. The setting up of any of these automated systems in a laboratory would appear justified when a large number of samples needs to be run routinely and specificity is demonstrated adequate for the type of samples to be analyzed.

C. Oxido-Reduction Methods Involving Iodine and Bromine

Barakat et al. (48) introduced the technique of titration of ascorbic acid with N-bromosuccinimide: after ascorbic acid was totally oxidized to dehydroascorbic acid with N-bromosuccinimide, which was irreversibly reduced to succinimide with the formation of hydrogen bromide, excess N-bromosuccinimide produced a second selective oxidation of potassium iodide liberating iodine which, in presence of starch, yielded a blue color indicating the end point. Reductones, reductic acid, and iron salts did not interfere with this titration (48). Evered (49) modified this procedure by extracting the liberated iodine in an organic solvent to avoid interference from highly colored solutions with end point detection. Hardesty (50) avoided the masking of end points by titrating ascorbic acid with N-bromosuccinimide in presence of potassium iodide with potentiometric detection using two platinum electrodes with a polarizing current. Sarwar et al. (51) found that the method of Barakat et al. (48) gave unsatisfactory results with samples of preserved juices and squashes containing metabisulfite as a preservative, because sulfite oxidation preceded that of ascorbic acid; to overcome this difficulty, they complexed bisulfite with acetone before the titration.

Murty and Roe (52) recently reviewed the determination of ascorbic acid with iodine, potassium iodate, potassium bromate, and iodine monochloride. Starch was not considered a suitable indicator because it decreased the reaction rate between ascorbic acid and iodine; other means that had been proposed included Variamine blue, and carbon tetrachloride or chloroform extraction in the presence of mercuric chloride (52). Instead of these, Murty and Roe (52) proposed using naphthol blue black, amaranth, or Brilliant Ponceau 5R as indicators. They also proposed a procedure based on the principle that potassium dichromate, when added to the titration mixture, first reacts with potassium iodide, which in turn oxidizes ascorbic acid; the end point was detected by potentiometric measurements or visually using one of the above indicators (52).

Varma and Gulati (53) used chloramine T, which in the presence of acidified potassium iodide or potassium bromide liberated iodine or bromine to oxidize ascorbic acid; the end point was detected by a starch iodine blue color or by the bleaching of methyl red with bromine. Iron did not interfere, and sulfite and sulfhydryl compounds were rendered nonreducing by a prereaction with acrylonitrile (53).

In general, these titrations involving iodine or bromine do not appear to offer much advantage over 2,6-dichloroindophenol titrations since there are modifications of the latter that can avoid or reduce interference from colors, iron, reductones, and reductic acid.

D. Oxidation-Reduction Methods Involving Iron, Copper, Mercury, and Selenious Acid

Reduction of ferric ions by ascorbic acid and colorimetric measurements of the resulting ferrous ions has been the basis of simple and sensitive methods for measuring ascorbic acid (54–61). Sullivan and Clark (54) measured the red-orange color produced by the α,α-dipyridyl complex with ferrous iron. Other reducing substances such as reductones were inhibited by the presence of orthophosphate and a high degree of acidity at pH 1–2; glutathione, cysteine, uric acid, and reductic acid gave no reaction by this procedure which was applied to the determination of ascorbic acid in urine, orange juice, and honey (54). Maickel (55) adapted this procedure to the determination of ascorbic acid in animal tissue. Zannoni et al. (56) described a micromodification applicable to human plasma and animal tissues and reported that glucose, fructose, sucrose, glutathione, and cysteine did not interfere. Vann (57) proposed an even more sensitive method for the determination of ascorbic acid in urine by formation of a colored complex of ferrous ions with bathophenanthroline and extraction of the complex into chloroform. Przyborowski (58) determined ascorbic acid in pharmaceutical preparations by titration of ferrous ions with EDTA in the presence of xylenol orange. Day et al. (59) preferred to react the ferrous ion resulting from the reduction of ferric ions by ascorbic acid with 2,4,6-tripyridyl-s-triazine (TPTZ) and applied this procedure to the routine assay of ascorbic acid in serum and plasma after deproteinizing with trichloroacetic acid; the interference due to reduction of ferric iron with uric acid was decreased by carrying the reaction in presence of an acetate buffer of high molarity. Day et al. (59) reported that glucose, urea, and cysteine did not interfere, but potassium oxalate decreased the ascorbic acid and EDTA gave a complete inhibition. Another variant of methods based on the reduction of ferric ions by ascorbic acid consisted in utilizing ferrozine for measuring the resulting ferrous ions (60). Citric acid and tartaric acid retarded the reaction but this effect could be removed by chelation with aluminum or lanthanium; that procedure was found applicable to citrus fruit juices but not to cranberry juice, which developed color changes with time (60). Removal of ferrous ions from extracts of samples with a cation-exchange resin was required to avoid falsely elevated ascorbic acid values (60). The above methods (54–60) do not measure dehydroascorbic acid, but recently Okamura (61) determined ascorbic acid and dehydroascorbic acid in blood plasma with the α,α-dipyridyl method after reducing dehydroascorbic acid with dithiothreitol at pH 6.5–8 and removing excess dithiothreitol with N-ethylmaleimide; this compound blocked most of the reducing power of glutathione and cysteine naturally present, and thus decreased their interference. Since iron determinations per se usually require great precautions to avoid contaminations from glassware, such contaminations and the iron naturally present in samples could cause interferences. Ferric ions arising from contamination or from the sample could be reduced to ferrous ions simultaneously to oxidation of ascorbic acid into dehydroascorbic acid even before initiating the determination of ascorbic acid; but ferrous ions naturally present could be producing falsely elevated vitamin C values. Consequently, vitamin C determination would require both removal of iron from samples extracts (60) and reduction of dehydroascorbic acid (61) before performing the analysis, but none of the above methods (54–61) combines these two features.

Recently a method was proposed (62) on the basis of the reduction of cupric-2,2-biquinoline complex to a cuprous-2,2-biquinoline complex by ascorbic acid and measurement of the resulting purple color at 540 nm. Interference from ferrous ions required their removal with a cation-exchange resin; other interfering substances included sodium thiosulfate and sulfhydryl compounds, such as cysteine (62).

Kum-Tatt and Leong (63) determined L-ascorbic acid in urine by reduction of mercuric chloride to mercurous chloride at pH 3.5–5.0; the insoluble mercurous salt was separated by centrifugation, dissolved with an iodine–potassium iodide solution and back-titrated with sodium thiosulfate. Ferrous salts, sodium sulfite, uric acid, and glucose did not interfere (63).

Ascorbic acid in food extracts could be determined by measuring the turbidity (reddish suspension) due to the formation of selenium produced by the reaction of selenious acid with ascorbic acid (27); the presence of stannous ions caused a reaction with selenious acid and required an independent analysis to correct for its presence (27).

E. Polarographic Analysis Involving Electrochemical Oxidation

Polarographic analysis can be employed for the quantitative determination of ascorbic acid on the basis of the electrochemical oxidation of ascorbic acid on a dropping mercury electrode and by observing the anodic wave arising from the diffusion current. The oxidation process of L-ascorbic acid has been described in detail by Ruitz et al. (64); it involves a two electrons transfer and obeys the overall reaction:

$$AH_2 \longrightarrow B + 2e + H^+$$

Lento et al. (65) measured total vitamin C by polarographic analysis after reducing dehydroascorbic acid with homocysteine and removing the interference of excess homocysteine and naturally occurring sulfhydryl compounds with N-ethylmaleimide. The vitamin C values of several foods by polarographic analysis compared well with those by the 2,4-dinitrophenylhydrazine procedure of Roe et al. (66,67). The polarographic method was found applicable to colored samples (65), but the interference from reductones required pretreatment of samples with formaldehyde (68). By applying a rapid alternating current polarographic procedure, Ratzkowski and Korol (69) were able to differentiate simultaneously L-ascorbic and D-isoascorbic acids in foods; malic acid, citric acid, and sodium chloride did not interfere. As judged by the rarity of papers published about polarographic analysis involving electrochemical oxidation of L-ascorbic acid, this type of method has not gained popularity; a possible explanation could be that polarographic apparatus has not become standard equipment in most analytical laboratories and that thorough studies of the specificity and precision of vitamin C determinations by polarographic analysis are not available.

F.   Methods Requiring Oxygen $\pm$ Ascorbic Acid Oxidase

Blanks for the determination of ascorbic acid from its absorbance at 265 nm were prepared by destroying ascorbic acid upon exposure to air at 90°C (70); this method was applied to a few fruits including tomatoes and cherries and gave values slightly lower than by 2,6-dichloroindophenol titration.

Air exposure of blood plasma to destroy ascorbic acid provided blanks for a very sensitive spectrofluorometric method where the nonfluorescent 1,2-naphthoquinone-4-sulfuric acid was quantitatively reduced by ascorbic acid to 1,2-dihydroxynaphthane-4-sulfuric acid fluorescing at λ ex $= 330$ nm and λ em $= 465$ nm (71).

Ascorbic acid oxidase obtained from the cell sap of cucumber fruits by precipitation with ammonium sulfate was utilized to provide sample blanks for the spectrophotometric measurement of ascorbic acid at 265 nm (72); total vitamin C was measured after reduction of dehydroascorbic acid with homocysteine. This procedure was applied only to a few plant tissues and the extent of possible interference from reductones and reductic acid and other substances has not been discussed (72).

Purified ascorbic acid oxidase (E.C. 1.10.33) has been utilized by Marchesini et al. (73) for ascorbic acid determination by measuring in a special cell the oxygen uptake during the enzymatic oxidation of ascorbic acid; total vitamin C determination required reduction of dehydroascorbic acid with homocysteine. Marchesini et al. (73) did observe the presence of reductic acid upon analysis of spinach subjected to heat treatment and concluded to the specificity of their procedure for ascorbic acid.

Beutler and Beinstingl (74) oxidized ascorbic acid with ascorbic acid oxidase to provide blanks for a colorimetric procedure based on the reduction of the tetrazolium salt [3-(4,5-dimethylthiazolyl-2)-2,5-diphenyl tetrazolium bromide] in presence of the electron carrier 5-methylphenazinium methyl sulfate at pH 3.5 to a formozan absorbing at 578 nm; total vitamin C determinations required reduction with homocysteine. D-isoascorbic acid was not differentiated. The interference of sulfur dioxide required treatment with formaldehyde, and color interference from dark juices was removed by decolorization with 1% polyvinylpolypyrrolidone before filtration (74). Sorbitol, alcohols, and oxalate above certain limits inhibited the ascorbic acid oxidase. However, the effect of oxalate could be removed by adding a slight excess of calcium ions (74). That method has been applied to a variety of foods (74) and a reagent test combination is available (Cat. No. 409677) from Boehringer Mannheim Biochemicals (Indianapolis, Indiana).

An amperometric sensor for L-ascorbic acid was constructed by Matsumoto et al. (75) by immobilizing ascorbate oxidase in the reconstituted collagen membrane and mounting on a Clark oxygen electrode. The enzyme responded to D-isoascorbic acid, but there was no significant interference from glucose, cupric and ferric ions, EDTA, and citric acid (75).

G. 2,4-Dinitrophenylhydrazine Coupling with Ketonic Groups of Dehydroascorbic Acid and Diketogluonic Acid

The determination of total vitamin C on the basis of coupling of 2,4-dinitrophenylhydrazine (DNPH) with the ketonic groups of dehydroascorbic acid (DHAA) and diketogluonic acid (DKGA) has been widely used for all kinds of samples since the publication by Roe and Kuether (66) of a procedure applicable to blood and urine. In the preparation of samples for analysis, trichloroacetic acid was used to precipitate proteins, and aliquots of the filtrates were shaken with acid-washed charcoal (Norit) and filtered. The charcoal served to clarify the solutions and oxidized all the vitamin C to DHAA. Ascorbic acid (AA) was not oxidized quantitatively by charcoal unless the solution contained a reagent such as acetic, trichloroacetic, and oxalic acids to prevent absorption of DHAA on the charcoal (76). Thiourea was added prior to DNPH to produce a mildly reducing medium because oxidants were found to produce unspecific coloration of DNPH during the 3-hr incubation at 37°C (66). The osazones were dissolved by adding 85% sulfuric acid drop by drop to the test tubes in an iced bath and the absorbance of the resulting red solution was measured at 545 nm (66).

Roe et al. (67) adapted the original method (66) to the differential determination of DKGA, DHAA, and AA in the same tissue extract. In that case, vitamin C was extracted with a metaphosphoric acid–stannous chloride solution and there was no charcoal treatment. AA in one aliquot was oxidized with bromine to DHAA, and excess bromine was expelled with air or nitrogen; the DNPH reaction gave a composite determination for AA, DHAA, and DKGA. In a second aliquot, DHAA was reduced to AA with H_2S, and excess H_2S was removed by bubbling CO_2 after adding thiourea to the sample; this DNPH reaction determined DKGA only. A third aliquot was neither reduced nor oxidized, so that DNPH reacted only with DHAA (67). The greatest disadvantage with that method is the use of H_2S presenting risks of toxicity and flammability and the difficulty of removing excess H_2S (65); bromine also requires special precautions to avoid breathing of vapors and contact with skin.

With the method using oxidation with charcoal to measure total vitamin C (66), the major disadvantages is the complexity of the addition of sulfuric acid for color development and, to a lesser extent, the charcoal treatment.

Roe (77) later proposed a method for determining the specificity of the DNPH procedure by comparing the coupling reaction for 3 hr at 37°C with 17 hr at 15°C. Since DHAA and DKGA had much faster coupling rates than interfering compounds, the slower-reacting compounds were expected to produce nonmeasurable amounts of osazones at the lower temperature; this effect was demonstrated by the analysis of tomato juice, which gave vitamin C values about 18% lower at the lower temperature (77). Roe (77) suggested that the interference of high concentrations of sugars could be rendered negligible by further diluting the samples, but it has not been demonstrated how this could affect the precision for lower vitamin C levels.

According to Pelletier and Brassard (78), the interference from high concentrations of sugars can be rendered negligible after incubation at 15°C (77) by measuring the absorbance 75 min after the addition of sulfuric acid instead of 30 min, as in the original method.

Roe (76) has rebutted some proposals to simplify the original procedure (66). Roe (76) objected to the use of 2,6-dichloroindophenol to oxidize ascorbic acid instead of charcoal which provided clarification of extracts. Incubation with DNPH for 10 min at 100°C was found to cause too great additive errors as compared with incubations at 15°C or 37°C in presence of interfering substances such as glucuronic acid, fructose, and glucose (76).

The use of several acid mixtures that had been proposed for replacing the tedious dropwise addition of sulfuric acid has been discussed by Pelletier (79). Glacial acetic acid and phosphoric and hydrochloric acid mixtures were considerably less sensitive than sulfuric acid; nitric acid diluted with water was found to produce nitrous oxides readily with spontaneous discoloration of DNPH and osazones (79). Pelletier (79) proposed a nitric acid–phosphoric acid mixture that did not produce nitrous oxides unless humidity was high and droplets would stick on the walls of test tubes not scrupulously clean (78). By using a nitric and citric acid mixture, the problem of nitrous oxides formation was completely eliminated (78).

Since reductones and reductic acid may be found in certain preserved and cooked foods because of the high-temperature exposure (23), Roe (76) proposed separation of these components from vitamin C by paper chromatography (80) before the DNPH reaction. The DNPH osazones due to vitamin C may be separated from interfering osazones by paper chromatography (81,82), thin-layer chromatography (83,84), column chromatography (85), and column chromatography followed by thin-layer chromatography (86) to differentiate AA from D-isoascorbic acid (IAA). Recently a high-performance liquid chromatography (HPLC) method has been used to separate the vitamin C osazone from aqueous humor (87). It would be advantageous to be able to separate the vitamin C osazones from those due to sugars, reductones, and reductic acid, but there are no indications if the reported procedure (87) could achieve that separation.

Pelletier (79) incorporated other principles into the original DNPH vitamin C methods (66,67) to provide a more accurate and simpler determination; oxidation of ascorbic acid could be made with 2,6-dichloroindophenol instead of activated charcoal which absorbed interfering pigments. The measurement of vitamin C with DNPH was improved by using blanks that measured the nonspecific absorbance contributed to the total measurement. The blank test consisted in the reduction of DHAA to AA with homocysteine and formation of a complex of AA with boric acid to prevent formation of DNPH osazone due to vitamin C. In the total test, the osazones due to AA and DHAA were formed after oxidizing AA to DHAA with 2,6-dichloroindophenol and after complexing DHAA with boric acid to prevent reduction to AA by the presence of homocysteine. Interfering substances yielded the same amount of osazones in both the blank and total test because sugars and DKGA were unaffected by homocysteine, whereas dehydroreductone types of compounds were reduced to the same extent in both the blank and total test. To determine AA and differentiate it from DHAA, a different blank was used where DHAA was first complexed with boric acid to prevent its reduction in presence of homocysteine. Initially, Pelletier (79) recommended solubilizing the osazone with nitric and phosphoric acid, but to avoid occasional problems with nitrous oxide formation, a mixture of nitric and citric acids was later utilized (78). The latter procedure also reduced the number of reagents additions by combining some of them; applicability to a wide variety of foods was demonstrated (78). These principles (78,79) form the basis of the manual DNPH procedure described in Section I of this chapter and the automated discrete sampling methods described in the chapter on automated methods.

Utilizing the same principles, but incubating at two different temperatures (32°C and 52°C) for 80 min, it was also possible to quantitatively differentiate AA from IAA (88); such a procedure is described in this chapter (Section II).

The DNPH methods for total vitamin C (78,79) have been adapted to automated flowthrough analysis (89–91) for application limited to certain samples such as serum, animal tissues, and pharmaceutical preparations, because the temperature above 37°C required to achieve sufficient sensitivity can considerably increase the formation of osazones from sugars and glucuronic acid (76). The automated discrete sample analysis method (78) described in the chapter on automated vitamin analysis does not have the temperature limitations of flowthrough analysis and is thus applicable to a variety of materials, including serum, with the same accuracy as the manual method.

H. Vitamin C Determinations by Direct Coupling with Compounds Other Than 2,4-Dinitrophenylhydrazine

Several colorimetric methods based on the coupling of ascorbic acid with aniline diazonium salts have been described (92–97). These salts produce purplish or blue reaction products with ascorbic acid in alkaline solutions. Schmall et al. (92) utilized diazotized 4-methoxy-2-nitroaniline for coupling with ascorbic acid in acid medium in the presence of ethanol or isopropanol and developed the reaction product to a purplish color in alkaline medium. There was no interference from ferrous and stannous salts, dehydroascorbic acid, and diketogluonic acid, but reductones and reductic acid required formaldehyde condensation to avoid erroneously high vitamin C values (92). Davidek and Davidkova (98) found that the method of Schmall et al. (92) gave erroneously low values in presence of flavanoids and pectic substances. Crossland (93) modified the method of Schmall et al. (92) to remove interfering substances from natural products and foodstuff by chromatography on a cellulose column. Even after chromatographic purifications, interfering colors from beet root extracts still remained, and a colorless substance from apples produced a reddish interfering color; sulfur dioxide decreased the ascorbic acid values but its interference could be removed by bubbling carbon dioxide (93). The method of Schmall et al. (92) has been adapted to automated flowthrough analysis of multivitamin preparation (94), serum, and urine (95). Weeks and Deutsch (96) modified the method of Schmall et al. (92) by substituting the more sensitive diazotized p-nitroaniline to determine ascorbic acid in pharmaceuticals. The presence of p-aminobenzoic acid produced an intense interfering color with p-nitroaniline, and protein and cysteine interfered by coupling with the diazonium cation (96). Michaelsson and Michaelsson (97) evaluated the sensitivity of 22 stabilized diazonium salts as reagents for ascorbic acid determination and found that diazotized 4-nitroaniline-2:5-dimethoxyaniline produced the most intense color. The color of the reaction product in an alkaline solution was stabilized with dyphilline in an aqueous medium instead of alcohol to avoid precipitation of plasma proteins; blanks were made by oxidizing ascorbic acid in plasma with copper before performing the reaction 97).

Formation of fluorescent product by condensation of o-phenylenediamine with dehydroascorbic acid following oxidation of ascorbic acid with Norit and the blocking of dehydroascorbic acid with boric acid in the blank are the basis of the method of Deutsch and Weeks (99) and the AOAC official method (100). Egberg et al. (101) reported that o-phenylenediamine reacted with diketogulonic acid to yield a fluorescent product that was cancelled by the blanks in the manual method (99), but no fluorescence was observed due to diketogulonic acid by the automated flowthrough method (101), which is described in the chapter on automated vitamin analysis. According to Bourgeois and Mainguy (102), the manual procedure of Deutsch and Weeks (99) works well with samples that are rather pure, but it is subject to fluorescence quenching by impurities; dehydroreductic acid, dehydroreductones, and alloxan interfere by producing fluorescence which is blocked in the blank but not the total test (102). Augustin et al. (103) obtained unrealistically high vitamin C values with the fluorometric method (100) in the analysis of processed potato products.

Zieghenhagen and Zobel (104) described a procedure for isolating the *o*-phenylenediamine derivative of dehydroascorbic acid from interfering compounds by paper chromatography and determining its absorbance at 342 nm following elution.

Bourgeois and Mainguy (102) replaced *o*-phenylenediamine by 4-nitro-1,2-phenylenediamine to obtain a product suitable for colorimetric measurement at 375 nm. Their method included purification of sample extracts with an anionic Sephadex column from which ascorbic acid was eluted by oxidation to dehydroascorbic acid with *p*-benzoquinone; for total vitamin C determination, dehydroascorbic acid was first reduced to ascorbic acid with dimercaptopropanol and excess of this reagent was removed by ether extraction before chromatography (102). After completion of the reaction of dehydroascorbic acid with 4-nitro-1,2-phenylenediamine, excess reagent was extracted with ethyl acetate before measuring the absorbance (102). This procedure appears quite specific since compounds such as pyruvic acid and dehydroxy-fumaric acid are not eluted from the column, and the interference of the reaction products of reductones and reductic acid was removed by ethyl acetate extraction (102). Obviously, the procedure has the disadvantage of being very complex and laborious.

Polarographic analysis of the condensation product of dehydroascorbic acid with *o*-phenylenediamine, after oxidation of ascorbic acid with silver nitrate, has been the basis of a vitamin C method introduced by Wasa et al. (105); there were three characteristic reduction waves corresponding to three different types of condensation products with dehydroascorbic acid. Davidek et al. (18) obtained one dominant wave for dehydroascorbic acid by using equimolar or lower concentrations of *o*-phenylenediamine. The presence of reduced sulfhydryl compounds, reductones, and diketogulonic acid caused no interference with the vitamin C determination (18). This method, originally devised for meat and meat products, was applied to a few fruits and vegetables; the interference from coloring substances was eliminated by separation on polyamide or Dowex 50W columns (18). The latter procedure was subsequently modified to oxidize ascorbic acid with 2,6-dichloroindophenol instead of silver nitrate before condensation of the resulting dehydroascorbic acid with *o*-phenylenediamine for vitamin C determinations of orange drinks (17), preserved fruits (19), and cooked fried potatoes (20). Steele et al. (22) found that amino acids–sugars interaction products produced during the process of preparation of dehydrated potatoes caused pseudo-vitamin C increases with the polarographic method of Wasa et al. (105) and extracted these interferences with chloroform before the cathodic wave polarography (21,22). According to Augustin et al. (103), this method (21) turned out unrealistically high vitamin C values in the analysis of processed potato products. Apparent limited usage of polarographic analysis of the condensation products of dehydroascorbic acid with *o*-phenylenediamine for measuring vitamin

C might be due to limited availability of polarographic apparatus in many laboratories and to the need to remove interfering compounds by chromatography or by solvent extraction before performing the analysis.

I. Gas-Liquid Chromatographic Determination

Gas-liquid chromatography (GLC) of trimethylsilyl derivatives of ascorbic acid has been used for the quantitative determination of ascorbic acid in brain tissues (106) and in a few foods (107). These methods required special precautions to prevent losses of ascorbic acid during sample preparation for trimethylsilylation. Allison and Stewart (106) lyophilized tissue samples at −20°C in preparation for derivatization. They allowed silylation to proceed for 48 hr at room temperature in a dessicator, and upon completion of silylation, stored the solutions at −85°C until the time of analysis. Schlack (107) devised a procedure in which ascorbic acid was extracted in ethanol and precipitated with lead acetate in presence of Celite 545. The precipitate was washed with 95% ethanol, followed by ether and drying at 100°C; after addition of a few Diedrite chips, trimethylsilyl derivatives were regenerated from the lead salt (107). Since GLC following trimethysilyl derivatization yielded several peaks from tissues (106) and foods (107), the specificity of these methods would require evaluation by mass spectrometry.

J. High-Performance Liquid Chromatographic Determinations

Normal bonded (nonpolar) columns with alkyl chemically bonded to silica support have been used with mobile phases that were acidic (108,109) or comprised modifiers for ion pairing (103,110–116) for determining vitamin C by HPLC. Detection was usually done by measuring absorbance at 254 nm or 265 nm, but also by electrochemical monitoring.

Wagner et al. (108) used 0.8% metaphosphoric acid as the mobile phase for determining ascorbic acid in urine without interference from uric acid. Miki (109) used 1% phosphoric acid as the mobile phase for ascorbic acid determinations in tomato products without interference from reductones. A possible drawback with these methods (108,109) is that column life may be shortened since it is known that acidic solutions slowly dissolve silicates; furthermore, detailed studies would be required to ascertain the specificity of these determinations for ascorbic acid.

Tridecylammonium formate was one of the reagents incorporated in water–methanol solutions at pH 5.0 (110) or 4.5 (103) for determining ascorbic acid in the reversed-phase, ion-pairing mode. By this HPLC mode, ascorbic acid determinations of a few fruits and vegetables gave values that were generally lower than the 2,6-dichloroindophenol values, and were comparable only in the case of lemon and asparagus (110). In the analysis of potatoes and potato products, Augustin et al. (103), reported that their procedure eliminated interfering substances that gave unrealistically high vitamin C values with certain processed potato products when analyzed by visual titration using 2,6-dichloroindophenol, by fluorometric (100) and polaragraphic analysis (21). However, with either of these two ion-pairing techniques (103,110), the separated interfering substances were not identified and it has not been demonstrated that there are no other UV-absorbing substances eluting at the same time as ascorbic acid.

Tetrabutylammonium phosphate was utilized in a similar fashion as tridecylammonium formate (103,110) by Wills et al. (111) and by Ruckerman (112,113). Ascorbic acid was separated from other water-soluble vitamins (111), and there was no interference from reductones, cysteine, and the reduced iron and zinc ions (112,113). These HPLC techniques were used to determine ascorbic acid in a variety of fruits and vegetables with UV detection (112), and in milk-replacing feed formulas with electrochemical detection (113).

Pachla and Kissinger (114) used tridecylamine in 15% methanol with an acetate buffer at pH 4.0 for ion pairing to analyze ascorbic acid by amperometric detection in foods including milk samples. Finley and Duang (115) found that tri-n-butylamine, in presence of a disodium phosphate-buffered solution, was preferable to tetrabutylammonium phosphate (PIC-A, Waters Assoc.) that yielded a high UV background. Ascorbic, dehydroascorbic, and diketogulonic acid were separated, not only in pure solution, but also in orange juice and a few other plant extracts; by increasing the pH above 3.5, D-isoascorbic acid was separated from L-ascorbic acid (115). A separation of these two acids was also obtained by using cetyltrimethylammonium in water-methanol solutions containing a phosphate buffer (116).

The ion-pairing HPLC determinations of ascorbic acid (103,110–116) appear promising, but it remains to be demonstrated which one gives the most specific values with most types of samples.

A moderately polar column (CN bonded to silica support) with 2% acetic acid methanol (19+1) as mobile phase has been used by Carnevale (117) to determine ascorbic, sorbic, and benzoic acid in citrus juice by HPLC followed by spectrophotometric measurement.

Several HPLC procedures used highly polar columns (NH_2 bonded to silica support) and mobile phases that included solutions containing various proportions of acetonitrile in presence of dilute phosphate buffers, or methanol in presence of citric acid or phosphate buffers, or simply an aqueous solution of citric acid. Ascorbic acid and isoascorbic acid were separated from samples of fruit juices with a mobile phase containing acetonitrile (118–120) but not with a mobile phase containing methanol and citric acid (121). Using a mobile phase composed of acetonitrile and dilute KH_2PO_4 (75+25), Doner and Hicks (119) demonstrated the separation of not only ascorbic and isoascorbic acids, but also dehydroascrobic, dehydroisoascorbic, diketogulonic, and diketogluconic acids; total vitamin C could be determined by reducing dehydroascorbic acid with dithiothreitol before chromatography; other ultraviolet-absorbing substances in orange juice and urine were resolved but most of them were not characterized. With a mobile phase comprised of acetonitrile and dilute KH_2PO_4 solution (50+50), Rose and Nahrwold (122) determined ascorbic acid and dehydroascorbic acid by monitoring ultraviolet absorbance at 254 nm and 210 nm respectively for the analysis of foods, biological samples, and pharmaceutical preparations. Using methanol and dilute KH_2PO_4 (50+50) as the mobile phase and electrochemical detection Mason et al. (123) determined ascorbic acid in plasma and urine by HPLC after precipitating proteins with trichloroacetic acid; urine and serum also presented additional unidentified peaks, some of them eluting much later than ascorbic acid. After reducing dehydroascorbic acid with homocysteine, Dennison et al. (124) determined total vitamin C in orange drink by using 50+50 methanol–0.25% KH_2PO_4 as the mobile phase and monitoring the absorbance at 244 nm. Using 80+20 methanol–0.125% citrate in water as the mobile phase, and monitoring the UV absorbance at 254 nm, Wills et al. (111) separated ascorbic acid from other water soluble vitamins; one of the authors (Day) commented in a nonpublished communication that citrates have the disadvantage of causing voids in the column. With the NH_2-bonded columns, separations that include acetonitrile as the mobile phase are the most documented, but that solvent requires special precautions to avoid breathing of vapors and absorption through the skin.

Columns packed with anion exchange particles consisting of–NR_3^+ groups bonded to silica gel particles have been used for HPLC determinations of vitamin C (125,126). One method utilized a sodium acetate solution buffer as the mobile phase and electrochemical detection to determine vitamin C in marine animal tissues (125). In another method (126), a similar mobile phase, utilized in conjunction with chemiluminescence measurements, gave a separation of ascorbic acid from glucose, gluconic acid, and creatinine; the method has been applied only to vitamin C tablets.

Another type of anion exchange columns filled with bonded pellicular packings (–NR_3^+ bonded on a layer of silica covering micro glass beads) has been used (127,128). In one method (127), the mobile phase consisted of 0.01 M NaH_2PO_4, and ascorbic acid was measured in brain tissue by electrochemical detection against an internal standard. With a similar column, but a slightly different buffer and UV monitoring at 254 nm, Liebes et al. (128) identified and quantitated ascorbic acid in extracts of human lymphocytes.

Columns packed with anion exchange resin, mechanically bonded on pellicular packings, were also utilized for vitamin C determination by HPLC (129–131). Williams et al. (129) determined ascorbic acid in presence of other water-soluble vitamins by using 0.005 M NaH_2PO_4 as the mobile phase and UV detection as 254 nm. Pachla and Kissinger (130) used a dilute acetate buffer as the mobile phase and monitored the ascorbic acid with an amperometric electrochemical detector for the analysis of foodstuff, pharmaceuticals, and body fluids; uric acid and ascorbic acid were shown to be well separated. Tsao and Salimi (131) adapted this method (130) for the measurement of ascorbic acid in plasma and white blood cells; by this procedure, the ascorbic acid content of human samples was systematically about 10% lower than by the method of Roe et al. (66,67).

Recently, Obata et al. (132) demonstrated the separation of L-ascorbic acid, reductic acid, and triose reductones by HPLC with an anion exchange resin utilizing 0.1 M $NaNO_3$ as the mobile phase, and UV detection at 260 nm: by using cyclopentanone as an internal standard, ascorbic acid was determined in orange juice, and triose reductones in heated skimmed milk.

HPLC with anion exchangers (125–132) appears as promising as ion-pairing HPLC (103,106–110) for the determination of ascorbic acid, but in both cases it remains to be demonstrated which methods have the accuracy and precision required for general applicability.

ANALYTICAL METHODOLOGY—SAMPLING AND EXTRACTION: GENERAL CONSIDERATIONS

The importance of the proper handling of samples for vitamin C determinations cannot be overemphasized. Procedures for preserving and sampling the material under examination, and for extracting the vitamin C must be done in such way that no significant change in vitamin C takes place before analysis.

A. Vitamin C Stability

Although vitamin C is usually quite stable in pharmaceutical preparations and fairly stable in canned or bottled fruits and their juices, and in dry powdered products, a gradual loss can occur after a container is opened (16,40) and even more so after reconstitution of dry powdered products such as fruit drinks (16,40). Direct reconstitution of dehydrated samples in a suitable extracting acidic medium could prevent some loss occurring after normal reconstitution but would not reflect the exact nutritive value. Although the vitamin C content of fresh fruits and vegetables available commercially is not expected to change rapidly with refrigeration, it is always preferable to avoid the risk of spoilage and to carry as soon as possible the vitamin C extraction with a stabilizing acid such as metaphosphoric acid, or to freeze the samples in liquid nitrogen (133). Ulrich and Departe (134) have reviewed the effects of various storage conditions of fruits on the stability of their ascorbic acid content. It has been reported that the slow decrease in fully prepared dishes can be stopped effectively by storing them deep-frozen in tight-closing containers for several days; but even greater protection is obtained by freezing the samples with metaphosphoric acid (86). After raw materials are cut, bruised, or chopped, they must be handled very rapidly and blended with stabilizing acid as quickly as possible to prevent undue oxidation of the vitamin. This is particularly true of raw products high in ascorbic acid oxidase activity. As much of the comminution as possible should be conducted in the presence of a stabilizing acid such as metaphosphoric acid. When handling numerous biological materials such as animals' organs, if it is not possible to extract the vitamin C immediately, the excised tissue should be placed immediately on dry ice and the vitamin C extracted within 24 hr with a cold metaphosphoric solution (88). Vitamin C is degraded rapidly in serum at room temperature (89,135), but can be stored with little change for periods up to 3 weeks at $-70°C$ without a preservative (133), or at $-10°$ to $-15°C$ in presence of metaphosphoric acid (89).

B. Extracting Media

Metaphosphoric acid, first suggested as an extracting medium by Fujita and Itawaka (136), possesses several advantages. Metaphosphoric acid retards the oxidation by inactivating the catalytic effect of ascorbic acid oxidase and copper. In addition, it is a protein precipitant and thereby aids in the removal of enzymatic oxidase and facilitates clarification of the extracts. Ponting (137) compared a large number of potential extractants and concluded that meta-phosphoric and oxalic acids were the most suitable. However, oxalic acid is not a protein precipitant and therefore is inapplicable for use with animal tissues. In these tissues, the existence of a protein oxidizing agent as, for example, oxyhemoglobin makes the use of a protein precipitant mandatory.

C. Combination of Metaphosphoric Acid with Other Media

The effectiveness of metaphosphoric acid solution can be improved by combining it with other reagents depending on the type of samples. Egberg et al. (138) reported that with cereals, the addition of methanol with the metaphosphoric acid solution avoided colloidal suspensions and it was only necessary to let the material settle for 1 min to obtain a clear supernatant. Randall et al. (133) also reported that ethanol was suitable as a slurrying medium before stabilization with metaphosphoric acid for total vitamin C determinations in frozen vegetables. Since metaphosphoric acid can be precipitated in presence of alcohol, it would be important in such cases to proceed with the determination of vitamin C without delay to avoid losses due to oxidation. Reemers (139) treated meta-phosphoric acid extracts of chips and French-fried potatoes with ethanol to remove starch and avoid possible inhibition of the formation of vitamin C osazones with DNPH. The presence of alcohol is compatible with the DNPH reaction (89,133,139) but Pelletier et al. (140) obtained suitable extracts from potatoes prepared in various ways by filtering through glass wool. Incorporation of 25% acetone into a solution containing 3% metaphosphoric acid and 8% acetic acid has also been found useful for extracting vitamin C from cooked potatoes by providing a satisfactory separation of solid and liquid phases (141). An additional benefit from acetone could be the formation of a complex with me-tabisulfite (51) added in the processing of certain foods (e.g., dehydration).

D. Incorporation of Ethylenediaminetetraacetic Acid Into the Extracting Media

Jager (142) had recommended the use of small amount of EDTA in addition to the metaphosphoric acid. In this mixture, he found ascorbic acid to be stable for 8 days in the presence of copper. EDTA is a very effective chelating agent but its effectiveness depends on the extracting medium; although it was found quite effective in stabilizing ascorbic acid in trichloroacetic acid extracts of plant material, it was not as good with metaphosphoric acid and was inefficient with oxalic acid (29). EDTA was also found effective to stabilize ascorbic acid in presence of citric acid for HPLC determinations (143). Pelletier and Morrison (26) made use of the chelating capacity of EDTA during aerial oxidation of ferrous and stannous ions in presence of an acetate buffer at pH 0.65 to remove the interference of these ions with the 2,6-dichloroindophenol titration of ascorbic acid. An extracting solution containing only acetic acid will decrease the interference of iron with the 2,6-dichloroindophenol titration but will result in low recoveries of ascorbic acid in presence of copper salts (41) and oxidative enzymes. Solution composed of a mixture of acetic and metaphosphoric acids do not remove the interference of ferrous salts (41) but can efficiently extract ascorbic acid from evaporated or condensed milk while precipitating proteins and other reducing materials (42).

E. Compatibility of Extracting Medium With the Analytical Method

The choice of an extracting medium is limited by is compatibility with the method of analysis. While formation of dehydroascorbic acid during extraction in a acidic medium such as metaphosphoric acid is not a problem with methods that measure total vitamin C (e.g., DNPH procedures), it is obviously a serious problem with methods based on oxido-reduction, on UV absorbance measurements, and on direct coupling with ascorbic acid. For those reasons, it would appear more practical to analyze samples presenting stability problems, with a method capable of determining total vitamin C.

I. DETERMINATION OF ASCORBIC ACID AND TOTAL VITAMIN C (ASCORBIC AND DEHYDROASCORBIC ACIDS) WITH 2,4-DINITROPHENYLHYDRAZINE

A. Scope

The procedure is applicable to a wide variety of foods, food products, biological materials, and pharmaceuticals.

B. Principle

The determination of total vitamin C is based on the oxidation of AA to DHAA followed by coupling with DNPH to give red-colored osazones. Because certain materials contain nonspecific substances that couple with DNPH, a "blank test" must be performed to subtract the nonspecific contribution from the "total test."

1. *Basis of the Total Test.*
   (a) Oxidation of AA to DHAA with 2,6-dichloroindophenol.

(b) Complex formation between DHAA and boric acid to block any reduction of DHAA by homocysteine.

(c) Formation of DNPH osazones due to total vitamin C and to DKGA and other nonspecific substances originally present in the sample.

(d) Development of osazone color with nitric or sulfuric acid and measurement of absorbance at 520 nm.

2. *Basis of Blank Test For the Total Vitamin C Determination.*

(a) Reduction of DHAA to AA with homocysteine.

(b) Complex formation between AA and boric acid to block possible oxidation of AA.

(c) Formation of DNPH osazones due to DKGA and to other nonspecific substances originally present in the sample.

(d) Development of osazone color with nitric or sulfuric acid and measurement of absorbance at 520 nm.

3. *Basis of Blank Test For the Determination Only of AA.*

(a) Complex formation between DHAA and boric acid to block any reduction of DHAA by homocysteine.

(b) Formation of DNPH osazones due to DHAA and to DKGA and other nonspecific substances originally present in the sample.

(c) Development of osazone color with nitric or sulfuric acid and measurement of absorbance at 520 nm.

C. Equipment

In addition to general laboratory glassware and equipment, the following items are required.

1. *Blender.*   The cutting blades and bowl must be of material that does not yield metallic ions capable of oxidizing ascorbic acid.

2. *Vortex Mixer or Equivalent.*

3. *Spectrophotometer.*   A Bausch and Lomb Spectronic 100 equipped with a micro flowthrough sample compartment including a micro flowthrough cell (1-cm path length) or equivalent instrumentation.

4. *Waterbath.*   Polystyrene water bath ($L \times W \times H = 100 \times 7.0 \times 15$ cm) maintained at 15°C with a refrigerating unit (Beckman, Model 1818 or equivalent) and a circulating pump (Haake, model E51 or the equivalent).

5. *Test Tubes.*   Disposable test tubes 15 × 85 mm (RTU, Beckton and Dickenson Co. or equivalent) with appropriate test tube holder to hold 100 tubes for immersion into water bath.

6. *Pipettes.*   'Cornwall' 1-mL and 2-mL pipettes (Fisher Scientific Co. B) and Plastipack 1-mL and 3-mL disposable syringes (Beckton and Dickenson Co.), or any combination of pipettes capable of delivering rapidly and accurately, the volumes specified for the total and blank tests.

D. Reagents

The chemicals for preparing reagents should be reagent grade and the water should be "copper free." For this reason, it is preferable to utilize water that has been glass distilled and deionized through an ion exchange resin.

1. *17% Metaphosphoric Acid Solution.*   Without heating, dissolve 250 g pellets containing 34% HPO_3 and 59% $NaPO_3$ in H_2O and dilute to 500 mL. Store at 3°C and prepare weekly since HPO_3 in solution is slowly hydrolyzed in H_3PO_4.

2. *0.85% Metaphosphoric Acid Solution.*   Dilute 50 mL 17% HPO_3 to 1 L with H_2O. Prepare fresh daily.

3. *10% Glucose and 5% Fructose Solution.*   Dissolve 10 g glucose and 5 g fructose in 0.85% HPO_3 and dilute to 100 mL with 0.85% HPO_3. Prepare only when required for assaying samples with high sugar content.

4. *Ascorbic Acid Standard.*   Dissolve 100 mg in 0.85% HPO_3 and dilute to 100 mL. Dilute to 10 mL of the above solution to 100 mL with 0.85% HPO_3. Pipette 2, 4, 6, 8, and 10 mL, respectively, of this second dilution into separate 100-mL volumetric flasks and dilute to volume with 0.85% HPO_3. These diluted standards contain 2, 4, 6, 8, and 10 μg/mL, respectively. Prepare fresh weekly and store at 3°C.

For determining vitamin C in sample with a high sugar content, add 10 mL of Reagent 3 per 100 mL of final dilution of standards.

5. *0.1% 2,6-Dichlorophenolindopheonol Solution.*   Dissolve 200 mg sodium salt of 2,6-dichloropheonolindophenol (sodium salt of 2,6-dichlorobenzenoneindophenol, Eastman) in approximately 150 mL of hot H_2O, cool, dilute with H_2O to 200 mL and filter. Keep in the refrigerator when not in use. The solution is stable up to 2 weeks at 3°C.

6. *5% Boric Acid.*   Dissolve 50 g boric acid in H_2O and dilute to 1 L. Prepare every 2 weeks and store at room temperature.

7. *3.33% Boric Acid Solution.*   Dilute 66.6 mL 5% H_3BO_3 to 100 mL with H_2O. This solution is stable for 2 weeks at room temperature. Filter before using.

8. *45% Potassium Phosphate Dibasic Solution.*   Dissolve 45 g K_2HPO_4 in H_2O and dilute to 100 mL. Prepare fresh weekly and store at room temperature.

9. *2,6-Dichloroindophenol and Boric Acid Solution.*   Into a 100-mL volumetric flask add 13.3 mL of 0.1% 2,6-dichloroindophenol solution, 66.6 mL of 5% H_3BO_3 and dilute volume with H_2O. Prepare daily and filter.

10. *Homocysteine and K_2HPO_4 Solution.*   Dissolve 210 mg DL-homocysteine (U.S. Biochemicals Corp.) in 50 mL H_2O, add 85 mL 45% K_2HPO_4 and mix. Prepare fresh daily and filter. To test quality of new lot of homocysteine, add about 10 mg to 5 mL 2,6-dichloroindophenol solution; if suitable, it will rapidly decolorize the dye.

11. *1.5% DNPH.*   Dissolve 1.5% g DNPH in 9 N H_2SO_4 and dilute to 1 L with 9 N H_2SO_4. This solution is stable for 2 weeks if refrigerated.

12. *1.2% DNPH Plus 3% Thiourea.*   Dissolve 6 g thiourea in 30 mL 9 N H_2SO_4, add 160 mL 1.5% DNPH and dilute to 200 mL with 9 N H_2SO_4. Prepare daily and filter.

13. *Nitric and Citric Acids Mixture.*   Dissolve 50 g citric acid in methanol to make 100 mL. To this solution add slowly while stirring 150 mL concentrated HNO_3. Mix well. Let cool to room temperature before use. Use within 90 min after preparation.

14. *85% Sulfuric Acid.*   Required only for analysis of samples having a high sugar concentration.

15. *Nitrogen Gas.*   Prepurified grade.

E. Procedure

1. *Extraction.*

(a) General guidelines.   Extract and dilute a representative portion of sample with a sufficient amount of 17% HPO_3 and H_2O to obtain a final optimal vitamin C concentration of 3–8 μg/mL in 0.85% HPO_3. For samples with a relatively high concentration of sugars such as certain noncitrus fruits with an expected vitamin C content less than 10 mg/100 g, incorporate 10 mL of Reagent 3 in each 100 mL of final dilution in 0.85% HPO_3. Up to three times the amount of glucose and up to nine times the amount of fructose incorporated give a constant increase (about 8%) in vitamin C response, thus eliminating the interference within that range.

For most purposes, when only the total vitamin C is required, some conversion of AA to DHAA during extraction will not affect the final values. HPO_3 will prevent aerial oxidation of AA to DHAA in most types of samples except those containing traces of cupric and ferric ions or oxidative enzymes. The enzymatic oxidation in certain plant and animal tissue will be retarded by keeping the temperature to less then 5°C during the extraction. See pages 321–323 for further general considerations on sampling and extraction.

(b) Application to samples other than blood, serum, and urine.   Dilute liquid food samples (e.g., fruit drinks) with HPO_3 as described in Section E.1(a), mix, and filter through Whatman No. 2 filter paper. Grind multivitamin tablets to a fine powder before blending. Blending of samples will vary from 30 sec for a small volume with a small blender to 3 min for a large volume with a large blender. Filter through Whatman No. 2 filter paper except for potato products (glass wool filter) and small animal tissues (Whatman glass fiber filter).

(c) Blood and serum.   Vitamin C is stable for about an hr after blood has been withdrawn, so proceed with the extraction promptly. Obtain serum by allowing blood to clot about 45 min. Centrifuge without delay. Since vitamin C is rapidly destroyed in serum, proceed promptly with the extraction. Prepare extracts by adding 2 mL of sample to 6 mL of 1.12% HPO_3 (6.6 ml of 17% HPO_3 diluted to 100 mL), mix well with Vortex, and centrifuge at

7000 x*g* for 5 min to obtain a clear supernatant. Metaphosphoric acid will stabilize vitamin C in serum for about 3 weeks in a freezer at $-10°$ to $-15°C$, but vitamin C from whole blood would not be expected to be stable because it is oxidized to DHAA in the extraction process. Vitamin C in isolated white cells can be stabilized for 2 weeks by freezing as pellets or in presence of metaphosphoric acid (144).

(d) Urine samples.   Collect urine samples over HPO_3 pellets (34% HPO_3) to obtain 1.70% HPO_3 in the final volume to be made up with H_2O up to two folds the initial urine volume. Keep this at 5°C and assay within 24 hr or freeze until the time of assay. Samples from subjects on a vitamin C daily intake over 100 mg can usually be analyzed directly after dilution to an expected vitamin C concentration of 3–7 $\mu g/mL$ in 0.85% HPO_3. Eliminate interfering substances from other samples by passing a 5-mL aliquot through a column (1–1.5 cm i.d.) containing 2 g Amberlite IR-20 (H^+) over a pledget of glass wool: collect effluent and H_2O washings into a 25-mL volumetric flask containing 1.0 mL 17% HPO_3 to provide final concentration of 0.85% HPO_3.

2. *Preparation of Tests for Total Vitamin C.*   Into two sets of test tubes (one for the total test and one for the blank test), place 1.0-mL aliquots of the following solutions: 0.85% HPO_3 (reference), first series of standards (2, 4, 6, 8, and 10 $\mu g/mL$), reference, second series of standards, reference, standard of 8 $\mu g/mL$ and samples in series of 15 each being followed by a reference and a standard of 8 $\mu g/mL$. Serum samples should be run in duplicate and food samples with high sugar content but less than 2 μg vitamin C/mL should be run in triplicate. The aliquots of standards and samples may be added with any pipette known to give high reproducibility. When large volumes of extracts are available, a Cornwall pipette (not equipped with a filling outfit) using Plasti-pack disposable syringes can be used, after rinsing the syringe by discarding twice before making additions. A Cornwall pipette equipped with a filling outfit may also be used for delivering reagents. Add the reagents in the prescribed sequences and within the time limits specified (Table 12.1). Mix with a Vortex after each addition except for the solutions containing nitric acid which can be mixed by bubbling nitrogen. (*Note*: Wear goggles for the steps involving nitric or 85% sulfuric acid.)

TABLE 12.1   Sequences of Addition of Reagents for Total Vitamin C

Reagents	Sequence	Blank Test	Total Test
10	1	0.5 mL	—
9	2	—	0.5 mL
10	3	—	0.5 mL
7	4	0.5 mL	—
12	5	1.0 mL	1.0 mL
13 or 14	6	2.0 mL	2.0 mL

Sequence 1.   Add Reagent 10 to all blank test tubes and note time to proceed with Sequence 4 in about 1.5 hr.

Sequence 2.   Proceed without delay after Sequence 1 by adding Reagent 9 to all total test tubes that can be handled in about 2 min and follow immediately with Sequence 3.

Sequence 3.   Add Reagent 10 about 2 min after the addition of the previous reagent in the same test tube and let stand about 1.5 hr before proceeding with Sequence 5.

Sequence 4.   Add Reagent 7 only to blank test tubes about 1.5 hr after the first addition in Sequence 1 and in the same order.

Sequence 5.   Add Reagent 12 to all tubes starting with blank tests. Hold tubes in a water bath at room temperature for 3 hr or at 15°C for 17 hr. The latter temperature is less subject to interference from high sugar concentrations by producing lower blanks, but it also yields about 30% less response to vitamin C.

Sequence 6.   Wear safety goggles. Add Reagent 13 to all tubes, which must be cooled to 15°C, and mix gently by bubbling nitrogen. For noncitrus fruits having a high sugar concentration and less than 10 mg vitamin C/100 g, more accurate results will be obtained by replacing Reagent 13 by 14, which must be added to each tube (including calibration standards) slowly from a burette (20 sec per addition) while keeping the tubes in an ice water bath. Mix gently by bubbling nitrogen during and after each addition of 14. Remove all tubes to room temperature for the period of time required for the spectrophotometric measurements.

3. *Preparations of Tests For Determination of AA Only and Excluding DHAA.*   Proceed in the same way as in the above Section 2 with the following exceptions. Proceed with total test as in Table 12.1, and prepare a DHAA blank by following the total test sequence by replacing Reagent 9 by Reagent 7 in Sequence 2.

4. *Spectrophotometric Measurements.*   Read absorbance at 520 nm, 30–90 min after completion of Sequence 6 (Section 2 or Section 3) when using Reagent 13 or 75 min following the addition of Reagent 14. Adjust spectrophotometer reading to 0 absorbance with one reagent reference tube treated in same way as all other tubes. Reading 75 min following the addition of sulfuric acid allows the turbidity due to sugar osazones to disappear and renders the absorbance contribution due to fructose and glucose equivalent in the blanks and total tests.

5. *Calculations.*   From the mean net absorbance (y) for each of the five consecutive levels of standards (x) in μg/mL, calculate the slope (b) and intercept (a) according to the following equation:

$$y = a + bx$$

Calculate the vitamin C concentration (X') in the diluted sample by the following formula:

$$X' = \frac{F(y' - a)}{b}$$

where y' = the net absorbance of the sample (test reaction minus test blank); a = the intercept; b = the slope of the standard curve; and F = a correction factor for possible changes in sensitivity during the course of analysis.

$$F = 2\ As/(AB + Aa)$$

where As = the absorbance of the fourth higher level of standard in the standard curve, and Ab and Aa = the absorbance of the same standard placed before and after each group of samples.

II. DIFFERENTIAL DETERMINATION OF D-ISOASCORBIC ACID AND L-ASCORBIC ACID WITH 2,4-DINITROPHENYLHYDRAZINE

A. Scope

This procedure is applicable to animal tissues. Although its applicability to foods has not been studied, it should be applicable to foods with a low sugar content.

B. Principle

Differentiation of D-isoascorbic acid (IAA) and L-ascorbic acid (AA) is based on the different rates of osazones formation of dehydro-L-ascorbic acid (DHAA) and dehydro-D-isoascorbic acid (DHIA) with DNPH following oxidation with 2,6-dichloroindophenol. The various steps of the procedure to eliminate the effect of other interfering substances is described in Section I.B. The concentration of each isomer can be calculated on the basis of a minimal difference in osazones production between the two isomers at 52°C for 80 min, and a maximum difference at 32°C for the same time.

C. Equipment

The same equipment as described in Section I.C but with two water baths regulated at 32°C and 52°C.

D. Reagents

The same reagents as described in Section I.D except that isoascorbic acid standards are also required and there should be sufficient materials to conduct duplicate determinations (one at 32°C and one at 52°C). After linearity of absorbance versus concentration has been established, it is only necessary to make separate dilutions of AA and IAA at 8 μg/mL.

E. Procedure

1. *Extraction.*   Extract as in Section I.E.

2. *Determination.*   Proceed with AA and IAA standards as in Section I.E.2 but prepare additional set of all tubes to incubate one set at 32°C for 80 min and another set of 52°C in Sequence 5. After the linearity of the standard curves has been established, only the 8 μg levels need to be determined. It is recommended to make duplicate determinations of each standard and sample of each temperature and to use the mean of each for calculations.

3. *Calculations.*   Calculate the concentrations of AA and IAA according to the following equations:

$$(1)\ \mu g\ AA/mL\ \text{sample} = 8[f(c/d) - e]/[b(c/d) - a]$$

$$(2)\ \mu g\ IAA/mL\ \text{sample} = 8[e - (aq/8)]/c$$

where *a-f* refers to absorbances: *a*, 8 μg AA at 52°C; *b*, 8 μg AA at 32°C; *c*, 8 μg IAA at 52°C; *d*, 8 μg IAA at 32°C; *e*, sample at 52°C; *f*, sample at 32°C; and *q* is the result obtained by Equation (1).

III.   2,6-DICHLOROINDOPHENOL TITRATION METHOD OF ASCORBIC ACID IN ABSENCE OF INTERFERING SUBSTANCES

A. Scope

The procedure is applicable only to the determination of ascorbic acid and not dehydroascorbic acid. It is not applicable in presence of copper, iron, and stannum salts, thiosulfate, reductones, reductic acid, tannins, betanin, and sulfhydryl compounds such as cysteine and glutathione. Products to which the method is applicable include pharmaceutical products that do not contain copper and iron, fresh fruits, and vegetables containing sufficient ascorbic acid to yield not less than 1 mg ascorbic acid/100-mL extract. Because of its simplicity, the method has been and still is very popular especially when the composition of the sample is known to be devoid of interfering ompounds.

B. Principle

Since ascorbic acid exhibits reducing properties, it may be quantitatively determined by reacting with 2,6-dichloroindophenol. In the absence of interfering substances that can reduce the dye or oxidize ascorbic acid during sample preparation, the capacity of an extract of sample to reduce a standardized dye solution as determined by titration, is directly proportional to the ascorbic acid content. A general discussion regarding the use of 2,6-dichloroindophenol for the determination of ascorbic acid can be found on pages 305-309.

C. Equipment

In addition to general laboratory equipment, including glassware, the following items are required:

1. *Mortar and Pestle.* Of size suitable for grinding multivitamin tablets.

2. *Waring Blender or its equivalent.* The cutting blades of the blender bowl must be well plated to eliminate copper contaminations.

3. *Microburet, 10 mL, graduated to 0.05 L.*

4. *Volumetric transfer pipettes.* Assorted sizes including 1, 5, 10, 20, and 25 mL.

5. *Coleman Junior II Spectrophotometer.* With adaptor for 25 × 105-mm cuvettes, or comparable fast-response instrument with large cuvettes.

D. Reagents

All chemicals should meet ACS specifications or be of Reagent Grade. The distilled water used in making acid solutions for extraction of samples should be "copper-free." For this reason it may be desirable to redistill certain lots of distilled water from an all-glass still.

1. *2% Metaphosphoric Acid Solution.* Without heating, dissolve 60 g clear sticks or pellets containing 34% HPO_3 and 59% $NaPO_3$ in 900 mL of H_2O (glass distilled) and dilute to 1 L. Filter and store at 3°C when not in use. On standing in solution, HPO_3 is slowly hydrolyzed to H_3PO_4; hence, a fresh solution should be prepared every 2 weeks.

In many instances it is not clear in the literature if the percentage metaphosphoric acid refers to pellets or HPO_3 per se. For example, Lugg (7) referred to the pellets per se as "metaphosphoric acid." In reality, 6 g of metaphosphoric pellets (vitreous sodium acid metaphosphate) per 100 mL is not a 6% HPO_3 solution, but a 2% HPO_3 solution.

2. *1% Metaphosphoric Acid Solution.* Dilute 500 mL of the above 2% HPO_3 solution to 1 L with H_2O.

3. *Ascorbic Acid Standard Solution.* Accurately weigh 100 mg of USP L-ascorbic acid reference standard which has been dried in the dark over sulfuric acid in a dessicator for 24 hr. Transfer to a 500-mL volumetric flask and make to volume with 1% HPO_3. Prepare fresh daily, and use to standardize the dye.

4. *0.025% 2,6-Dichlorophenolindophenol Solution.* Dissolve approximately 50 mg of the sodium salt of 2,6-dichlorophenolindophenol (sodium 2,6-dichlorobenzenoneindophenol, Eastman, or equivalent) in approximately 150 mL of

warm H_2O containing 42 mg $NaHCO_3$; cool and dilute with water to 200 mL. Place in a brown bottle and store at 3°C, renewing once a week.

5. *Ethylene Dichloride.* Required for the analysis of oily capsules.

6. *Source of Nitrogen.* A cylinder of N_2 with facilities for saturating the gas with moisture.

7. *Acetone.* Required to eliminate the effect of SO_2.

E. Procedure

1. *Standardization of 2,6-Dichloroindophenol.* Standardize daily in triplicate as follows. Dilute a 5-mL aliquot of the standard ascorbic acid solution (contining 1 mg ascorbic acid) with 5 mL of 1% HPO_3. Titrate with the dye solution to a pink color which persists for 10 sec, as compared with titration of a blank containing 10 mL 1% HPO_3. Subtract these blank values from the titration values of the standards and average the net titration values which should agree within 2%. Since the net volume of dye represents 1 mg of ascorbic acid, the ascorbic acid equivalent (T) of 1 mL of dye solution is equal to 1 divided by the volume in mL of the dye solution used in this titration.

2. *Extraction.* Perform the extraction rapidly to avoid oxidation of ascorbic acid. See pages 321–323 of this chapter for general considerations on sampling and extraction.

(a) Multivitamin tablets. Grind from 5 to 10 tablets in a mortar and dissolve in 1% HPO_3. Transfer to a volumetric flask and make the necessary dilutions with extracting agent so that each mL contains approximately 0.1 mg of ascorbic acid. Filter if necessary, discarding the first few mL of filtrate.

(b) Vitamin capsules. Place from 5 to 10 capsules in a 250-mL beaker and add approximately 75 mL of 1% HPO_3 and 2 mL of ethylene dichloride. If necessary, warm slightly with continuous stirring until complete disintegration occurs. Transfer to a volumetric flask of suitable volume and make the necessary dilutions with extracting agent such that each mL contains 0.1 mg ascorbic acid. Filter if necessary, discarding the first few mL of filtrate.

(c) Liquid materials. Dilute an aliquot with 2% HPO_3 and H_2O or 1% HPO_3 so that each mL will contain about 0.1 mg ascorbic acid in 1% HPO_3.

(d) Fruits and vegetables. Blend equal weights (200–300 g) of the sample and 2% HPO_3 as necessary (usually less than 3 min) to obtain a homogeneous slurry. An inert atmosphere has been suggested for use during the blending of fresh biological material containing large amounts of oxidative catalysts. Such a step would minimize contact with atmospheric oxygen. A simple means of conducting this step is to introduce N_2 through a glass tube extending into the blender bowl under the surface of the liquid extractant. If N_2 is bubbled into the bowl for 15–30 sec before starting the blender, the possibility of oxidation by catalysts or enzymes that are liberated with the breaking of the sample tissues is somewhat lessened. This is particularly true if the extracting medium does not completely inactivate these catalysts. Another way to retard the oxidation consists in conducting the extraction with solutions at 3°C.

If the expected concentration of ascorbic acid in the slurry is less than 3 mg/100 mL, centrifuge and/or filter. If more than 3 mg/100 g slurry is expected, weigh an amount of slurry sufficient to yield not less than 1 mg but optimally 10 mg ascorbic acid, transfer to a 100-mL volumetric flask, and dilute to volume with 1% HPO_3. It may be necessary to add a drop of caprylic alcohol to break foam, which may cause difficulty in ascertaining the proper liquid level in the volumetric flask. In the case of products that were sulfited during dehydration, the effect of SO_2 can be eliminated readily by adding 20 mL acetone before dilution to the mark.

3. *Visual Titration of Ascorbic Acid.*   Pipette 10-mL aliquots of extract into three Erlenmeyer flasks and titrate with standardized 2,6-dichloroindophenol to a pink end point lasting for at least 10 sec. In the case of extracts with an expected ascorbic acid content between 0.03–0.05 mg/mL, aliquots of 20 mL should be used for titration; for expected concentrations of less than 0.03 mg, aliquots of 30 mL should be used. Comparison on the titration stand of the flask being titrated with the two other containing aliquots of the same sample sometimes makes detection of the end point easier. When using aliquots greater than 10 mL, a reagent blank of the same volume should be titrated. The net value for calculations is the average of three titrations minus the average blank value.

4. *Spectrophotometric Titration of Ascorbic Acid.*   With colored samples in which visual detection of the end point is difficult and sometimes impossible, the titration may be done by judging the end point by the change in percent transmittance at 545 nm. Set the colorimeter to approximately the center of the scale with a 25-mm-diameter cuvette containing at least a 12-mL volume. Determine a rough end point by adding the dye in 0.5-mL increments and observing the transmittance; the latter will first increase due to dilution because the dye is completely and rapidly decolorized by ascorbic acid, but at the end point the excess dye will cause a decrease in the transmittance. Determine the end point more accurately with another aliquot by adding the dye one drop at a time when near the rough end point.

The final volume in the cuvette must be more than the minimum required for the particular instrument being used. Adjustment in the volume of extract used may be necessary so that sufficient dye can be added and good mixing is achieved.

5. *Calculations.*   Calculate the ascorbic acid concentration according to the following formula:

$$T \times V \times D = mg\ ascorbic\ acid\ per\ g,\ mL,\ tablet,\ or\ capsule$$

where T = ascorbic acid equivalent of dye solution
expressed as mg/mL of dye;

V = net mL dye used for titration of aliquot
of diluted sample;

D = dilution factor.

As an example of calculations:

300 g product,
300 g extracting acid,
30 g slurry diluted to 100 mL,
10 mL filtrate used for analysis,
3.3 mL dye required for titration,
0.125 mg ascorbic acid/mL dye.

$$0.125 \times 3.3 \times \frac{1}{10} \times \frac{100}{30} \times \frac{600}{300} = 0.275 \; mg/g$$

IV. 2,6-DICHLOROINDOPHENOL TITRATON OF ASCORBIC ACID IN PRESENCE OF FERROUS AND STANNOUS SALTS

A. Scope

The procedure is applicable to multivitamin preparations and to canned fruit juices and drinks with the following limitations. It eliminates the interference of ferrous and stannous ions but not that of ferric and cupric ions which can cause oxidation of ascorbic acid during the process of sample extracts preparation.

B. Principle

Because ferrous and stannous ions can be oxidized by 2,6-dichloroindophenol, their interference with the titration of ascorbic acid is removed by selective oxidation by air in presence of an acetate buffer (pH 0.65) and EDTA in sufficient quantity to chelate the oxidized ions. The possibility of incorporating EDTA into the acetate buffer before extraction to prevent oxidation of ascorbic acid in the presence of copper ions has not been investigated.

C. Equipment

In addition to the items listed under Section III.C, two units of a suction apparatus are needed. Each unit consists of four 50-mL Erlenmeyer flasks equipped with side arm for suction and fitted with a rubber stopper through which 5-mm i.d. glass tubing is inserted so that it extends approximately 5 mm into the solution in the flask. The four flasks are connected with rubber tubing of equal length to 2 "Y" tubes leading to another "Y" connected directly to water aspirator or a vacuum pump. The air flow through the system is adjusted so that air will bubble moderately in each flask.

D. Reagents

The reagents specifications are as in Section III.D.

1. *EDTA Solution.*   Add 20 g of EDTA to 200 mL of H_2O. Add 14 mL of 10 N NaOH and shake or stir until dissolved. If necessary, adjust the pH to 6.0 ± 0.05. Dilute to 250 mL with H_2O.

2. *0.025% 2,6-Dichloroindophenol Solution.* (Same as Section III.D.4.)

3. *Buffer.* To 1200 mL H_2O add 77 mL concentrated HCl and 500 mL 1.0 N sodium acetate. Mix well and adjust to pH 0.65 if necessary with either 1.0 N HCl or 1.0 N sodium acetate, as required. Dilute to 2 L with H_2O.

4. *Ascorbic Acid Standard Solution.* Accurately weigh 50 mg USP L-ascorbic acid reference standard which has been dried in the dark in a dessicator over sulfuric acid for 24 hr. Transfer to 100-mL volumetric flask and dilute to volume with buffer. Prepare fresh daily.

5. *Ferrous Sulfate Solution.* Weigh 250 mg $FeSO_4 \cdot 7H_2O$ and dilute to 100 mL with buffer.

E. Procedure

1. *Sample Preparation.*

(a) Multivitamin tablets and capsules. Prepare as in Section III.E.2(a) and (b), respectively, but using buffer instead of HPO_3 and diluting to an expected ascorbic acid concentration of not less than 0.08 mg/mL. Into a 100-mL volumetric flask, add an aliquot containing 4–7 mg ascorbic acid; add buffer to 50 mL and make to volume with H_2O.

(b) Juices and fruit drinks. Into a 100-mL volumetric flask, add 50 mL of buffer and an amount not exceeding 50 mL of juice or fruit drink containing 4–7 mg ascorbic acid. Dilute to 100 mL with H_2O. Filter if necessary, discarding the first few mL of filtrate.

2. *Visual Titration.* Add 1.0 mL of standard solution to each of two Erlenmeyer flasks with side arm and label as "A." Add 1.0 mL of buffer to two similar flasks and label as "B." Add 10 mL of sample solution to each flask. Add approximately 1 mL of 0.25% $FeSO_4 \cdot 7H_2O$ to each flask. For samples containing a large quantity of ferrous ions, a smaller quantity of $FeSO_4 \cdot 7H_2O$ should be added. The amount to be added can be determined as follows. Take 10 mL of diluted sample solution, add about 100 mg metaphosphoric acid, and titrate with 0.05% aqueous solution of methylene blue to a blue end point. Similarly titrate 1.0 mL of 0.25% $FeSO_4 \cdot 7H_2O$ plus 4 mL of buffer and 5 mL H_2O. The volume (mL) of $FeSO_4 \cdot 7H_2O$ to be added is calculated as follows:

$$\frac{\text{Titration } FeSO_4 \cdot 7H_2O - \text{titration of sample}}{\text{Titration } FeSO_4 \cdot 7H_2O}$$

Add 5 mL of EDTA solution to each "A" and "B" flasks, mix by swirling, and simultaneously bubble air by suction for 10 min. Wash glass tube with 1–2 mL H_2O. Titrate each flask with 2,6-dichlorophenolindophenol to a permanent end point, that is, one that persists for at least 30 sec.

Prepare reagent blanks ("C") similarly, omitting sample and ascorbic acid, using 7 mL of buffer including the $FeSO_4$ solution, 5 mL H_2O, and 5 mL of EDTA.

3. *Spectrophotometric Titration.* (See Section III.E.4.)

4. *Calculations.* Calculate the ascorbic acid according to the following formula where D is the dilution factor:

$$0.05 \times D \times \frac{\text{titrations } B - C}{\text{titrations } A - B} = mg/mL, \text{ tablet, or capsule}$$

As an example:

5 tablets (50 mg ascorbic acid/tablet),
250 mL buffer in first dilution,
5 mL from preceding dilution made up to 100 mL final dilution,
mL (average) dye utilized: A (10.2), B (5.2), C (0.2).

$$0.05 \times \frac{250}{5} \times \frac{100}{5} \times \frac{5.2 - 0.2}{10.2 - 5.0} = 50 \text{ mg/tablet}$$

V. 2,6-DICHLOROINDOPHENOL TITRATION OF ASCORBIC ACID UTILIZING BLANKS WITH FORMALDEHYDE CONDENSATION OF ASCORBIC ACID

A. Scope

This procedure is applicable to the determination of ascorbic acid in enriched evaporated or condensed milk. The applicability of this procedure to other types of samples has not been investigated but might be limited by the amount of reductone-like substances present in the samples (7,23,32). See pages 305–309 for further discussion on this and other interfering materials.

B. Principle

The ascorbic acid content of enriched evaporated or condensed milk is determined by titrating with 2,6-dichlorophenolindophenol after removal of other reducing substances in enriched evaporated or condensed milk by precipitation with an acetic and metaphosphoric acid solution. Traces of interfering reducing substances still present after precipitation and filtration are corrected by using formaldehyde blanks. Formaldehyde condenses readily with ascorbic acid at pH 3.5 whereas reductones do not condense appreciably.

C. Equipment

The same equipment as in Section III.C except that 125-mL Erlenmeyer flasks are required instead of 50-mL flask.

D. Reagents

The reagents specifications are as in Section III.D.

1. *Acetic Acid–Metaphosphoric Acid Solution.* Dissolve with shaking or stirring and without applying heat 160 g metaphosphoric acid pellets containing 34% HPO_3 and 59% $NaPO_3$ in 800 mL H_2O. Add 530 mL glacial acetic acid and dilute to 2 L with H_2O. Filter rapidly and store in a refrigerator to prevent metaphosphoric acid being converted to orthophosphoric acid. Prepare every 2 weeks.

2. *Ascorbic Acid Standard Solutions.* Accurately weigh 67 mg USP L-ascorbic acid reference standard which has been dried in the dark over sulfuric acid in a dessicator for 24 hr. Transfer to a 100-mL volumetric flask and dilute with acetic acid–metaphosphoric acid extractant. Prepare fresh daily and further dilute 10 mL to 100 mL with the same extractant; this solution contains 0.067 mg ascorbic acid/mL.

3. *Sodium Acetate 2.5 M Solution.* Dissolve 205 g sodium acetate or 340 g sodium acetate trihydrate in H_2O and dilute to 1 L.

4. *0.025% 2,6-Dichloroindophenol Solution.* (Same as Section III.D.4.)

5. *Hydrochloric Acid, 5.0 N Solution.*

6. *Formaldehyde.* 37% Formaldehyde solution.

E. Procedure

1. *Standarization of 2,6-Dichloroindophenol.* Pipette 15.0-mL aliquots of standard ascorbic acid solution containing 0.067 mg/mL into each of four 125-mL Erlenmeyer flasks. To each flask, add 15 mL H_2O and mix. Promptly titrate contents of two of the flasks with the dye solution until a pink color persists for at least 10 sec. To each of the two remaining flasks (blanks) add 5 mL 2.5 M sodium acetate, 10 mL 37% formaldehyde, mix, and let stand for 4 min. Add 2.0 mL 5.0 N HCl, mix, and immediately titrate. Subtract the blank values from the titration values of the standards and average the net titration values, which should agree within 2%. Since the net volume of dye represents 1.005 mg of ascorbic acid, the ascorbic acid equivalent (T) of 1 mL of dye solution is equal to 1.005 divided by the volume in mL of the dye solution used in this titration.

2. *Extraction.* Measure 50-mL aliquots samples in a 50-mL volumetric flask; transfer to a 500-mL Erlenmeyer flask. Add 100 mL acetic acid–metaphosphoric acid to the Erlenmeyer flask and mix thoroughly. Rinse flask with 50 mL H_2O, add rinse to the 500-mL Erlenmeyer flask, and mix again. Filter through fluted filter paper (Whatman No. 12), discarding the first 10 mL of filtrate.

3. *Titration.* Pipette 30 mL of filtrate into each of four 125-mL Erlenmeyer flasks. Promply titrate two of the flasks with the dye solution until a pink color persists for at least 10 sec. To each of the two remaining flasks (blanks), add 5 mL 2.5 M sodium acetate, 10 mL 37% formaldehyde, mix, and let stand 4 min. Add 2.0 mL 5.0 N HCl, mix, and immediately titrate. Subtract the blank values from the titration values of the first two flasks and average.

4. *Calculations.* Calculate the ascorbic acid concentration in condensed or evaporated milk as follows:

$$T \times V \times 13.33 \times F = \text{mg ascorbic acid/100 mL sample}$$

where T = ascorbic acid equivalent of dye solution expressed as mg/mL of dye;

V = net mL of dye used (e.g., 2.4 mL) for titration of aliquot of diluted sample;

F = correction factor to adjust the dilution factor 13.33 for volume occupied by precipitated proteins.

Calculate F as follows:

$$F = \frac{\text{total wt (g)} - \text{dry wt (g) of precipitate}}{\text{specific gravity of filtrate} \times 200}$$

where the total weight is that of 50 mL milk, 50 mL H_2O, and 100 mL acetic metaphosphoric acid solution. The dry weight of precipitate can be obtained by collecting the precipitate on a filter paper, washing with H_2O, and drying for 24 hr in a drying oven at 120°C. The weight of paper is obtained from a paper treated as above except for the addition of milk.

VI.   FLUOROMETRIC DETERMINATION OF TOTAL VITAMIN C (ASCORBIC AND DEHYDROASCORBIC ACIDS) WITH o-PHENYLENEDIAMINE (99)

A.   Scope

The procedure is applicable to the determination of total vitamin C without differentiating ascorbic and dehydroascorbic acids. It is not applicable to certain processed foods containing dehydroreductones and dehydroreductic acids and can produce unrealistically high vitamin C values in the analysis of deep-fat fried products such as potato chips and French fries. The method has been demonstrated to be applicable to pharmaceutical preparations, fruit juices, fruit drinks, and enriched cereal products.

B.   Principle

The formation of a fluorescent product by the reaction of dehydroascorbic acid with o-phenylenediamine is the basis of vitamin C determination following oxidation of ascorbic acid. Blanks to differentiate vitamin C from possible interfering substances are prepared by forming a boric acid–dehydroascorbic acid complex to prevent the reaction of dehydroascorbic acid with o-phenylenediamine.

C.   Equipment

Besides general laboratory equipment and glassware for preparation of reagents, the following special equipment is required:

1. *Blender.*   The cutting blades and the bowl must be of a material that does not yield metallic ions capable of oxidizing ascorbic acid.

2. *Vortex Mixer or Equivalent.*

3. *Fluorometer.* The Aminco Fluoro-Microphotometer equipped with lamp F4T4/BL, primary filters Corning Nos. 7380 and 5860, secondary filters Corning Nos. 5113 and 3389, standardized cuvets 18 × 150 mm, and cuvet adaptor No. B12-63019, or equivalent equipment.

4. *Automatic Pipette.* Any pipette capable of delivering accurately and rapidly up to 5.0 mL of solutions.

D. Reagents

The chemicals for preparing reagents should be reagent grade and the H_2O should be deionized through an ion-exchange resin.

1. *Acetic–Metaphosphoric Acid Solution.* Dissolve with shaking or stirring and without applying heat 30 g metaphosphoric acid pellets containing 34% HPO_3 and 59% $NaPO_3$ in 80 mL glacial acetic acid and 500 mL H_2O, and dilute to 1000 mL. Filter rapidly and store in a refrigerator to prevent metaphosphoric acid being converted to orthophosphoric acid. Prepare every 2 weeks.

2. *Acetic–Metaphosphoric–Hydrochloric Acids Solution.* Prepare as in Section VI.D.1, replacing H_2O by 0.3 N H_2SO_4.

3. *Ascorbic Acid Standard Solutions.* Accurately weigh 100 mg USP L-ascorbic acid reference standard which has been dried in the dark over sulfuric acid in a dessicator for 24 hr. Transfer to a 100-mL volumetric flask and dilute with the acid sollution (Reagent 1). Prepare fresh daily and further dilute 10 mL to 100 mL with the same solution. This solution contains 10 mg ascorbic acid/100mL.

4. *Sodium Acetate Solution.* Dissolve 500 g sodium acetate trihydrate in H_2O and dilute to 1 L.

5. *Boric Acid–Sodium Acetate Solution.* Dissolve 3 g boric acid in 100 mL sodium acetate solution. Prepare fresh daily.

6. *0.02% o-Phenylenediamine Hydrochloride Solution.* Weigh 20 mg o-phenylenediamine hydrochloride (Eastman Kodak Co.) for each 100 mL solution required and dilute to volume with H_2O immediately before use.

7. *0.04% Thymol Blue pH Indicator.* Dissolve 0.1 g thymol blue by triturating with 10.75 mL 0.02 N NaOH and dilute to 250 mL with H_2O.

8. *Acid-Washed Norit.* Place 200 g Norit (Matheson, Coleman & Bell) in a large flask, add 1 L diluted HCl (one part concentrated HCl and 9 parts H_2O) and stir well. Heat to boiling and filter with suction. Remove the cake of Norit to a large beaker, add 1 L H_2O, stir thoroughly and filter. Repeat washing with H_2O and filtering. Dry overnight in an oven at 100 ± 5°C. Avoid heating above the recommended temp.

E. Procedure

1. *Extraction.* A sufficient amount of each sample that is not liquid or cannot be liquified must be ground to a fine powder to have at least two representative

portions. A representative portion must contain sufficient vitamin C to provide for a final volume of at least 100 mL containing optimally about 10 mg vitamin C. Test the pH of one powdered portion of sample mixed with about 25 mL metaphosphoric–acetic acid solution, or a liquid portion mixed with an equal volume of metaphosphoric–acetic acid. A drop of thymol blue in presence of a few drops of homogeneous sample will indicate that the sample contains an appreciable amount of basic substances when pH is above 1.2 (transition range: 2.8 yellow–1.2 red). Extract and dilute a representative portion of sample containing no appreciable amount of basic substance with a sufficient amount of acetic acid–metaphosphoric acid solution (Reagent 1) to obtain a final vitamin C concentration of about 10 mg/10 mL. Dilute samples difficult to filter to about 5 mg/100 mL but in that case, also dilute the ascorbic acid standard to 5 mg/100 mL. Samples containing an appreciable amount of basic substances require the preliminary addition of the acetic–metaphosphoric–hydrochloric acid solution (Reagent 2) to adjust pH to about 1.2; for the remainder, use the acetic–metaphosphoric acid solution (Reagent 1). Blend nonliquid samples for periods ranging from 30 sec (small volume in a small blender) to 3 min (large volume in large blender). Filter through Whatman No. 2 folded filter paper.

2. *Determination.*   Perform the following steps without delay.

(a) Norit Treatment.   Place 100 mL of ascorbic acid standard solution (containing 10 mg or 5 mg to match the sample's concentration) and 100 mL of the sample's extract into separate 300—mL Erlenmeyer flasks. Add 2 g of acid-washed Norit, shake vigorously, and filter through Whatman No. 12 paper (or the equivalent) discarding the first few mL of filtrate.

(b) Determination. Pipette 5 mL of each filtrate into separate 100-mL volumetric flasks containing 5 mL boric acid–sodium acetate solution and let stand 15 min with occasional swirling. Designate these as "blank" solutions.

During the waiting period, pipette 5 mL-aliquots of the filtrates into another set of 100—mL volumetric flasks containing 5 mL sodium acetate solution and about 75 mL H₂O, and designate as "test" solutions. Dilute each test solution to 100 mL with H_2O and pipette 2 mL of each into three test tubes.

After the 15 min waiting period, dilute the blank solutions to 100 mL with H_2O and pipette 2 mL of each into three separate test tubes.

With the autopipette, add 5 mL o-phenylenediamine solution to all tubes and vortex. Protect from light and let stand 35 min at room temperature before transferring to fluorescence-reading cuvets.

3. *Measurements.*   Measure the fluorescence of all tubes matching each blank and test of the appropriate standard and sample. Subtract each blank value from the corresponding test value for each standard and sample and average the net value for each standard (X) and sample (Y).

Calculate the vitamin C concentration according to the following formula:

$$\text{mg per g, mL, capsule, or table} = \frac{Y}{X} \times \frac{\text{STD}}{100} \times D$$

where STD refers to either 10 or 5 mg ascorbic acid standard/100 mL (depending on the standard used for the determination) and D is the dilution factor of the sample (e.g., 200/5 in the case when 5 g was diluted to 200 mL with acetic acid-metaphosphoric acid).

LITERATURE CITED

1. Chatterjee, I. B. "Ascorbic acid metabolism." *World Rev. Nutr. Diet.* **30**, 69 (1978).

2. King, C. G. "Present knowledge of ascorbic acid (vitamin C)." In *Present Knowledge in Nutrition.* The Nutrition Foundation, New York, 76–79 (1967)

3. Barnes, M. J. "Function of ascorbic acid in collagen metabolism." *Ann. N.Y. Acad. Sci.* **258**, 264 (1975).

4. Irwin, M. I. and Hutchins, B. K. "A conspectus of research on vitamin C requirements of man." *J. Nutr.* **106**, 821 (1976).

5. Mattok, G. L. "The mechanism of reduction of adenochrome by ascorbic acid." *Chemical Soc. J.* 4728–4735 (1965).

6. Lopez, A., Krerhl, W. A., and Good, E. "Influence of time and temperature on ascorbic acid stability." *J. Am. Diet. Assoc.* **50**, 303 (1967).

7. Lugg, J. W. H. "The use of formaldehyde and 2,6-dichlorophenolindophenol in the estimation of ascorbic acid and dehydroascorbic acid." *Australian J. Explt. Biol. Med. Sci.* **20**, 273 (1942).

8. Huelin, F. E. "Investigations on the stability and determination of dehydroascorbic acid." *Austral. J. Sci. Res. Series B Biol. Sci.* **19**, 346 (1949).

9. Linkswiller, H. "The effect of ingestion of ascorbic acid and dehyroascorbic acid upon the blood levels of these two components in human subjects." *J. Nutr.* **64**, 43 (1958).

10. Jackson, S. F., Chichester, C. O., and Joslyn, M.A. "The browning of ascorbic acid." *Food Res.* **4**, 484 (1960).

11. Pelletier, O. and Godin, C. "Vitamin C activity of D-isoascorbic acid for the guinea pig." *Can. J. Physiol. Pharmacol.* **47**, 985 (1969).

12. Sherman, H. C., LaMer, V. K., and Campbell, H. L. "The quantitative determination of the antiscorbutic vitamin (vitamin C)." *J. Am. Chem. Soc.* **44**, 165 (1922).

13. Burns, J. J., Fullmer, H. M., and Dayton, P. G. "Observations on vitamin C activity of D-ascorbic acid." *Proc. Soc. Expl. Biol Med.* **101**, **46** (1959).

14. Pelletier, O. "Turnover rates of D-isoascorbic acid and L-ascorbic acid in guinea pig organs." *Can. J. Physiol. Pharmacol.* **47**, 993 (1969).

15. Tillmans, J. "The antiscorbutic vitamin." *Z. Lebensm. Unters. Forsch.* **60**, 34 (1930).

16. Pelletier, O., Brassard, R., and Madine, R. "Vitamin C in fruit drinks prepared in various ways." *Can. Med. Assoc. J.* **108**, 1483 (1973).

17. Davidek, J., Velisek, J., and Janicek, G. "The stability of vitamin C in orange drink." *Lebensm.-Wiss.-Technol.* **7**, 285 (1974).

18. Davidek, J., Grundova, K., Velisek, J., and Janicek, G. "Determination of L-dehydroascorbic acid in foods." *Lebensm.-Wiss.-Technol.* **5**, 213 (1972).

19. Grundova, J., Davidek, J., Velisek, J., and Janicek, G. "Determination of L-ascorbic acid and L-dehydroascorbic acids in plant materials and preserved foods." *Lebensm.-Wiss.-Technol.* **6**, 11 (1973).

20. Domah, A. A. M. B., Davidek, J., and Velisek, J. "Changes of L-ascorbic acid and L-dehydroascorbic acids during cooking and frying of potatoes." *Z. Lebensm. Unters. Forsch.* **154**, 270 (1974).

21. Jadhav, S., Steele, L., and Hadziyev, D. "Vitamin C losses during production of dehydrated mashed potatoes." *Lebensm.-Wiss.-Technol.* **8**, 222 (1975).

22. Steele, L., Jadhav, S., and Hadziyev, D. "The chemical assay of vitamin C in dehydrated mased potatoes." *Lebensm.-Wiss.-Technol.* **9**, 239 (1976).

23. Mapson, L. W. "Vitamin methods VI. The estimation of ascorbic acid in the presence of reductones and allied substances." *J. Soc. Chem. Ind.* **62**, 223 (1943).

24. Kuusi, T. "Reductone interference in the assay of ascorbic acid—A comparative study of different methods of analysis." *Suomen Kemistilehti* B **33**, 139 (1960).

25. Brown, F. and Adam, W. B. "The determination of ascorbic acid in the presence of ferrous salts, with particular reference to canned foods." *J. Sci. Food Agric.* **1**, 50 (1950).

26. Pelletier, O. and Morrison, A. B. "Determination of ascorbic acid in the presence of ferrous and stannous salts." *J. Assoc. Off. Anal. Chem.* **49**, 800 (1966).

27. Ralls, J. W. "Turbidimetric determination of ascorbic acid in foods." *Agric. Food Chem.* **23**, 609 (1975).

28. Sommers, G. F., Kelly, W. C., Thacker, E. J., and Redder, A. M. "Erroneous ascorbic acid values resulting from interference by anthocyanins." *Science* **110**, 17 (1949).

29. Freebairn, H. T. "Determination and stabilization of reduced ascorbic acid in extracts from plant materials." *Anal. Chem.* **31**, 1850 (1959).

30. King, C. G. "Chemical methods for the determination of vitamin C." *Ind. Eng. Chem., Anal. Ed.* **13**, 225 (1941).

31. Bessey, O. A. "Vitamin C methods of assay and dietary sources." *J. Am. Med. Assoc.* **111**, 1290 (1938).

32. Hughes, R. E. "The use of homocysteine in the estimation of dehydroascorbic acid." *Biochem. J.* **64**, 203 (1956).

33. Hughes, R. E. "Use of cation-exchange resin in the determination of urinary ascorbic acid." *Analyst* **89**, 618 (1964).

34. Howard, A. N. and Constable, B. J. "The use of homocystein in the estimation of ascorbic acid in urine." *Clin. Chim. Acta.* **13**, 387 (1966).

35. Gero, E. and Candido, A. "Une technique chimique du dosage de l'acide ascorbique total par une réaction d'oxido-reduction." *Internat. J. Vit. Res.* **39**, 259 (1969).

36. Bhattacharya, H. and Ganguly, S. K. "Estimation of vitamin C in pharamceutical preparations coloured with edible dyes." *Ind. J. Pharmacy.* **26**, 200 (1964).

37. Robinson, W. B. and Stotz, E. "The indophenol-xylene extraction method for ascorbic acid and modifications for interfering substances." *J. Biol. Chem.* **160**, 217 (1945).

38. Gero, E. "Mise au point d'une nouvelle technique de dosage de l'acide ascorbique." *Bull. Sté. Chim. Biol.* **31**, 825 (1949).

39. Nadkarni, B. Y. "Determination of ascorbic acid in coloured extracts: A new modification of the indophenol technique." *Mikrochim. Acta.* **1**, 21 (1965).

40. Pelletier, O. and Morrison, A. B. "Content and stability of ascorbic acid in fruit drinks." *J. Am. Diet. Assoc.* **47**, 401 (1965).

41. Chapman, D. G., Rochon, O., and Campbell, J. A. "Estimation of ascorbic acid in pharmaceuticals with particular reference to interfering substances." *Anal. Chem.* **23**, 1113 (1951).

42. Pelletier, O. "Determination of ascorbic acid in enriched evaporated milk." *J. Assoc. Off. Anal. Chem.* **50**, 817 (1967).

43. Owen, J. A. and Iggo, B. "The use of *p*-chloromercuribenzoic acid in the determination of ascorbic acid with 2,6-dichlorophenolindophenol." *Biochem. J.* **62**, 675 (1966).

44. Nesset, B. L., Windsor, B. L., Humphrey, R. R., and Callantine, M. R. "Automated determination of ascorbic acid." *Anal. Biochem.* **19**, 89 (1967).

45. Beyer, W. F. "Automated determination of rat adrenal ascorbic acid in the bioassay of corticotropin." *J. Pharm. Sci.* **56**, 526 (1967).

46. Gary, P. J., Owen, G. M., Lashley, D. W., and Ford, P. C. Automated analysis of plasma and whole blood ascorbic acid." *Clin. Biochem.* **7**, 131 (1974).

47. Saindelle, A., Ruff, F., and Parrot, J. L. "Automatisation du dosage de l'acide ascorbique dans le sang total, les urines et les tissues." *Bull. Soc. Chim. Biol.* **51**, 621 (1969).

48. Barakat, M. Z., El-Wahab, M. F. A., and El Sadr, M. M. "Action of *N*-bromosuccinimide on ascorbic acid. New titrimetric method for estimation of vitamin C." *Anal. Chem.* **27**, 536 (1955).

49. Evered, D. F. "The determination of ascorbic acid in highly colored solutions with N-bromosuccinimide." *Analyst* **85**, 515 (1960).

50. Hardesty, W. S. "Potentiometric determination of vitamin C in highly colored products." *J. Assoc. Off. Agric. Chem.* **47**, 754 (1964).

51. Sarwar, M., Igbal, Z., and Zaidi, S. "Modified method for the estimation of ascorbic acid from preserved juices and squashes." *Mikrochim. Acta (Wien)* **2**, 699 (1975).

52. Murty, N. K. and Rao, K. R. "Vitamin C (ascorbic acid)." *Methods in Enzymol.* **62**, 12 (1979).

53. Verma, K. K. and Gulati, A. K. "Determination of vitamin C with chloramine-T." *Anal. Chem.* **52**, 2336 (1980).

54. Sullivan, M. X. and Clarke, H. C. N. "A highly specific method for ascorbic acid." *J. Assoc. Off. Agric. Chem.* **38**, 514 (1955).

55. Maickel, R. P. "A rapid procedure for the determination of adrenal ascorbic acid. Application of the Sullivan Clarke method to tissues." *Anal. Biochem.* **1**, 498 (1960).

56. Zannoni, V., Lynch, M., Goldstein, S., and Sato, P. "A rapid micromethod for the determination of ascorbic acid in plasma and tissues." *Biochem. Med.* **11**, 41 (1974).

57. Vann, L. S. "A rapid method for determination of ascorbic acid in urine by ferric reduction." *Clin. Chem.* **11**, 979 (1965).

58. Przyborowski, L. "Kompleksometryczne oznaczenie kwasu askorbowego." *Dissertationes Pharmaceuticae et Pharmacologicae* **18**, 505 (1966).

59. Day, B. R., Williams, D. R., and Marsh, C. A. "A rapid manual method for routine assay of ascorbic acid in serum and plasma." *Clin. Biochem.* **12**, 22 (1979).

60. Jaselskis, B., and Nelapy, J. "Spectrophotometric determination of microamounts of ascorbic acid in citrus fruits." *Anal. Chem.* **44**, 379 (1972).

61. Okamura, M. "An improved method for the determination of L-ascorbic acid and dehydro-L-ascorbic acid in blood plasma." *Clin. Chim. Acta.* **103**, 259 (1980).

62. Shieh, H. H. and Sweet, T. R. "Spectrophotometric determination of ascorbic acid." *Anal. Biochem.* **96**, 1 (1979).

63. Kum-Tatt, L. and Leong, P. C. "A new method for the determination of ascorbic acid in urine." *Clin. Chem.* **10**, 575 (1964).

64. Ruiz, J. J., Aldaz, A., and Dominguez, M. "Mechanism of L-ascorbic acid oxidation and dehydro-L-ascorbic acid reduction on a mercury electrode—I. Acid medium." *Can. J. Chem.* **55**, 2799 (1977).

65. Lento, H. G., Daugherty, C. E., and Denton, A. E. "Polarographic determination of total ascorbic acid in foods." *Agric. Food Chem.* **11**, 22 (1963).

66. Roe, J. H. and Kuether, C. A. "The determination of ascorbic acid in whole blood and urine through the 2,4-dinitrophenylhydrazine detrivative of dehydroascorbic acid." *J. Biol. Chem.* **147**, 399 (1943).

67. Roe, J. H., Mills, M. B., Oesterling, M. J., and Damron, C. M. "The determination of diketo-1-gulonic, dehydro-L-ascorbic acid and L-ascorbic acid in the same tissue extract by the 2,4-dinitrophenylhydrazine method." *J. Biol. Chem.* **174**, 201 1948).

68. Hove, E. L. "Conference on vitamin C methodology: A summary report." *J. Assoc. Off. Agric. Chem.* **48**, 991 (1965).

69. Ratzkowski, C., and Korol, J. "The quantitative, differential determination of ascorbic acid and erythorbic acid in foods by polarography." *Can. Inst. Food Sci. Technol.* **10**, 215 (1977).

70. Baczyk, S., and Swidzinska, K. "Méthode spectrophotométrique directe du dosage simultané de l'acide, L-ascorbique et de l'acide déhydro-L-ascorbique." *Mikrochim. Acta. (Wien)* **2**, 259 (1975).

71. Hubmann, B., Monnier, D., and Roth, M. "Une méthode de dosage rapide et précise de l'acide ascorbique; application à la mesure des taux plasmitiques." *Clin. Chim. Acta.* **25**, 161 (1969).

72. Heweitt, E. J. and Dickes, G. J. "Spectrophotometric measurements of ascorbic acid and their use for the estimation of ascorbic acid and dehydroascorbic acid in plant tissues." *Biochem. J.* **78**, 384 (1961).

73. Marchesini, A. Montuori, F., Muffato, D., and Maestri, D. "Application and advantages of the enzymatic method for the assay of ascorbic acid and dehydroascorbic acid and reductones." *J. Food Sci.* **39**, 568 (1974).

74. Beutler, H. O. and Beinstingl, G. "Bestimmung von L-Ascorbinsäure in Lebensmittelin." *Deutsche Lebensmittel-Rundschau* **76**, 69 (1980).

75. Matsumoto, K., Yamada, K., and Osajirma, Y. "Ascorbate electrode for determination of L-ascorbic acid in food." *Anal. Chem.* **53**, 1974 (1981).

76. Roe, J. H. "Appraisal of methods for the determination of L-ascorbic acid." *Ann. N.Y. Acad. Sc.* **92**, 277 (1961).

77. Roe, J. H. "Comparative analyses for ascorbic acid by the 2,4-dinitrophenylhydrazine method with coupling reaction at different temperatures: A procedure for determining specificty." *J. Biol. Chem.* **236**, 1611 1961).

78. Pelletier, O. and Brassard, R. "Determination of vitamin C (L-ascorbic acid and dehydroascorbic acid) in food by manual and automated photometric methods." *J. Food Sci.* **42**, 1471 (1977).

79. Pelletier, O. "Determination of vitamin C in serum, urine, and other biological materials." *J. Lab. Clin. Med.* **72**, 674 (1968).

80. Chen, Y. T., Isherwood, F. A., and Mapson, L. W. "Quantitative estimation of ascorbic acid and related substances in biological extracts by separation on a paper chromatigram." *Biochem. J.* **55**, 821 (1953).

81. Szoke, K. "Ein Beitrag zur quantitativen Bestimmung von Vitamin C in wärmebehandelten Substanzen." *Die Nahrung* **9**, 825 (1960).

82. Zloch, Z. "Bestimmung des Vitamin C in kleinen Mengen tierischer Gewebe und im Blutserum mittels Ringpapierchromatographie." *Microchim. Acta. (Wien)* 753 (1969).

83. Beljaars, P. R., Horrocks, W. V. S., and Rondags, T. M. "Assay of L-ascorbic acid in buttermilk by densitometric transmittance measurement of dehydroascorbic acid osazone." *J. Assoc. Off. Anal. Chem.* **57**, 65 (1974).

84. Zloch, Z. "Bestimmung des Vitamin C in kleinen Mengen Harn mittels zweidimensionaler Dünnschicht-Chromatographie." *Microchim. Acta (Wien)* 213, (1975).

85. Mapson, L. W. "A note on the estimation of dehydro-L-ascorbic acid in plant tissues by the Roe & Kuether procedure." *Biochem. J.* **80**, 459 (1961).

86. Vuilleumier, J. "Analytische Probleme bei der Bestimmung von Vitamin C im Zusammenhang mit Ernährungserhebungen." *Internat. J. Vit. Res.* **37**, 504 (1967).

87. Garcia-Castineiras, S., Bonnet, V. D., Figueroa, R., and Miranda, M. "Ascorbic acid determination by hydrophobic liquid chromatography of the osazone derivative. Application to the analysis of aqueous humor." *J. Liq. Chromatogr.* **4**, 1619 (1981).

88. Pelletier, O. "Differential determination of D-isoascorbic acid and L-ascorbic acid in guinea pig organs." *Can. J. Biochem.* **4**, 449 (1969).

89. Pelletier, O. and Brassard, R. "A new automated method serum for vitamin C." *Adv. Automat. Anal. Technicon Int. Congr.* **9**, 73 (1973).

90. Pelletier, O. and Brassard, R. "Automated analysis of vitamin C in pharmaceutical products." *J. Assoc. Off. Anal. Chem.* **58**, 104 1975).

91. Behrens, W. A. and Madere, R. "Improved automated method for determining vitamin C in plasma and tissues." *Anal. Biochem.* **92**, 510 (1979).

92. Schmall, M. Pifer, C. W., and Wollish, E. G. "Determination of ascorbic acid by a new colorimetric reaction." *Anal. Chem.* **25**, 1486 (1953).

93. Crossland, E. "Chromatographic determination of ascorbic acid." *Act. Chem. Scand.* **14**, 805 (1960).

94. Geller, M., Weber, O. W. A., and Senkowski, B. Z. "Automated determination of ascorbic acid in multivitamin preparations." *J. Pharm. Sci.* **58**, 477 (1969).

95. Wilson, S. S. and Guillan, R. A. "The automated measurement of ascorbic acid in serum and urine." *Clin. Chem.* **15**, 282 (1969).

96. Weeks, C. E. and Deutsch, M. J. "Assay of ascorbic acid in pharmaceuticals: A modified colorimetric procedure using p-nitroaniline." *J. Assoc. Off. Agric. Chem.* **48**, 1245 1965).

97. Michaelsson, G. and Michaelsson, M. "A new diazo method for the determination of ascorbic acid in blood plasma." *Scand. J. Clin. Lab. Inv.* **20**, 97 (1967).

98. Davidek, J. and Davidkova, E. "Einfluss der Flavonoide auf die kolorimetrische Bestimmung der L-Ascorbinsäure mit 4-methoxy-2-nitranilin." *Die Nahrung* **3**, 515 (1959).

99. Deutsch, M. J. and Weeks, C. E. "Microfluorometric assay for vitamin C." *J. Assoc. Off. Agric. Chem.* **42**, 1248 (1965).

100. Association of Official Analytical Chemists. *Official Methods of Analysis,* 13th ed. Washington, D.C. 746–757, (1980).

101. Egberg, D. C., Potter, R. H., and Heroff, J. C. "Semiautomated method for the fluorometric determination of total vitamin C in food products." *J. Assoc. Off. Anal. Chem.* **60**, 126 (1977).

102. Bourgeois, C. F. and Mainguy, P. R. "Determination of vitamin C (ascorbic and dehydroascorbic acids) in food and feeds." *Internat. J. Vit. Nutr. Res.* **45**, 70 (1975).

103. Augustin, J., Beck, C., and Marousek, G. I. "Quantitative determination of ascorbic acid in potatoes and potato products by high performance liquid chromatography." *J. Food Sci.* **46**, 312 (1981).

104. Ziegenhagen, D. and Zobel, M. "Modifizierung der photometrischen Gesamt Vitamin C—Bestimmungsmethode mit papierchromatographischer Trennung nach Imhoff." *Lebensm. Unters. Forsch.* **140**, 110 (1969).

105. Wasa, T., Takagi, M., and Ono, S. "Polarographic investigation of vitamin C, III." *Bull. Chem. Soc. Japan* **34**, 518 (1961).

106. Allison, J. H. and Stewart, M. A. "Quantitative analysis of ascorbic acid in tissues by gas-liquid chromatography." *Anal. Biochem.* **43**, 401 (1971).

107. Schlack, J. E. "Quantitative determination of L-ascorbic acid by gas-liquid chromatography." *J. Assoc. Off. Anal. Chem.* **57**, 1346 (1974).

108. Wagner, E. S., Lindley, B., and Coffin, R. D. "High performance liquid chromatographic determination of ascorbic acid in urine." *J. Chromatogr.* **163**, 225 (1979).

109. Miki, N. "High performance liquid chromatographic determination of ascorbic acid in tomato products." *Nippon Shokuhin Kogyo Gakkaiski* **28**, 264 (1981).

110. Sood, S. P., Sartori, L. E., Wittmer, D. P., and Haney, W. G. "High pressure liquid chromatographic determination of ascorbic acid in selected foods and multivitamin products." *Anal. Chem.* **48**, 796 (1976).

111. Wills, R. B. H., Shaw, C. B., and Day, W. R. "Analysis of water soluble vitamins by high pressure liquid chromatography." *J. Chromatogr. Sci.* **15**, 262 (1977).

112. Ruckemann, H. "Methoden zur Bestimmung von L-Ascorbinsäure mittels Hochleistungs-Flüssigchromatographie (HPLC). I Bestimmung von L-Ascorbinsäure in Obst and Gemüse." *Z. Lebensm. Unters. Forsch.* **171**, 357 (1980).

113. Ruckermann, H. "Methoden zur Bestimmung von L-Ascorbinsäure mittels Hochleistungs-Flüssichromatographie (HPLC). II. Bestimmung von L-Ascorbinsaure in Milchaustauschfuttermitteln." *Z. Lebensm. Unters. Forsch.* **171**, 446 (1980).

114. Pachla, L. A. and Kissinger, P. T. "Analysis of ascorbic acid by liquid chromatography with amperometric detection." *Methods in Enzymol.* **62**, 15 (1979).

115. Finley, J. W. and Duang, E. "Resolution of ascorbic acid, dehydroascorbic acid and diketugulonic acids by paired ion reversed-phase chromatography." *J. Chromatogr.* **207**, 449 (1981).

116. Coustard, J. M. and Sudraud, G. "Séparation des acides ascorbique et isoascorbique par chromatographie de paires d'ions sur phase inverse." *J. Chromatogr.* **219**, 338 1981).

117. Carnevale, J. "Determination of ascorbic, sorbic and benzoic acids in citrus juices by high-performance liquid chromatography." *Food Technol. Australia* **32**, 302 (1980).

118. Bui-Nguyen, M. H. "Application of high-performance liquid chromatography to separation of ascorbic acid from isoascorbic acid." *J. Chromatogr.* **196**, 163 (1980).

119. Doner, L. D. and Hicks, K. B. "High-performance liquid chromatographic separation of ascorbic acid, erythorbic acid, dehydroascorbic acid, diketogluonic acid, and diketogluconic acid." *Anal. Biochem.* **115**, 225 (1981).

120. Geigert, J., Hirano, D. S., and Neidleman, S. L. "High-performance liquid chromatographic method for the determination of L-ascorbic acid and D-isoascorbic acid." *J. Chromatogr.* **206**, 396 (1981).

121. Archer, A. W., Higgins, V. R., and Perryman, D. L. "Determination of ascorbic and erythorbic acid by high performance liquid chromatography." *J. Assoc. Pub. Analyst* **18**, 99 (1980).

122. Rose, R. C. and Nahrwold, D. L. "Quantitative analysis of ascorbic acid and dehydroascorbic acid by high-performance liquid chromatography." *Anal. Biochem.* **114**, 140 (1981).

123. Mason, W. D., Amick, E. N., and Heft, W. "Analysis of ascorbic acid in human plasma and urine by HPLC with electrochemical detection." *Anal. Letters* **13**, 817 (1980).

124. Dennison, D. B., Troy, G. B., and Hunter, L. D. "Rapid high-performance liquid chromatographic determination of ascorbic and combined ascorbic acid-dehydroascorbic acid in beverages." *J. Agric. Food Chem.* **29**, 927 (1981).

125. Carr, R. C. and Neff, J. M. "Determination of ascorbic acid in tissues of marine animals by liquid chromatography with electrochemical detection." *Anal. Chem.* **52**, 2428 (1980).

126. Veazey, R. L. and Nieman, T. A. "Chemiluminescence high-performance liquid chromatographic detector applied to ascorbic acid determinations." *J. Chromatogr.* **200**, 153 (1980).

127. Thrivikraman, K. V., Refshauge, C., and Adams, R. N. "Liquid chromatographic analysis of nanogram quantities of ascorbate in brain tissues." *Life Sci.* **15**, 1335 (1974).

128. Liebes, L. F., Kuo, S., Krigel, R., Pelle, E., and Silber, R. "Identification and quantitation of ascorbic acid in extracts of human lymphocytes by high-performance liquid chromatography." *Anal. Biochem.* **118**, 53 (1981).

129. Williams, R. C., Baker, R. D., and Schmit, J. A. "Analysis of water soluble vitamins by high-speed ion-exchange chromatography." *J. Chromatogr. Sci.* **11**, 618 (1973).

130. Pachla, L. A. and Kissinger, P. T. "Determination of ascorbic acid in foodstuffs, pharmaceuticals and body fluids by liquid chromatography with electrochemical detection." *Anal. Chem.* **48**, 364 (1976).

131. Tsao, C. S. and Salimi, S. L. "Ultramicromethod for the measurement of ascorbic acid in plasma and white blood cells by high-performance liquid chromatography with electrochemical detection." *J. Chromatogr.* **224**, 477 (1981).

132. Obata, H., Tsuchihashi, W., and Tokuyama, T. "Determination of reductones by high-pressure liquid chromatographic method." *Agric. Biol. Chem.* **44**, 1435 (1980).

133. Randall, V. G., Pippen, E. L., Plotter, A. L., and McGready, R. M. "Determination of total ascorbic acid in vegetables from alcoholic slurries." *J. Food Sci.* **40**, 894 (1975).

134. Ulrich, R. and Delaporte, N. "L'acide ascorbique dans les fruits conservés par le froid, dans l'air et en atmosphère controllée." *Ann. Nutr. Alim.* **24**, B287 (1970).

135. Bradley, D. W. Emery, G., and Maynard, J. E. "Vitamin C in plasma: A comparative study

of the vitamin stabilized with trichloroacetic acid or metaphosphoric acid and the effects of storage at $-70°$, $-20°$, $4°$ and $25°$ on the stabilized vitamin." *Clin. Chim. Acta.* **44**, 47 (1973).

136. Fujita, A. and Itawaka, D. "The determination of vitamin C with 2,6-dichlorophenolindophenol." *Biochem. Z.* **277**, 293 (1935).

137. Ponting, J. D. "Extraction of ascorbic acid from plant materials, relative suitability of various acids." *Ind. Eng. Chem., Anal.* **15**, 389 1943).

138. Egberg, D. C., Larson, P. A., and Honold, G. R. "Automated determination of vitamin C in fortified foodstuffs." *J. Sci. Food Agric.* **24**, 789 (1973).

139. Remmers, P. A. J. F. "The vitamin C level of potato products heated in oil." *Internat. J. Vit. Nutr. Res.* **38**, 392 (1968).

140. Pelletier, O., Nantel, C., Leduc, R., Tremblay, L., and Brassard, R. "Vitamin C in potatoes prepared in various ways." *J. Inst. Can. Sci. Technol. Aliment.* **10**, 138 (1977).

141. Cooke, J. R. "The chemical estimation of vitamin C." In *Vitamin C: Recent Aspects of Its Physiological and Technological Importance*, Wiley, New York, 31–39 (1974).

142. Jager, H. "Beitrag zur Frage der Stabilisierung wässriger Ascorbinsäurelösungen." *Pharmazie* **3**, 536 (1948).

143. Archer, A. L. "Stability of aqueous solutions of ascorbic acid prepared for analysis by high performance liquid chromatography." *J. Assoc. Publ. Analysts* **19**, 91 (1981).

144. Marchand, C. M. and Pelletier, O. "Studies with an improved white cell isolation method to assess the vitamin C status in surveys." *Internat. J. Vit. Nutr. Res.* **47**, 836 (1977).

13 Thiamin

Wayne C. Ellefson

GENERAL CONSIDERATIONS (1–13)

Studies finally leading to the isolation and characterization of thiamin* as a vitamin began about 1890, when it was first recognized that beriberi was caused by lack of a food essential, later shown to be thiamin. Thiamin deficiency is characterized by loss of appetite and weight. Polyneuritis, involving degeneration of the peripheral nerves, along with increased concentrations of pyruvate and lactate in the blood, can occur in the latter stages of deficiency. However, beriberi, the common name for this condition, occurs infrequently. Subclinical deficiencies are more common.

Thiamin hydrochloride, also known as vitamin B_1, thiamin chloride, thiamin, aneurin, antineuritic vitamin, or the antiberiberi vitamin, has the structural formula:

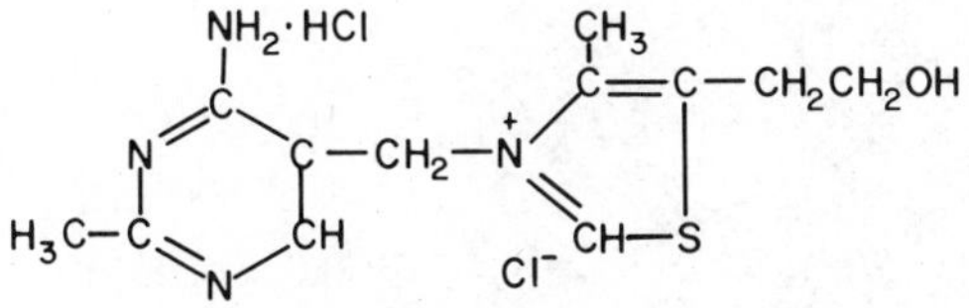

Thiamin is a white crystalline powder with a yeast-like odor and a salty, nut-like taste. It can be crystallized from alcoholic aqueous solutions as colorless monoclinic crystals of the hemihydrate. The crystals are hygroscopic, absorbing up to one mole of water. Ultraviolet absorption curves are shown in Figure 13.1.

*The term thiamin refers to thiamin chloride hydrochloride.

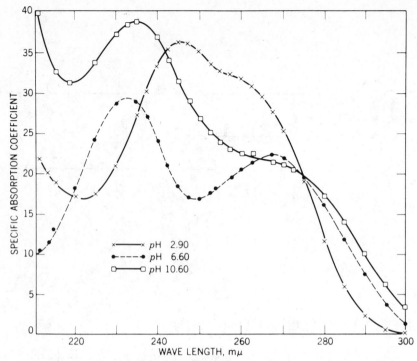

FIGURE 13.1 Ultraviolet absorption curves for thiamine in aqueous solution.

Other physical properties are listed below:

Empirical formula	$C_{12}H_{18}ON_4SCl_2$
Molecular weight	337.26
Melting point	246–250°C (decomposition)
pH of a 1% solution in water	3.13
pH of a 0.1% solution in water	3.58
Optical rotation	Absent
Solubility	
Water	100 g/100 mL
Ethanol, 95%	1 g/100 mL
Ethanol, 100%	0.3 g/100 mL
Glycerol	5 g/100 mL
Ethyl ether	Insoluble
Acetone	Insoluble
Benzene	Insoluble
Hexane	Insoluble
Chloroform	Insoluble

Thiamin is rapidly destroyed in neutral or alkaline solutions. It can withstand sterilization at 120°C for one-half hour when in acid solution. Sulfites will cause a cleavage of the molecule in acid solution. Thiaminase, which occurs in certain plants and fish, also destroys thiamin.

In dry form, thiamin is very stable and is not sensitive to atmospheric oxidation. In solution, thiamin is very sensitive to oxidation and reduction. A dihyro-compound, devoid of vitamin activity is formed by mild reduction. Mild oxidation can yield a disulfide with biological activity equal to that of thiamin. Thiochrome, which is biologically inactive, is formed by in vitro oxidation of thiamin. Prolonged standing of thiamin in alcoholic solutions yields very small amounts of thiochrome.

Thiamin can occur in a variety of forms: as free thiamin, as a protein complex, as mono-, di-, or triphosphate esters, or as a phosphorous protein complex. In foods, the amount of any of these forms varies considerably. Phosphate esters may account for up to 20–25% of the thiamin in nuts. Phosphorolytic enzymes can be used to release thiamin from its phosphate esters. Products such as nuts, pork, yeast, and cereal germs are especially rich in this vitamin.

METHODS AVAILABLE

Many methods have been used over the years for the analysis of thiamin. Each method has advantages and disadvantages.

The first assays developed were animal assays, since the vitamin nature of thiamin was first detected by observing the failure of man or animals to thrive on thiamin-deficient diets. These assays are of importance in determining the thiamin available to an animal. Growth measurements and curative tests were the most common animal assays. One of the principal disadvantages of these biological procedures is time consumption. The growth test requires 6–8 weeks, whereas the rat curative procedure is slightly shorter. The need for large groups of animals and carefully prepared diets, along with the time required, make these assays very expensive. Like all biological data, the results vary considerably, depending on the particular group of animals or upon the techniques employed. It has been demonstrated that bacteria in the intestinal tract can synthesize thiamin and make it available to the animal. This further complicates evaluation of the data obtained by biological methods. Since the object of most thiamin assays is to determine the amount available for metabolism, the biological assays are used as a measure of physiologically available thiamin.

Microbiological methods have also been used in the determination of thiamin. Various procedures have been used, including fermentation and the growth of or acid production by bacteria, yeasts, molds, or fungi. Some of these bacteria are reportedly very specific for thiamin (14,15). These methods consume much less time, are less expensive, and yield more reproducible results than animal assays. From 4 hours to 3 days are required to complete an assay. In these procedures, other substances, such as breakdown products of thiamin may respond in the same manner as thiamin. Blanks and correction factors may improve the accuracy. The use of thiaminase to effect a blank has been reported (15). Reproducibility of results may be a problem, although some report success in this regard (15).

Chemical assays are much more prevalent at this time. They can be carried out rapidly and economically and consequently are more applicable to routine determinations. Precision is generally improved with chemical procedures. Chemical procedures can be split into two groups: manual and automated. In both groups, the thiochrome procedure, or a variation of it, is predominant.

The manual thiochrome procedure is applicable to most any sample matrix including foods, feeds, and pharmaceuticals. This method involves oxidation of thiamin to thiochrome after purification of the extract by ion-exchange chromatography (1,16,17). Some analysts have automated the thiochrome reaction and the fluorimetry sections of this analysis (18). Others also include a thiochrome inhibition step as a blank in the semi-automated procedure (19).

Advantages of the thiochrome procedure are good precision, rapid analyses, and a wide range of applicability. A major disadvantage at this time is the difficulty in locating an enzyme that will consistently release thiamin from its phosphate esters. Although thiamin phosphates are converted to thiochrome phosphates, they are not soluble in isobutyl alcohol and are therefore undetectable in the assay (20).

Recently, the use of chromatographic systems notably in the form of high-performance liquid chromatography (HPLC) has received increased attention. Several developments have emerged recently using HPLC determination of thiamin or thiochrome, either singly or simultaneously with other water-soluble vitamins (21–25). The various phosphate esters of thiamin may also be separated by HPLC (26). Seifert and Mung determined thiamin in pinto beans by gas liquid chromatography of its sulfite cleavage product 5-(L-hydroxyethyl)-4-methyl thiazole (27).

ANALYTICAL METHODOLOGY

THIOCHROME METHOD

A.   Principle

Thiochrome procedures depend upon the oxidation of thiamin to thiochrome, which fluoresces in ultraviolet light. Under standard conditions and in the absence of other fluorescing substances, the fluorescence is proportional to the thiochrome present, and hence to the thiamin. The thiamin may be freed from interfering substances by use of ion-exchange chromatography if necessary.

B. Equipment

In addition to general glassware and equipment associated with analytical laboratory work the following items are required:

1. *Chromatography Columns.* With a 25–30-mL reservoir and a column 6–8 mm $\times$ 15 cm long drawn into a capillary fitted with an extra coarse frit or a small wad of glass wool.

2. *Photofluorometer 365/435 nm Excitation/Emission Filters.*

C. Reagents

All chemicals should meet ACS specifications or be of Reagent Grade. Cork or rubber stoppers should not be used because contact of reagents with these materials may contribute fluorescing substances that will interfere with the assay.

1. *Anhydrous Sodium Sulfate.* Granular.

2. *15% Sodium Hydroxide Solution.* Dissolve 15 g NaOH in H_2O and dilute to 100 mL.

3. *1.0% Potassium Ferricyanide Solution.* Dissolve 1.0 g $K_3Fe(CN)_6$ in H_2O and dilute to 100 mL. Store refrigerated in a brown bottle.

4. *Alkaline Potassium Ferricyanide Solution.* Dilute 3 mL of 1.0% $K_3Fe(CN)_6$ solution to 100 mL with 15% NaOH solution. Prepared fresh just prior to use. Keep protected from UV light.

5. *0.14 N Hydrochloric Acid Solution.* Slowly add 210 mL of concentrated HCl to H_2O and dilute to 18 L.

6. *2.5 M Sodium Acetate Solution.* Dissolve 205 g anhydrous $NaC_2H_3O_2$ or 345 g $NaC_2H_3O_2 \cdot 3H_2O$ in H_2O and dilute to 1 L.

7. *Acid 25% Potassium Chloride Solution.* Dissolve 250 g KCl in H_2O, add 8.5 mL concentrated HCl and dilute to 1 L with H_2O.

8. *Isobutyl Alcohol (Burdick & Jackson, distilled in glass or equivalent).* Isobutyl alcohol should be checked by reading in a fluorometer to assure that no extraneous fluorescence is present. Alternatively, the isobutyl alcohol may be redistilled using all glass apparatus.

9. *Enzyme Solution.*

(a) Prepare fresh daily using a suitable phosphatase. Suspend, with vigorous shaking, 6 g of enzyme in a 2.5 M sodium acetate solution (Reagent 6) and dilute to 100 mL with additional 2.5 M sodium acetate. The enzyme should be checked to ensure that it is thiamin-free.

(1) The suitability of an enzyme can be determined by making a thiamin phosphate standard and treating it with the enzyme. Comparison with thiamin reference standard will then reveal the effectiveness of an enzyme. Generally, 80–90% recovery of thiamin from its phosphate forms is good (17).

(2) Takadiastase (Pfaltz and Bauer, Stamford, Connecticut) and α-amylase (Miles Laboratories) have been determined to be effective.

10. *Ion-Exchange Resin.*

(a) Bio-Rex 70, 50–100 mesh, (BioRad Laboratories) or equivalent (17).

(1) Bio-Rex 70 (Na form) has a pH of 10.8 when suspended in H_2O (17). This alkaline pH will destroy thiamin. Therefore the resin must be converted to the hydrogen form.

(b) Add 300 mL of 2N HCl to 50 g of Bio-Rex 70 (Na form). Stir for 15 min, decant acid. Repeat.

(c) Add 300 mL H_2O and stir for 1 min and decant. Repeat H_2O washes until excess acid has been removed.

(1) These H_2O washings should also be used to decant excess "fines" away from the resin. This will improve the flow rate.

11. *Stock Thiamin Solution.*   Use USP reference standard thiamin. Dry thiamin over P_2O_5 in a dessicator for 24 hr, or at 100°C for 2 hr. Dissolve 0.1000 g of thiamin in 25% ethanol or in 0.14 normal HCl and dilute to 1 L with the same. Store in a refrigerator. This solution is stable several months to 1 year.

12. *Intermediate Thiamin Solution.*   Dilute 5 mL of stock thiamin solution to 100 mL (or 250 mL if a more sensitive fluorometer is used) with H_2O.

13. *Working Thiamin Solution.*   To a 100-mL flask add 4 mL of intermediate thiamin to 5 mL of sodium acetate solution (Reagent 6) and 45 ml 0.14 N HCl and dilute to 100 mL. This gives a final concentration of 0.2 μg/mL. If a more sensitive instrument is employed, add 5 mL of intermediate thiamin that was made to 250 mL to a 100-mL volumetric flask containing 45 mL of 0.14 N HCl and 5 mL of sodium acetate solution. Dilute to volume to obtain a final concentration of 0.1 μg/mL.

14. *Stock Quinine Sulfate Solution.*   Dissolve 100 mg of USP quinine sulfate in 0.1 N H_2SO_4 and dilute to 1 L with the same. This solution is stable indefinitely if stored in a dark brown bottle. If the solution becomes turbid, discard and prepare anew.

15. *Working Quinine Sulfate Solution.*   Dilute 3 mL of stock quinine solution to 1 L with 0.1 N H_2SO_4 to give a final concentration of 0.3 mg/L. Fluorescent glass standards are also available for use.

D. Procedure

The following procedure is a composite of several published methods (1,16,17,28–47) and/or unpublished modifications. Variations suitable to specific products may be required.

1. *Extraction.*

(a) Accurately weigh an appropriately prepared sample, containing 10–20 μg of thiamin, if possible, into a 400-mL beaker. Add 50 mL of 0.14 N HCl and heat for 30 min in a boiling water bath.

(1) The sample may be autoclaved 15 min at 15 lb psi instead of heating in a water bath.

(2) The function of extraction is twofold: (a) The use of an acid extraction effects a practically complete solution of the various forms of thiamin that may be present in the product, and (b) the pH of the acid extract is such that the thiamin is very stable. In the past both HCl and H_2SO_4 have been used for the extraction of thiamin. There is some suggestion that in some samples, insoluble sulfates are formed that absorb thiamin (31). For this reason, HCl is the preferred acid. In case different acid concentrations are used, the amount of sodium acetate used in the next step must also be adjusted so the final pH will be 4.5–5.0.

(3) Smaller quantities of thiamin can be determined, but precision and accuracy will suffer accordingly.

(4) With some samples, it is advisable to add part of the acid to the beaker before adding the sample in order to prevent the sample from sticking to the beaker.

(b) Cool the extract to 50°C or lower and add 5 mL of freshly prepared enzyme suspension. Incubate at 45–50°C for 2 hr or longer.

(1) This step is necessary for the conversion of bound thiamin to its free form. The phosphatase will hydrolyze any phosphate esters of thiamin present thus liberating the thiamin. This is important because the thiochrome phosphates are not soluble in isobutyl alcohol (32,39,43,47).

(2) The enzyme will also hydrolyze the starch present in food samples.

(3) 4 M sodium acetate may be substituted for the 2.5 M reagent. The former has a lesser tendency to support mold growth. The volume added may need to be altered as the pH must be 4.5–5.0.

(4) Two hrs is sufficient for most samples. Occasionally longer digestions give higher results. When working with unfamiliar material, it is well to extend the period to 3 hr or more. It is frequently convenient to allow samples to stand overnight at 37–50°C (34,43).

(5) For the assay of top yeast and animal tissues, treatment of the sample with thioglycolic acid or cysteine at pH 4.5–5.0 is recommended to reduce any reversibly oxidized thiamin that may be present (48). The oxidized form is not assayable by the thiochrome procedure.

(6) This step may be omitted for pharmaceuticals and many products where all thiamin is in the free form, provided that the product will be filterable (34–36,49). The pH must still be adjusted with 5 mL of 2.5 M sodium acetate.

(7) Milk samples may need to be treated with a proteolytic enzyme such as papain in order to release bound thiamin (37). Others indicate that this treatment may not be necessary with all varieties of milk (13).

(c) Cool to room temperature, transfer to a 100-mL volumetric flask with water and dilute to 100 mL. Mix thoroughly and filter.

(1) If the filtrate is turbid, refilter. Some samples may not be able to be clarified. If this happens, high-speed centrifugation may be tried. Continue on to the next step, even if filtrate is turbid.

(2) If much fat is present, the volume should be adjusted to 100 mL exclusive of the fat, which contains insignificant quantities of thiamin.

(3) If the assay cannot be finished in 1 day, this is a convenient stopping point if the filtrate is held refrigerated.

2. *Purification.*

(a) Fill each chromatography column with H_2O. Transfer the ion-exchange resin (prepared as in Section C.10 above) to the column, allowing the resin to fall in place by gravity. The column should be packed to a height of 7–10 cm. Allow excess H_2O to drain.

(1) Preparation of the column in the described manner gives a free-flowing column. This also prevents air pockets from forming.

(b) Pipette 5–25 mL of filtrate onto the column. Allow it to pass through by gravity flow. Discard the filtrate. Wash the reservoir and column with three successive 10-mL portions of hot H_2O, discarding the washings. Place 10 mL of acid KCl on the column, collecting the eluate in a 25-mL volumetric flask. Add a second 10-mL portion when the first has totally entered the resin, collecting the eluate in the same 25-mL flask. A third portion of 2–3 mL may be added to the column, again collecting in the 25-mL flask. Dilute contents of the 25-mL flask to volume with acid KCl solution and mix.

(1) A properly prepared resin will adsorb thiamin from solution, separating it from many substances which might interfere in later steps. Treatment of the column with acid KCl replaces the adsorbed thiamin with potassium ions. The thiamin then is usually pure enough to permit accurate quantitation.

(2) Bio-Rex 70 (hydrogen form) resin can adsorb thiamin at a capacity greater than or equal to Decalso, which was formerly used, and recoveries of thiamin through the resin are greater than what was generally possible with Decalso (17).

(3) Depending on the capability of the instrument available for reading, the aliquot taken should contain approximately 1–5 μg of thiamin.

(4) The aliquot for adsorption, the H_2O used for washing, and the acid KCl may all be heated before introduction to the column. This will yield faster flow rates through the column. The acid KCl should not be heated to a temperature greater than 70°C or losses may occur (50).

(5) Some investigators prefer adjusting the pH of the filtrate to 3.5 before adsorption on the column.

(6) With certain sample matrices, the purification step may be omitted provided the blanks are not more than 1.5 times the standard blank. Preliminary experimentation should be done to determine whether purification is necessary. The purification step may be eliminated on such

matrices as milk, certain pharmaceuticals, vitamin concentrates, products fortified at a high level, and certain meat products (32,34,42,45,46,49,51). Inclusion of the purification step eliminates some of the errors caused by interfering substances (52).

(7) Extraction of interfering substances with isobutanol prior to purification may sometimes be necessary (53,54).

(8) If the tip of the chromatography column fits tightly into the volumetric flask, an air pocket may form in the flask causing overflow and loss of eluate. This can be avoided by adjusting the column height so that the tip barely touches the inside top of the flask.

(9) The eluate is stable for several days if refrigerated.

(c) Repeat steps a and b with a new column, using 25 mL of working thiamin standard containing 0.1 or 0.2 μg/mL of thiamin.

(1) Concentration of the standard again depends upon the instrument available and the preference of the analyst.

(2) The elution of a working thiamin solution provides a standard for use in calibrating the instrument.

(3) The working thiamin solution adsorbed and eluted can be checked against one that has bypassed the purification step. The fluorescence of both solutions can be compared and the recovery through the resin determined. Recoveries of 97–100% are normal. Recoveries of 95% are acceptable (17). *Caution:* All remaining steps should be carried out in subdued lighting as thiochrome is unstable to UV light.

3. *Conversion to Thiochrome.*

(a) Pipette 3–5 mL of the acid KCl eluate into a reaction vessel.

(1) The size of the aliquot can be varied depending on the sensitivity of the fluorometer used.

(b) To the vessel add 3 mL of alkaline ferricyanide solution with gentle swirling. Immediately add 15 mL of isobutyl alcohol. Shake vigorously for 90 sec.

(1) Thiamin is oxidized by potassium ferricyanide in the presence of strong alkali, yielding thiochrome (8,28,29,32):

Thiochrome is soluble in isobutyl alcohol. The yield is not quantitative but is very constant under standardized conditions (39). When irradiated with ultraviolet light, thiochrome fluoresces, emitting a blue light. Thiochrome has absorption maxima at 358 nm and 375 nm (8) and excitation maxima at 365 nm and emission maxima at 430 nm (16,55).

(2) Some investigators claim that speed is of the utmost importance in the thiochrome step (50,56). Others maintain that the solutions may stand for several minutes after the addition of alkaline ferricyanide solution and before shaking with isobutyl alcohol without altering the assay value. One investigator suggests addition of the KCl eluate to the alkaline ferricyanide solution rather than in the usual reverse manner (57). Whatever technique is employed should remain constant for all standards and unknowns. The reaction vessels should be arranged so that several may be shaken simultaneously.

(3) Extraction of thiochrome with isobutyl alcohol may also be effected by bubbling a stream of air or nitrogen through the reaction vessels instead of shaking them (58).

(4) Hematin accelerates the destruction of thiochrome in alkaline solutions. The precipitation of proteins will remove hematin from most solutions in which it may occur (59). The assay of blood requires special techniques and precautions (50).

(5) Excesses of iron are to be avoided, as iron will combine with the ferricyanide and inhibit the oxidation of thiamin to thiochrome.

(6) Separate 3-mL pipettes should be used for the alkaline ferricyanide solution and for the NaOH solution used for blanks. This prevents high blanks from occurring due to the presence of small amounts of ferricyanide.

(7) Caution is necessary regarding the use of any lubricant in the stopcocks of an automatic buret for isobutyl alcohol, if such equipment is used. Vaseline, Lubriseal, or other similar lubricants are dissolved by isobutyl alcohol and will contribute to the fluorescence. Silicone, glycerol, or orthophosphoric acid have been reported to be acceptable for use.

(8) Some investigators use stronger alkali and more ferricyanide whereas others have shown no difference in assay values when the alkali is increased (29,39,40,50,57). Some have advocated addition of the alkaline ferricyanide solution dropwise until a faint yellow color persists. This avoids any great excess of ferricyanide (41). Regardless of the procedure used, the yellow color should persist for at least 15 sec.

(9) Whichever of the many techniques possible is chosen, each analyst should standardize the technique. Each sample and standard should consistently receive exactly the same treatment.

(c) Repeat steps (a) and (b) using the working thiamin KCl eluate.

4. *Separation of Thiochrome Solution.*

(a) Centrifuge the reaction vessels 1–3 min.

(b) Siphon out the aqueous lower layers and add 2–3 g of anhydrous, granular Na_2SO_4 to the alcohol solution. Shake for 30 sec.

(1) A siphon bottle may be used for removal of the aqueous layer.

(2) The Na_2SO_4 need not be weighed. If the purification step is omitted, more Na_2SO_4 may be necessary (34). Roughly equal amounts should be added to all vessels to carry out this drying procedure, because large variance in the amount used may produce variation in the readings. The Na_2SO_4 may be checked for background fluorescence by shaking 2–3 g with 15 mL of isobutyl alcohol and comparing the reading with that of the alcohol alone. If the difference is more than 2–3% transmission, the lot should be rejected.

(3) Some analysts prefer to use 1 mL of ethanol instead of Na_2SO_4 (51).

(c) Centrifuge for 1 min.

(1) Centrifuging increases the amount of isobutyl alcohol recoverable from the Na_2SO_4 and minimizes the possibility of decanting Na_2SO_4 particles into the cuvet or reading tube.

5. *Preparation of Blank.*

(a) Place a second aliquot of the acid KCl eluate into a reaction vessel. Treat it identically, except that 15% NaOH is added rather than alkaline ferricyanide.

(1) Samples and blanks should be run simultaneously.

(2) In some samples nonthiamin fluorescent substances are affected differently by the alkaline ferricyanide and the NaOH solutions. In such cases, blanks prepared with NaOH are not valid. In some matrices, it has been shown (58) that much of this interference can be eliminated by adding 0.50 mL of a mixture of equal parts of concentrated HCl and 85% H_3PO_4 to the reaction vessels containing the assay solution and the blank solution before shaking with isobutyl alcohol.

(3) An alternative blank may be used by adding one drop of concentrated HCl to the cuvet or reading tube after the initial reading has been made. Mix and determine the fluorescence again. The fluorescence of thiochrome is quenched in this manner. Collaborative studies have shown this to be a valid blank procedure on cereal products (36). The applicability of this procedure to a wide range of matrices has not been completely investigated.

6. *Measurement of Thiochrome.*

(a) Decant 10 mL of the clear colorless isobutyl alcohol solutions into matched cuvets or standardized reading tubes.

(1) Colored isobutyl alcohol solutions may cause erroneous readings. Recovery experiments must be conducted before reliance can be placed on the analysis of such solutions.

(2) The amount of isobutyl alcohol solution used for fluorescence measurement is dependent upon the instrument used (60). The volume used for this need not be accurately measured except to guarantee that the minimum necessary for the instrument is used.

(b) Determine the fluorescence of isobutyl alcohol solutions, operating the fluorometer according to the manufacturer's instructions. Check the fluorometer between readings with a glass standard or with the working quinine solution.

(1) Since ultraviolet light destroys thiochrome, readings should be made rapidly. The maximum exposure should be 10–15 sec.

(2) All solutions should be at room temperature.

(3) Although thiochrome is stable in isobutyl alcohol, readings should be made promptly.

7. *Calculation.*

(a) The thiamin content, calculated as thiamin hydrochloride, in

$$\mu g/g = \frac{S - SB}{ST - STB} \times \frac{C}{A} \times \frac{25}{V} \times \frac{100}{SW}$$

where S = % transmittance of the sample;

         SB = % transmittance of the sample blank;

         ST = % transmittance of the standard;

    STB = % transmittance of the standard blank;

         C = concentration of the standard;

         A = aliquot taken;

        25 = final volume of eluate;

         V = volume used in purification step;

     100 = volume original sample was made up to;

      SW = sample weight.

(1) This calculation assumes the same size aliquot for samples and standard. If different size aliquots are used, the calculation must be adjusted.

(2) If the thiamin present is in a form other than thiamin hydrochloride, the calculation may also need to be adjusted (e.g., if thiamin mononitrate is present, multiply the thiamin hydrochloride results by 0.97).

(3) Providing that a homogeneous sample can be obtained, the precision on duplicate analyses made on separate days should be ±2.5–5.0% of the mean depending on the skill of the analyst.

Application of Method

This method is applicable to a wide range of sample matrices. Among these are meats, cereals and grain products, milk and dairy products, fresh and dehydrated fruits and vegetables, poultry, animal feeds, pet foods, pharmaceuticals and vitamin concentrates, processed foods, "health" foods, snack foods, diet supplements, etc.

1. The procedure has been applied to almost any matrix imaginable (13). Minor modifications may be necessary in some cases.

2. On certain matrices, some steps in the procedure may be omitted (e.g., on pharmaceuticals and vitamin concentrates, the 2-hr enzyme incubation and the chromatography steps may be omitted). On most products it is advisable for the analyst to determine by proper experimentation whether any of the steps in the procedure may be eliminated.

LITERATURE CITED

1. Freed, M. *Methods of Vitamin Assay*, 3rd ed. Interscience, New York, 123–145 (1966).
2. *The Merck Index*, 9th ed., Merck, Rahway, N.J., 9029 (1976).
3. *CRC Handbook of Chemistry and Physics*, 62nd ed. CRC Press, Inc., Boca Raton, Fla. C-570 (1981–1982).
4. *Lange's Handbook of Chemistry*, 12th ed. McGraw-Hill, New York (1979).
5. Williams, R. R. and Spies, T. D. *Vitamin B_1 and Its Use in Medicine*. MacMillan, New York (1938).
6. Williams, R. R. "The chemistry of thiamine (vitamin B_1), Chapter VII." *The Vitamins*: "A symposium arranged under the auspices of the Council on Pharmacy and Chemistry and the Council on Foods of the American Medical Association." The American Medical Association, Chicago, Il. (1939).
7. *Annotated Bibliography, Vitamin B_1*. Merck, Rahway, N.J. (1941).
8. Rosenberg, H. R. *Chemistry and Physiology of the Vitamins*. Interscience, New York, 99–150 (1942).
9. Beadle, B. W., Greenwood, D. A., and Kraybill, H. R. "Stability of thiamine to heat." *J. Biol. Chem.* **149**, 339 (1943).
10. Elvehjem, C. A. "The water soluble vitamins, Chapter XI." *Handbook of Nutrition*: "A symposium prepared under the auspices of the Council on Foods and Nutrition of the American Medical Association." The American Medical Association, Chicago, Ill. (1943).
11. Williams, R. R. and Cline, J. K. "Synthesis of vitamin B_1." *J. Am. Chem. Soc.* **58**, 1504 (1936).
12. Melnick, D., Hochberg, M., and Oser, B. L. "Physiological availability of the vitamins—2. The effect of dietary thiaminase in fish products." *J. Nutr.* **30**, 81 (1945).
13. Hazleton Raltech, Inc., Unpublished.
14. Sebrell, W. H., Jr. and Harris, R. S. "Thiamine." In *The Vitamins: Chemistry, Physiology, Pathology, and Methods*. Academic Press, New York, 98 (1967).
15. Defibaugh, P., Smith, J. S., and Weeks, C. E. "Assay of thiamine in foods, using manual and semiautomated fluorometric and microbiological methods." *J. Assoc. Off. Anal. Chem.* **60**, 522 (1977).
16. Association of Official Analytical Chemists. *Official Methods of Analysis*, 13th ed. Washington, D.C., 43.024–43.029 and 750 (1980).

17. Ellefson, W. C., Richter, E., Adams, M., and Baillies, N. T. "Evaluation of ion exchange resins and various enzymes in thiamine analysis." *J. Assoc. Off. Anal. Chem.* **64**, 1336 (1981).

18. Association of Official Analytical Chemists. *Official Methods of Analyses*, 13th ed. Washington D.C., 43.013 and 741 (1980).

19. Soliman, A. M. "Comparison of manual and benzenesulfonyl chloride—semiautomated thiochrome procedures for the analysis of thiamine in food." Abstract 94th Annual Meeting, Association of Official Analytical Chemists, 32 (1980).

20. Kinnersley, H. W. and Peters, R. A. "Note upon the preparation of crude cocarboxylase from vitamin B$_1$ by yeast." *Biochem. J.* **32**, 697 (1938).

21. Ang, C. Y. W. and Mosley, Frederick A. "Determination of thiamin and riboflavin in meat and meat products by high-pressure liquid chromatography." *J. Agric. Food Chem.* **28**, 483 (1980).

22. Roser, R. L., Andrist, A. H., and Harrington, W. H. "Determination of urinary thiamin by high-pressure liquid chromatogrphy." *J. Chromatogr.* **46**, 43 (1978).

23. Fellman, J. K., Artz, W. E., Tassinari, P. J., Cole, C. L., and Augustin, J. "Simultaneous determination of thiamin and riboflavin in selected foods by high performance liquid chromatography." *J. Food Sci.* **47**, 2048 (1982).

24. Roser, R. L., Andrist, A. H., Harrington, W. H., Naito, H. K., and Lonsdale, D. "Determination of urinary thiamine by high pressure liquid chromatography utilizing the thiochrome fluorescent method." *J. Chromatogr.* **140**, 43 1976).

25. Kamman, J. F., Labuza, T. P., and Warthesen, J. J. "Thiamin and riboflavin analysis by high performance liquid chromatography." *J. Food Sci.* **45**, 1497 (1980).

26. Ishii, K., Sarai, K., Sanemori, H., and Kawasaki, T. "Analysis of thiamine and its phosphate esters by high-performance liquid chromatography." *Anal. Chem.* **97**, 191 (1979).

27. Seifert, R. M. and Mung, C. F. "Analysis of thiamine in pinto beans by gas chromatography of its sulfite cleavage products *S*-(2-hydroxyethyl)-4-methyl thiazole." *J. Assoc. Off. Anal. Chem.* **56**, 1273 (1973).

28. Kinnersley, H. W., O'Brien, J. R., and Peters, R. A. "The properties of blue fluorescent substances formed by oxidation of vitamin B$_1$ (quinochromes)." *Biochem. J.* **29**, 2369 (1935).

29. Jansen, B. C. P. "A chemical determination of aneurin by the thiochrome reaction." *Rec. Trav. Chim.* **55**, 1046 1936).

30. Bechtel, W. G. and Hollenbeck, C. M. "A revised thiochrome procedure for the determination of thiamine in cereal products." *Cereal Chem.* **35**, 1 (1958).

31. McRoberts, L. H. "Determination of thiamine in enriched cereal and bakery products." *J. Assoc. Off. Anal. Chem.* **43**, 47 (1960).

32. Hennessy, J. D. J. and Cerecedo, L. R. "The determination of free and phosphorylated thiamine by a modified thiochrome assay." *J. Am. Chem. Soc.* **61**, 179 (1939).

33. *Determination of Thiamine Hydrochloride by the Thiochrome Method, with the Adaptation of the Hennessy and Cerecedo Procedure, as Carried out in the Laboratories of Merck and Co., Inc., Rahway, N.J.* Merck & Co., Inc., Rahway, N.J. (1941).

34. Andrews, J. S. and Nordgren, R. "The application of the thiochrome method to the thiamine analysis of cereals and cereal products." *Cereal Chem.* **18**, 686 (1941).

35. Booth, R. G. "Estimation of aneurine—the aneurine content of wheats." *J. Soc. Chem. Ind.* **59**, 181 (1940).

36. McRoberts, L. H. "Determination of thiamine in enriched flour, comparison of fluorometric methods." *J. Assoc. Off. Agric. Chem.* **37**, 757 (1954).

37. Halliday, N. and Denel, H. J. "Free and combined thiamine in milk." *J. Biol. Chem.* **140**, 555 (1941).

38. McRoberts, L. H. "Report on the determination of thiamine in enriched cereal and bakery products." *J. Assoc. Off. Agric. Chem.* **37**, 837 (1953).

39. Conner, R. T. and Straub, G. J. "Determination of thiamine by the thiochrome reaction." *Ind. Eng. Chem., Anal. Ed.* **13**, 380 (1941).

40. McFarlane, W. D. and Chapman, R. A. "An improved thiochrome method for estimation of vitamin B_1." *Can. J. Res.* **19B**, 136 (1941).

41. Wang, Y. L. and Harris, L. J. "Vitamin methods. I. An improved procedure for estimating vitamin B_1 in foodstuffs and biological materials by the thiochrome test including comparisons with biological assays." *Biochem. J.* **33**, 1050 (1941).

42. Ministry of Food. "Vitamin B_1 (aneurine) assay in white flour." *Analyst* **67**, 15 (1942).

43. Clausen, D. F. and Brown, R. E. "Determination of thiamine in bread by the thiochrome method." *Ind. Eng. Chem., Anal. Ed.* **15**, 100 (1943).

44. Hoffer, A., Alcock, A. W., and Geddes, W. F. "A rapid method for the determination of thiamine in wheat and flour." *Cereal Chem.* **20**, 717 (1943).

45. Glick, D. "Simplified procedures for the determination of thiamine in wheat flours and bread by the thiochrome method." *Cereal Chem.* **21**, 119 (1944).

46. Rice, E. E. and Beuk, J. F. "Reaction rates for decomposition of thiamine in pork at various cooking temperatures." *Food Res.* **10**, 99 (1945).

47. Rinde, G. and deGiuseppe, L. "A new chromatographic method for the determination of thiamine and its mono-, di-, and triphosphates in animal tissues." *Biochem. J.* **78**, 602 (1960).

48. Hennessy, D. J. and Bonvicino, G. "Behavior of the disulfide form of thiamine in the thiochrome assay for thiamine." *Abstr., 116th Meeting, Amer. Chem. Soc.* **63C** (Sept., 1949).

49. *The United States Pharmacopeia,* 20th ed. Mack Printing, Easton, Penn., 928 (1980).

50. Friedemann, T. E. and Kmieciak, T. C. "The determination of thiamine in blood." *J. Lab. Clin. Med.* **28**, 1262 (1943).

51. Hinman, W. F., Halliday, E. G., and Brookes, M. H. "Thiamine in beef muscles." *Ind. Eng. Chem., Anal. Ed.* **16**, 116 (1944).

52. Domange, L. and Longuevalle, S. "The separation of vitamin B_1 from other interfering fluorescent substances." *Pharm. Weekblad.* **90**, 119 (1955); in *Chem. Abstr.* **49**, 7810 (1955).

53. Cleland, J. B. "Effect of salicylates on the estimation of thiamine by the thiochrome method." *Austral. J. Exptl. Biol. Med. Sci.* **21**, 153 (1953).

54. Organ, J. G. and Workes, F. "Vitamin B_1 in unmalted and maled cereals and malt extracts." *J. Soc. Chem. Inc.* **63**, 165 (1944).

55. Burch, H. A., Bessey, O. A., Love, R. H., and Lowry, O. "The determination of thiamine and thiamine phosphates in small quantities of blood and blood cells." *J. Biol. Chem.* **198**, 477 (1952).

56. Brown, E. B., Hamm, J. C., and Harrison, H. E. "Comparison of thaimine values by chemical and bioassay methods." *J. Biol. Chem.* **151**, 153 (1943).

57. Watson, H. A. "Study of some factors influencing the oxidation of thiamine to thiochrome." *Cereal Chem.* **23**, 166 (1946).

58. Mickelsen, O., Condiff, H., and Keys, A. "The determination of thiamine in urine by means of the thiochrome technique." *J. Biol. Chem.* **160**, 361 (1945).

59. Owen, P. S., Weissman, N., and Ferrebee, J. W. "Effect of hematin upon stability of thiochrome in solutions of alkaline ferricyanide." *Proc. Soc. Exptl. Biol. Med.* **52**, 59 (1943).

60. Loofbourow, J. R. and Harris, R. S. "The evaluation of fluorophotometers to be used in the thiochrome assay for vitamin B_1." *Cereal Chem.* **19**, 151 (1943).

14 Riboflavin

Jitendra J. Shah

GENERAL CONSIDERATIONS

Riboflavin (synonymous with vitamin B$_2$, lactoflavin, vitamin G, hepatoflavin, 7,8-dimethyl-10-(1′-ribityl) isoalloxazine is a yellow-green, fluorescent, water-soluble pigment widely distributed in plant and animal cells (1–6). It has the following structural formula:

Riboflavin or 7,8-dimethyl-10-(1′-ribityl) isoalloxazine

It crystallizes from absolute alcohol and is a yellow-orange, needle-shaped crystal cluster. Other properties are:

Empirical formula	C$_{17}$H$_{20}$N$_4$O$_6$
Molecular weight	376.37
Melting point	271–293°C (decomposition)
Solubility:	
Water (25°C)	0.012 g/100 mL
Ethanol (100%) (27.5°C)	0.0045 g/100 mL

Ethyl ether, acetone, benzene,   Insoluble
and chloroform
Optical rotation$[\alpha]_D^{20}$ $-114°$ (in 0.1 N NaOH)
Redox potential -0.21 V (pH 7.0)

The melting point variation is due partly to polymorphism of riboflavin crystals. The lower melting form(s) of riboflavin are about 10 times as soluble in water as the higher melting form. The fully reduced form (flavohydroquinone) is much less soluble (7).

Riboflavin is relatively stable in dry form under normal lighting. Riboflavin is stable in strong mineral acids even at elevated temperatures, and toward most oxidizing agents (H_2O_2, Br_2H_2O, concentrated HNO_3), but it is oxidized by chromic acid. It is also destroyed by $KMnO_4$ in 0.1 N acetic acid in 10 min at room temperature; but at pH 4.5 there is less than 10% destruction by $KMnO_4$ in 10 min (8). Although stable in the presence of H_2O_2, it is decomposed by H_2O_2 in the presence of ferrous ion (9). It is unstable in alkaline solutions. Riboflavin is reversibly reduced to a lencobase, a dehydro compound, by active hydrogen, sodium hydrosulfite, stannous and titanous chloride, and alkaline sulfides. Irradiation of alkaline solutions yields lumiflavin (6,7,9-trimethylisoalloxazine) and in acid solutions lumichrome (6,7-dimethyl alloxazine) is formed, which is characterized by a blue fluorescence.

It is very sensitive to both visible and ultraviolet light (10,11). All manipulations with riboflavin or riboflavin-containing materials should be carried out in subdued light or in low-actinic glassware. Even subdued daylight may be destructive but artificial light of an intensity of 6 candles per square feet or less is permissible (12).

Lumiflavin   Lumichrome

One of the distinguishing properties of riboflavin is its yellow-green fluorescence in neutral solutions which reaches a minimum at pH 6.7–6.8.

Riboflavin in aqueous solution shows four major bands centered around 220, 267, 373, and 447 nm that vary somewhat depending on the nature of the environment of the flavin chromophore. The 373-nm band is the most affected by solvent, generally shifting to shorter wavelengths with decreasing solvent polarity (7).

Based on the similarity between the action spectrum for phototropism and the spectrum of riboflavin in castor oil Galston (14) suggested flavins in a hydrophobic environment to be involved in phototropism in plants. The UV-visible spectra of 20 different samples of riboflavin in dilute acetic acid solution consist of three major bands around 266, 371, and 444 nm. Since these bands are associated with the isoalloxazine portion of the molecule, they cannot be taken as proof of identity, but such constants have value in control work on pharmaceutical preparations.

Riboflavin shows an intense fluorescence at about 530 nm for emission and a fluorescence quantum yield $\pi f = 0.25$ for riboflavin in water. When flavins are bound to proteins, there is generally a dramatic quenching of fluorescence. Recent studies of flavin analog binding and fluorescence (16) as Shethna flavoprotein suggest that the hydroxyl groups of the ribityl side chains play a role in fluorescence quenching (17). Modifications of the riboflavin molecule by shifting the methyl group from position 7 to 8 destroy the vitamin and coenzyme activity. At least one of the methyl groups in position 6 or 7 is required for vitamin activity in a flavin molecule. So far as the side chain is concerned, only D-ribityl or to a lesser extent L-arabityl groups attached to the nitrogen atom in position 9 have thus far been demonstrated to be associated with vitamin activity of flavins.

In living cells, riboflavin generally occurs combined either with phosphoric acid or with phosphoric acid and adenylic acid, both of which may be combined with specific proteins to form oxidative enzymes. In some products, like milk, riboflavin is reported to be in part in a free, dialyzable form. In most analytical procedures for riboflavin, it is necessary to treat natural products with acid or enzymes to get maximal values. This insures the liberation of riboflavin from its protein combination and makes it more readily extractable.

METHODS AVAILABLE

The methods that are available for the determination of riboflavin are animal and microbiological, as well as physical and chemical.

Animal assays (20–25) using rats or chicken were developed prior to the other methods. The rat assay (20) was the original standard for other methods. The Bourguin-Sherman rat diet for riboflavin assays, however, does not permit as great a rate of growth as a similar diet supplemented with additional thiamin, pyridoxine, calcium, pantothenate, and choline. Values obtained by the use of this rat diet tend to be too high because of the presence of additional amounts of these B vitamins in the food analyzed (26). Animal assays are the most time-consuming, expensive, and the least accurate. Their main advantage is that they best reflect riboflavin bioavailability.

The most commonly used microorganism for the analysis of riboflavin is *Lactobacillus casei.* The two other microorganisms that have also been used for the determination of this vitamin—*Leuconostoc mesenteroides* (27) and the protozoan *Tetrahymena pyriformis* (28) have not found widespread acceptance. *T. pyriformis* has the advantage of reacting to riboflavin specifically whereas the other microorganisms respond not only to riboflavin but to some of its analogs, which are devoid of biological value as well (27, 29).

The spectrophotometric measurement of riboflavin is often satisfactory for assaying pharmaceutical preparations. However, because of its low sensitivity and the presence of interfering substances, it is not used as an assay method in foods.

The fluorometric method (18,19) is probably most commonly used for the determination of riboflavin. Because of its high sensitivity, it is applicable to many food systems. Problems can arise with this method due to the presence of interfering fluorescent substances, for example, nonenzymatic browning reaction compounds. Such problems can often be solved by the conversion of riboflavin to lumiflavin and its subsequent fluorescence determination.

Recently, HPLC has been reported as a method of riboflavin assay, either by itself (30–34) or in conjunction with the simultaneous determination of multiple water-soluble vitamins (35–40). Details on multivitamin analyses by HPLC are outlined in Chapter 4.

A comparison of the rat-growth, microbiological, and fluorometric methods for the determination of riboflavin in pharmaceutical products has been made (41,42). The three methods gave similar and reproducible results on samples of high potency. Greater differences were observed in low-potency samples.

Another comparative study (43) was made of the rat, chick, microbiological, and fluorometric methods for the estimation of riboflavin in dried milk products. Good agreement was obtained between the fluorometric and microbiological assays when fat-soluble factors were removed before applying the latter procedure. The rat and chick assays gave more variable and inconclusive results, usually yielding much higher values than the fluorometric and microbiological methods.

The microbiological and chemical methods lend themselves to semiautomation. Details on these are outlined in Chapters 3 and 5.

ANALYTICAL METHODOLOGY

I.   MICROBIOLOGICAL METHOD
   (*LACTOBACILLUS CASEI* SUBSP. *RHAMNOSUS* ATCC 7469)

A.   Principle

See page 43

B.   Equipment

See page 50

C. Reagents

Reagents 8, 28, 29, 33, 34, 35, 36, and 37 as listed on pages 53–58 are required. In addition, the following reagents will be needed for this method:

38. *0.1 N Hydrochloric Acid.*   Dilute 8.5 mL concentrated HCl to 1 L with H₂O.

39. *Riboflavin Stock.*   Solution A (25 μg riboflavin/mL in 0.02 N acetic acid). Weigh accurately 50 mg USP reference standard riboflavin which has been dried in a vacuum desiccator or oven over conc H_2SO_4 for 24 hr, and transfer quantitatively to a 2-L volumetric flask. Add about 1500 mL H_2O, 2.4 mL glacial acetic acid, and warm to aid solution. After cooling to room temperature, make to volume with H_2O. Preserve under toluene, protected from light, in a refrigerator. When the more concentrated stock solution of 100 μg/mL heretofore recommended by most authors (44) is cooled in a refrigerator, riboflavin crystallizes from solution (45).

40. *Stock Riboflavin Solution B (10μg riboflavin/mL in 0.002 N acetic acid).*   Dilute 40 mL of stock riboflavin solution A to 100 mL with H_2O. Preserve under toluene, protected from light, in a refrigerator.

41. *Riboflavin Working Standard (0.1 μg/mL).*   Dilute 1 mL of stock riboflavin B to 100 mL with H_2O. Prepare immediately before use.

42. *Alkali-Treated Peptone Solution.*   Dissolve 40 g peptone (Difco Bacto or Wilson's is suitable) in 250 mL H_2O, and 20 g of NaOH in 250 mL H_2O. Mix the two solutions. Allow to stand for 18–24 hr, then neutralize with glacial acetic acid (approximately 25 mL). Add 14 g of anhydrous sodium acetate (or 23.2 g $NaC_2H_3O_2 \cdot 3H_2O$) and sufficient H_2O to make to 800 mL. Preserve under toluene in a refrigerator.

43. *0.1% Cystine Solution.*   Suspend 1 g of *l*-cystine in 20 mL H_2O and add concentrated HCl until the crystals are dissolved. No more than 10 mL should be required. Add sufficient H_2O to make a volume of 1 L. Keep under toluene at room temperature.

44. *Yeast Supplement Solution.*   Dissolve 100 g of yeast extract or autolyzed yeast (Difco is suitable) in 500 mL H_2O, and 150 g of basic lead acetate in 500 mL of H_2O. Mix the two solutions, adjust the pH to red phenolphthalein with concentrated NH_4OH, and filter through a Buchner funnel. Adjust the filtrate to pH 6.5 with glacial acetic acid, precipitate the excess lead with H_2S, and refilter. Evaporate about 200 mL H_2O under vacuum to remove the dissolved H_2S. Preserve with toluene and chloroform in the refrigerator. An alternate method of preparing riboflavin-free yeast solution involves the use of Florisil, which quantitatively absorbs riboflavin at a pH of 4.5. Dissolve 20 g of yeast extract in a beaker with 150 mL H_2O. Adjust the pH to 4.5 with acetic acid and add 10 g of Florisil. Stir for 30 min. Filter. Adjust the pH to 4.5 and repeat the treatment with 10 g of additional Florisil. Filter and adjust the pH to 6.8 with 1 N NaOH and make to 200 mL with H_2O.

45. *Basal Medium Stock Solution.*

Quantity	Reagent	Reagent No.
100 mL	Alkali-treated peptone solution	42
100 mL	0.1% Cystine solution	43
20 mL	Yeast supplement solution	44
10 mL	Metals mix A (Reagent 8)	8
10 g	Glucose, anhydrous	

Dissolve the glucose in the mixture of the solutions, adjust the pH to 6.8 with 1 N NaOH, and add sufficient H_2O to make 500 mL.

An entirely different basal medium for the estimation of riboflavin has been proposed by Roberts and Snell (46). Although a total of 18 constituents need to be weighed or measured out, the authors point out how these may be combined into three stock solutions and thus the preparation of the medium greatly simplified. A dehydrated medium is available from Difco.

46. *Culture Medium for Growing Inoculum.* To 250 mL of basal medium stock solution (Reagent 45), add 5 mL stock riboflavin solution B (Reagent 40) and H_2O to 500 mL. Mix well. Add approximately 10 mL to test tubes, plug with appropriate cover, autoclave at 15 psi for 15 min, and store in a refrigerator. This medium contains 1 μg riboflavin in 10 mL. Dehydrated Bacto Lactobacillus Broth (Difco) may be substituted for this reagent.

D. Procedure

The following procedure represents a composite of several published methods. (44,47–55) and unpublished modifications, all of which are adaptations of the original microbiological method of Snell and Strong (56). Note the time relationships (p. 58–60) which must be observed.

1. *Preparation of Stock Culture, L. casei ATCC 7469.* Stock cultures of *L. casei* ATTC 7469 are prepared by stab inoculation of Bacto-Lactobacilli Agar (Reagent 29). Incubate at 35–37°C for 24–48 hr and store tubes in the refrigerator. The culture should be transferred at 2–4-week intervals for maintenance. Fresh stab cultures less than 1 week old are used for inoculum preparation.

2. *Preparation of Inoculum.*

(a) Transfer cells from stock culture to sterile tubes containing 10 mL of Reagent 46 on Bacto-Lactobacilli Broth. Incubate overnight at 35–37°C. Under aseptic conditions, centrifuge culture and decant supernatant. Wash cells with 10-mL portions of sterile 0.9% NaCl solution. Cells should be washed at least one time. The cells are resuspended in 10 mL of sterile 0.9%

NaCl solution. One drop of the dilution is used to inoculate each of the assay tubes.

(1) AOAC procedure requires that cells be washed three times with 10-mL portions of sterile 0.9% NaCl solution. The cells are then suspended in 10 mL of sterile 0.9% NaCl solution. Preparation of the inoculum can be varied to conform to the needs of the investigator's laboratory. Assay controls should produce insignificant growth with the *L. casei* assay.

3. *Preparation of Sample.*   Extraction and hydrolysis.

(a) Into a 125-mL Erylenmeyer flask, weigh a homogeneous sample containing 10 or more μg riboflavin, add 50 mL 0.1 N HCl, and autoclave at 15 psi for 15 min.

(1) When the concentrations of the various members of the B complex (thiamin, riboflavin, niacin, and biotin) are wanted on the same sample or samples, the following general enzymatic digestion procedure has been used for their simultaneous release from plant and animal tissue. Dilute approximately 1 g of finely minced tissue with 8 mL of 0.2 N sodium acetate buffer having a pH of 4.5 to 4.7. Add 1 mL of a freshly prepared enzyme suspension containing 20 mg of papain and 20 mg of Takadiastase/ mL. To prepare the enzyme suspension, mix 20 mg of papain with one drop of glycerine, add 20 mg of Takadiastase, and make to 1 mL with H_2O. In practice, when several samples are assayed simultaneously, a suitable multiple of these quantities is used. After mixing the enzyme with the sample, add a few drops of benzene or toluene, cover loosely, and incubate for 24 hr at 37–45°C (57).

Since papain and Takadiastase contain varying amounts of riboflavin (1–8 μg/g), it is important, especially with low-potency samples, that the vitamin content of each lot of enzyme be determined and proper correction made in the calculation.

Heat the samples in flowing steam or autoclave for 10 min. Add a level teaspoonful (about 1 g) of Filter Cel or equivalent filter aid (must not absorb riboflavin), shake, and filter through a Whatman No. 40 paper. Collect the filtrate in a volumetric flask of suitable size. Wash the residue with small amounts of H_2O and collect the washings with the filtrate. Finally, dilute the extracts so that the riboflavin concentration is between 0.05 and 0.5 μg/mL. If the samples are to be stored, transfer to brown bottles, add a few drops of toluene, and refrigerate.

(b) Cool to room temperature, adjust the pH to 4.5, transfer to a 100-mL volumetric flask, make to volume, and filter.

(1) For most samples, filtration at pH 4.5 is effective in removing growth stimulants and inhibitors, such as starch, fatty acids, and phospholipids. Some workers find that the stimulating effect of starch may be avoided, and lower and more uniform values can be obtained with cereal products if, after autoclaving in 0.1 N HCl, the samples are digested at

50°C for one-half hr with 5 mL of 6% Takadiastase in 2.5 N sodium acetate prior to pH adjustment and filtration. Also, some find that fat has a stimulating effect. In the case of high-fat materials such as cheese, liver meal, and fish meal, the difficulty is overcome by ether extraction (48). After autoclaving with 0.1 N HCl, adjust to pH 4.5, make to volume and filter. Extract a 50-mL aliquot of the filtrate three times with 30-mL portions of ether. Then adjust to pH 6.8 and dilute to 100 mL.

(2) When urine is assayed without dilution as is sometimes necessary when the riboflavin concentration is extremely low, care should be taken that the urea concentration does not exceed 20 μg per tube. If more than this amount is present, the growth of the organism is inhibited. If it is possible to keep the urea concentration below this level, a formula to correct the result has been devised (58).

(c) Measure 50 mL (or an aliquot containing about 5 μg riboflavin) of the filtrate into a 100-mL volumetric flask, adjust the pH to 6.8 and dilute to 100 mL.

4. *Preparation of Standard Tubes.*

(a) To duplicate tubes, add 0.0-, 0.5-, 1.0-, 1.5-, 2.0-, and 3.0-mL quantities of the riboflavin working standard (Reagent 41).

(1) See Section D.3(a),

(b) Add sufficient H_2O to bring the volume in each tube to 5.0 mL.

(c) To each of these tubes add 5.0 mL of the basal medium stock solution (Reagent 45).

5. *Preparation of Assay Tubes.*

(a) To duplicate tubes add five levels of the sample extract ranging from 0.05 to 0.25 μg riboflavin. Volumes of unknown should vary by not less than 0.5 mL. Volumes greater than 5 mL cannot be used.

(1) See Section D.4(a),

(b) Add sufficient H_2O to bring the volume 5.0 mL.

(c) To each of these tubes, add 5.0 mL of basal medium stock solution (Reagent 45). Reagent 24 (page 56) or a commercially prepared dehydrated medium available from Difco may also be used.

6. *Sterilization.*   See page 59.

7. *Inoculation and Incubation.*   See page 59.

8. *Determination.*   See page 60.

9. *Calculation.*   See page 62.

(a) From the titration values of the standard riboflavin tubes, prepare a standard curve plotting mL 0.1 N NaOH against micrograms of riboflavin. Values for a typical standard are shown in the accompanying table. In a similar manner, standard curves can be obtained by plotting transmittance or absorance against micrograms of riboflavin.

Standard (mL)	µg per tube	0.1 N NaOH (mL)
0.0	0.0	0.5
0.0	0.0	0.5
0.5	0.05	2.3
0.5	0.05	2.3
1.0	0.10	4.0
1.0	0.10	4.0
1.5	0.15	5.9
1.5	0.15	5.9
2.0	0.20	8.2
2.0	0.20	8.1
2.5	0.25	9.0
2.5	0.25	9.0
3.0	0.30	10.2
3.0	0.30	10.0

(b) Using this curve, determine the riboflavin content corresponding to the titration value of each tube or to the average value of duplicate tubes. Divide the riboflavin content per tube by the volume of the sample aliquot added to it getting the concentration of riboflavin in terms of µg/mL sample extract. Riboflavin values of less than 0.05 µg or more than 0.30 µg per tube cannot be used, since they are beyond the useful range of the standard curve.

(1) Except for the most precise work, if the titrations for duplicate check within 0.2 mL, the values may be averaged before calculating the content per milliliter. Titrations above 10 mL may be averaged if they do not differ by more than 0.5 mL.

(c) Determine the average concentration of riboflavin per mL of sample extract, using only those values that do not differ from the average by more than 10%.

(1) The term "upward drift" is applied to data in which the calculated values for µg riboflavin/mL of test solution consistently increase as the size of the sample is decreased. Downward drift relates to a corresponding progressive decrease.

The cause of upward drift is the presence in the sample of some growth factor which is inadequately supplied in the basal medium. The remedy is to enrich the basal medium. For this purpose, the use of 14 g of anhydrous sodium acetate in the preparation of the alkali-treated peptone and 10 g of glucose/250 mL of basal medium has been recommended. The above procedure specifies such a medium. Some workers find that this is all that is necessary. Others prefer to enrich their medium further with 6 mL of 1% asparagine, 25 µg of pantothenic acid/250 mL of medium, and to double the amount of cystine. Still others use 1 mg of niacin/250 mL of medium as the only enrichment. Some workers use as much as 15 g of glucose in the preparation of the medium, but this is not desirable because caramelization during autoclaving makes subsequent titration difficult. As little as 5 g of glucose may be used.

Downward drift may be due to some toxic or inhibitory factor in the sample. In these cases, the remedy is to remove these factors; for examples, see references (58–60). Downward drift may also be due to some factor that stimulates at low but not at high concentration of sample. The nature of some of these growth promoters and inhibitors and methods for removing them are discussed in Section 3.b(1) under Extraction and Hydrolysis. This problem of stimulation and inhibition, and enrichment of media, has been ably discussed by Strong (61).

(d) Calculate the riboflavin content of the sample from the formula:

$$\mu g/g = \frac{\text{Average } \mu g/mL \text{ of extract} \times \text{volume}}{\text{Weight of sample}} \times \text{dilution factor.}$$

(1) For samples of potencies such that the procedure can be followed exactly, the volume is 100 mL, Section D.3(b), and the dilution factor is 100/50, Section D.3(c). Effectively, this is equivalent to setting the volume equal to 200 mL. This will simplify calculations somewhat. A sample of 4 g meat scraps was treated with 80 mg of Takadiastase, 80 mg of papain, 30 mL of 0.1 N sodium acetate (pH 4.6), incubated 24 hr at 37°C, autoclaved 30 min at 15 psi, cooled to room terperature, and filtered. The filtrate was adjusted to pH 6.8 with alkali and made up to 200 mL with H_2O.

Sample (mL)		0.1 N NaOH (mL)	μg per tube	μg/mL
0.5		1.5	0.030	
0.5		1.8	0.036	0.072
1.0		3.1		
1.0		3.0		
	Avg. =	3.05	0.076	0.076
1.5		4.3		
1.5		4.3		
	Avg. =	4.3	0.110	0.074
2.0		5.4		
2.0		5.6		
	Avg. =	5.5	0.147	0.073
2.5		7.5		

Sample (mL)	0.1 N NaOH (mL)	μg per tube	μg/mL
2.5	7.6		
Avg. =	7.55	0.185	0.074
		Avg. =	0.074

$$\frac{0.074 \times 100}{4} \times \frac{100}{50} = 3.7 \ \mu g/g \ \text{sample, uncorrected}$$

The riboflavin content of the quantity of enzymes used was 0.8 μg, corresponding to a correction of 0.2 μg/g of sample. The corrected value, therefore, is:

$$3.7 - 0.2 = 3.5 \ \mu g/g.$$

II. FLUOROMETRIC METHOD

A. Principle

Riboflavin fluoresces in light of wavelength 440–550 nm. The yellowish-green fluorescence of riboflavin in UV light is dependent upon the pH of the solution as well as the concentration. Maximum intensity of fluorescence is between pH 6 and 7. The fluorescence is not, however, usually measured in this pH range, but in the range pH 3–5 where the intensity is constant and apart from the effect of salt concentration. Iron content, and concentration of sugars, depends only on the concentration of riboflavin. The intensity of fluorescence is proportional to the concentration of riboflavin in dilute solutions. Riboflavin is measured in terms of the difference between the fluorescence before and after chemical reduction.

B. Equipment

1. *Photofluorometer.*   Any photofluorometer capable of accurately measuring riboflavin concentrations of 0.05–0.2 μg/mL with an excitation filter of about 440 nm and an emission filter of about 565 nm is acceptable.

C. Reagents

All chemicals should meet ACS specifications or be of Reagent Grade. Insofar as possible, contact of reagents and solutions with cork or rubber should be avoided because these materials may contribute fluorescing substances that will interfere with the assay.

1. *0.1 N Hydrochloric Acid.*   Dilute 8.9 mL concentrated HCl to 1 L with H$_2$O.

2. *0.1 N Sodium Hydroxide.*   Dissolve 4 g NaOH pellets in sufficient H_2O to make 1 L.

3. *Glacial Acetic Acid.*

4. *3% Potassium Permanganate.*   Dissolve 3 g $KMnO_4$ in sufficient H_2O to make 100 mL. Prepare fresh daily.

5. *3% Hydrogen Peroxide.*   Prepare this at the time of use by diluting 30% H_2O_2 1 + 9 with H_2O.

6. *Riboflavin Stock Solution (25 μg Riboflavin/mL).*   See Reagent 39, page 369.

7. *Riboflavin Working Standard (0.5 μg Riboflavin/mL).*   Dilute 1 mL stock solution to 50 mL with H_2O. Prepare immediately before use. It may be necessary to test different concentrations of the working standard with the particular instrument to be used, because the various instruments differ in sensitivity.

8. *Sodium Hydrosulfite (Dithionite) $Na_2S_2O_4$.*

D.   Procedure

The following procedure represents a composite of several published methods (62–78) or unpublished modifications but is principally the procedure (79). The analyst who uses modifications of the regular procedure must establish the reliability of deviations from accepted procedures. Pigments and other interfering substances present in the sample must be considered, as well as potency in deciding what steps are necessary or optional.

The fluorometric method is not applicable to samples that contain high concentrations of iron unless it is removed or to those that have been heated so that interfering colors like caramel may be present. Since riboflavin is light-sensitive and is most readily destroyed by light in the blue and violet regions, it is necessary to perform all operations in the absence of strong light. The use of red or amber glassware or a darkened room is advantageous. *The higher the pH of the solution, the greater will be the destruction of riboflavin in the presence of light.*

1. *Extraction.*

(a) Weigh a sample estimated to contain a 5–10 μg of riboflavin and transfer to a 125-mL Erlenmeyer flask. After adding 50 mL of 0.1 N HCl to the flask, autoclave for 30 min at 15 psi.

(1) When a sample solution contains a high concentration of inorganic iron, this iron may be removed immediately after autoclaving by the addition of an excess of phosphoric acid, sodium phosphate, or potassium phosphate and precipitating and filtering at pH 4.5–6.6.

(2) Some materials such as dry mineral–vitamin feed supplements may contain enough basic substances to neutralize or more than neutralize 50 mL of 0.1 N HCl. Where an appreciable amount of basic substances is present, an excess of dilute HCl should be added. For many types of

samples, even after adjustment to proper acidity, it has been found necessary that the volume of 0.1 N HCl be equal in mL to not less than 10 times the dry weight of the sample in grams (80).

(3) If an autoclave, pressure retort, or pressure cooker is not available, extraction may be accomplished in a boiling water bath agitating every 5 min for 1 hr.

(4) An acid-acetone extraction has been used by some workers (81) to eliminate troublesome cloudiness that occurs with some samples. The acetone flocculates colloidal suspensions and prevents the absorption of riboflavin from solution by proteins.

2. *Precipitation of Interfering Impurities.*

(a) After autoclaving, cool the sample and adjust to pH 6.0 with NaOH. Since riboflavin is unstable in alkaline solution, the extract should be swirled constantly during the addition of alkali to prevent local areas of high pH. Immediately add 1 N HCl to bring the pH to 4.5.

(1) Some workers prefer to add sufficient 2.5 M sodium acetate to bring the pH to 4.5 without any preadjustment to pH 6.0 (81). However, this procedure may not be as effective as precipitation in the pH range of 4.5–6.0.

(2) It is necessary to remove interfering substances by precipitation through a pH range of 4.5–7.0 followed by oxidation at an acid pH. In some products, it may be necessary to include further purification steps; it is better to use the microbiological procedure for the analysis of samples that are highly colored or difficult to purify. Absorption and elution techniques have been used for this purpose (65).

(3) After autoclaving, cool the sample, add 15 mL of 2% Takadiastase in 2.5 M sodium acetate. Incubate overnight at 37°C.

(b) Dilute the solution to 100 mL with H_2O and filter.

(c) To a 50-mL aliquot of the filtrate, add 1 N HCl dropwise until no more precipitate forms. Follow by an approximately equal number of drops of 1 N NaOH with constant shaking. Dilute the aliquot to 100 mL with water and filter again if necessary.

(1) Care must be taken not to add an excess of NaOH so that the pH is raised above 6.6. If an equal number of drops of HCl and then NaOH are added, no such difficulty should be encountered.

3. *Acidification of Extract.*

(a) Add 10 mL of sample solution and 1 mL H_2O to each of two test tubes and mix.

(1) The addition of 1 mL H_2O compensates for the extra dilution of the sample by the standard in the following step and thus simplifies the calculation by eliminating the volume correction.

(b) Add 10 mL of sample solution and 1 mL of riboflavin working standard (0.5 µg/mL) to each of two other test tubes and mix.

(1) This and the preceding step may be carried out directly in the cuvettes. If test tubes are used, transfer the contents to cuvettes prior to the measurement of fluorescence. The oxidation and fluorometry are carried out in duplicate for each sample.

(c) Add 1 mL of glacial acetic acid to all four tubes and mix.

4. *Oxidation.*

(a) Add 0.5 mL of 3% $KMnO_4$ to each tube, mix, and allow to stand for exactly 2 min.

(1) Removal of the interfering fluorescent substances and pigments that occur in extracts may also be accomplished by treatment with $SnCl_2$ and $Na_2S_2O_4$. These reagents reduce the interfering fluorescent substances and the riboflavin to the nonfluorescent form. Shaking in the presence of air oxidizes the riboflavin and the fluorescence may then be measured.

(b) After 2 min add 0.5 mL of 3% H_2O_2 and mix thoroughly. The red color should disappear within 10 sec.

(1) Sufficient H_2O_2 should be added to just decolorize the tubes. Avoid an excess of H_2O_2 because bubbles will form and interfere with the reading of the fluorescence and the use of $Na_2S_2O_4$ for reading the blank.

(2) A fine precipitate, MnO_2, may be formed at this point. Centrifugation will settle this precipitate and result in a clear solution. Usually, however, solutions are clear.

5. *Fluorometry.*

(a) Measure fluorescence of the extract containing added H_2O (reading "A"). Add with mixing approximately 20 mg of $Na_2S_2O_4$ and measure fluorescence within 10 sec (reading "C").

(1) Sufficient mixing may be accomplished by tapping the cuvette against the finger. Care should be taken not to scratch the cuvet if a stirring rod is used.

(2) Excessive quantities of $Na_2S_2O_4$ should be avoided since high salt concentrations may change the fluorescent properties of the blanks. Since the blank may change on standing, it should be read immediately after the addition of the $Na_2S_2O_4$.

(3) Instead of solid $Na_2S_2O_4$, 0.5 mL of a 5% solution prepared by dissolving 5 g of $Na_2S_2O_4$ in 100 mL of an ice-cold $NaHCO_3$ solution (2 g of $NaHCO_3/100$ mL) may be used. The addition of the solution instead of the solid prevents use of an excess of $Na_2S_2O_4$. With care, however, an excess can be avoided even with the solid. The use of the solution has two disadvantages—it is stable for only 2–4 hr even in an ice bath and corrections for a change in volume are necessary.

(4) During the fluorescence measurements, care should be taken to avoid excess exposure of the solution to the ultraviolet light, which causes rapid destruction of riboflavin.

(b) Measure fluorescence of the extracts containing added riboflavin (reading "B").

6. *Calculation.*

(a) Calculate the riboflavin content of the sample from the following formula:

$$\frac{A-C}{B-A} \times \frac{\text{riboflavin increment}}{10 \text{ mL aliquot}} \times \text{dilution factor} \times \frac{1}{\text{sample weight}} = \mu g/g$$

(1) The factor $\dfrac{A-C}{B-A} \times$ riboflavin increment equals μg per 10-mL aliquot. This divided by 10 equals concentration per mL. If the dilutions recommended above can be used the formula will reduce to:

$$\frac{A-C}{B-A} \times \frac{0.5}{10} \times \frac{100}{50} \times 100 \times \frac{1}{\text{weight}} = \frac{A-C}{B-A} \times \frac{10}{\text{weight}} = \mu g/g$$

(2) The following example illustrates the method of calculation suggested. Two grams of feed were extracted yielding 100 mL of assay solution after precipitation and filtration. During the procedure, a 50-mL aliquot was diluted to 100 mL and a 10-mL aliquot of this solution was pipetted into the cuvets.

	Fluorometer Reading		
Reading	Dup. I	Dup. II	Average
A 10 mL filtrate + 1 mL H_2O	65.3	64.8	65.0
B 10 mL filtrate + 0.5 μg riboflavin	86.5	85.5	86.0
C Blank of filtrate	2.2	2.2	2.2

$$\frac{65.0-2.2}{86.0-65.0} \times \frac{0.5}{10} \times \frac{100}{50} \times 100 \times \frac{1}{2} = 15.0 \ \mu g/g$$

(3) Calculation by the increment technique compensates for the variations that may occur in the fluorescence of riboflavin in the presence of interfering substances. Theoretically, these interfering substances will affect both standard and sample fluorescence similarly, thus correcting for the effect of salt content, extraneous color, and solvent concentration. With certain extracts, it is possible to determine the riboflavin content by direct comparison of an aliquot with that obtained for a standard riboflavin solution carried through the identical procedure. The advantage of this method over that of the increment technique lies in the fact that only one value need be determined for the standard of a whole series of extracts, thus eliminating the numerous readings made in the increment technique

and also minimizing variations in the reading of the standard. In such cases the calculation becomes:

$$\frac{\text{Sample} - \text{sample blank}}{\text{standard blank}} \times \mu\text{g in standard} \times \frac{\text{dilution factor}}{\text{weight of sample}} = \mu\text{g}/\text{g}$$

This method is applicable only to those extracts having low blanks and little, if any, interfering fluorescent substances. Whenever it is employed for a new product, the results should be checked by the increment technique.

(4) These calculations do not take into account the possibility of loss of riboflavin during the procedure. If such corrections are desired, treat 6 mL of stock riboflavin solution exactly as the sample including extraction, precipitation, oxidation, and fluorometry as described in Sections D.2, D.3, D.4, and D.6. Calculate the percent recovery, and, to correct values for the loss of riboflavin during the procedure, divide each by this percentage.

(5) All three readings may be made on one aliquot by first taking reading A, adding 1 mL of standard, mixing and taking reading B, followed by addition of $Na_2S_2O_4$ and taking reading C. In this case, the calculation is identical except that readings B and C must be multiplied by $^{11}/_{10}$ to correct for changes in volume.

LITERATURE CITED

1. Kuhn, R., Reinemund, K., Weygard, F., and Strobele, R. "Uber die Synthese des Lactoflavins (Vitamin B_2)." *Ber.* **68**, 1765 (1935).

2. Karrer, P. and Meerwein, H. F. "Eine verbesserte Synthese des Lactoflavins und 6,7-Dimethyl-9-(1'-arabity)-isoalloxazins." *Helv. Chim. Acta* **19**, 264 (1936).

3. Booher, L. E. "Chemical aspects of riboflavin, Chapter 13." *The Vitamins*: "A symposium arranged under the auspices of the Council on Pharmacy and Chemistry and the Council on Foods of the American Medical Association." American Medical Association, Chicago (1939). Figure 14.1 reproduced from p. 265, courtesy Dr. Booher and the Amer. Med. Assoc.

4. Rosenburg, H. R. *Chemistry & Physiology of Vitamins.* Interscience, New York, 153–194 (1942).

5. Merck & Company, Inc. *Annotated Bibliographies—Riboflavin.* Rahway, New Jersey (1941) (1942).

6. Elvehjem, C. A. "The water soluble vitamins, Chapter XI." *Handbook of Nutrition*: "A symposium prepared under the auspices of the Council on Foods and Nutrition of the American Medical Association." American Medical Association, Chicago (1943).

7. Rivlin, R. S. *Riboflavin.* Plenum Press, New York, 2–3 (1975).

8. Strong, F. M., Kruger, E. O., and Lerner, E. Private communication.

9. Leviton, A. "The microbiological synthesis of riboflavin—a theory concerning its inhibition." *J. Am. Chem. Soc.* **68**, 835 (1946).

10. Williams, R. R. and Cheldelin, V. H. "Destruction of riboflavin by light." *Science* **96**, 22 (1942).

11. DeMerre, L. J. and Brown, W. S. "Effect of various lighting conditions on riboflavin solutions." *Arch. Biochem.* **5**, 181 (1944).

12. Ottes, R. T. and Roberts, F. "Protection of riboflavin from destructive light rays during analysis." *J. Assoc. Off. Agric. Chem.* **32**, 797 (1949).

13. Penzer, G. R. and Radda, G. K. "The chemistry and biological function of isoalloxazines (flavines)." *Quant. Rev. Biol.* **21**, 43 (1967).

14. Galston, A. W. "Regulatory systems in higher plants." *Am. Science* **55**, 149 (1967).

15. Trus, B. L., Wells, J. L., and Johnstone, R. M. "Crystal structure of the yellow 1:2 molecular complex lumiflavin-bisnaphthalene-2,3-diol." *Chem. Commun.* 751 (1971).

16. Edmondson, D. E. and Tollin, G. "Chemical and physical characterization of the shethna flavoprotein and apoprotein and kinetics and themodynamics of flavin analogue binding to the apoprotein." *Biochem.* **10**, 124 (1971).

17. McCormick, D. B. "Nature of the intramolecular complex of flavin adenine dinucleotide in molecular associations in biology." In B. Pullman, Ed., *Molecular Associations in Biology. Academic Press, New York, 377 (1978).*

18. Bursch, H. B. "Fluorometric assay of FAD, FMN and riboflavin." In S. P. Colowick and N. O. Kaplan, Eds., *Methods in Enzymology,* Vol. 3. Academic Press, New York, 960 (1957).

19. Association of Official Analytical Chemists. *Official Methods of Analysis,* 13th ed. Washington, D.C. 774 (1980).

20. Bourquin, A. and Sherman, H. C. "Quantitative determination of vitamin G (B_2)." *J. Am. Chem. Soc.* **53**, 3501 (1931).

21. Clark, M. F. "Biological assay of riboflavin." *J. Nutr.* **20**, 133 (1940).

22. Wagner, J. R., Axelrod, A. E., Lipton, M. A., and Elvehjem, C. A. "A rat assay method for the determination of riboflavin." *J. Biol. Chem.* **136**, 357 (1940).

23. Street, H. R. "Studies on the rat growth assay method for riboflavin." *J. Nutr.* **22**, 399 (1941).

24. Wilgus, H. S., Jr., Norris, L. C., and Heuser, G. F. "The relative protein efficiency and relative vitamin G content of common prosupplements used in poultry rations." *J. Agric. Res.* **51**, 383 (1935).

25. Herman, V. and Carver, J. S. "The relative flavin (vitamin G) content of dried skim milk, dried whey and dried buttermilk." *Poultry Sci.* **16**, 434 (1937).

26. Cassner, L. B. and Schuck, C. "Suitability of the Bourquin-Sherman diet for riboflavin assays and results obtained in the assay of evaporated milk." *J. Nutr.* **35**, 725 (1948).

27. Pearson, W. N., Bliss, C. I., and Gyorgy, P. "Riboflavin." In P. Gyorgy and W. N. Pearson, Eds., *The Vitamins,* Vol. 7, 2nd ed. Academic Press, New York, 99–136 (1967).

28. Baker, H. and Frank, O. *Clinical Vitaminology—Methods and Interpretation.* Interscience, New York (1968).

29. Langer, B. W., Jr. and Charoensin, S. "Growth response of lactobacillus casei (ATCC 7469) to riboflavin." *Proc. Soc. Exptl. Biol. Med.* **122**, 151 (1966).

30. Ang, Y. C. W. and Moseley, F. A. "Determination of thiamin and riboflavin in meat and meat products by high-pressure liquid chromatography." *J. Agric. Food Chem.* **28**, 483 (1980).

31. Wittmer, D. P. and Haney, W. G. "Analysis of riboflavin in commercial multivitamin preparations by high speed liquid chromatography." *J. Pharm. Sci.* **63**, 588 (1974).

32. Van de Weedrdjof, J., Wiersum, M. C., and Reissenwebber, A. "Application of liquid chromatography to food analysis." *J. Chromatogr.* **83**, 455 (1973).

33. Rhys, T., Williams, R., and Slavin, W. "Determination of B_2 in milk and urine using HPLC with fluorescent detection." *Chromatogr. Newsletter,* **5**, 9 (1977).

34. Richardson, P. J. Favell, D. J., and Gidley, G. C. "Critical comparison of the determination of B_2 in foods by HPLC." *Proc. Anal. Div. Chem. Soc.* **15**(2), 53 (1978).

35. Callmer, K. and Davies, L. "Separation and determination of vitamin B_1, B_2, B_6 and niacin in

commercial vitamin preparations using high performance cation exchange chromatography." *Chromatographia* **7**, 664 (1974).

36. Rueckemann, H. and Ranifft, K. "Methods for determination of vitamins by means of HPLC." *Z. Lebensm. Unters. Forsch* **166**, 151 (1978).

37. Vinchmeier, R. L. and Upton, R. P. "Simultaneous determination of niacin, niacinamide, pyridoxine and riboflavin in multivitamin blends by ion-pair high-pressure liquid chromatography." *J. Pharm. Sci.* **67**, 1444 (1978).

38. Kamman, J. F., Labuza, T. P., and Warthesen, J. J. "Thiamin and riboflavin analysis by high-performance liquid chromatography." *J. Food Sci.* **45**, 1497 (1980).

39. Skurray, G. R. "A rapid method for selectively determining small amounts of niacin, riboflavin and thiamin in foods." *Food Chem.* **7**, 77 (1981).

40. Fellman, J. K., Artz, W. E., Tassinari, P. D., Cole, C. L., and Augustin, J. "Simultaneous determination of thiamin and riboflavin in selected foods by high-performance liquid chromatography." *J. Food Sci.* **47**, 2048 (1981).

41. Emmett, A. D., Bird, O. D., Brown, R. A., Peacock, G., and Vanderbelt, J. M. "Determination of vitamin B$_2$ (riboflavin). Comparison of bioassay, microbiological and fluorometric methods." *Ind. Eng. Chem., Anal. Ed.* **13**, 219 (1941).

42. Daniel, L. and Norris, L. C. "Riboflavin content of milk and milk products." *Food Res.* **9**, 312 (1944).

43. Sullivan, R. A., Beaty, A., Bloom, E., and Reeves, E. "Determining riboflavin in dried milk products—3. A comparison of methods of assay." *Arch. Biochem.* **2**, 333 (1943).

44. *The United States Pharmacopeia*, 14th ed. Mack Printing, Easton, Penn. 752–755 (1950).

45. Hanson, S. W. F. and Weiss, A. F. "Standard solutions for the estimation of riboflavin." *Analyst* **70**, 48 (1945).

46. Roberts, E. C. and Snell, E. E. "An improved medium for microbiological assays with *Lactobacillus casei.*" *J. Biol. Chem.* **163**, 499 (1946).

47. Scott, M. L., Randall, F. E., and Hessel, F. H. "A modification of the Snell and Strong microbiological methods for determining riboflavin." *J. Biol. Chem.* **141**, 325 (1941).

48. Strong, F. M. and Carpenter, L. E. "Preparation of samples for microbiological determination of riboflavin." *Ind. Eng. Chem. Anal. Ed.* **14**, 909 (1942).

49. Wegner, M. I., Kemmerer, A. R., and Fraps, G. S. "Some factors that affect the microbiological method for riboflavin." *J. Biol. Chem.* **144**, 731 (1942).

50. Andrews, J. S., Boyd, H. M., and Terry, D. E. "Riboflavin analysis of cereals." *Ind. Eng. Chem. Anal. Ed.* **14**, 271 (1942).

51. Arnold, A. "Report of the 1944–45 committee on riboflavin assay." *Cereal Chem.* **22**, 455 (1945).

52. Kremmerer, A. R. "Report on riboflavin." *J. Assoc. Off. Agric. Chem.* **29**, 25 (1946).

53. Yamada, Masoko. "Microbiological assay method for B$_2$ by the cup-plate technique using lactobacillus casei as the test organism." *Vitamin* **42**(55), 294 (1970—Japan).

54. Chatterje, K. P. and Ghose, N. "Microbiological assay of vitamin B$_2$." *Sci. Culture* **36**(12), 656 (1970).

55. Bell, J. G. "Microbiological assay of vitamins of the B group in foods." *Lab. Pract.* **23**(5), 235 (1974).

56. Snell, E. E. and Strong, F. M. "A microbiological assay of riboflavin." *Ind. Eng. Chem. Anal. Ed.* **11**, 346 (1939).

57. Cheldelin, V. H., Eppright, M. A., Snell, E. E., and Guirard, B. M. "Enzymatic liberation of B vitamins from plant and animal tissues." University of Texas Publication 4237, p 15 (1942).

58. Isbell, H., Woodey, J. G., and Fraser, H. F. "The inhibiting effect of urea on the microbiological assay of riboflavin." *U.S. Publ. Health Rep.* **56**, 282 (1941).

59. Eckardt, R. E., Gyorgy, P., and Johnson, L. V. "Presence of a factor in blood which enhances bacterial growth activity of riboflavin." *Proc. Soc. Exptl. Biol. Med.* **46**, 405 (1941).

60. Chattway, F. W., Happold, F. C., and Sandford, M. "The microbiological assay of riboflavin. The influence of inorganic constituents and unknown growth factors." *J. Biochem.* **37**, 298 (1943).

61. Strong, F. M. "The microbiological determination of riboflavin." In *Biol. Symposia*, Vol. 12. Jacques Cattell, Lancaster, Penn. 143–165 (1947).

62. Cohen, F. H. "Eine objektive Methode zur Bestimmung der Flourescenz mit spezieller Anwendung auf die Bestimmung des vitamin B₂." *Acta Brevia Neerland Physiol. Pharmacol Microbiol.* **5**, 18 (1935).

63. Hodson, A. Z. and Norris, L. C. "A fluorometric method for determining the riboflavin content of foodstuffs." *J. Biol. Chem.* **131**, 621 (1939).

64. Supplee, G. C., Bender, R. C., and Jensen, O. G. "Determining riboflavin, a Fluorometric and biological method." *Ind. Eng. Chem., Anal. Ed.* **11**, 495 (1939).

65. Conner, R. T. and Straub, G. J. "Combined determination of riboflavin and thiamin in food products." *Ind. Eng. Chem., Anal. Ed.* **13**, 385 (1941).

66. Kemmer, A. R. "Report on riboflavin." *J. Assoc. Off. Agric. Chem.* **25**, 459 (1942).

67. Andrews, J. S. "Report of the 1943–44 methods of analysis subcommittee on riboflavin assay." *Cereal Chem.* **21**, 398 (1944).

68. Hoffer, A., Alcock, A. W., and Geddes, W. F. "Some factors affecting the determination of riboflavin by the fluorometric method." *Cereal Chem.* **21**, 515 (1944).

69. Rubin, S. H. DeRitter, E., Schuman, R. L., and Bauernfeind, J. C. "Determination of riboflavin in low-potency foods and feeds." *Ind. Eng. Chem., Anal. Ed.* **17**, 136 (1945).

70. Peterson, W. J., Brady, D. E., and Shaw, A. O. "Fluorometric determination of riboflavin in pork products." *Ind. Eng. Chem., Anal. Ed.* **15**, 634 (1943).

71. McLaren, B. A., Cover, S., and Pearson, P. B. "A simplified flurometric method for riboflavin in meat." *Arch. Biochem.* **4**, 1 (1944).

72. Hoffer, A., Alcock, A. W., and Geddes, W. F. "A rapid method for the determination of riboflavin in wheat and wheat products." *Cereal Chem.* **21**, 524 (1944).

73. Sakharov, B. P. and Gordinenko, V. I. "Quantitative determination of riboflavin." Otkrytiya, Izobret, Prom, Obraztsy, Tovarhye, Znaki, **46**(13), 110 (1969).

74. Venkata Rao, E. and Narayanan, M. N. "A colorimetric method for the estimation of riboflavin." *Indian J. Pharm.* **30132**, 70–1 (1968).

75. Woodrow, I. L. and Tome, K. M. "Determination of B₂ in dried milk products." *Can. Inst. of Food Tech. J.* **2**, 120 (1969).

76. DeRitter, E. "Collaborative study of extraction methods for fluorometric assays of riboflavin." *J. Assoc. Off. Anal. Chem.* **53**, 542 (1970).

77. Moszczyhski, P. "Determination of some B group vitamins in multi-vitamin preparations and premixes. I. Determination of riboflavin." Zesz, Nauk, Politech, Lodz. *Chem. Spozyw* **17**, 83 (1970 —Pol).

78. Mueller, V. and Von Lengerlan, M. "Easy method for the determination of riboflavin in premixes and initiation of active principle." *Die. Nahrung* **16**, 375 (1972).

79. Loy, H. W., Jr. "Report on riboflavin." *J. Assoc. Off. Agric. Chem.* **32**, 461 (1949).

80. Loy, H. W., Jr. Private communication.

81. Scott, M. L., Hill, F. W., Norris, L. C., and Heuser, G. F. "Chemical determination of riboflavin." *J. Biol. Chem.* **165**, 65 (1946).

15 Niacin

*Ronald R. Eitenmiller
and Selwyn De Souza*

GENERAL CONSIDERATIONS

Niacin (nicotinic acid or nicotinamide) was one of the first water-soluble vitamins to be isolated and characterized. Chemically, nicotinic acid is pyridine-3-carboxylic acid and nicotinamide is pyridine-3-carboxylic acid amide. Nicotinic acid is readily converted to the physiologically active nicotinamide. Nicotinamide functions metabolically as a component of the coenzymes, nicotinamide adenine dinucleotide (NAD), and nicotinamide adenine dinucleotide phosphate (NADP). These coenzymes act in many oxidation-reduction reactions and function as hydrogen acceptors or donors. Some of the most understood metabolic processes that involve niacin are glycolysis, fatty acid synthesis, and respiration (1). Structures of niacin and its coenzymes are presented in Figure 15.1.

Nicotinic acid and nicotinamide occur as white, needle-shaped crystals or as white crystalline powders. Nicotinamide is more water soluble (100 g/100 mL) than nicotinic acid (1.67 g/100 mL) (2). Both are odor free; however, nicotinamide exhibits a bitter flavor. Some of the more important chemical and physical properties of the two niacin forms are shown in Table 15.1.

Nicotinic acid and nicotinamide are stable in the dry form and in aqueous solutions. They are unaffected by light or pH extremes. Nicotinamide hydrolyzes easily in acid or alkali media, forming nicotinic acid (2). Nicotinic acid is relatively stable to oxidizing agents. Niacin in aqueous solution is stable to heat. Because of its good thermal stability, autoclaving is usually the method of choice for extraction prior to quantitation.

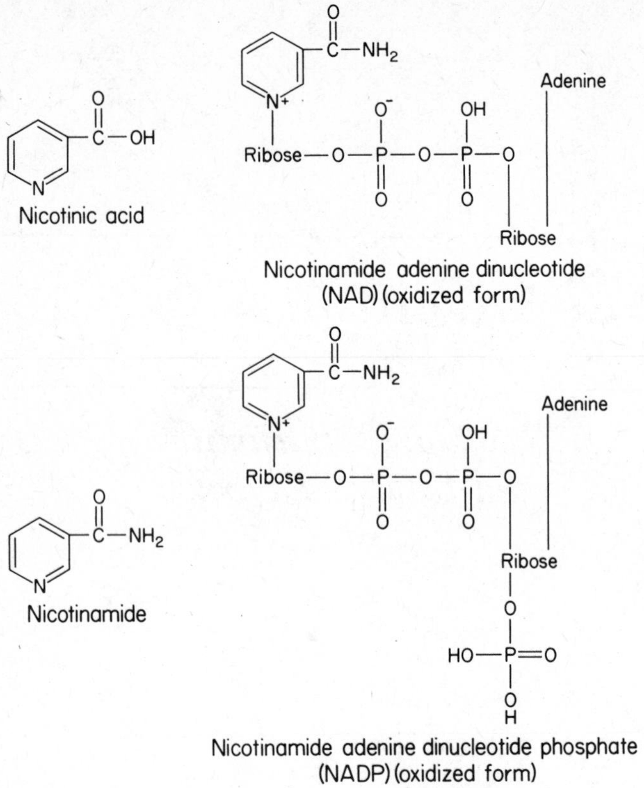

FIGURE 15.1 Structure of niacin and its coenzymes.

TABLE 15.1 Chemical and Physical Properties of Niacin

Properties	Nicotinic Acid	Nicotinamide
Appearance	Colorless needles	Colorless needles
Taste	Tart	Bitter
Empirical formula	$C_6H_5O_2N$	$C_6H_6ON_2$
Molecular weight	123.11	122.12
Melting point	235.5–236.5°C	128–131°C
Boiling point	Sublimes	150–160°C at 5×10^{-4} mm
Hygroscopicity	Nonhygroscopic	Slightly hygroscopic
Absorption maximum	361 nm	361 nm
pH of 1% solution	3.0	6.0
Solubility:		
Water at 25°C	1.67 g/100 mL	100 g/100 mL
Ethyl alcohol	0.73 g/100 mL	66.6 g/100 mL
Ethyl ether	Insoluble	Very slightly soluble
Glycerine at 25°C		10 g/100 mL

Niacin is widely available in the food supply. Average diets in the United States supply 16–34 mg of niacin equivalents per day (3). Although most foods contain fair amounts of niacin, the richest sources are meat and yeast extracts. Because of the contribution of tryptophan, foods containing balanced protein are important to total niacin equivalent intake. For this reason, milk and eggs are considered to be good sources, although the actual niacin content of bovine milk and eggs is somewhat low.

A significant amount of the niacin in unenriched cereal products exists in a bound form. Without further treatment of the products, the bound vitamin is unavailable to man. Hepburn (4) reported that approximately 50% of the niacin in unenriched wheat and wheat products was bound. Treatment of corn with alkali is known to liberate bound niacin, making it biologically available (5). The association of pellagra in man with cereal diets is related to such biologically unavailable forms. Likewise, the alkali treatment of tortilla flour in Central and South America frees bound niacin and prevents pellagra in these areas (6).

Bound forms of niacin in cereals have never been fully characterized. Studies indicate that niacin is bound to carbohydrates or peptides (7,8,9). Recent work by Koetz et al. (10) identified 3-O-nicotinoyl-O-glucose as an acid hydrolysis product of wheat bran (Figure 15.2). It was proposed that the ester linkage between nicotinic acid and the 3-position of glucose establishes one form of bound niacin. Amide linkages between an amino group and the carboxyl group of nicotinic acid provide another potential bonding mechanism, although such structures have not been isolated and characterized.

METHODS AVAILABLE

Several methods are currently available for the determination of niacin in foods, biological fluids, and pharmaceuticals. Regulatory methods at the present time rely on chemical procedures based on the classical Konig reaction in which nicotinic acid reacts with cyanogen bromide to form colored complexes that are measured colorimetrically or by microbiological assay techniques using *Lactobacillus plantarum* ATCC 8014. Semiautomated continuous flow techniques have been successfully applied to the cyanogen bromide method for niacin (11,12) and in many laboratories microbiological assay procedures have been partially automated. The semiautomated method for niacin in food products gives results comparable to both the microbiological and manual colorimetric method results

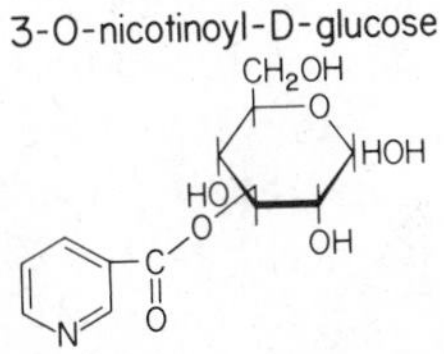

FIGURE 15.2   3-O-nicotinoyl-D-glucose.

(11). A radiometric assay based on the *L. plantarum* microbiological method was recently developed for the determination of niacin in biological fluids (13). The method is reported to have several advantages over the turbidimetric assay including enhanced specificity, lack of interference from colored or turbid sample extracts, and adaptability to automation.

Generally, microbiological assay procedures are applicable to a wider variety of material without modification than are chemical methods. Microbiological assays are not well suited for an occasional assay because the test organism requires frequent attention to maintain continuity in the assay. Chemical methods require fewer reagents and are simpler insofar as the initial preparation is concerned. However, they are somewhat less sensitive than microbiological methods, which makes it more difficult to apply the chemical methods to materials containing low amounts of vitamin. The chemical methods are less specific than microbiological procedures, being influenced by biologically inactive materials occurring naturally or produced during extraction. On the other hand, all microbiological assays are subject to error induced by growth-stimulating or growth-depressing materials in the extract. Microbiological assays must be closely monitored to detect drift from linear response.

In addition to the *L. plantarum* assay, other microorganisms including *Tetrahymena thermophila* (previously *Tetrahymena pyriformis*) and *Leuconostoc mesenteroides* have been successfully applied to niacin quantitation. Use of the protozoan *T. thermophila* permits a wider assay range and more comprehensive response than does *L. plantarum* (14,15). *T. thermophila* utilizes nicotinic acid and nicotinamide, but when they are added together at the same concentration, the growth increment may not equal the sum of the increments when the two forms are added separately (14). Voigt et al. (16) showed niacin levels in low-acid foods to be consistently higher when determined by *T. thermophila* compared with determination by *L. plantarum*.

L. mesenteroides responds only to nicotinic acid. Picolinic acid, isonicotinic acid, quinolinic acid, and nicotinic acid diethylamide are inactive for *L. plantarum* and *L. mesenteroides* assays (17).

At present, officially accepted methods, even with the application of automation, are time consuming, suffer from interference from other materials sometimes present in the extract, often lack sensitivity required for low-concentration products, and, as is the case for the chemical procedure for niacin, require the use of toxic reagents. Microbiological procedures, while sensitive and usually specific, are highly labor intensive.

Problems inherent to existing methods in use for water-soluble vitamin analysis have led investigators to search for new and better methodology. Considerable success has been achieved in adapting high-performance liquid chromatography (HPLC) procedures to water-soluble vitamin analyses. HPLC offers speed, sensitivity, and a high degree of specificity. HPLC methods have been developed for niacin either by itself (18,19,20) or in conjunction with other vitamins (21,22,23) and applied to a variety of foods and biological fluids. Detailed procedures for the microbiological and chemical determination of niacin are given in the following sections. These procedures are based upon currently approved methodology of the Association of Official Analytical Chemists (24) and the American Association of Cereal Chemists (25).

ANALYTICAL METHODOLOGY

I.   MICROBIOLOGICAL METHOD FOR NIACIN AND NIACINAMIDE   (*LACTOBACILLUS PLANTARUM* ATCC 8014)

A.   Principle

See page 43.

B.   Equipment

See page 50.

C.   Reagents

Reagents 1, 2, 3, 4, 5, 6, 7, 8, 9, 28, 29, 33, 34, 35, 36, and 37 which are/or may be needed for this method are listed on pages 51–58. In addition, the following reagents are required for the analysis of niacin:

38. *1N Sulfuric Acid.*   It is usually advantageous to prepare large volumes of this reagent since it is used in extracting the niacin from most materials. Mark a glass carboy at the 18-L mark and fill about three-quarters full of H_2O. Add 500 mL concentrated H_2SO_4 and make to the mark with H_2O, giving an approximately 1N solution.

39. *Working Niacin Standard (0.1 μg/mL).*   Dilute 1 mL of the standard niacin stock solution (Reagent 7) to 1 L with H_2O. This working standard is prepared on the day it is used.

40. *Basal Medium for Niacin Assay.*   Add 1 mL calcium pantothenate (Reagent 5) and 4 mL of a 1:500 dilution of biotin (Reagent 6) stock solutions to 500 mL of the basal medium stock solution (Reagent 9). Mix. A commercially prepared dehydrated niacin medium is available from Difco.

D.   Procedure

The microbiological method described is similar to the procedures outlined by the AOAC and the AACC (24,25). Comments made regarding microbiological procedures made in Section D, Chapter 3, apply for niacin determinations as well.

1. *Preparation of Stock Culture, L. plantarum* ATCC 8014. Prepare stock cultures of *L. plantarum* ATCC 8014 by stab inoculation of Bacto-Lactobacilli Agar AOAC or Bacto-Micro Assay Culture Agar (26). Incubate at 35–37°C for 24–48 hr and store tubes in the refrigerator. The culture should be transferred at 2–4-week intervals for maintenance. Fresh stab cultures less than 1 week old are used for inoculum preparation.

2. *Preparation of Inoculum.*

(a) Transfer cells from stock culture to sterile tubes containing 10 mL of Bacto-Lactobacilli Broth AOAC or Bacto-Micro Inoculum Broth. Incubate overnight at 35–37°C. Under aseptic conditions, centrifuge culture and decant supernatant. Wash cells with 10-mL portions of sterile 0.9% NaCl solution. Cells should be washed at least one time. The cells are resuspended in 10 mL sterile 0.9% NaCl solution. The cell suspension is then diluted 1:100 with 0.9% NaCl solution. One drop of the dilution is used to inoculate each of the assay tubes.

(1) AOAC procedure requires that cells be washed three times with 10-mL portions of sterile 0.9% NaCl solution. The cells are then suspended in 10 mL of sterile 0.9% NaCl solution. Preparation of the inoculum can be varied to conform to the needs of the investigator's laboratory. Assay controls should produce insignificant growth with the *L. plantarum* assay.

3. *Preparation of Samples.*

(a) Weigh sufficient material to contain approximately 0.1 mg of niacin into a 250-mL flask.

(1) In choosing the quantity of material to be extracted, the degree of homogeneity with respect to niacin should be considered. In general, samples smaller than 2.0 g should be avoided. With high-potency material, take 2.0 g and then dilute the extract obtained in Section 3(d) sufficiently to give a niacin concentration of 0.05–0.1 μg/mL.

(b) Add 100 mL of 1 N H_2SO_4 and mix thoroughly.

(1) Dilute acids and H_2O extract less niacin from cereal products than do dilute alkali products (27). Extraction with 1 N H_2SO_4 gives practically the same values for niacin in cereals, animal products, and pharmaceuticals as does extraction with alkali from 0.05 to 1.0 N. Weak acids do not free niacin from the bound forms common in cereals.

(2) AOAC procedures recommend that 1 N H_2SO_4 be added in amounts greater than 10 times the dry weight of dry or semidry samples. If a dry or semidry sample is strongly basic, the pH should be adjusted to 5.0–6.0 with dilute H_2SO_4 and an amount of H_2O 10 times greater than the dry weight of sample is added; 10 mL of 10 N H_2SO_4/100 mL is added to this mixture.

(3) For liquid samples, adjust to pH 5.0–6.0 with dilute H_2SO_4 or dilute NaOH; 10 mL of 10 N H_2SO_4 should be added per 100 mL of pH adjusted liquid.

(c) Autoclave the mixture at 15 psi for 30 min and cool.

(d) Adjust pH to 6.8 with dilute NaOH. Dilute with H_2O to final volume such that 1 mL of extract contains 0.05–0.1 μg niacin/mL. Filter or centrifuge to clarify, if necessary.

(1) If dissolved protein is present, the pH should be adjusted to 6.0–6.5 with NaOH solution and immediately adjusted to pH 4.5 with dilute HCl or until no further protein precipitation is evident. Adjust mixture to a known volume with H_2O and filter or centrifuge. The clarified extract should be adjusted to pH 6.8 with dilute NaOH and adjusted to final volume with H_2O. If cloudiness occurs, the extract can be refiltered or centrifuged.

4. *Preparation of Standard Curve.*   The following determination is based on the turbidimetric quantitation of niacin. Titrimetric methods can be used according to procedures given in the AOAC or AACC (24,25).

(a) To duplicate 16 $\times$ 150—mm tubes, add 0.0, 0.5, 1.0, 1.5, 2.0, 2.5, 3.0, 4.0, and 5.0 mL of the working niacin standard solution. Extra tubes should be set up at the 0.0 level for the uninoculated blank and at the highest standard for use in determining time of maximum growth.

(1) At levels above 0.25–0.30 μg niacin per tube, the growth response as measured turbidimetrically becomes nonlinear. Investigators might find the use of more levels in the lower range of the standard curve useful.

(b) Add sufficient H_2O to bring the volume in each tube to 5.0 mL.

(c) To each of these tubes add 5.0 mL Reagent 40.

(1) Adding the basal medium to the extract and water gives better mixing of the two solutions than adding the extract and water to the basal medium. Better mixing can be attained in this step by allowing part of the basal medium to run down the side of the tube and part to fall directly on the liquid surface. An automatic, 5-mL pipette or pipetting machine is a valuable time saver in this step.

(2) The required number of tubes for both the standard and samples should be placed in a rack and identified either by labeling to withstand autoclaving or by noting their positional arrangement in numbered ranks.

5. *Preparation of Assay Tubes.*

(a) To duplicate tubes add 0.5-, 1.0-, 2.0-, and 3.0-mL aliquots of the sample extract.

(1) The extract is used at four levels so that several tests will fall on the standard curve. The best index of the validity of the assay is agreement of the calculated results at different test levels.

(b) Add sufficient H_2O to bring the volume to 5.0 mL.

(c) To each tube, add 5.0 mL Reagent 40.

6. *Sterilization.*   See page 59.

(a) Mix contents of each tube thoroughly by vortexing each tube.

(b) Cap each tube.

(c) Autoclave 10 min at 15 psi at 121°C. Oversterilization of the medium will lead to erratic assay results. The final reaction of the medium will be pH 6.8 at 25°C.

(d) Cool tubes to 37°C or below.

(1) All tubes must be the same temperature all the way through the rack. Allow the culture tube rack to stand in a water bath or at room temperature until there is no question that the temperature is uniform.

7. *Inoculation and Incubation.*   See page 59.

(a) Aseptically inoculate each tube with one drop of the cell suspension prepared in Section 2(a).

(b) Incubate at 35–37°C for 16–18 hr until maximum turbidity is reached. Maximum turbidity is obtained as indicated by lack of significant change (1–2% T) during an additional 2 hr of incubation in tubes containing highest level of standard when measured against the inoculated blank which is set at 100% T (24).

8. *Determination.*   See page 60.

(a) Thoroughly mix contents of each tube and determine % transmittance of the inoculated blank at any specific wavelength between 540 nm and 660 nm. Use the uninoculated blank to set the spectrophotometer at 100% T.

(1) Many investigators prefer to use absorbance measurements.

(b) Reset T at 100% using the inoculated blank and determine % T of each tube.

(c) Prepare standard curve by plotting % T readings for each standard level against niacin concentration.

(d) Determine the amount of vitamin for each level of sample extract by interpolation from the standard curve.

(e) Discard any values which show more than 0.45 μg or less than 0.025 μg of niacin per tube.

(f) Calculate the niacin content per mL extract in the remaining tubes. Determine the mean and the range of ±10%. Discard any values that fall outside ±10% of the mean and use the remainder of the values to calculate the mean μg/mL of extract.

9. *Calculation.*   Use the following formula to calculate niacin content of the sample:

$$\mu\text{g/g} = \frac{\text{Mean } \mu\text{g/mL} \times \text{initial volume of extract}}{\text{Weight of sample (g)}} \times \text{dilution factor}$$

(1) All calculations including best fit of the standard curve using regression techniques can be completed by computer.

II. COLORIMETRIC METHOD FOR NIACIN AND NIACINAMIDE

A. Principle

The colorimetric determination of niacin is based upon the reaction of nicotinic acid with cyanogen bromide to give a pyridinium compound (Figure 15.3). The latter undergoes rearrangement yielding derivatives that couple with aromatic amines to produce colored compounds (28). Under proper conditions, the density of the color produced is proportional to the niacin present and may be measured spectrophotometrically. Factors that must be controlled for the method to produce reliable results are reaction temperature and pH, choice of an aromatic amine that will give a maximum stable color, and preparation of blank corrections (29). The manual procedure for the chemical determination of niacin is presented in the following section. The manual procedure follows AOAC methodology (24). The semiautomated method based on the AACC-AOAC Official First Action method (12) is discussed in the Automated Methods chapter.

B. Equipment

In addition to the general glassware and equipment associated with analytical laboratory work, a UV/vis spectrophotometer is required.

C. Reagents

1. *Standard Niacin Stock Solution (100 µg/mL).* Dissolve 50 mg USP niacin reference standard that has been dried to constant weight and stored in dark over P_2O_5 in a desiccator in 25% alcohol and make to 500 mL with 25% alcohol. Store in the dark, refrigerated. Stock niacin solution should be allowed to equilibrate to room temperature before diluting to volume.

2. *Niacin Working Standard Solution 1 (10 µg/mL).* Dilute 10 mL niacin stock solution to 100 mL with H_2O.

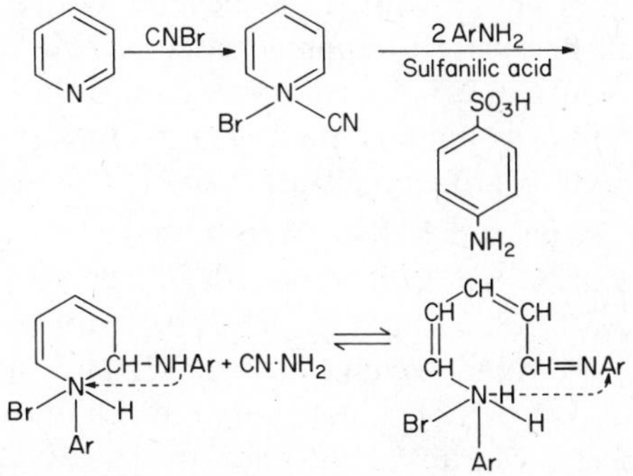

FIGURE 15.3 Colorimetric reaction for niacin determination.

3. *Niacin Working Standard Solution 2 (4 μg/mL).* Dilute 2 mL stock solution to 50 mL with H_2O.

4. *Dilute Ammonium Hydroxide.* Dilute 5 mL concentrated NH_4OH to 250 mL with H_2O.

5. *Dilute Hydrochloric Acid.* Dilute 100 mL concentrated HCl with 500 mL H_2O.

6. *Phosphate Buffer Solution (pH 8.0).* Dissolve 60 g $Na_2HPO_4 \cdot 7H_2O$ and 10 g KH_2PO_4 in warm H_2O. Dilute to 200 mL.

7. *10% Cyanogen Bromide Solution.* Prepare 10% CNBr solution under hood by warming 370 mL of H_2O to 40°C in a 1000-mL flask, add 40 g CNBr. Shake until dissolved and cool. Dilute to 400 mL and store refrigerated.

CAUTION!!! CNBr is extremely poisonous. All operations involving this reagent should be carried out in an efficient hood. Do not breathe any vapors, and, if solution comes in contact with the skin, wash immediately with H_2O.

8. *10% Sulfanilic Acid Solution.* Add concentrated NH_4OH in 1-mL portions to mixture of 20 g sulfanilic acid and 170 mL H_2O until the acid dissolves. Adjust to pH 4.5 with 5 N HCl and dilute to 200 mL. The solution should be almost colorless.

9. *55% Sulfanilic Acid Solution.* Add 27 mL H_2O and 27 mL concentrated NH_4OH to 55 g sulfanilic acid and shake until dissolved. The solution may be warmed if the acid does not dissolve readily. Adjust to pH 7.0 with a few drops of NH_4OH or 5 N HCl and dilute to 100 mL. Store in the dark.

D. Procedure

1. *Sample Preparation.*

(a) Pharmaceuticals. Prepare sample containing at least five tablets or capsules by dispersing in small volume of H_2O with heating. Tablets may be ground before dispersing in H_2O. Cool and transfer to volumetric flask and dilute to volume so that final solution contains 50–200 μg of niacin/mL. Pipette 10 mL aliquot into 250-mL Erlenmeyer and add 10 mL concentrated HCl. Evaporate on hot plate to approximately 2 mL, cool, and add 25–50 mL of H_2O. Adjust pH to 2.5–4.5 with 40% NaOH or KOH. Adjust volume with H_2O so that final volume contains approximately 4 μg niacin/mL. If the solution is cloudy, clarify by filtration or centrifugation.

(b) Noncereal foods and feeds. Weigh approx 25–30 g of sample into 1000-mL Erlenmeyer flask and disperse with 200 mL of 1 N H_2SO_4. Autoclave for 30 min at 15 psi, cool, and adjust pH to 4.5 with 10 N NaOH. Dilute to 250 mL with H_2O and filter. Weigh 17 g of $(NH_4)_2SO_4$ into 50-mL volumetric flask and pipette in 40 mL of sample solution. Dilute to volume with H_2O and shake vigorously. Clarify by filtration or centrifugation and use 1 mL for niacin quantitation.

Prepare standard by pipeting 40 mL of working Solution 2 (4μg/mL) into 50-mL volumetric flask containing 17 g of $(NH_4)_2SO_4$ and dilute to volume with H_2O.

(c) Cereal products.   Add 1.5 g $Ca(OH)_2$ to each of six 250-mL Erlenmeyer flasks. Add 0, 5, 10, 15, 20, and 25 mL of working Solution 1 (10 μg/mL) to each flask, respectively. Weigh approximately 2.5 g of sample into another flask containing 1.5 g $Ca(OH)_2$. Add H_2O to each flask so that volume is approximately 90 mL, mix, and autoclave at 15 psi for 2 hr. Mix while hot, cool to 40°C, and transfer to 100-mL volumetric flasks. Dilute to volume with H_2O.

(1) Whenever it is necessary to prepare a larger number of samples than can be handled in 1 day, the analysis may be interrupted at this point. Extracts may be stored in the refrigerator for a period up to 1 week.

Transfer approximately 50 mL from each flask to centrifuge tubes and place in ice bath for 15 min or in refrigerator for at least 2 hr. Centrifuge at 2000–5000 rpm for 15 min and pipette 20 mL of supernatant from each tube into separate centrifuge tubes containing 8 g of $(NH_4)_2SO_4$ and 2 mL of phosphate buffer. Dissolve by shaking and warm to 55–60°C. Clarify by centrifuging or filtering through Whatman No. 12 paper or equivalent.

2. *Determination.*

(a) Pharmaceuticals and noncereal foods and feeds.   Add 10% sulfanilic acid solution and CNBr solution under hood from burets or automatic pipette. A separate sample blank should be prepared for each sample.

Standard Blank	Sample Blank
1.0 mL Reagent 2 or 3	1.0 mL Sample solution
5.0 mL H_2O	5.0 mL H_2O
0.5 mL Reagent 4	0.5 mL Reagent 4
2.0 mL Reagent 8	2.0 mL Reagent 8
0.5 mL Reagent 5	0.5 mL Reagent 5

Standard Solution	Sample Solution
1.0 mL Reagent 2 or 3	1.0 mL Sample solution
0.5 mL Reagent 4	0.5 mL Reagent 4
5.0 mL Reagent 7	5.0 mL Reagent 7
2.0 mL Reagent 8	2.0 mL Reagent 8
0.5 mL H_2O	0.5 mL H_2O

(a) Mix contents of each tube thoroughly by vortexing each tube.

Pipette working standard 2 (4 μg/mL) and sample solution into respective tubes and add 5 mL of H_2O for standard blank and sample blank. Add all subsequent solutions to tube and read color before proceeding with next tube.

Starting with standard blank, swirl tube to give rotary motion in liquid, and immediately add dilute NH_4OH. Swirl again, and add sulfanilic acid and swirl. Immediately add 0.5 mL dilute HCl, mix, and place in spectrophotometer and adjust instrument to 0 absorbance at any specific wavelength between 430 nm and 450 nm within 30 sec after addition of sulfanilic acid solution.

For standard solution, add dilute NH_4OH with same technique as used for the standard blanks. Immediately swirl tube, and add CNBr solution, and swirl again. Wait 30 sec, swirl tube, and add the sulfanilic acid solution and swirl again. Immediately add 0.5 mL H_2O, mix, and stopper. With instrument set at 0 absorbance for standard blank, read A of standard at maximum absorbance.

(1) Color reaches maximum at approximately 1.5 min after addition of the sulfanilic acid solution. The color will remain at maximum for about 2 min before starting to fade.

Determine absorbance of solutions in a similar manner. Niacin content is proportional to absorbance if standard and sample solutions are approximately the same concentration.

(b) Cereal products. Prepare the following tubes for each standard and sample: Two tubes containing 5.0 mL of standard solution prepared in Section D.1(c) and two tubes containing 5.0 mL of sample solution. Prepare one tube containing 5.0 mL of H_2O for use as the reagent blank. To one standard tube and one sample tube to be used as their respective blanks, add 10 mL H_2O. Let all tubes stand 30 min in ice bath, preferably in the refrigerator.

To remaining sample and standard tubes and to the reagent blank, consecutively add 10 mL of cold CNBr, followed in 30 sec by 1.0 mL of 55% sulfanilic acid solution. Swirl each tube immediately after the addition of each reagent. Stopper the tubes containing CNBr and place all tubes back in the ice bath. To standard and sample blanks, add 1.0 mL of 55% sulfanilic acid solution.

Set spectrophotometer to 0 absorbance at 470 nm with standard blank [0 standard prepared in Section D.1(c)] and read A of other tubes 12–15 min after the addition of sulfanilic acid.

(1) Uniform cooling of the tubes is necessary. Wipe each tube dry before placing in spectrophotometer. If tubes fog, dip momentarily in hot H_2O and wipe before reading.

Construct a standard curve by plotting A of standard corrected for the reagent blank against niacin concentration in μg/mL. Use A of sample corrected to determine concentration, C, from the standard curve. The following formula can be used to determine niacin concentration of the sample:

$$\text{mg Niacin}/100\text{ g sample} = \frac{C(\mu g/mL)}{\text{sample weight (g)}} \times 10$$

ACKNOWLEDGMENT

The authors wish to thank Dr. A. M. Soliman of the Atlanta Center for Nutrient Analysis, Food and Drug Administration, for advice given in preparation of this manuscript.

LITERATURE CITED

1. Goodhart, R. S. and Shils, M. E. *Modern Nutrition in Health and Disease.* Lea & Febiger, Philadelphia (1976).

2. Peterson, M. S. and Johnson, A. H. *Encyclopedia of Food Science.* Avi, Westport, Conn. (1978).

3. Committee on Dietary Allowances, Food and Nutrition Board. *Recommended Dietary Allowances.* National Academy of Sciences, Washington, D.C. (1980).

4. Hepburn, F. N. "Nutrient composition of selected wheats and wheat products—7. Total and free niacin." *Cereal Chem.* **48**, 369 (1971).

5. Kodicek, E., Braude, R., Kon, S. K., and Mitchell, K. G. "The availability to pigs of nicotinic acid in tortilla baked from maize treated with lime-water." *Brit. J. Nutr.* **13**, 363 (1959).

6. Kreutler, P. A. *Nutrition in Perspective.* Prentice-Hall, Englewood Cliffs, N.J. (1980).

7. Mason, J. B. and Kodicek, E. "The analysis of *o*-amino phenol and *o*-aminophenyl glucose in wheat bran." *Cereal Chem.* **50**, 646 (1973).

8. Mason, J. B., Gibson, N., and Kodicek, E. "The chemical nature of the bound nicotinic acid of wheat bran: studies of nicotinic acid-containing macromolecules." *Brit. J. Nutr.* **30**, 297 (1973).

9. Das, M. L. and Guha, B. C. "Isolation and chemical characterization of bound niacin (niacinogen) in cereal grains." *J. Biol. Chem.* **235**, 2971 (1960).

10. Koetz, R., Amado, R., and Neukom, H. "Nature of the bound nicotinic acid in wheat bran." *Lebensm.-Wiss. and Technol.* **12**, 346 (1979).

11. Egberg, D. C. "Semiautomated method for niacin and niacin-amide in food products: Collaborative study." *J. Assoc. Off. Anal. Chem.* **62**, 1027 (1979).

12. Association of Official Analytical Chemists. "Changes in methods." *J. Assoc. Off. Anal. Chem.* **64**, 522 (1981).

13. Kertcher, J. A., Guilarte, T. R., Chen, M. F., Rider, A. A., and McIntyre, P. A. "A radiometric microbiologic assay for the biologically active forms of niacin." *J. Nucl. Med.* **20**, 419 (1979).

14. Baker, H. and Frank, O. *Clinical Vitaminology.* Interscience New York. Chapter 4, 31–40 (1968).

15. Voigt, M. N., Eitenmiller, R. R., and Ware, G. O. "Vitamin assay by microbial and protozoan organisms: Response to vitamin concentration, incubation time and assay vessel size." *J. Food Sci.* **43**, 1418 (1978).

16. Voigt, M. N., Eitenmiller, R. R., and Ware, G. O. "Comparison of protozoan and conventional methods of vitamin analysis." *J. Food Sci.* **44**, 729 (1979).

17. Strohecker, R. and Henning, H. M. *Vitamin Assay: Tested Methods.* Verlag Chemie, GMBH, Weinheim/Bergstr, Germany (1966).

18. Hengen, N., Seiberth, V., and Hengen, M. "High performance liquid chromatographic determination of free nicotinic acid and its metabolite, nicotinuric acid in plasma and urine." *Clin. Chem.* **24**, 1740 (1978).

19. Tyler, T. A. and Shrago, R. R. "Determination of niacin in cereal samples by HPLC." *J. Liq. Chromatogr.* **3**, 269 (1980).

20. De Vries, J. X., Gunthert, W., and Ding, R. "Determination of nicotinamide in human plasma and urine by ion-pair reversed-phase high-performance liquid chromatography." *J. Chromatogr.* **221**, 161 (1980).

21. Toma, R. B. and Tabekhia, M. M. "High performance liquid chromatographic analysis of B-vitamins in rice and rice products." *J. Food Sci.* **44**, 263 (1979).

22. Skurray, G. R. "A rapid method for selectively determining small amounts of niacin, riboflavin and thiamine in foods." *Food Chemistry* **7**, 77 1981).

23. Kirchmeier, R. L. and Upton, R. P. "Simultaneous determination of niacin, niacinamide, pyridoxine, thiamine and riboflavin in multivitamin blends by ion-pair high pressure liquid chromatography." *J. Pharm. Sci.* **67**, 1444 (1978).

24. Association of Official Analytical Chemists. *Official Methods of Analysis,* 13th ed. Washington, D.C. (1981).

25. Approved Methods Committee. *Approved Methods of the AACC,* Vol. 2. American Association of Cereal Chemists, St. Paul, Minn. (1976).

26. *DIFCO Supplementary Literature,* DIFCO Laboratories, Detroit, Mich. (1968).

27. Melnick, D. "Collaborative study of the applicability of microbiological and chemical methods to the determination of niacin in cereal products." *Cereal Chem.* **19**, 553 (1942).

28. Harris, L. J. *Vitamins in Theory and Practice.* Cambridge University Press, 93 (1955).

29. Goldsmith, G. A. and Miller, D. N. "Niacin." In P. Gyorgy and W. N. Pearson, Eds, *The Vitamins.* Academic Press, New York, 137–164 (1967).

16 Pantothenic Acid

Bonita W. Wyse, Won O. Song,
Joan H. Walsh, and
R. Gaurth Hansen

GENERAL CONSIDERATIONS

In 1933, Williams (1) reported the isolation of a growth factor from yeast that was an acidic substance with wide distribution in biological tissues; this substance was named pantothenic acid. When two research groups (2–3) simultaneously and independently reported that the yeast growth factor was identical with the chick antidermatitis factor, the status of pantothenic acid as a vitamin for animals was established.

At the molecular level, pantothenic acid is the vitamin moiety of coenzyme A and phosphopantetheine (Figure 16.1), both of which carry acyl groups through thioester bonds. These S-acyl derivatives are formed on oxidation of aldehydes, on oxidative decarboxylation of α-keto acids, and from organic acids activated by ATP or GTP. The activated acyl groups may be transferred to other acceptors, or modified by oxidative-reduction, carboxylation-decarboxylation, hydration-dehydration, racemization, carbon skeleton rearrangement, or formation of new carbon to carbon bonds. The versatility of these acylated coenzymes arises in part from the configuration of pantetheine and in part from the reactivity conferred by the thioester bond.

Abiko (4) has listed more than 70 catalytic reactions that involve coenzyme A or phosphopantetheine as cofactors. Generally, the pantothenate derivatives mediate the metabolism of carbohydrates, lipids, and amino acids (Figure 16.2). Specifically, in the tricarboxylic acid cycle, coenzyme A functions as an acyl acceptor for the pyruvate and α-ketoglutarate dehydrogenase complexes, forming

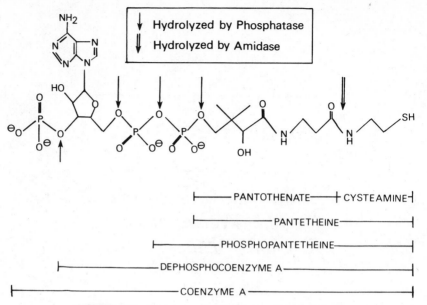

FIGURE 16.1   Structure of pantothenic acid and derivatives.

acetyl coenzyme A and succinyl coenzyme A, respectively. These coenzyme A thioesters are also formed on oxidative degradation of several amino acids. The acetyl coenzyme A is the carbon source for the biosynthesis of fatty acids, prostaglandins, ketone bodies, cholesterol, steroid hormones, and other compounds. Succinyl coenzyme A is an essential precursor for porphyrins and hence, hemoglobin and cytochromes. For fatty acid synthesis and degradation, pantothenate coenzymes carry the acids as acyl groups through repetitive synthetic or degradative steps. A coenzyme A thioester is a necessary intermediate in the degradation of cholesterol to bile acids. Phosphopantetheine has been implicated in the synthesis of peptide antibiotics (5,6) through and oligopeptide synthetic system that may be an evolutionary forerunner of modern ribosomal protein synthesis (7).

Some of the physical and chemical properties of pantothenic acid are shown in Table 16.1.

As expected from its molecular function, pantothenic acid is widely distributed in biological tissues and in foods. Pantothenic acid values are available for approximately 800 food items (8–10). Foods that are good sources of pantothenic acid include milk, chicken, beef, potatoes, oat cereals, tomato products, and whole grains. Relatively low amounts of pantothenic acid are found in many processed foods, including products made from refined grains, fruit products and fat- or cereal-extended meats and fish (8).

Meyer et al. (11) reported that 89% of pantothenic acid was retained in the meat of an oven roasted beef loin, and 56% of the vitamin was retained in the muscle of an oven-braised round. In both cases, most of the pantothenic acid

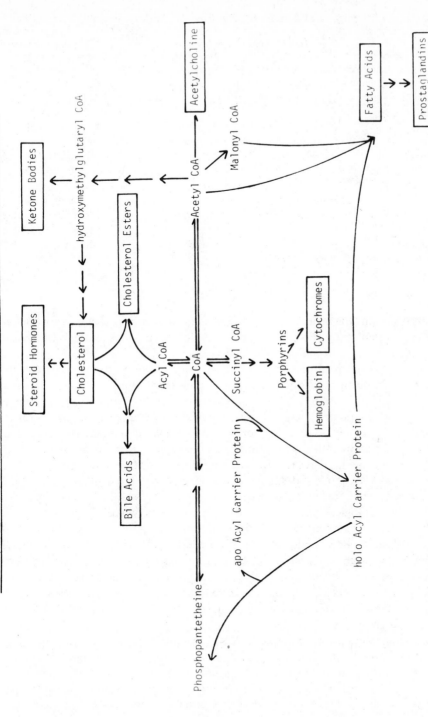

Some Important Compounds Whose Synthesis is Catalyzed by Pantothenate Derivatives

FIGURE 16.2 Some important compounds whose synthesis is catalyzed by pantothenate derivatives.

TABLE 16.1   Physical and Chemical Properties of Pantothenic Acid and Its Salts

Property	Pantothenic Acid	Ca Pantothenate	Na Pantothenate
Physical appearance	Viscous oil	White crystal	White crystal
Empirical formula	$C_9H_{17}O_5N$	$(C_9H_{16}O_5N)_2Ca$	$C_9H_{16}NNaO_5$
Molecular weight	219.23	476.53	241.22
Solubilities:			
Water	Readily soluble	Readily soluble	Readily soluble
Ethyl acetate	Readily soluble	Moderately soluble	Insoluble
Dioxane	Readily soluble	Insoluble	Moderately soluble
Glacial acetic acid	Readily soluble	Readily soluble	Readily soluble
Ether	Moderately soluble	Insoluble	Moderately soluble
Amyl alcohol	Moderately soluble	Moderately soluble	Moderately soluble
Benzene	Insoluble	Moderately soluble	Moderately soluble
Chloroform	Insoluble	Insoluble	Moderately soluble
Optical rotation	$[\alpha]_D^{25} + 37.5°$	$[\alpha]_D^{25} + 28.2°$	$[\alpha]_D^{25} + 27.1°$

was recovered in the meat drippings. Cooking of frozen vegetables can result in a 10–40% loss of pantothenic acid, and cooking frozen meats and fish can cause losses of up to 15% of pantothenic acid (12).

Concerns about pantothenic acid requirements in human led to the attempts to measure pantothenic acid in tissue, blood, and serum. Blood contains relatively high levels of pantothenic acid. Serum is known to contain only free pantothenic acid in small amounts whereas the majority of the vitamin in erythrocytes is present as coenzyme A or other forms (13–17). Blood samples collected and held at room temperature will autolyze spontaneously to free the bound form of pantothenic acid, giving rise to false high values for free pantothenic acid in whole blood (18). To avoid such possible errors, measurement of total blood pantothenic acid is recommended unless the timing is well controlled. Because of the methodological difficulties and variation in enzymatic hydrolysis, pantothenic acid levels reported in the literature range from 59 ng/mL to 2622 ng/mL for whole blood and range from 137 ng/mL to 1830 ng/mL for serum.

Due to the large variation in the data, estimation of vitamin adequacy differs among researchers. Sauberlich et al. (16) suggest that a total level of less than 1000 ng/mL of whole blood be considered as low or inadequate status, while Baker and Frank (17,19) suggest a level of less than 160 ng/mL of whole blood as a hypovitaminosis.

A few controlled studies (8,20–23), where both dietary intake and urinary excretion are determined, indicate that urinary excretion of pantothenic acid is related to dietary intake. The studies suggest that little or no bound pantothenic acid appears in urine. The pantothenate excretion can be expressed either as total pantothenate in 24 hr of urine collection or pantothenate per gram of creatinine.

METHODS AVAILABLE

The conventional pantothenate determinations measure either "free" (no previous enzymatic hydrolysis) or "total" (measurement after enzyme treatment) pantothenate. Most of the pantothenic acid in biological materials exist as coenzyme A and other bound forms (24). Enzymatic treatment to release the bound form is essential for pantothenic acid measurement (Figure 16.1). Ives and Strong (25) first recommended that Mylase P be used. Later, Neilands and Strong (26) and Novelli (24) reported increased pantothenic acid release with a double-enzyme treatment that used pigeon liver extract and alkaline phophatase. The pigeon liver extract used to break the amide bond of pantetheine, however, contained large amounts of endogenous pantothenic acid, and most of the pantothenic acid measured in the assay was from the liver extract, rather than from the sample (26). Various avian livers and mammalian kidneys have been substituted for the pigeon liver extracts (27). Novelli and Schmetz (28) reported that anion exchange treatment could be used to reduce the amount of pantothenic acid in the liver extract, yet leave the enzyme in an active form. Dupre et al. (29) and Dupre and Cavallini (30) have recently purified "pantetheinase" from horse kidney, but have not applied it to pantothenic acid assay. A pantetheinase with a low endogenous pantothenic acid content has been partially purified and characterized from hog kidneys by Wittwer et al. (31) (see purification procedure).

In light of current knowledge, even when specific pantetheinase and alkaline phosphatase are applied, pantothenate in acyl carrier protein will not be released. In acyl carrier protein, phosphopantetheine is linked to serine via a phosphodiester bond (32).

The Association of Official Analytical Chemists (AOAC) attempted to develop a standard procedure for assaying pantothenic acid. The first step was to conduct a collaborative study, involving eight laboratories, using the microbiological assay for free pantothenic acid (33). Fairly good agreement was obtained among the laboratories on four unknown samples containing free pantothenic acid. The AOAC (34) then proposed a collaborative study for release of bound pantothenic acid employing both the liver extract and the phosphatase. The study progressed slowly, and problems arose. Dried yeast, which has a high but variable percentage of bound pantothenic acid, was assayed by four different laboratories each using five different levels of liver extract. Since the results are variable, no statement on optimum enzyme levels for freeing pantothenic acid was made. The referee for the procedure recommended "that collaborative studies be inactivated. When sufficient information on the specific enzyme activity is available, it may be desirable to reactivate collaborative studies" (35). The 13th edition of AOAC (36) includes a microbiological method applicable only to materials containing calcium pantothenate or other free forms of pantothenic acid.

Methods for measuring pantothenic acid can be divided into two main categories: (1) animal and microbiological bioassays and (2) chemical and/or physical procedures. Bird and Thompson (37) have published a thorough review of this literature. For the animal bioassays, a basal ration deficient in pantothenic acid or supplemented with metabolic antagonist is fed to induce vitamin deficiency symptoms. The diet with materials containing unknown amounts of pantothenic acid is then supplemented and its curative or prophylactic effect of deficiency symptoms is determined. Chicks (38–41) and rats (42–44) have been commonly used for the bioassays.

Microbiological procedures have mostly replaced the animal assays for pantothenic acid. These have employed a number of microorganisms and protozoans including *Saccharomyces cerevisiae* (1), *Saccharomyces carlsbergensis* (45), *Lactobacillus casei* (46), *Lactobacillus plantarum* (47), *Tetrahymena pyriformis* (48), *Proteum morganii* (49), *Streptococcus faecalis* (50), and *Lactobacillus fermenti* (51). Among these *L. plantarum* seems to yield reasonable recovery of pantothenic acid added to biological materials with the best general reproducibility (18) and is therefore the most widely used assay organism for pantothenic acid (36).

Other chemical and physical procedures are also available for pantothenate determination. Tesmer and Hotzel (52,53) have used gas chromatography for measuring pantothenic acid in food. Schulze zur Weische et al. (54) also have used gas chromatography for the vitamin determination in urine. The method quantitates pantolactone formed from pantothenic acid by acid hydrolysis and extracted from the aqueous phase by dichloromethane.

Spectrophotometric (55,56) and fluorometric methods (57) have been used for determination of panthenol and calcium pantothenate in pharmaceutical products. Spectrophotometric procedure is based on the reaction of a hydrolysis product of pantothenate with 1,2-naphthoquinone-4-sulfonate. In the fluorometric procedure, samples treated with magnesium trisilicate and ion-exchange chromatography are hydrolyzed in an alkaline medium and reacted with a mixture of o-phthalaldehyde and 2-mercaptoethanol in boric acid solution. The fluorescence is due to the formation of a fluorogenic compound measured at 455 nm.

In 1979 Wyse et al. (58) reported the development and validation of a radioimmunoassay (RIA) for free pantothenic acid. The assay is based on the binding specificity of an antibody specific for pantothenic acid. The measurement depends on competitive binding between the unlabeled antigen (sample) and radioactive antigen by antibody. The assay has proved to be specific, sensitive, precise, and convenient. Results of RIA and those of microbiological assay with *L. plantarum* were highly correlated in blood (20,58), in urine (20), and in foods (8,59).

An enzyme-linked immunosorbent assay (ELISA) for pantothenate has recently been developed (60). In the procedure, antibodies specific for pantothenate are convalently linked to alkaline phosphatase with glutaraldehyde. An immobilized pantothenate substrate is obtained by attaching human serum albumin-pantothenate conjugate to the surface of polystyrene culture tubes by passive adsorption. The binding of the enzyme-linked antibody to immobilized substrate is inhibited by free pantothenate in standards or samples. The binding ratio is determined by the absorbance at 405 nm from the hydrolysis of p-nitrophenyl phosphate. A standard curve plotting known amounts of pantothenic acid on log-logit paper is linear from 2 ng to 1000 ng pantothenate. Initial experiments have shown that the ELISA may be useful in assessing pantothenate in appropriately deproteinized blood samples and food extracts.

Among the methods described above, microbiological and radioimmunoassays have been most commonly used recently (8,15,20,58,59,61–64). Both assays are sensitive to free pantothenic acid only and have been validated for the vitamin in foods and biological samples. The two assays produce comparable results, thus confidence can be placed in the results of either assay.

The choice of an assay method depends on such factors as physical properties of the sample, equipment, and expertise available. Given similar conditions, the RIA uses more expensive chemicals and reagents, but labor costs are lower. Using the microbiological assay, data can be obtained in 24–26 hr with 6–8 hr of actual labor by the technician. In the same situation, one will require 6–7 hr to get the results of RIA with 2.5–3 hr of actual labor.

Besides the glassware, disposable pipette tips, Vortex, test tube rack, the RIA requires a scintillation counter, whereas the microbiological assay uses autoclave, spectrophotometer, and incubator. Both assays require great attention to detail and painstaking pipetting; however, the RIA requires fewer operations than the microbiological assay, and thus has better reproducibility and is easier for a technician to master.

ANALYTICAL METHODOLOGY

I.   SAMPLE PREPARATION

The following sample preparation steps are common to both the microbiological and the radioimmunoassay.

A.   Foods

1. Homogenize a representative sample in a suitable blender with sufficient H_2O of known volume to produce a pourable slurry, then transfer into a suitable, sealable, and vapor-impermeable container, freeze, and store at $-10°C$ until analysis.

(a) An alternate way of sample preparation is to freeze samples by immersion into liquid nitrogen and follow by freeze-drying and grinding.

2. Thaw frozen slurry at 5°C and adjust pH to 6.5–7.5, and then dilute to a known volume with H_2O.

3. After thorough mixing, weigh out 10 g and autoclave at 121°C for 10 min.

4. Weigh out exactly 1–2 g of the autoclaved slurry and transfer to assay tube. It is advisable to run samples in triplicate.

5. To each tube, add 1 mL of the following and mix:

(a) 26 units bovine intestine alkaline phosphatase, type VII (E.C.3.1.3.1, Sigma Chemical Co.); 1 unit hydrolyses 1.0 μM p-nitrophenylphosphate per min at pH 10.4 and 37°C.

(b) 4 × 10^{-3} units pantetheinase (purification procedure see page 411–414); 1 unit hydrolyses 1.0 μM pantetheine per min as determined by the mercaptide assay (31).

(c) 0.4 mL 1 M Tris (pH 8.3) and

(d) H_2O to 1.0 mL.

6. Incubate 12–15 hr at 37°C in a shaker bath.

7. Transfer each sample quantitatively into a Spectrapor (Fisher Scientific Co.) or equivalent 6-mm diameter dialysis tube and dialyze against approximately 80 mL H_2O at 5°C for at least 8 hr.

8. Following dialysis discard tube and its contents and use the H_2O extract for the microbiological and/or the radioimmunoassay.

B. Blood and Tissues

1. Collect blood samples in vacuum tubes containing sodium heparin as an anticoagulant and hemolyze by three freeze-thaw cycles.

(a) Tissue samples are homogenized in two volumes H_2O, and then centrifuged.

2. To 0.5 mL hemolyzed blood, or tissue homogenate add the following:

(a) 10 units bovine intestine alkaline phosphatase, type VII (E.C.3.1.3.1, Sigma Chemical Co.).

(b) 0.1 units pantetheinase.

(c) 0.1 mL 1 M Tris buffer (pH 8.3) and

(d) H_2O to a total volume of 1 mL.

3. Incubate at 37°C for 7–8 hr.

4. Deproteinize the samples according to the method of Somogyi (65) as follows. To each sample add 5% $ZnSO_4$ and 0.3 N $Ba(OH)_2$ in equimolar concentration [see step (a) below], and centrifuge at 4000 × g for 10 min.

(a) The volume of $Ba(OH)_2$ required to neutralize $ZnSO_4$ is determined with phenolphthalein as an indicator.

(b) For tissues other than blood, where the pantothenic acid content is much higher, the precipitation step may not be necessary. In this case the enzyme-digested extract is centrifuged immediately after incubation and used directly following proper dilution.

5. Dilute the supernatants appropriately and use for either the microbiological and/or radioimmunoassay.

C. Urine

Since urine appears to contain only free pantothenic acid (20,21), the enzyme treatment is not necessary, and thus requires merely the following preparation for further assaying:

Thaw frozen urine samples and centrifuge at approximately 4000 $\times$ g for 5 min, then dilute the supernatant 1:20 with H_2O.

II. MICROBIOLOGICAL METHOD
(*LACTOBACILLUS PLANTARUM* ATCC 8014)

A. Principle

See page 43.

B. Equipment

See page 50.

C. Reagents

Reagents 1, 2, 3, 4, 5, 6, 7, 8, 9, 28, 29, 33, 34, 35, 36, and 37 which are and/ or may be needed for this method are listed on pages 51–58. In addition the following reagents are required for the analysis of pantothenic acid:

38. *Calcium Pantothenate Working Solution.* Dilute Reagent 5 1:5000 with H_2O to obtain a concentration of 20 ng/mL.

39. *Basal Medium for Calcium Pantothenate Assay.* Add 4 mL of a 1:5000 of biotin stock solution (Reagent 6) and 1 mL of the niacin stock solution (Reagent 7) to 500 mL of the basal medium stock solution (Reagent 9) and mix. The commercially available dehydrated medium Bacto-Pantothenate Medium AOAC USP (Difco) can be used instead and is to be prepared according to label directions.

D. Procedure

The microbiological method described below is similar to the procedure outlined by the AOAC (36) as modified by Walsh et al. (59). Comments regarding microbiological procedures presented in Section D in Chapter 3 apply for determination of calcium pantothenate as well.

1. *Preparation of Stock Culture.* Inoculate a pure culture of *Lactobacillus plantarum* (ATCC 8014) on two or more agar stock culture tubes. Incubate at 35–37°C for 24–48 hr, and store at −20°C until used. Alternatively, the incu-

bated stab cultures can be stored in the refrigerator. Such cultures should be transferred at 2–4-week intervals for maintenance. If used for the preparation of the inoculum, fresh stab cultures less than 1 week old must be used.

2. *Preparation of Inoculum.* Transfer cells from thawed frozen or refrigerated stock culture aseptically to a sterile tube(s) containing 10 mL Bacto-Lactobacilli MRS broth or Bacto-Lactobacilli Broth. Incubate overnight at 35–37°C, then centrifuge for 1 min, decant supernatant, and resuspend cells in 0.9% saline solution. Repeat the centrifugation and resuspension steps two to three times.

3. *Preparation of Standard Tubes.*

   (a) To duplicate tubes add standard working solution (Reagent 38) and H_2O, as outlined below:

Tubes	Reagent 39 (mL)	H_2O (mL)	Reagent 29 (mL)	ng PA/Tube
1, 2	0.5	4.5	5	10
3, 4	1.0	4.0	5	20
5, 6	1.5	3.5	5	30
7, 8	2.0	3.0	5	40
9, 10	2.5	2.5	5	50
11, 12	3.0	2.0	5	60
13, 14	3.5	1.5	5	70
15, 16	4.0	1.0	5	80
17, 18	4.5	0.5	5	90
19, 20	4.0	0	5	100
21, 22	0.55	4.45	5	11
23, 24	0.60	4.40	5	12
25, 26	0.65	4.35	5	13
27, 28	0	5.0	5	0

   (b) To each tube add 5.0 mL of basal medium (Reagent 39) and mix.

4. *Preparation of Assay Tubes.*

   (a) To duplicate tubes add 1.0-, 2.0-, 3.0-, 4.0-, and 5.0-mL aliquots to sample extract.

   (b) Add H_2O to a volume of 5.0 mL to each tube.

   (c) Add 5.0 mL of the pantothenic acid basal medium to each tube.

5. *Sterilization.* See page 59.

6. *Inoculation and Incubation.* See page 59.

7. *Titrimetric or Turbidimetric Determination.* See page 60. Figure 16.3 shows a typical standard curve using the turbidimetric method. Paralleling this curve are values obtained with three different food samples which are assayed

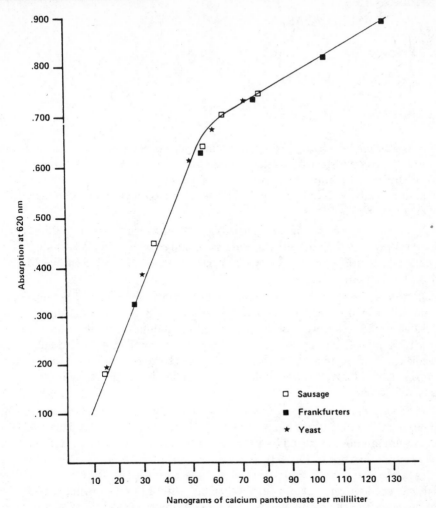

FIGURE 16.3 Parallelism of three food samples to microbiological assay samples to microbiological assay standard curve.

at different concentration levels. Parallelism in this case signifies the test organisms' growth dependence on the presence of pantothenic acid in the samples, and indicates the absence of any growth stimulating or inhibiting factors in these samples.

8. *Calculation.*

$$\text{ng/g sample} = \frac{\text{ng/mL} \times \text{volume}}{\text{weight of sample}} \times \text{dilution factor}$$

Appropriate stoichiometric corrections are necessary if results are to be recorded as pantothenic acid, as opposed to calcium pantothenate.

III.   RADIOIMMUNOASSAY (RIA)

A.   Principle

See page 409–500.

B.   Antibody Formation

1. D-*Pantothenic Acid.*   Add equivalent amounts of oxalic acid to an aqueous solution of calcium pantothenate (Sigma Chemical Co.), then separate calcium oxalate by centrifugation. Concentrate the supernatant to a viscous oil in a rotary evaporator under reduced pressure. Take up the oil in ethyl acetate and dehydrate by exposure to Na_2SO_4.

2. *Bromoacetyl Pantothenate.*   Mix 63 g D-pantothenic acid with 25 μL bromoacetyl bromide in 5 mL ethylacetate containing 200 mL $MgCO_3$ at 4°C. After 3 min, add 2 mL aqueous 0.5 M phosphate buffer (pH 7.8). Remove $MgCO_3$ by centrifugation.

3. *Bovine Serum Albumin.*   The denaturation and reduction of bovine serum albumin is accomplished by the method of Iyer and Klee (66) as modified by Wyse et al. (58). Dissolve 18 mg bovine serum albumin at room temperature in 10 mL 50 mM phosphate buffer (pH 7.8) containing 1 mM/L disodium ethylenediaminetetraacete and 8 mM/L urea. Add 11 mg dithiothreitol dissolved in approximately 1 mL 1 mM disodium ethylenediaminetetraacetate and allow to react for 30 min.

4. *Preparation of Antigen.*   Synthesize the pantothenic acid–bovine serum albumin conjugate by combining bromoacetyl pantothenate and denatured bovine serum albumin followed by pH adjustment to 7.3 with 2 M Na_2HPO_3. Hold the reaction mixture in the dark at room temperature for 24 hr, then dialyze at 4°C against 0.5 M NaCl and 1 mM phosphate buffer (pH 7.0). Concentrate the dialyzed product on a Diaflo filter (Amicon) with an exclusion limit of 10,000 daltons. Sterilize the conjugate by passing it through a 0.45 μm Millipore filter, and lyophilize.

5. *Antibody Induction.*   Inject into each foot pad of several New Zealand rabbits, each weighing approximately 4 kg, 0.1 mL (0.25 mg) of the antigen in Complete Freund's adjuvant (Difco). Repeat this series of injections first after 2 weeks and then weekly thereafter for 8 weeks. Sample blood from the peripheral ear vein in the animals and allow it to clot. Store the resulting antiserum at −40°C, and use without any further treatment in each assay.

C.   Procedure

This procedure described below was developed by Wyse et al. (58) and is outlined with some unpublished modification made by this group.   .

1. *Determination of Binding Capacity of Antiserum.*   For each batch of antibody, determine the amount of antiserum needed to provide approximately

50% binding of added radiolabeled pantothenate in the absence of unlabeled pantothenic acid. To ascertain this level, add a fixed amount of sodium [1-^{14}C]D-pantothenate (approximately 5000 cpm) to increasing amounts of antiserum diluted with a 1% solution of rabbit albumin in 10 mM phosphate buffer (pH 7.0). In most instances, a 1:100 dilution results in about 50% binding.

2. *Sample Assay.*   Pipette 0.5 mL sample extract into a 4 mL (1.2 × 5.5 cm) Omni-vial (Wheaton), add 0.5 mL diluted antiserum, 50 μL radiolabeled sodium [1-^{14}C]D-pantothenate (5000 cpm), and incubate for 15 min at room temp.

To each vial add 1 mL neutral, saturated $(NH_4)_2SO_4$ solution, then centrifuge at 12,000 × g for 12 min at 2°C. Wash the precipitate once with 0.5 mL 50% $(NH_4)_2SO_4$ and recentrifuge. Dissolve the washed precipitate containing the antibody-bound pantothenic acid in 0.3 mL Soluene (Packard Instruments), and then add 3.0 mL Dimilume-30 scintillation cocktail (Packard Instruments), and measure radioactivity in a liquid scintillation counter.

3. *Preparation of Standard Curve.*   To duplicate vials add 0.5 mL calcium pantothenate standard solutions using seven different concentrations ranging from 10 to 200 ng/vial. Treat standard samples identically to the sample extracts.

4. *Calculation.*   Calculate percent binding as B/B_o × 100 where B and B_o represent the cpm values obtained with and without unlabeled pantothenate respectively. Plot these values against the amounts of unlabeled standard pantothenate added on probits paper as shown in Figure 16.4.

Determine the amount of pantothenate in each unknown by reference to the standard curve.

Figure 16.4, besides representing a typical standard curve, also shows the parallelism that was obtained when determining the amount of pantothenic acid in a wheat germ sample using eight different dilution levels. Assays of this nature provide reliable indications on the presence or absence of interfering substances.

IV.   PARTIAL PURIFICATION OF PANTETHEINASE

A.   Pig Kidney Pantetheinase

This enzyme is purified according to the procedure developed by Wittwer et al. (31). All steps are to be performed at 4°C.

1. Obtain slices of cortex from fresh pig kidneys from a local slaughterhouse and freeze.

2. Homogenize about 275 g of thawed cortex in four volumes of ice cold H_2O in a Waring Blender or other suitable blender at high speed for 4 min.

3. Remove large particulate matter by centrifugation at 10,000 × g for 10 min.

4. Agglutinate the microsomes in the supernatant by adjusting the pH to 4.2 with the addition of 1 M formic acid.

5. Centrifuge at 20,000 × g for 10 min, resuspend the precipitate in approximately 400 mL H_2O, and homogenize briefly.

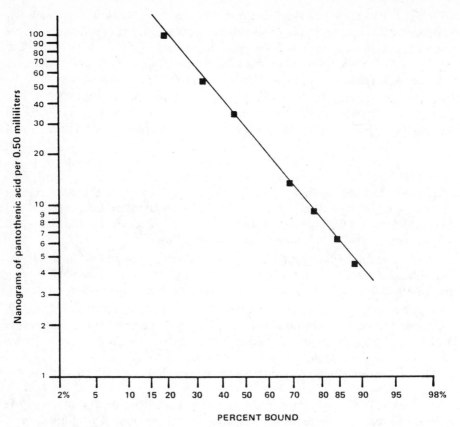

FIGURE 16.4 Parallelism of wheat germ sample to RIA standard curve.

6. Adjust pH to 5.75 with 0.5 M Tris-HCl (pH 9.0) and add 1.5 volumes of *n*-butanol, homogenize briefly, then centrifuge at $10,000 \times g$ for 10 min.

7. Immediately remove the butanol from the aqueous phase containing the solubilized enzyme by passing the solution through a 5.5×65-cm Sephadex G-25 column (Pharmacia Fine Chemicals) that was previously equilibrated with 0.02 M phosphate (pH 7.0).

8. Adjust the pH of the eluate to 5.0 with 1 M formic acid.

9. Warm in a 75°C water bath to 70°C, and hold at 70°C for 2 min, then cool rapidly and centrifuge at $20,000 \times g$ for 10 min.

10. Treat the supernatant solution with $(NH_4)_2SO_4$ to 55% saturation (32.6 g/100 mL) and centrifuge at $20,000 \times g$ for 15 min. Render the eluting supernatant solution 70% saturated with $(NH_4)_2SO_4$ (9.3 g/100 mL), and centrifuge at $20,000 \times g$ for 30 min. Dissolve the precipitate in a small volume of 0.02 M Tris-HCl (pH 8.2) and remove the $(NH_4)_2SO_4$ by dialysis or gel filtration.

The above procedure yields a 150-fold purification with 35% recovery of enzymatic activity. Assays are available to monitor pantetheine hydrolysis conveniently (31). A unit of enzyme activity is defined as the amount of enzyme that hydrolyzes 1 μM of pantetheine/min under the conditions of the mercaptide assay (31). A total activity of approximately 35 units is produced from 275 g kidney. The specific activity achieved is 0.4 units/mg protein (67).

The enzyme preparation is stable indefinitely if frozen at $-20°C$, or for at least 30 hr at 25°C when kept between pH 6.5 and pH 8.5. Its pantothenate blank is negligible.

B. Liver Pantetheinase

Pigeon or chicken liver enzyme acetone powders (Sigma Chemical Co.) however, contain high levels of pantothenic acid that need to be removed prior to the enzyme's usage (27). All steps are to be performed at 4°C.

1. Homogenize approximately 6 g liver acetone powder in 60 mL 0.02 M $KHCO_3$ for 1 min, then centrifuge.

2. Transfer the supernatant into a beaker containing 60 g 50–100-mesh Dowex 1×4, chloride form (Bio-Rad Laboratories) which was previously rinsed three times with H_2O, and filled to 125 mL with H_2O.

3. Adjust pH to 8.0 with 1.0 M Tris-HCl (pH 8.3).

4. Stir for 15 min, allow the resin to settle, then transfer the supernatant to a second beaker containing Dowex resin, which was prepared identically as described above, and stir for 5 min.

5. Remove supernatant and store at $-10°C$ in convenient aliquots of 5 mL or 10 mL for further use.

LITERATURE CITED

1. Williams, R. J., Lymann, C. W., Goodyear, G. H., Truesdail, J. H., and Holiday, D. "Pantothenic acid, a growth determinant of universal biological occurrence." *J. Am. Chem. Soc.* **55**, 2912 (1933).

2. Jukes, T. H. "Pantothenic acid and the filtrate (chick antidermatitis) factor. *J. Am. Chem. Soc.* **61**, 975 (1939).

3. Wooley, D. W., Waisman, H. A., and Elvehjem, C. A. "Studies on the structure of the chick antidermatitis factor." *J. Biol. Chem.* **129**, 673 (1939).

4. Abiko, Y. "Metabolism of coenzyme A." In D. M. Greenberg, Ed., *Metabolic Pathways,* Vol. 7. Academic Press, New York, 1–25 (1975).

5. Lee, S. G. and Lipmann, F. "Isolation of amino acid activating subunit-pantetheine protein complexes: Their role in chain elongation in tyrocidine synthesis." *Proc. Natl. Acad. Sci.* **74**, 2343 (1977).

6. Ishihara, H., Endo, Y., Abe, S., and Shimura, K. "The presence of 4'phosphopantetheine in the bacitricin synthetase." *FEBS Lett.* **50**, 43 (1975).

7. Lipmann, F. "Attempts to map a process evolution of peptide biosynthesis." *Science* **173**, 875 (1971).

8. Walsh, J. H., Wyse, B. W., and Hansen, R. G. "Pantothenic acid content of 75 processed and cooked foods." *J. Am. Dietet. Assoc.* **78**, 140 (1981).

9. Orr, M. L. "Pantothenic acid, vitamin B_6 and vitamin B_{12} in foods." *Home Economics Research Report No. 36.* USDA, Washington, D.C. (1969).

10. Posati, L. P. and Orr, M. L. "Composition of foods—dairy and egg products." *Agriculture Handbook No. 8-1,* USDA Washington, D.C. (1976).

11. Meyer, B. H., Mysinger, M. A., and Wodarski, L. A. "Pantothenic acid and vitamin B_6 in beef." *J. Am. Dietet. Assoc.* **54**, 122 (1969).

12. Fennema, O. "Effects of freeze-preservation on nutrients." In R. S. Harris and E. Karmas, Eds., *Nutritional Evaluation of Food Processing,* 2nd ed. Avi, Westport, Conn., 281 (1975).

13. Ishiguro, K., Kobayashi, S., and Kaneta, S. "Pantothenic acid content of human blood." *Tohoku J. Exptl. Med.* **74**, 65 (1961).

14. Ishiguro, K. "Blood pantothenic acid content of pregnant women." *Tohoku J. Exptl. Med.* **78**, 7 (1962).

15. Ishiguro, K. "Aging effect of blood pantothenic acid content in female." *Tohoku J. Exptl. Med.* **107**, 367 (1972).

16. Sauberlich, H. E., Dowdy, R. P., and Skala, J. H. *Laboratory Tests for the Assessment of Nutritional Status.* 88–91 (1974).

17. Baker, H. and Frank, O. *In Clinical Vitaminology: Methods and Interpretations.* Chapter 6, "Pantothenic acid." Interscience, New York (1968).

18. Hatano, M. "Microbiological assay of pantothenic acid in blood and urine." *J. Vitaminol.* **8**, 134 (1962).

19. Baker, H., Frank, O., Feingold, S., Christakis, G., and Ziffer, H. "Vitamins, total cholesterol and triglycerides in 642 New York City school children." *Am. J. Clin. Nutr.* **20**, 850 (1969).

20. Srinivasan, V., Christensen, N., Wyse, B. W., and Hansen, R. G. "Pantothenic acid nutritional status in the elderly—institutionalized and noninstitutionalized." *Am. J. Clin. Nutr.* **34**, 1736 (1981).

21. Fox, H. M. and Linkswiler, H. "Pantothenic acid excretion on three levels of intake." *J. Nutr.* **75**, 451 (1961).

22. Cohenour, S. H. and Calloway, D. H. "Blood, urine and dietary pantothenic acid levels of pregnant teenagers." *Am. J. Clin. Nutr.* **25**, 512 (1972).

23. Lews, C. M. and King, J. C. "Effect of oral contraceptive agents on thiamin, riboflavin, and pantothenic acid status in young women." *Am. J. Clin. Nutr.* **33**, 832 (1980).

24. Novelli, G. D., Kaplan, N. O., and Lipmann, F. "The liberation of pantothenic acid from coenzyme A." *J. Biol. Chem.* **177**, 97 (1949).

25. Ives, M. and Strong, F. M. "Preparation of samples for the microbiological assay of pantothenic acid." *Arch. Biochem.* **9**, 251 (1946).

26. Neilands, J. B. and Strong, F. M. "The enzymatic liberation of pantothenic acid." *Arch. Biochem.* **19**, 287 (1948).

27. Schweigert, B. S. and Guthneck, B. T. "Liberation and measurement of pantothenic acid in animal tissues." *J. Nutr.* **51**, 283 (1953).

28. Novelli, G. D. and Schmetz, F. J. "An improved method for the determination of pantothenic acid in tissues." *J. Biol. Chem.* **192**, 181 (1951).

29. Dupre, S., Graziani, M. T., Rosei, M. A., Fabi, A., and Del Grosso, E. "The enzymatic breakdown of pantethine to pantothenic acid and cystamine." *Eur. J. Biochem.* **16**, 571 (1970).

30. Dupre, S. and Cavallini, D. "Purification and properties of pantetheinase from horse kidney." *Methods in Enzymol.* **6**, 262–267 (1979).

31. Wittwer, C., Wyse, B. W., and Hansen, R. G. "Assay of the enzymatic hydrolysis of pantetheine." *Anal. Biochem.* **122**, 312 (1982).

32. Majerus, P. W., Alberts, A. W., and Vagelos, P. R. "Acyl carrier protein— 4. The identification of 4'-phosphopantetheine as the prosthetic group of the acyl carrier protein." *Proc. Natl. Acad. Sci.* **53**, 410 (1965).

33. Loy, H. W. "Report on pantothenic acid, microbiological method." *J. Assoc. Off. Agric. Chem.* **35**, 722 (1952).

34. Loy, H. W. "Report on pantothenic acid, microbiological method." *J. Assoc. Off. Agric. Chem.* **37**, 779 (1954).

35. Toepfer, E. W. "Microbiological assay for total pantothenic acid." *J. Assoc. Off. Agric. Chem.* **43**, 28 (1960).

36. Association of Official Analytical Chemists. *Official Methods of Analysis,* 13th ed. Washington, D.C. 43:126–43:133, 43:159–43.167 (1980).

37. Bird, O. D. and Thompson, R. Q. "Pantothenic acid," In P. Gyorgy and W. N. Pearson, Eds., *The Vitamins,* Vol. 7, 2nd ed. Academic Press, New York, 209–241 (1967).

38. Jukes, T. H. "The biological and microbiological assay of pantothenic acid." *Biol. Symposia.* **12**, 253 (1947).

39. Hegsted, D. M. and Lipmann, F. "The pantothenic acid content of coenzyme A by chick assay." *J. Biol. Chem.* **174**, 89 (1948).

40. Coates, M. E., Kon, S. K., and Shepheard, E. E. "The use of chicks for the biological assay of members of the vitamin B complex—1. Tests with pure substances." *Brit. J. Nutr.* **4**, 203 (1950).

41. Coates, M. E., Ford, J. E., Harrison, G. F., Kon, S. K., Shepheard, E. E., and Wilby, F. W. "Use of chicks for the biological assay of members of the vitamin B complex—2. Tests on natural materials and comparison with microbiological and other assays." *Brit. J. Nutr.* **6**, 75 (1952).

42. Bacon, J. S. D. and Jenkins, G. N. "A biological method for estimation of pantothenic acid with rats in which wheat germ is included in the basal diet." *Biochem. J.* **37**, 492 (1943).

43. King, T. E., Strong, F. M., and Cheldelin, V. H. "Pantothenic acid studies: The influence of a pantothenic acid conjugate (PAC) upon growth and citrate formation in rats." *J. Nutr.* **42**, 195 (1950).

44. Lih, H., King, T. E., Higgens, H., Baumann, C. A., and Strong, F. M. "Growth-promoting activity of bound pantothenic acid in the rat." *J. Nutr.* **44**, 361 (1951).

45. Atkin, L., Williams, W. L., Schultz, A. S., and Frey, C. N. "Yeast microbiological methods for determination of vitamins." *Ind. Eng. Chem. Anal. Ed.* **16**, 67 (1944).

46. Pennington, D., Snell, E. E., and Williams, R. J. "An assay for pantothenic acid." *J. Biol. Chem.* **135**, 213 (1940).

47. Skeggs, H. R. and Wright, L. D. "The use of *Lactobacillus arabinosis* in the microbiological determination of pantothenic acid." *J. Biol. Chem.* **156**, 21 (1944).

48. Baker, H., Frank, O., Pasher, L., Dinnerstein, A., and Sobotka, H. "An assay for pantothenic acid in biological fluids." *Clin. Chem.* **6**, 36 (1960).

49. Pelczar, M. J. and Porter, R. J. "A microbiological assay technique for pantothenic acid with the use of *Protus morganii.*" *J. Biol. Chem.* **136**, 111 (1941).

50. Kocher, V. "*Streptococcus faecalis,* a new test organism for the microbiological estimation of riboflavin and pantothenic acid." *Z. Vitaminforsch.* **6**, 113 (1945).

51. Craig, J. A. and Snell, E. E. "The comparative activities of pantethine, pantothenic acid and coenzyme A for various microorganisms." *J. Bact.* **61**, 283 (1951).

52. Tesmer, E. and Hotzel, D. "Pantolacton aus Coenzyme A Bestimmung von Pantothensaure." *Z. Anal. Chem.* **277**, 124 (1975).

53. Tesmer, E., Leinert, J., and Hoetzel, D. "Gaschromatographic determination of pantothenic acid in foods." *Die Nahrung* **24**, 697 (1980).

54. Schulze zur Wiesch, V. E., Hesse, C., and Hotzel, D. "Gaschromatographische Bestimmung von Pantothensäure in Urin." *Z. Klin. Chem. Klin. Biochem.* **12**, 498 (1974).

55. Panalaks, T. and Campbell, J. A. "Preliminary solvent extraction for the spectrophotometric determination of panthenol in pharmaceutical products." *Anal. Chem.* **33**, 1038 (1961).

56. Panalaks, T. and Campbell, J. A. "Solvent extraction and anion exchange chromatography for the spectrophotometric determination of calcium pantothenate in pharmaceutical products." *Anal. Chem.* **34**, 64 (1962).

57. Roy, R. B. and Buccafuri, A. "Automated Fluorometric analysis of calcium pantothenate in multivitamin preparations." *J. Assoc. Off. Anal. Chem.* **61**, 720 (1978).

58. Wyse, B. W., Wittwer, C., and Hansen, R. G. "Radioimmunoassay for pantothenic acid in blood and other tissues." *Clin. Chem.* **25**, 108 (1979).

59. Walsh, J. H., Wyse, B. W., and Hansen, R. G. "A comparison of microbiological and radioimmunoassay methods for the determination of pantothenic acid in foods." *J. Food. Biochem.* **3**, 175 (1980).

60. Smith, A. H., Wyse, B. W., and Hansen, R. G. "The development of an ELISA for pantothenate." Abstract No. 3886. *Fed. Proc.* **40**, 915 (1981).

61. Schroeder, H. A. "Losses of vitamins and trace minerals resulting from processing and preservation of foods." *Am. J. Clin. Nutr.* **24**, 562 (1971).

62. Baker, H., Frank, O., Thompson, A. D., Langer, A., Munves, D. E., de Angelis, B., and Kaminetzky, H. A. "Vitamin profile of 174 mothers and newborns at parturition." *Am. J. Clin. Nutr.* **28**, 56 (1975).

63. Ellestad-Sayed, J. J., Nelson, R. A., Addson, M. A., Palmer, W. M., and Soule, E. H. "Pantothenic acid, coenzyme A and human chronic ulceratic and granulomatous colitis. *Am. J. Clin. Nutr.* **29**, 1333 (1976).

64. Srinivasan, V. and Belavady, B. "Nutritional status of pantothenic acid in Indian pregnant and nursing women." *Internat. J. Vit. Nutr. Res.* **46**, 433 (1976).

65. Somogyi, M. "Determination of blood sugar." *J. Biol. Chem.* **160**, 69 (1945).

66. Iyer, K. S. and Klee, W. A. "Direct spectrophotometric measurement of the rate of reduction of disulfide bonds. *J. Biol. Chem.* **248**, 707 (1973).

67. Lowry, O. H., Rosebrough, N. J., Farr, A. L., and Randall, R. J. "Protein measurement with the Folin phenol reagent." *J. Biol. Chem.* **193**, 265 (1951).

17 Vitamin B₆*

Marilyn M. Polansky, Robert D. Reynolds and Joseph T. Vanderslice

GENERAL CONSIDERATIONS (1)

Vitamin B_6 is a water-soluble vitamin found in all foods of both animal and plant origin. Its occurrence in free form is limited and the major portion is associated with amino acids (2) and proteins (3). It does not appear to be bound to various fibers (4), but at least one form has been reported to be naturally bound to glucose (5). The vitamin exists in the six forms whose structures are given below, and may be interconvertable, depending upon the enzymatic complement present in the cells (Figure 17.1).

Pyridoxine was the form first isolated in 1938 (6). In the early literature, the term "pyridoxine" was used synonymously with the term "vitamin B_6." The pyridoxal and pyridoxamine forms were described in 1944 (6), and the phosphorylated forms in 1947–1951. The predominant forms found in biological samples are pyridoxine, pyridoxal, pyridoxal 5'-phosphate, and pyridoxamine 5'-phosphate. The term "pyridoxine" should be used only to denote the alcohol form. Due to the nearly equivalent biopotency, as opposed to bioavailability of the various forms, the term "vitamin B_6" may be used in a generic sense to denote structural nonspecific biological activity for the various forms of the vitamin.

---

* Vitamin B_6 compounds have been abbreviated according to published recommendations (IUPAC-IUB Commission on Biological Nomenclature, 1970) as follows: PN, pyridoxine; PL, pyridoxal; PM, pyridoxamine; PNP, pyridoxine 5'-phosphate; PLP, pyridoxal 5'-phosphate; PMP, pyridoxamine 5'-phosphate.

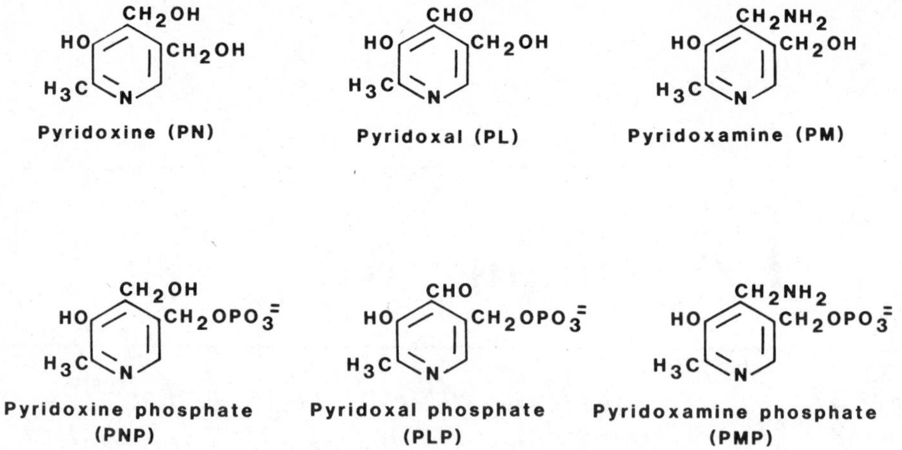

FIGURE 17.1   Structure of B$_6$ vitamers.

Table 17.1 summarizes some of the more pertinent physical characteristics and properties of several of the forms of vitamin B$_6$.

Other properties of vitamin B$_6$ include instability to near-UV light, stability in acid solution, instability of PN and PLP in basic solutions, and a possible instability of PLP to oxygen in solution (9). Interconversions of the different vitamers does not occur in a solution of standards, but can occur in biological samples (6).

The need for vitamin B$_6$ is well established in all living systems. Plants and most microoranisms can synthesize it, but most animals require a dietary source of the vitamin. The coenzyme forms, predominantly PLP and occasionally PMP, participate in transamination, decarboxylation, deamination, transsulfuration, desulfhydration, and racemization of amino acids (6). In humans, insufficient dietary intake results in infantile convulsive seizures, altered electroencephalograms, loss of body weight, anorexia, angular stomatitis, glossitis, and scaly dermatitis (6,10). Under normal dietary conditions, the vitamin is excreted in the urine along with its principle metabolite, 4-pyridoxic acid. Although the vitamin has a relatively low toxicity in vivo, massive intakes have been reported to cause gradual paralysis and eventual death in dogs (11) and an alteration in behavior and a loss of curiosity in rats (12).

METHODS AVAILABLE

There have been many methods reported for the separation, detection, and quantitation of standard compounds. Most of these methods are of limited usefulness with the more complex biological samples most often encountered and will not be discussed here. The methods that have been demonstrated to be most applicable to biological samples are animal growth assays, microbiol-

TABLE 17.1 Physical Characteristics and Properties of the Forms of Vitamin B_6[a]

	PN	PN · HCl	PL · HCl	PM · 2HCl	PMP	PLP
Physical form	Colorless crystalline powder	White prisms	White rhomboid crystals	White deliquessent platelets	White prisms and crystals	White crystals
Molecular weight	169	205.7	203.6	241.1	248.2 (hydrate 284.2)	247.1 (hydrate 265.1)
Melting point	160	204–6[b]	165[b]	226–27[b]	—	Oxime 229–30[b]
pH of aqueous sol.	—	3.2	2.7	2.4	—	—
Solubility						
Water	Readily soluble	22.2 g/100 mL	50 g/100 mL	50 g/100 mL	Soluble	Soluble
Ethyl alcohol	Readily soluble	1.1 g/100 mL	1.7 g/100 mL 95%	0.65 g/100 mL 95%	—	Slightly soluble
Acetone	Readily soluble	Slightly soluble	—	—	—	Insoluble
Ether	Slightly soluble	Insoluble	—	—	—	Insoluble
Absorption maxima						
0.1 N HCl	—	291	288	293	—	293,334
pH 7.0	—	254,324	318	253,325	254,327	330,388
0.1 N NaOH	—	244,309	240,300,390	245,308	244,312	305,388

[a]Data from Refs. 1,7,8.
[b]Melts with decomposition.

ogical growth assays, and high-performance liquid chromatography (HPLC). The animal growth assays are expensive, of long duration (several weeks per sample), and relatively imprecise in quantitation. They are, however, the only method that can determine the actual amount of the vitamin that is biologically avialable to the animal for its utilization. The animals most commonly used for these assays have been chicks and rats (13,14).

The most commonly used assay method has been the microbiological growth assay. Recently, improved separation and detection technologies have allowed the successful utilization of HPLC as a major method for the assay of vitamin B$_6$. These two methods will be discussed in detail. Simplification of certain aspects of these methods can be employed to measure only pure standards, if desired, but the basic principles are the same as those used for the assay of the vitamin in more complex biological samples. Chemical detection methods have been recently reviewed (15) and will not be presented here.

ANALYTICAL METHODOLOGY

I. MICROBIOLOGICAL METHOD
(*SACCHAROMYCES UVARUM* ATCC 9080)

A. Principle

See page 43

B. Equipment

The limiting factor in the assay method is the capacity or the number of tubes that can satisfactorily be arranged in the shaking machine. The list of equipment, unique to the assay for vitamin B$_6$, is based on the needs of the standards and 32 samples at five levels in triplicate, requiring 600 assay tubes.

1. *Incubating-Rotary Shaking Machine.* Capable of (repeated) steady operation for 22 hr at a rate of about 200 rpm, having a capacity of 600 16 $\times$ 150-mm screw-capped glass culture tubes and fitted with a means of securing the racks. (A rotary shaker in a constant temperature room is satisfactory.) The incubator or constant temperature room must maintain a constant and uniform temperature of 30°C.

2. *Oven.* Capable of maintaining 260° for 2 hr and holding 750 clean assay tubes and glass beads.

3. *Beads.* Solid glass spherical to withstand high temperatures, 4-mm diameter.

4. *Screw-Cap Glass Culture Tubes.* 16x150-mm with plastic caps with 1/8-inch hole drilled through top.

5. *Glass Columns.* Approximately 20 $\times$ 400-mm (diameter $\times$ length), with stopcock or similar flow-control device at bottom.

C. Reagents

WORK IN SUBDUED LIGHT WITH ALL SOLUTIONS CONTAINING ANY FORM OF VITAMIN B_6, AND OTHER LIGHT-SENSITIVE VITAMINS.

1. *Potassium Acetate Buffer, 1 M.* Dissolve 98.1 g potassium acetate in H_2O and make to 1 L.

2. *Potassium Acetate Buffer, 0.01 M (pH 4.5).* Put 10 mL 1 M potassium acetate solution (Reagent 1) in approximately 800 mL H_2O, adjust pH to 4.5 with acetic acid, and make to 1 L.

3. *Potassium Acetate Buffer, 0.02 M (pH 5.5).* Put 20 mL 1 M potassium acetate solution (Reagent 1) in approximately 800 mL H_2O, adjust pH to 5.5 with acetic acid, and make to 1 L.

4. *Potassium Acetate Buffer, 0.04 M (pH 6.0).* Put 40 mL 1 M potassium acetate solution (Reagent 1) in approximately 750 mL H_2O, adjust pH to 6.0 with acetic acid, and make to 1 L.

5. *Potassium Acetate, 0.1 M (pH 7.0).* Put 100 mL 1 M potassium acetate solution (Reagent 1) in approximately 700 mL H_2O, adjust pH to 7.0 with acetic acid or KOH, and make to 1 L.

6. *Potassium Chloride–Potassium Phosphate Solution (pH 8.0).* Dissolve 74.6 g KCl and 17.4 g K_2HPO_4 in approximately 800 mL H_2O, adjust pH to 8.0 with acetic acid solution, and make to 1 L.

7. *Ion-Exchange Resin.* Dowex AG 50W-X8, 100–200 mesh. (Bio-Rad Laboratories).

8. *Vitamin Assay Casamino Acids (Difco) or Acid-Hydrolyzed Casein.* For acid-hydrolyzed casein, mix 100 g vitamin-free casein with 500 mL of constant-boiling HCl (about 5 N HCl, 208 mL concentrated HCl made to 500 mL with H_2O) and reflux 8 hr. Remove the HCl from the mixture by distillation under vacuum until a very thick syrup remains, keeping the temperature of the water bath below 80°C. Dissolve the syrup in H_2O and concentrate again in the same manner. Redissolve the syrup in H_2O. Adjust to pH 4 with 40% NaOH, add H_2O to bring the volume to 600 mL, add 40 g of activated charcoal of the Darco G-60 type, stir 4 hr, and filter with vacuum through a Buchner funnel with a thin pad of HCl-washed Filtercel. If filtrate is not clear, add 20 g of Darco to the filtrate, stir for 1 hr, and refilter.

Repeat with a fresh 10 g portion Darco and filter. When solution is clear and colorless, make to 1 L with H_2O. Two to 3 mL 6 N HCl may be added before making to volume to lengthen the time before microbial growth occurs. Store in refrigerator. (1 mL equals 100 mg hydrolyzed casein.)

9. *Vitamin Solution I.* Dissolve 10 mg thiamin and 1 g inositol in 200 mL H_2O, and make to 1 L. Store in refrigerator. (1 mL equals 10 μg thiamin and 1 mg inositol.)

10. *Vitamin Solution II.* Dissolve 10 mg biotin in 100 mL 50% alcohol–H_2O. Store in refrigerator. (1 mL equals 100 μg biotin.) Dissolve 200 mg calcium

pantothenate and 200 mg niacin in 200 mL H$_2$O; add 8 mL of the above biotin solution; make to 1 L with H$_2$O. Store in refrigerator. (1 mL equals 200 μg each calcium pantothenate and niacin, 0.8 μg biotin.)

11. *Salt Solution I.*   Dissolve 17 g KCl, 10.3 g MgSO$_4$·7H$_2$O, 100 mg FeCl$_3$·6H$_2$O, and 100 mg MnSO$_4$·H$_2$O in about 800 mL H$_2$O. Add 2 mL concentrated HCl. Dissolve 5 g CaCl$_2$·2H$_2$O in about 100 mL H$_2$O; add to the first solution and make to 1 L with H$_2$O. Store in refrigerator. (1 mL equals 17 mg KCl, 5.03 mg MgSO$_4$, 50 μg FeCl$_3$, 89.3 μg MnSO$_4$, and 3.77 mg CaCl$_2$.)

12. *Salt Solution II.*   Dissolve 22 g KH$_2$PO$_4$ and 40 g (NH$_4$)$_2$HPO$_4$ in H$_2$O and make to 1 L. Store in refrigerator. [1 mL equals 22 mg KH$_2$PO$_4$ and 40 mg (NH$_4$)$_2$HPO$_4$.]

13. *"Tween 80" Solution.*   Weigh 2.5 g of "Tween 80" in a small beaker. Transfer with warm (45°) H$_2$O and make to 500 mL volume. Store in refrigerator. (1 mL equals 5 mg "Tween 80".)

14. *1 + 1 Citric Acid Solution.*   Dissolve 50 g of citric acid in 50 mL of H$_2$O. Store at room temperature in a bottle with a plastic stopper.

15. *1 + 2 Ammonium Phosphate Solution.*   Dissolve 25 g (NH$_4$)$_2$HPO$_4$ in 50 mL H$_2$O. Store at room temperature in a bottle with a plastic stopper.

16. *PN Standard Solutions.*

(a) Stock solution, 100 μg/mL.   Dissolve and dilute 12.16 mg USP PN·HCl reference standard (previously dried 5 days over P$_2$O$_5$) to 100 mL with 1 N HCl. Store in a red, glass-stoppered bottle in a refrigerator.

(b) Intermediate solution, 1.0 μg/mL.   Dilute 2 mL stock solution [Reagent 16(a)] to 200 mL with H$_2$O. Prepare fresh for each assay.

(c) Working Solution 1.0 ng/mL.   Dilute 1 mL intermediate solution [Reagent 16(b)] to 1 L. Prepare fresh for each assay.

17. *PL Standard Solutions.*

(a) Stock solution, 100 μg/mL.   Prepare as for PN [Reagent 16(a)] except use 12.18 mg PL·HCl of high purity.

(b) Intermediate solution, 1.0 μg/mL.   See Reagent 16(b).

(c) Working solution, 1.0 ng/mL.   See Reagent 16(c).

18. *PM Standard Solutions.*

(a) Stock solution, 100 μg/mL.   Prepare as for PN [Reagent 16(a)] except use 14.34 mg PM·2HCl of high purity.

(b) Intermediate solution, 1.0 μg/mL.   See Reagent 16(b).

(c) Working solution, 1.0 ng/mL.   See Reagent 16(c).

19. *Mixed PN, PL, PM Standard Solution.*

(a) Intermediate solution, 0.33 μg/mL each PN, PL, PM.   Dilute 0.667 mL each of PN stock solution [Reagent 16(a)], PL stock solution [Reagent 17(a)], and PM stock solution [Reagent 18(a)] to 200 mL with H$_2$O. Prepare fresh for each assay.

(b) Working solution, 0.33 ng/mL each PN, PL, PM. Dilute 1 mL of mixed intermediate solution [Reagent 19(a)] to 1 L. Prepare fresh for each assay.

20. *Mixed PN, PL, PM Solution for Liquid Broth Culture.* Dilute 6 mL of mixed intermediate solution [Reagent 19(a)] to 1 L with H_2O.

21. *Citrate Buffer Solution.* Dissolve 100 g potassium citrate and 20 g citric acid and make to 1 L with H_2O. Store in refrigerator. (1 mL equals 100 mg potassium citrate and 20 mg citric acid.)

22. *Basal Medium Stock Solution.*

Reagent	Reagent Number	For 180 Tubes	For 600 Tubes
H_2O	—	400 mL	1400 mL
Citrate buffer	21	100 mL	320 mL
Casamino acids or casein solution	8	10 g or 100 mL	32 g or 320 mL
Vitamin solution I	9	50 mL	160 mL
Vitamin solution II	10	25 mL	80 mL
Salt solution I	11	50 mL	160 mL
Salt solution II	12	50 mL	160 mL
Glucose	—	100 g	320 g
dl-Tryptophan*	—	22 mg	70.4 mg
l-Histidine*	—	27 mg	86.4 mg
dl-Methionine*	—	100 mg	320 mg
dl-Isoleucine*	—	216 mg	691.2 mg
dl-Valine*	—	256 mg	819.2 mg
"Tween 80"	13	20 mL	64 mL
Final volume		1000 mL	3200 mL

*Place together in a small beaker, dissolve in a small amount of 10% HCl before adding to the media.

Add the reagents to the H_2O in the order listed. Dissolve the glucose in the liquids with vigorous stirring. Adjust to pH 4.5 with citric acid (Reagent 14) or $(NH_4)_2HPO_4$ (Reagent 15). Make to final volume in cylinder or marked beaker with H_2O; store in Pyrex bottle plugged with cotton in refrigerator. Prepare not longer than 24 hr before use. When ready, steam for 10 min and cool.

Pyridoxine-Y medium is not recommended for assay of foods or biological samples as less growth response was obtained for both the assay inoculum and the assay standards. Furthermore, equivalent growth response to PN, PL, and PM was not achieved when using Pyridoxine-Y medium (see also Section E, below).

23. *Test Organism.   Saccharomyces uvarum,* ATCC 9080.

24. *Agar Culture Medium (YM or Bacto-Wort, Difco).*   For YM agar, suspend 20.5 g YM agar in about 400 mL H$_2$O in a marked 500-mL wide-mouth Erlenmeyer flask. Plug with cotton, steam for about 10 min to dissolve the agar, adjust the volume to 500 mL. Pipette the hot agar in 10-mL amounts into 20 $\times$ 150-mm test tubes, plug with absorbent cotton and autoclave for 15 min at 15 psi. Tilt the hot agar tubes to form slants and cool in this position. For the Wort agar, suspend 25 g Bacto-Wort agar in about 400 mL H$_2$O in a marked 500-mL wide-mouth Erlenmeyer flask. Plug with cotton, steam for about 10 min to dissolve the agar, adjust the volume to 500 mL. Pipette the hot agar in 10-mL amounts into 20 $\times$ 150-mm test tubes, plug with absorbent cotton, and autoclave for 15 min at 15 psi. Inasmuch as this medium has an acid reaction, care should be taken to avoid overheating which will result in a softer medium. Tilt the hot agar tubes to form slants and cool in this position.

25. *Liquid Culture Medium.*   Pipette 5 mL of mixed solution (Reagent 20) for liquid broth culture tubes into 16 $\times$ 150-mm test tubes, containing two glass beads (4 mm), plug with absorbent cotton, and autoclave for 10 min at 15 psi. Add 5 mL steamed vitamin B$_6$-free basal medium (Reagent 22) under aseptic conditions. Store at about 4°C.

26. *Inoculum Rinse.*   Pipette 5 mL H$_2$O into test tubes, plug with abosorbent cotton, and autoclave for 10 min at 15 psi. Add 5 mL of steamed vitamin B$_6$-free basal medium (Reagent 22) under aseptic conditions. Store tubes at about 4°C.

D.   Procedure

The folllowing method is essentially that of Toepfer and Polansky (16). It must be emphasized constantly that vitamin B$_6$ is light-sensitive and that sufficient precautions must be taken through the procedure to minimize exposure of standard and test solutions. All work with solutions containing vitamin B$_6$ is performed in a darkened laboratory. The use of red or gold fluorescent light is suitable. Note the time relationship that must be observed in microbiological procedures. Active slants of the stock culture must be available for the preparation of inoculum. It is advisable to make daily agar transfers for several days before preparing the assay inoculum. The assay inoculum should be started from a fresh 24-hr slant of yeast cells. The assay inoculum should be grown in liquid broth 20 hr before it is used in the assay. The time of inoculation of the assay tubes should be planned so that reading of the absorbance can be carried out 22 hr later. It is advisable to extract the samples on Monday, chromatograph, if desired, and set up and sterilize the assay tubes on Tuesday, inoculate the assay tubes on Wednesday, and read the absorbance of the assay tubes on Thursday. If large numbers of samples are to be assayed and sufficient equipment and technical assistance are available, two sets can be run each week, by extraction of two sets of samples on Monday, chromatographing and setting up the second set of assay tubes on Wednesday, inoculating on Thursday, and reading on Friday. Care must be taken throughout the microbiological assay to prevent contamination from undesirable organisms.

1. *Culture Care.*   Maintain the *S. uvarum* culture by weekly transfers on YM agar slants (Reagent 24). Incubate these freshly seeded agar slants at 30° for 24 hr and then refrigerate.

2. *Assay Inoculum.*   Incubate cells of inoculum on agar at 30°C for 24 hr just before use. Transfer cells with loop under aseptic condition to liquid broth culture tubes (Reagent 25). Plug with absorbent cotton held in place with masking tape and place the tubes on the shaker at 30°C for 20 hr. Replace the cotton plugs aseptically with sterile rubber stoppers; centrifuge at 2500 rpm for 1.5 min. Decant the liquid and resuspend in 10 mL of inoculum rinse (Reagent 26). Separate by centrifugation at 2500 rpm for 1.5 min. Decant the liquid, resuspend in a second 10 mL of sterile inoculum rinse, centrifuge for 1.5 min, and decant. The cells suspended in the third 10 mL of inoculum rinse are the assay inoculum.

3. *Preparation of Exchange Resin and Column.*   To 250 g Dowex AG 50W-X8 (100–200 mesh) in the hydrogen form add excess 6 N KOH until the supernatant liquid is blue to litmus. Let settle, decant, and rinse the resin with H_2O until the supernatant liquid is clear. Add about 600 mL 3 N HCl, stir, and heat for one-half hr in a boiling water bath. Decant and repeat this treatment with 3 N HCl two more times. Rinse the resin until the rinse H_2O is neutral. Add 6 N KOH until pH is strongly basic and stir for 1 hr. Rinse with H_2O until rinse water is neutral. Suspend in 2 M potassium acetate and store at 4°C until needed. Just before use, wash resin with H_2O until pH is 7.0. The resin can be regenerated beginning with the 3 N HCl treatment.

Pour 30 ml of the prepared resin into 20 × 400-mm column with H_2O. After the resin settles in the column, place a plug of glass wool on top of the resin. Rinse the column with 50 mL hot H_2O followed by two 50-ml portions of hot 0.01 M potassium acetate (pH 4.5) (Reagent 2). The pH of the last buffer rinse from column should be 4.5; otherwise, more rinsing with Reagent 2 would be required. Do not permit the level of the liquid on the column to fall below the top glass wool plug at any time.

4. *Extraction.*

(a) Foods.   Fresh, frozen, or dried samples should be ground or in a finely divided state. Generally 1-g or 2-g samples are used for dry products and up to 20 g for fresh products. Place the weighed sample in a 500-mL, wide-mouth Erlenmeyer flask and suspend in 200 mL 0.44 N HCl for plant products; in 200 mL 0.055 N HCl for animal products; and 200 mL 0.2 N HCl for food composites. Autoclave the plant products at 15 psi for 2 hr. Autoclave the animal products and food composites for 5 hr at 15 psi. Cool to room temperature, adjust to pH 4.5 with 6 N KOH, bring to 250 mL volume in a volumetric flask, and filter through Whatman No. 40 filter paper.

(b) Serum or plasma.   Suspend 3–5 mL of serum or plasma in 200 mL of 0.055 N HCl in a 500 mL, wide-mouth Erlenmeyer flask and autoclave at

15 psi for 5 hr. Cool to room temperature, adjust to pH 4.5 with 6 N KOH, bring to 250 mL volume in a volumetric flask, and filter through Whatman No. 40 filter paper. If the volume of serum or plasma is limited and only total vitamin B$_6$ is desired, less sample volume may be used, but be sure to maintain the ratio of acid to serum or plasma at 50:1.

(c) Urine.   Suspend 1–5 mL of urine in 200 mL of 0.2 N HCl in a 500-mL, wide-mouth Erlenmeyer flask and autoclave at 15 psi for 5 hr. Cool to room temperature, adjust to pH 4.5 with 6 N KOH, bring to 250-mL volume in a volumetric flask, and filter through Whatman No. 40 paper.

For all of the above types of samples, to determine PN, PL, and PM individually, pass 40–200 mL of filtered aliquot through the resin column. If only total vitamin B$_6$ values are desired, the samples would not be chromatographed. They should be diluted according to expected vitamin B$_6$ concentration and added to the assay tubes.

5. *Chromatography.* (This step may be omitted if only total vitamin B$_6$ concentration is desired.) Put desired amount of the filtered extract on the ion-exchange column in approximately 50-mL portions and allow to pass completely through with no regulation of the flow. Wash the beaker and column three times with about 5-mL portions of hot 0.02 M potassium acetate pH 5.5 (Reagent 3) followed by a similar washing of the sides of the column. Wash the column with the same solution until a total of 100 ml of the 0.02 M potassium acetate pH 5.5 solution is used. PL is eluted with two 50-mL portions of boiling 0.04 M potassium acetate pH 6.0 (Reagent 4), collecting the eluate in a 100-mL volumetric flask. PN is eluted with two 50-mL portions of boiling 0.1 M potassium acetate pH 7.0 (Reagent 5) collecting the eluate in a 100-mL volumetric flask. The PM is eluted with two 50-mL portions of boiling KCl–K$_2$HPO$_4$ pH 8.0 (Reagent 6). Collect PM in a 250-mL beaker. Adjust pH to 4.5. Make eluates of PN and PL to 100-mL volume and PM to 200 mL unless otherwise desired.

For standard PN, PL, and PM, mix 5 mL each of 1.0 µg/mL standard solution [Reagents 16(b), 17(b), 18(b)], neutralize with KOH and make to pH 4.5 with acetic acid. This procedure provides a slight buffer capacity to the standard solutions. Put this solution on the column, wash, and elute the fractions according to the above procedure. Make the eluted PN and PL standards to 100 mL, and the eluted PM, after pH is adjusted to 4.5, to 200 mL. Dilute the eluted standards to contain 1.0 ng/mL.

6. *Microbiological Assay Procedure.*   Heat clean tubes and glass beads to 260°C for 2 hr. Place two 4-mm glass beads in each 16 × 150-mm screw-cap glass culture tube. For the standard curve, pipette in triplicate the appropriate freshly prepared standard [Reagents 16(c), 17(c), 18(c)] to give 0.0, 0.0, 0.5, 1.0, 2.0, 3.0, 4.0, 5.0 ng PN, PL, or PM per tube. Similarly prepare a set of tubes for the eluted standards, omitting the blanks. If only total vitamin B$_6$ values for biological samples are desired, include mixed PN, PL, PM [Reagent 19(b)] and omit the eluted standards. If pharmaceutical preparations are being assayed, use PN [Reagent 16(c)] for the standard. Dilute the samples or sample eluates from the chromatographic column to contain about 1 ng vitamin B$_6$ component/mL.

Pipette 1, 2, 3, 4, and 5 mL of the diluted eluates or samples into triplicate tubes. Pipette H_2O into all tubes to bring the volume to 5 mL per tube. Cap the tubes with plastic caps with a 1/8-inch hole through the top. Autoclave the entire set for 10 min at 15 psi. Cool the tubes to room temperature. Using an automatic pipette with sterilized delivery attachements, pipette 5 mL of the steamed medium (Reagent 22) through the hole in the cap. Cover the tubes with sterile cheesecloth and place in refrigerator.

Remove from refrigerator 1 hr before inoculation. Aseptically inoculate through the hole in the cap of each tube, except the first set of 0.0 level for the standard curves, with 1 drop of the assay inoculum of the suspended cells of *S. uvarum.* Take care to maintain a uniform suspension of the cells because they may settle out during the inoculation step. Incubate the tubes on a rotary shaker at 30° for 22 hr. Steam the tubes in the autoclave for 5 min, cool, and remove the caps. Read the absorbance at 550 nm on a spectrophotometer. To read the uninoculated blank, set at zero with H_2O. To read the inoculated blank, set at zero with the uninoculated blank. Mix the 9 or 12 inoculated blank tubes and with this mixture set the instrument at zero to read all other tubes.

7. *Calculations.*   Average the readings of the triplicate tubes and plot absorbance against nanograms of eluted standard PN, PL, or PM per tube or against the mixed PN, PL, and PM standard if only total vitamin B_6 is being determined. Determine by interpolation the amount of PN, PL, or PM or total vitamin B_6 per sample tube. Report µg of PN, PL, and PM or total vitamin B_6 per g or per mL sample. Figure 17.2 shows a typical set of standard curves for PN, PL, PM, and the standard mix.

E. Variations of the Method

Numerous other organisms have been used in the microbiological assay for vitamin B_6 such as *Neuospora sitophila* (17), *Streptococcus lactis* (18), *Lactobacillus casei,* and *Streptococcus faecalis* (19). For various reasons, *Saccharomyces uvarum* has been the most widely used. One problem with the microbiological assay using *S. uvarum* is the reported lower sensitivity of the microorganism to PM compared with PN and PL (20–24, Figure 17.2). The reason for the differential response is not known. This can result in a substantial calculated concentration error in certain foods that are high in PM if the chromatography step is omitted, but is of little or no concern in foods that are substantially fortified with PN or in pharmaceutical preparations containing PN. Recently, the use of *Kloeckera apiculata* (ATCC 9774) has been suggested as an alternative to achieve equivalent growth response from PM, PN, and PL (22). The microbiological growth assay has been modified further to produce a combined radiometric-microbiological growth assay in which L-[1-^{14}C]valine is added to the growth medium (25,26). The growth of the microorganisms, in response to the concentration of vitamin B_6 in the medium, is monitored by the detection of $^{14}CO_2$ which is generated from metabolism of the [1-^{14}C]valine. The use of *K. apiculata,* however, in two other laboratories has failed to yield equivalent growth response in the standard

GROWTH RESPONSE OF <u>SACCHAROMYCES</u> <u>UVARUM</u> TO PN, PL, PM.
(30°C, 22 HOURS, HN MEDIUM)

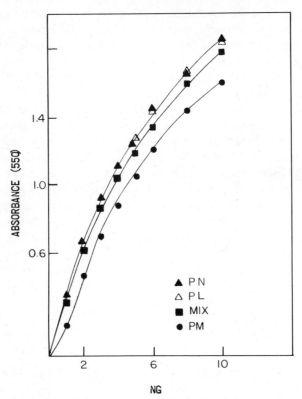

FIGURE 17.2   Typical growth-response curve with *S. uvarum* (25).

microbiological growth assay (23,24) and the radiometric-microbiological assay has not yet been confirmed in other laboratories. Thus, the use of organisms other than *S. uvarum* should be used with caution and should be confirmed in other laboratories prior to their acceptance as a standard test organism.

II.   HIGH-PERFORMANCE LIQUID CHROMATOGRAPHY METHOD

A.   Introduction

HPLC provides the opportunity of quantitating all six forms of vitamin B₆. This method, however, imposes severe constraints on the procedures used to extract the vitamers from samples in that interfering substances must be eliminated while the vitamers are being recovered without destruction. The methods described below (27–32) provide appropriate samples for analysis from many different biological samples and yield recoveries close to 100% for all vitamers. The method provides for the inclusion of an internal standard, 3-hydroxypyridine (HOP), which is added to the biological sample before extraction and analysis, thus correcting for any dilution errors and instrument variation. The described method has been checked (in-house) against the previously described microbiological method and satisfactory agreement was obtained for meat samples. Differences exist in values obtained between the two methods for fruits and vegetables which may be attributed to difficulties in extraction of these foods for HPLC analyses.

B. Equipment

The following instrumentation is required to set up the complete chromatographic system. For convenience, model numbers of certain manufacturers are specified, but in practically all cases, comparable models are available from other manufacturers.

1. *Pumps.* Milton Roy, Mini-Pump Model 396, 16–160 mL/hr (LDC/Milton Roy).

2. *Pressure Gauges.* Capable of reading to 500 psi, U.S. Gauge (Benchmark Technical Sales).

3. *Needle Valves.* SS-1SG, (Nupro Co.).

4. *Inject Valves (External Volume, 6 Port).* One manual model No. CV-6UHPa-HC; one automatic model No. AHCV-6UHPa-HC (Valco Instrument Company). Detailed instructions for assembly provided by Valco.

5. *Switching Valve (4 Port).* Model No. AHCV-4-UHPa-HC, (Valco Instrument Company).

6. *Chromatographic columns.* Two model No. 3202-6x3OUL, one model No. 3202-3x3OUL. Glenco Sci., Inc.

7. *Resins.* Bio-Rad Aminex A-25; Dowex AG 2-X8, 200–400 mesh (Bio-Rad Laboratories.) Columns should be packed according to instructions in Bio-Rad and Glenco catalogs. The Aminex A-25 should be checked to ensure separation of the phosphate from nonphosphate forms; recently, at least one lot of resin did not show characteristics of earlier lots of this resin.

8. *Water Baths.* One model No. FK-13-874-130 (−15–50°C), Haake Circulating; one model No. FS-13-874-114 (30–250°C), Haake Circulating (Fisher Scientific Co.).

9. *Computing Integrator with Relay Control Accessory.* Model No. A-221-16386-90 Chromatographic-R1A Recording Processor with relay control accessory A-221-17084-90 Programmer PRG-102A, (Shimadzu Scientific Instruments, Inc.). Instructions for calibration, writing time program and control of relays provided in Shimadzu manuals.

10. *Recorder.* Kipp and Zonen, model BD 40, (Preiser Scientific Company).

11. *Detector.* Perkin-Elmer model No. LS-5 Fluorescence Spectrophoto-

meter. This model can be programmed to automatically change excitation and emission wavelengths. It is not as sensitive as their model No. 650-40, but the latter must be controlled with an extra microcomputer (9,33)(Perkin-Elmer Corp.).

12. *Detector.*   Aminco Fluoromonitor with Corning 7-54 primary and Wratten 2E secondary filters. (American Instrument Co.).

13. *Solenoid Valves.*   Model No. 062-4E1-36 4-way single solenoid, (Humphrey Products).

14. *Homogenizer.*   Sorvall Omni-Mixer with 6-50-mL chamber assemblies, (DuPont Co.).

15. *Vortex Mixer.*   Model K-500-J, (Scientific Industries, Inc.).

16. *Centrifuge.*   Model J2-21, (Beckman Instruments Co.).

17. *Filters.*   0.45 μm Cat. No. HAWP 025 00; 0.22 μm Cat. No. GSWP 025 00, (Millipore Corp.).

18. *Swinnex Filter Holders.*   Cat. No. 5x00 025 00, (Millipore Corp.).

19. *"Swagelok" Nuts and Ferrules.*   ¹/₁₆-in. nut with front and back ferrules, SS-102-1, SS-103-1, SS-104-1 ⅛-in. nut with front and back ferrules, SS-202-1, SS-203-1, SS-204-1, (Crawford Fitting Co.).

20. *"Cheminert" Fittings.*   Unions UCI-16; unions UCI-8; adaptors, metal 107A76; tube ends TEF-107; couplings 107A3; plug 107A16; tees CJ-3031; glass adaptors G2-C; leur adaptors-female 107B8; adaptors, metal 107A20; pressure gauge adaptor kits PG-11-4CI; flaring tool FI-1.

21. *Tubing.*   Stainless Steel #304 ¹/₁₆-in. and ⅛-in. o.d., (Alltech Associates). Teflon - 26 AWG thick wall, (Penntube Plastics.) Teflon - 18 AWG, (Read Plastics).

22. *Air and Filter Trap.*   Inline filter TF-600 with No. 301 fitting, Discs-3130-D, (MER Chromatographic).

23. *Switching Valve (for reservoirs).*   3 port valve No. 1530 (MER Chromatographic).

C. Reagents

1. *pH 10 Buffer.*   0.4 M NaCl, 0.01 M glycine, 0.005 M semicarbazide; pH adjusted to 10 with 50% NaOH.

2. *pH 2.5 Buffer.*   0.4 M NaCl, 0.01 M glycine; pH adjusted to 2.5 with 1 M HCl.

3. *pH 11.5 Solution.*   0.4 M NaCl, 0.01 M glycine; pH adjusted to 11.5 with 50% NaOH.

4. *0.1 M HCl Mobile Phase Clean-up.*   83 mL concentrated HCl diluted to 1 L to make 1 M HCl. 100 ml 1 M HCl diluted to 1 L to obtain 0.1 M HCl.

5. *FeCl₃ Precolumn Clean-Up.*   2% FeCl₃, 0.1 M HCl (40 g FeCl₃ + 200 mL 1 M HCl diluted to 2 L).

6. *5% 5-Sulfosalicylic Acid Solution (SSA).*   12.5 g in 250 mL H₂O.

7. *Internal Standard Solutions.*   For solid samples, it is convenient to use a solution of 6 mg HOP in 100 mL H_2O. When preparing the 5% solution of SSA for deproteinization (Reagent 6), add 3 mL of 6 mg% HOP solution to this before diluting to 250 mL. For liquid samples, prepare a solution of 12 mg HOP in 100 mL H_2O. Ten μL of this solution is then added to 10 mL of sample immediately after the solid SSA (0.5 g) is added.

8. *Pyridoxine 5'-Phosphate.*   Synthesized according to the method of Peterson and Sober (34).

D. Analytical System

The liquid chromatographic system that will accept "clean" samples is assembled as shown in Figure 17.3 (28). The principal components are a depulsed positive-displacement pump (9,35), a pneumatically activated six-way external volume sample injection valve with a 0.5-mL sample loop, a pneumatically activated column switching valve, two columns packed with Bio-Rad Aminex A-25 resin, a fluorescence spectrophotometer, and a computing integrator with an external relay control box. All components are connected by 26 AWG thick-wall Teflon tubing and Cheminert fittings, except for the connections between the reservoir and pump, which is 18 AWG. Tubing lengths are kept as short as possible to avoid increasing the dispersion of the sample.

1. *Depulsing the Pump.*   The positive displacement pump is depulsed as detailed in Figure 17.4a. The gauges are inserted into the line by means of Cheminert three-way connectors. A needle valve is inserted between the two gauges and adjusted so that the pressure on the first gauge does not exceed 400 psi. This absorbs most of the pulsation from the positive displacement pump. The pulsation on the second gauge normally does not exceed 10–20 psi. Pressures throughout should never exceed 500 psi; otherwise, the tubing will rupture. The pump is attached to the system as shown in Figure 17.4b.

2. *Sample Injection and Switching Valve.*   These valves are controlled by relay-operated solenoid valves; the relays are controlled through a relay control box activated by appropriate programming of the computing integrator (Figure 17.3). The details of the air hook-up is shown in Figure 17.4c and details of sample loading and injection are illustrated in Figure 17.5.

3. *Chromatographic Columns.*   The first column is 6 mm $\times$ 24 cm and is slurry-packed with Bio-Rad Aminex A-25 resin. It is thermostated at 50°C as shown in Figure 17.3. The second column, similarly packed, is thermostated at 18°C. Since all column packings vary slightly, it may be necessary to vary the temperatures on the two columns slightly to achieve maximum separation.

4. *Detector.*   Fluorescence detection is recommended over ultraviolet absorption because of the relative greater sensitivity. The detector must have a flow cell compatible with HPLC systems and the capability of changing the excitation and emission wavelengths—either manually or automatically—at least four times during the course of an analysis. All high-quality detectors have

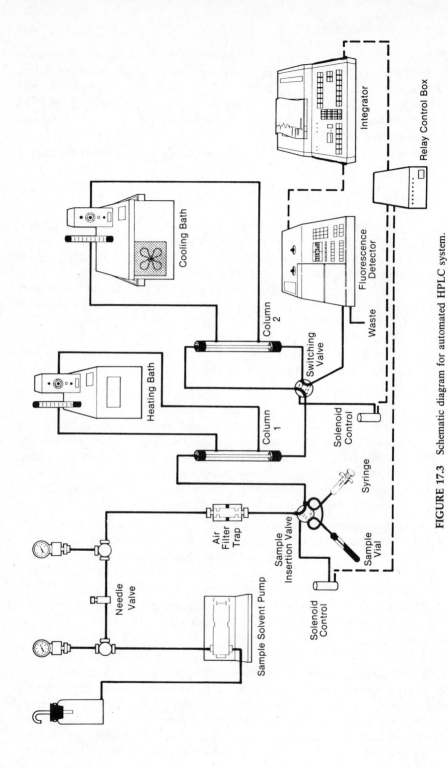

FIGURE 17.3 Schematic diagram for automated HPLC system.

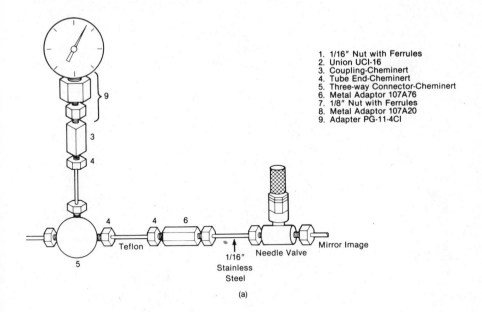

1. 1/16" Nut with Ferrules
2. Union UCI-16
3. Coupling-Cheminert
4. Tube End-Cheminert
5. Three-way Connector-Cheminert
6. Metal Adaptor 107A76
7. 1/8" Nut with Ferrules
8. Metal Adaptor 107A20
9. Adapter PG-11-4Cl

(a)

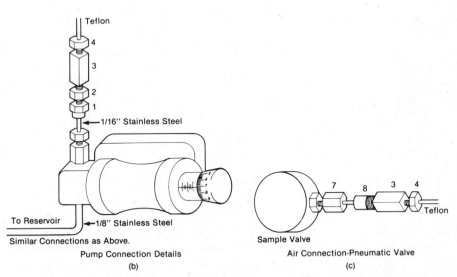

Pump Connection Details
(b)

Air Connection-Pneumatic Valve
(c)

FIGURE 17.4 a. Hook-up for depulsing of positive-displacement pump. b. Attachment of pump to HPLC system. c. Details of pneumatic valve hook-up.

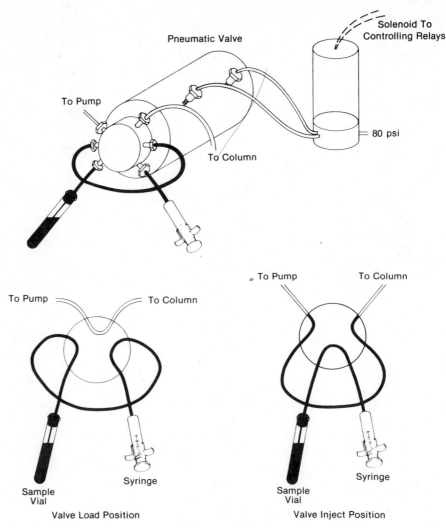

FIGURE 17.5   Details of sample loading and injection procedure.

different sensitivity ranges, signal suppressions, and damping constants. These different characteristics are useful in vitamin B$_6$ analyses because different samples vary in their vitamin content and the various excitation and emission wavelength settings on a particular instrument produce different background signals. To free the operator for other duties, it is preferable to automate the necessary excitation and emission wavelength changes of the detector. As mentioned earlier, instruments are now available that can be programmed to make these changes. However, if expertise is available, it is often possible to connect an inexpensive microcomputer to the detector keyboard and control the wavelength changes through the computer (9,33). In this manner, it has been possible to take advantage of the excellent sensitivity of the Perkin-Elmer Model 650-40 fluorescence spectrophotometer and to control automatically wavelength changes at minimal expense.

5. *Computing Integrator.* The computing integrator should not only produce a chromatographic trace during an analysis, but also be able to print out the concentrations of the different vitamers on the basis of observed peak areas, the known amount of added internal standard (HOP), and a previous calibration run on pure standards. The integrator must be capable of accepting integration instructions, as well as handling baseline irregularities. It must also have the capability of controlling at least the two external relays that operate the solenoid valves. All of the computing integrator packages that provide such capabilities include a detailed set of instructions on how to program the instrument to accomplish the above tasks.

E. Procedures

A single buffer is used in this procedure. It consists of 0.4 M sodium chloride, 0.01 M glycine, and 0.005 M semicarbazide adjusted to a pH of 10 with NaOH (Reagent 1). The flow-rate is 1.25 mL/min. For the first 23.4 min after injection, the buffer passes only through the first column at a pressure of 150 psi before entering the detector; during this time, PMP, PM, PNP, and PN are eluted and detected. The fluorescence excitation and emission wavelengths are set at 310 nm and 380 nm, respectively (all four forms are detected at these wavelengths). The switching valve then redirects the effluent from the first column through the second column before entering the detector; the working pressure is now 200 psi. At the same time, the excitation and emission wavelengths are changed to 280 nm and 487 nm, respectively, to detect PLP. After PLP has been eluted and detected (39.5 min), the wavelengths are switched back to 310 nm and 380 nm to detect the internal standard, HOP. At 52.4 min, the second column is switched out of the flow, the wavelengths are set at 280 and 487 nm, and PL is detected at 63.4 min as it elutes from the first column.

The sample injection and column switching are controlled by a time program previously incorporated into the computing integrator. This time program also directs the integrator on how to integrate the peak areas and how to cope with baseline irregularities due to sample injection or wavelength changes. A typical chromatographic trace for a sample of standard including an internal standard is shown in Figure 17.6.

1. *Calibration and Unknowns.* Before analyzing biological samples, the system must first be calibrated. The computing integrator time program is entered and the integrator is switched into its calibration mode. A solution of standards, including the internal standard, is prepared, the concentrations entered into the integrator, and a sample of the solution is injected into the mobile phase. (The concentrations in the standard solution should be comparable with these expected

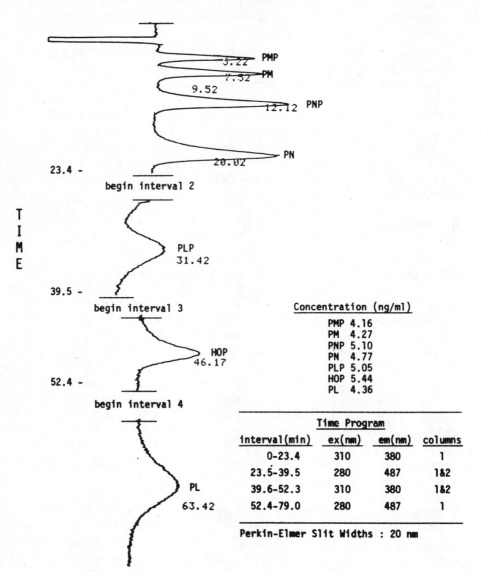

RELATIVE FLUORESCENCE

FIGURE 17.6 Typical trace of standard B$_6$ vitamers and internal standard.

in the unknown.) At the end of the run, the integrator upon instruction calibrates itself and stores the appropriate constants. After switching the integrator to the analysis mode, a series of unknowns can be injected; the concentrations are automatically determined and printed out at the end of each run. Normally, it is advisable to calibrate at least once each week. It has been our experience that the calibration varies only slightly from week to week. If there is a drastic change in the calibration parameters, then the results reported for the week should be suspect.

2. *Column Clean-Up.* It is advisable to clean the columns each week by flushing with a solution of 0.4 M sodium chloride and 0.01 M glycine, adjusted to pH 2.5 with HCl (Reagent 2). The solution is first passed through only the first column until it is clean as evidenced by a stable baseline and then is passed sequentially through both columns until another stable baseline is attained. At a flow rate of 1.25 mL/min, this process takes 4 hr. The columns are then reequilibrated at pH 10 (Reagent 1) for ½ hr before additional analyses are made.

F. Sample Preparation

The analytical system described above is capable of handling samples that do not contain compounds which would interfere with the analysis. The accurate analysis of biological samples also requires a procedure that extracts the different vitamers from complex matrices without loss and yields recoveries of approximately 100%. The following two sections describe a successful extraction procedure and a useful sample purification system (29–31).

1. *Extraction Procedures.* Solid and liquid samples are treated slightly differently. In both cases, however, sulfosalicylic acid is used as the deproteinating agent and the internal standard is added directly to the samples before any treatment.

(a) Solid samples. Add to a 2-g sample 10 mL of 5% (w/v) solution of SSA to which a known amount of the internal standard has been added (see recommended amounts in Section C.7). Homogenize the mixture in an Omni-mixer at medium speed for 10 min. Add 10 mL of methylene chloride to extract lipids and regrind the entire mixture for another 5 min. Centrifuge at 7500 × g for 10 min at 4°C; remove the upper water layer and filter through a 0.45 μm Millipore filter in a Swinnex holder and introduce an aliquot (0.5 mL) of the resulting solution into the sample purification system (see Section F.2 below).

(b) Liquid samples. To 10 mL of sample add 0.5 g SSA and 10 μL of an internal standard solution (12 mg/100 mL). Vortex the solution for 1 1/2 min; add 10 ml of methylene chloride and vortex for an additional 1 1/2 min. Centrifuge at 7500 × g for 10 min at 4°C; remove the upper H_2O layer and filter through a 0.45 μm Millipore filter as with solid samples. Introduce an aliquot into the sample purification system.

2. *Sample Purification System.* The sample purification system is shown in Figure 17.7 (31). It is a HPLC system with the same depulsed pump described earlier and a manual injection valve. Pack the 6-mm × 25-cm column with 200–400 mesh Dowex AG 2-X8 anion exchange resin and monitor the eluted peak a fluorescence detector (Aminco fluorimonitor) with Corning 7-54 primary filter and a Wratten 2E secondary filter. All components are again connected by 26 AWG thick-wall Teflon tubing in conjunction with Cheminert fittings

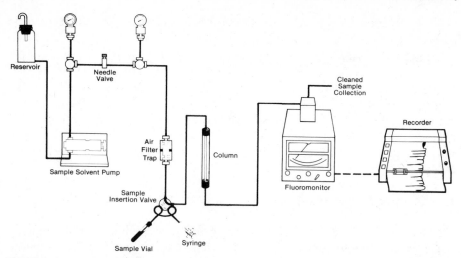

FIGURE 17.7 Sample purification system for removal of SSA prior to injection onto analytical system (Shown in Figure 17.3).

except for the reservoir-to-pump line which is 18 AWG. The signal output of the detector is monitored on a strip chart recorder. The mobile phase is 0.1 M HCl. Two min after injection, the extracted vitamers begin to elute from the columns at which time the effluent is collected for about 6 min until all vitamers (including the internal standard HOP) are eluted and baseline is reached. Adjust the pH of the solution to between pH 7 and 8, and inject the sample on the analytical column which separates and quantifies the vitamers. SSA and interfering compounds are normally retained on the Dowex precolumn.

Clean the precolumn after approximately 10 samples have been purified. This is done by passing the FeCl₃ clean-up solution (Reagent 5) *from bottom to top* through the Dowex column at a flow rate of 1.2 mL/min. When the deep purple color that is initially formed has disappeared (about 2 hr), the column is then flushed with 0.1 M HCl for 1/2 hr and is ready for reuse.

G. Sample Handling

A word of caution is in order when one is dealing with biological systems. Although in some samples, such as muscle tissue, enzymatic activity is at a minimum, there are cases such as rat liver, where the possibility of enzymatic activity is high and care must be exercised in the initial stages of sample handling (31). It has been observed that phosphatase activity can seriously influence the observed concentrations of the different vitamers if such activity is not inhibited (31). Interconversions and degradation do occur with time so it is necessary to inhibit enzyme activity soon after the tissue is excised from the animal. This problem is not unique for chemical assays but is also a problem for any microbiological assay. Phosphatase inhibitors such as 50 mM NaF (36) or 80 mM Na₂HPO₄ at pH 7.5 (37,38) can be added to the SSA extracting solutions.

In the initial investigations on any new biological matrix, it is recommended that the effect of sampling time, enzyme inhibition, and storage conditions be investigated before any results are treated with confidence.

H.   Helpful Hints

1. Always work under gold or red light and use actinic glassware whenever possible.

2. If the method of Peterson and Sober (34) is used to prepare PNP, the resin used to purify the compound, XE-64, is now identified as Amberlite IRP-64.

3. If the Rockwell AIM microcomputer is used to control the fluorescence spectrophotometer, it will be necessary to purchase one ROM Basic A65-020, one AIM 65 enclosure with power supply, and one AIM 65 with 4K RAM memory from, among others, Hamilton Avnet Electronics.

4. If the needle valve in the pump depulsing system tends to clog, insert an additional filter air trap in the line after the pump.

5. The buffer reservoirs and waste containers should be kept at the same level and both should be elevated above pump level.

6. All glassware and containers should be autoclaved routinely as part of the cleaning process.

7. If air bubbles develop in the line after the columns and before the detector, add a several meter length of 32 AWG tubing after the detector to increase the back pressure.

8. If air bubbles are trapped in the flow cell, flush out with methanol.

9. Check daily for gaps at top of column. If it becomes necessary to remove top fitting to add resin, continue pumping while slowly removing top.

10. When loading a sample, maintain pressure on syringe so no back flushing occurs. Pull at least 1 mL of sample through a 0.5-mL loop for adequate flushing.

11. After loading sample, flush out valve while it is in inject position.

12. If it becomes necessary to remove the column from the system, plug both ends so no air is introduced.

13. On the air lines to the pneumatic valves, introduce a 150-mL ballast volume close to the valve inlet. Model No. 304-HDF4, (Whitey Co).

14. After precolumn runs, flush pump to remove 0.1 N HCl. Leave main column pump overnight with pH 10 buffer (Reagent 1) in chamber.

15. In the described procedure, dilution of about 10 occurs. If less dilution is desirable, use a smaller precolumn but a fewer number of samples can then be run before column cleanup becomes necessary.

16. At concentrations of PLP less than 2 ng/mL, use degassed buffers (9).

17. In muscle tissue with high vitamin concentrations, it may be desirable to extract with 10% (w/v) SSA. Recovery studies on chicken breasts were significantly improved over the 5% SSA extraction.

18. The described procedures used on human breast milk yielded compounds that interfered with the PMP and PM determinations. However, there were only trace amounts of these vitamers present. The principal forms were PL and PLP for which no interferences occurred (32).

19. With smoked ham samples, the first column of the analytical system must be cleaned after only 10 runs. A solution of 0.4 M NaCl, pH 11.5 solution was the most effective. After the buffer front has passed and the signal starts to stabilize, shift to the pH 2.5 buffer solution (Reagent 2) and flush for 1 hr. Reequilibrate with the pH 10 buffer (Reagent 1) before renewing runs.

20. For high fiber fruits and vegetables, further clean up studies are required before this method can be routinely used.

21. For each new type of biological sample encountered, storage and recovery studies should be done as different procedures may be necessary for different samples. For example, it is possible to store overnight frozen SSA extracts of muscle tissue without detectable loss of vitamers. For human breast milk, this was not possible but frozen samples of the original milk could be kept overnight without loss. When enzymes are present in the sample, enzyme inhibitors should be added to the extracting medium (31,32).

22. *Plasma Preparation.* Blood (10 mL) is drawn into a syringe containing 10 mg sodium citrate dihydrate, 5.5 mg Na$_2$HPO$_4$, and 6.0 mg NaH$_2$PO$_4$. The collected blood samples are mixed gently for 1–2 min and centrifuged at 550 × g (max) for 30 min at 4°C. The plasma is removed and treated as a liquid sample.

23. If the Rockwell-AIM minicomputer is used to control the Perkin-Elmer 650-40 detector, it must be turned off and reloaded after the light source is activated. The radio frequencies generated may delete the Rockwell memory.

24. Don't forget to raise the pH of the solution obtained from the precolumn prior to injecting into the analytical system!!

I. Variations of the Method

Although the foregoing HPLC method for the separation and quantitation of the B$_6$ vitamers may appear complex, in reality, it is a relatively simple system. Both the cleanup and analytical chromatographic system use standard techniques that are well known and have proven to be reliable. The described procedure is the simplest one reported to date that separates and quantitates all six forms of the vitamin from biological samples in a single run. With respect to the detection methods available, due to the different fluorescence characteristics of the vitamers, no single set of detector parameters appears to be capable of detecting all forms at concentrations which occur in most biological samples. This, then necessitates the use of an adjustable detector during each analytical run.

If one wishes to determine the concentration of vitamin B$_6$ in fortified foods or in pharmaceutical preparations (predominantly PN), then the above described

HPLC system may be greatly simplified, eliminating the necessity of multiple columns and varying detector conditions. Gregory has described a system using a reverse-phase column for the quantitation of PN in fortified breakfast cereals (39) that uses fluorescence detection and yields quantitatible data in about 7 min. Another system has been described by Vandemark (40) for the separation of several water-soluble vitamins in pharmaceutical preparations. The results of this system have not yet been verified by other methods. Gregory has described a discrepancy between his HPLC method (39) and the microbiological growth assay using *S. uvarum*. His HPLC method generally yielded higher values than did the microbiological assay. This discrepancy may be the result of an inhibition of the microbiological growth assay by certain samples.

An alternative extraction method has been described involving hot acidification of a 95% ethanol extract of various plant products, followed by digestion with diastase and papain (41). Preliminary data (42) from utilization of this extraction procedure resulted in approximately 20% greater values for vitamin B_6, both by the standard microbiological and by HPLC analyses. This procedure must be further verified on many types of samples prior to its possible incorporation into an analytical system. Furthermore, the utilization of diastase to convert the phosphorylated to the nonphosphorylated forms prevents the quantitation of the biochemically important phosphorylated forms. More studies on the comparison of all assay and extraction methods currently used need to be performed.

LITERATURE CITED

1. Freed, M. *Methods of Vitamin Assay,* 3rd ed. Interscience, New York 209–221, (1966).
2. Gregory, J. F. and Kirk, J. R. "The bioavailability of vitamin B-6 in foods." *Nutr. Rev.* **39**, 1 (1981).
3. Anderson, B. B., Newmark, P. A., Rawlins, M., and Green, R. "Plasma binding of vitamin B-6 compounds." *Nature* **250**, 502 (1974).
4. Nguyen, L. B., Gregory, J. F., Burgin, C. W., and Cerda, J. J. "In vitro binding of vitamin B-6 by selected polysaccharides, lignin, and wheat bran." *J. Food Sci.* **46**, 1860 (1981).
5. Ogata, K., Tani, Y., Uchida, Y., and Tochikura, T. "Studies on transglycosidation to vitamin B-6 by microorganisms. I. Formation of a new vitamin B-6 derivative, pryridoxine glucoside, by *Sarcina lutea.*" *J. Vitaminol* **15**, 142 (1969).
6. Snell, E. E. "Vitamin B-6 analysis: Some historical aspects." In J. E. Leklem and R. D. Reynolds, Eds. *Methods in Vitamin B-6 Nutrition.* Plenum Press, New York 1–19 (1981).
7. Harris, S. A., Harris, E. E., and Burg, R. W. "Pyridoxine." *Kirk-Othmer Encycl. Chem. Tech.* **16**, 806 (1968).
8. Snell, E. E. "Vitamin B-6." *Comp. Biochem.* **2**, 48 (1963).
9. Vanderslice, J. T., Brown, J. F., Beecher, G. R., Maire, C. E., and Brownlee, S. G. "Automation of a complex high-performance liquid chromatography system. Procedures and hardware for a vitamin B-6 model system." *J. Chromatogr.* **216**, 338 (1981).
10. Sauberlich, H. E. "Vitamin B-6 status assessment: Past and present." In J. E. Leklem and R. D. Reynolds, Eds., *Methods in Vitamin B-6 Nutrition.* Plenum Press, New York 203–240 (1981).
11. Krinke, G., Schaumburg, H. H., Spencer, P. S., Suter, J., Thomann, P., and Hess, R. "Pyridoxine

megavitaminosis produces degeneration of peripheral sensory neurons (sensory neuronopathy) in the dog." *Neurotoxicol.* **2**, 13 (1980).

12. Driskell, J. A. and Lokar, S.F. "Behavioral patterns of female rats fed high levels of vitamin B-6." *Nutr. Reports Int.* **14**, 467 (1976).

13. Hegsted, D. M., Elvehjem, C. A., and Hart, E. B. "The vitamin B-6 requirement of the chick." *Poultry Sci.* **21**, 379 (1942).

14. Conger, T. W. and Elvehjem, C. A. "The biological estimation of pyridoxine (vitamin B-6)." *J. Biol. Chem.* **138**, 555 (1941).

15. Dakshinamurti, K. and Chauhan, M. S. "Chemical assays of pyridoxine vitamers." In J. E. Leklem and R. D. Reynolds, Eds., *Methods in Vitamin B-6 Nutrition.* Plenum Press, New York, 99–122 (1981).

16. Toepfer, E. W. and Polansky, M. M. "Microbiological assay of vitamin B-6 and its components." *J. Assoc. Off. Agric. Chem.* **53**, 546 (1970).

17. Stokes, J. L., Larson, A., Woodward, C. R., Jr., and Foster, J. W. "A Neurospora assay for pyridoxine (sitophila #299)." *J. Biol. Chem.* **150**, 17 (1943).

18. Snell, E. E. "The vitamin activities of 'pyridoxal' and 'pyridoxamine'." *J. Biol. Chem.* **154**, 313 (1944).

19. Snell, E. E. "The vitamin B-6 group—4. Evidence for the occurrence of pyridoxamine and pyridoxal in natural products." *J. Biol. Chem.* **157**, 491 (1945).

20. Parrish, W. P., Loy, H. W., and Kline, O. L. "A study of the yeast method for vitamin B-6." *J. Assoc. Off. Agric. Chem.* **38**, 506 (1955).

21. Parrish, W. P., Loy, H. W., and Kline, O. L. "Further studies on the yeast method for vitamin B-6." *J. Assoc. Off. Agric. Chem.* **39**, 157 (1956).

22. Guilarte, T. R., McIntyre, P. A., and Tsan, M.-F. "Growth response of the yeasts *Saccharomyces uvarum* and *Kloeckera brevis* to the free biologically active forms of vitamin B-6." *J. Nutr.* **110**, 954 (1980).

23. Polansky, M. "Microbiological assay of vitamin B-6 in foods." In J. E. Leklem and R.D. Reynolds, Eds., *Methods in Vitamin B-6 Nutrition.* Plenum Press, New York, 21–44 (1981).

24. Gregory, J. "Relative activity of the nonphosphorylated B-6 vitamers for *Saccharomyces uvarum* and *Kloeckera brevis* in vitamin B-6 microbiological assay." *J. Nutr.* **112**, 1643 (1982).

25. Guilarte, T. R. and McIntyre, P. A. "Radiometric microbiologic assay of vitamin B-6: Analysis of plasma samples." *J. Nutr.* **111**, 1861 (1981).

26. Guilarte, T. R., Shane, B., and McIntyre, P. A. "Radiometric microbiological assay of vitamin B-6: Application to food analysis." *J. Nutr.* **111**, 1869 (1981).

27. Vanderslice, J. T., Stewart, K. K., and Yarmas, M. M. "Liquid chromatographic separation and quantification of B-6 vitamers and their metabolite, pyridoxic acid." *J. Chromatogr.* **176**, 280 (1979).

28. Vanderslice, J. T. and Maire, C. E. "Liquid chromatographic separation and quantification of B-6 vitamers at plasma concentration levels." *J. Chromatogr.* **196**, 176 (1980).

29. Vanderslice, J. T., Maire, C. E., Doherty, R. F., and Beecher, G. R. "Sulfosalicylic acid as an extraction agent for vitamin B-6 in food." *J. Agric. Food Chem.* **28**, 1145 (1980).

30. Vanderslice, J. T., Maire, C. E., and Beecher, G. R. "B-6 vitamer analysis in human plasma by high performance liquid chromatography. A preliminary report." *Am. J. Clin. Nutr.* **34**, 947 (1981).

31. Vanderslice, J. T., Maire, C. E., and Beecher, G. R. "Extraction and quantitation of B-6 vitamers from animal tissues and human plasma: A preliminary report." In J. E. Leklem and R. D. Reynolds, Eds., *Methods in Vitamin B-6 Nutrition.* Plenum Press, New York 123–147 (1981).

32. Vanderslice, J. T., Brownlee, S. G., Cortissoz, M. E., and Maire, C. E. "Vitamin B-6 analysis: Sample preparation, extraction procedures and chromatographic separations." In A. P.

DeLeenheer and M. G. DeRutyer, Eds., *Modern Chromatography of Vitamins.* Marcel Dekker, New York (1983).

33. Brown, J. F., Vanderslice, J. T., Maire, C., Brownlee, S. G., and Stewart, K. K. "Control programming without language: Automation of vitamin B-6 analysis." *J. Automat. Chem.* **3**, 187 (1981).

34. Peterson, E. A. and Sober, H. A. "Preparation of crystalline phosphorylated derivatives of vitamin B-6." *J. Am. Chem. Soc.* **76**, 169 (1954).

35. Stewart, K. K. "Depulsing system for positive displacement pumps." *Anal. Chem.* **49**, 2125 (1977).

36. Ohishi, N. and Fukui, S. "Further study on the reaction products of pyridoxal and pyridoxal 5'-phosphate with cyanide." *Arch. Biochem. Biophys.* **128**, 606 (1968).

37. Loo, Y. H. and Badger, L. "Spectrofluorimetic assay of vitamin B-6 analogues in brain tissue." *J. Neurochem.* **16**, 801 (1969).

38. Takanshi, S., Matsunaga, I., and Tamura, Z. "Fluorometric determination of pyridoxal and its 5'-phosphate in biological materials." *J. Vitaminol.* **16**, 132 (1970).

39. Gregory, J. F., III "Comparison of high-performance liquid chromatographic and *Saccharomyces uvarum* methods for the determination of vitamin B-6 in fortified breakfast cereals." *J. Agric. Food Chem.* **28**, 486 (1980).

40. Vandemark, F. L. "A liquid chromatography procedure for determining water-soluble vitamins in pharmaceutical preparations." *Chromatogr. Newsletter* **8**, 27 (1980).

41. Wong, F. F. "Analysis of vitamin B-6 in extractives of food materials by high-performance liquid chromatography." *J. Agric. Food Chem.* **26**, 1444 (1978).

42. Augustin, J. Personal communication.

18 | Folacin

Microbiological and Animal Assays

Pamela M. Keagy

GENERAL CONSIDERATIONS

The term folacin refers to the group of compounds that qualitatively exhibit the biological activity of folic acid (1). Folic acid, or pteroylglutamic acid, has been the subject of many investigations involving several species of animals and microorganisms. Hence, the vitamin had a confusing roster of names before it was learned that the same or similar substances were being studied. Folic acid or folates are the general terms for a group of compounds based on the N-[(6-pteridinyl)methyl]-p-aminobenzoic acid skeleton conjugated with one or more L-glutamic acid units. Folacin is the generic descriptor for folic acid and related compounds exhibiting qualitatively the biological activity of folic acid. Folic acid is pteroylmonoglutamic acid (1).

A. History

As early as 1935, a nutritional deficiency in monkeys, now known to respond to folic acid, was described. This factor was called "vitamin M" (2). In 1939, Hogan and Parrott described an anemia in chicks due to a deficiency of an unknown factor, which they termed "vitamin B" (3). In 1941, Stokstad and coworkers reported a factor necessary in the nutrition of *Lactobacillus casei*, which they named "the *L. casei* factor" (4), and Mitchell, Snell, and Williams isolated a crystalline compound from spinach, which they called "folic acid" from the Latin term for leaf (folium) (5). These and several other factors were later shown to belong to the nutritionally and chemically related family of pteroylglutamic acid compounds.

445

The structure of pteroylglutamic acid was determined and its synthesis and isolation were completed by a large group of workers at Lederle Laboratories (6) and by a group at Parke, Davis and Company (7). It contains three subunits: 2-amino-4-hydroxy-6-methylpteridine (8), p-aminobenzoic acid, and glutamic acid (Figure 18.1).

B. Physical, Chemical, and Biochemical Properties

The enzymatically active forms are derivatives of pteroylglutamic acid reduced at the 5, 6, 7, and 8 positions. Reduction at position 6 creates optically active D and L diastereoisomers. The unnatural D isomers may be inactive or inhibitory for some folate enzymes (9).

Tetrahydrofolic acid functions biochemically as a carrier of single carbon fragments. These may be at three levels of oxidation corresponding to formate, formaldehyde and hydroxymethyl, they are carried at or between the N^5 and N^{10} positions and may be converted enzymatically one into the other. Successive molecules of glutamic acid may be attached to the first glutamic acid radical in γ-peptide linkages. Compounds with nine or more glutamic acid residues have been identified (9).

Pteroylglutamic acid (mol. wt. 441.42) crystallizes as yellow, spear-shaped platelets. The free acid is slightly soluble in H_2O (10 μg/mL at 0°C and more than 500 μg at 100°C) (10). It dissolves in dilute solutions of alkali carbonates and hydroxides and in dilute solutions of hot sulfuric and hydrochloric acids. It is insoluble in organic solvents such as alcohol, ether, and benzene. Pteroylglutamic acid is more stable in alkaline than acid media (11); thus, standards are made in basic solutions. Its characteristic ultraviolet absorption spectra

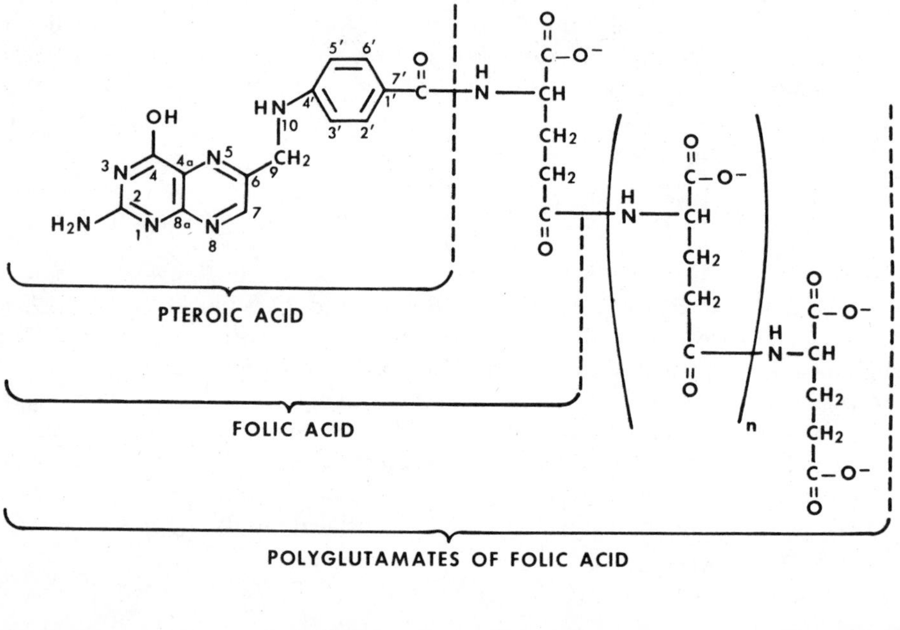

PTEROIC ACID

FOLIC ACID

POLYGLUTAMATES OF FOLIC ACID

exhibit maxima at 256, 283, and 365 nm in 0.1 N NaOH with corresponding E_{max} (mol) values of 24,500, 23,400, 8,500 (12,13). Other investigators have reported slightly different values which may be due in part to the degree of purity of the compounds that were used.

C. Stability

All of the folic acids are sensitive to light with cleavage at the C^9-N^{10} position (14). The reduced compounds are sensitive to molecular oxygen with the production of p-aminobenzoylglutamic acid and a number of pterins (12). In the presence of unlimited oxygen, destruction proceeds as a pseudo-first-order reaction where the rate constant is an exponential function of the temperature as described by the Arrhenius equation $k = Ae^{-Ea/RT}$. The rate constant increases with ionization of the 3,4 amide group (pKa = 10.8) (15,16). Ascorbic acid, 2-mercaptoethanol, and dithiothreitol are used to delay oxidation during analysis, with ascorbic acid being the most effective on a molar basis (17).

Table 18.1 illustrates the stability of several folacin compounds that have been identified in natural materials (17–19). The results were all obtained without ascorbic acid in the solution, and the data of Reed and Archer (19) were determined spectrophotometrically whereas the others were determined microbiologically. Pteroylglutamic acid and 5-formyltetrahydrofolic acid are the most stable. The substitution at the N^5 position limits access to the 4a carbon and stabilizes the structure. Tetrahydrofolic acid is the most labile of the folates and it is doubtful that it is completely retained in most extraction procedures. Ascorbic acid acts as a scavenger of molecular oxygen in folacin solutions and delays the initiation of oxidation. Addition of 0.1% ascorbic acid limited 5-methyltetrahydrofolic acid destruction to 20% after 3 hr at 100°C. Without ascorbate, 5-methyletrahydrofolic acid lost 90% of its activity after 65 min of heating under similar conditions (20). Copper at low concentrations accelerates oxidation, and chelating agents such as EDTA may improve stability by competing with impurities in some buffers. Phenol also will inhibit oxidation by breaking the free-radical chain process (15).

Neutral pH buffers are recommended for optimum stability during extraction. Table 1 shows increased destruction of most folates at pH 4.0 compared with pH 7.0. More alkaline pH conditions increase the stability under some circumstances but not all, and accelerate the rate of ascorbic acid destruction in the extraction buffers.

D. Folacin Polyglutamates and Conjugases

Most natural folates occur in the polyglutamate form. L. casei responds equally to mono-, di-, and triglutamates and much more slowly to longer-chain derivatives (21). The slow growth and steep slope of the response curves to tetra- and longer-chain polyglutamates produces positive drift in assays of free folate without conjugase treatment. Thus, free folate assays are technically invalid in most samples and the results are arbitrary functions of the extraction and assay conditions.

TABLE 18.1 Stability of Folacin Compounds

Compound[a]	Time Unit	Temp °C	Time for 50% Degradation			References
			pH4.0	pH 7.0	pH 10.0	
PteGlu	Hr	22°	56[b]	>700[b], 84[c]	>700[d,e]	(17)
		100°	22[g]	—	36.5[g]	(18)
5-CHO-H4PteGlu	Days	22°	23[b]	31[b], 32[c]	32[d], 20[e]	(17)
		100°	—	—	3[g]	(18)
10-CHO-H4PteGlu	Hr	22°	132[b]	108[b], 97[c]	>800[d], 64[e]	(17)
5-CH3-H4PteGlu	Hr	22°	28[b]	119[b], 98[c]	265[d], 7[e]	(17)
	Min	100°	3.35[g]	8.77[g]	3.45	(18)
H2PteGlu	Min	22°	>10	>10	>10	(17)
	Hr	30°		4.5[f]		(19)
H4PteGlu	Min	22°	28[b]	22[b], 21[c]	20[d]	(17)
		30°	60[f]	40[f]	2[f]	(19)
		100°	1.2[g]	4[g]	(16.5 @ pH 12)[g]	(18)

[a] PteGlu = pteroylglutamatic acid or folic acid; 5-CHO-H4PteGlu = 5-formyltetrahydrofolic acid; 10-CHO-H4PteGlu = 10-formyltetrahydrofolic acid; 5-CH3-H4PteGlu = 5-methyltetrahydrofolic acid; H2PteGlu = dihydrofolic acid, H4PteGlu = tetrahydrofolic acid.

[b] 0.05 M Citrate/phosphate buffer.

[c] 0.05 M Phosphate buffer.

[d] 0.05 M Carbonate/bicarbonate.

[e] 0.1 M Sodium hydroxide.

[f] 0.02 M Each citrate/phosphate/borate.

[g] Universal buffer.

Conversion of polyglutamates to mono- or diglutamates requires a γ-glutamyl-carboxypeptidase commonly referred to as conjugase. Most proteases are ineffective for this purpose because the glutamate residues are attached through the γ-carboxyl rather than the more common α-carboxyl linkage of most proteins. Conjugase enzymes are widely distributed in nature and must be rapidly inactivated if the research objective is the study of natural folacin forms.

Table 18.2 shows the sources and properties of the most frequently used or studied conjugase enzymes. Chick pancreas and hog kidney have been the traditional sources for analysts. Desiccated chick pancreas is commercially available (Difco). The enzyme is an exopeptidase with a pH optimum of 7.8 and produces a diglutamate end product (9,22). Hog kidney conjugase must be prepared by the investigator. It has a pH optimum of 4.5 and a monoglutamate end product (23,24) and is reported to be affected by inhibitors from plant sources whereas the chick pancreas enzyme is less affected (25). McMartin et al. (26) recently reported a marked loss of folate after incubation at pH 4.7 with crude hog kidney conjugase. At pH 6.0, adequate conversion of polyglutamates was obtained and the recovery of tetrahydrofolic acid and 5-methyltetrahydrofolic acid was improved to 60–80%. They suggested this was due to nonenzymatic binding to components in the enzyme preparation since the recovery of both folates was similar when incubated with a boiled conjugase preparation.

Other sources of conjugase are plasma, liver, and rat pancreas. The plasma and liver enzymes are important sources, as liver and whole blood samples are frequently prepared by activating the endogenous enzymes at pH 4.5. Lakshmaiah and Ramasastri (31) have used plasma directly as a conjugase source for food analysis. Its primary advantages are availability, low folacin content, and absence of need for purification. These authors have also reported adequate conjugase activity at pH 6.0 for a limited number of food samples. The ideal standardized conjugase treatment for all samples has not been developed and it is recommended that preliminary studies be used to determine the source, purity, and incubation conditions required for each sample type.

TABLE 18.2 Folacin Conjugase Sources

Source	Optimum pH	End Product Glutamate Residues	References
Chick pancreas	7.8	2	(9), (22)
Hog kidney	4.5	1	(23)
Rat pancreas	5.5–6.0	1	(27)
Human jejunum	4.5	1	(28)
	6.5	1	
Plasma	4.5	1	(29)
Liver	4.5	1	(9)
Cabbage	5.0	1 or 2	(30)
	8.0	3	

E. Nutritional Properties

Pteroylgutamic acid gives a significant reticulocyte response and increase in red blood cells in some human macrocytic anemias (32), including pernicious anemia (33,34) and sprue (35,36). The vitamin does not, however, cure the neurological lesions produced by pernicious anemia. Due to the risk of masking an undiagnosed B_{12} deficiency, vitamin supplements containing more than 400 μg folic acid require a prescription in the United States. Approximately 100 μg pure folic acid per day will maintain normal serum levels. Limited studies have suggested that 25–50% of dietary folacin is nutritionally available, therefore, the RDA is 400 μg folacin per day as measured by *L. casei* after conjugase treatment (37).

Folic acid and its derivatives participate in the synthesis of compounds involving a single carbon fragment. It mediates synthesis of purines (38), pyrimidines (39), pantothenic acid (40), and certain amino acids (41–43) by transferring "active formate" and "active formaldehyde." These compounds consist of formyl and hydroxymethyl groups bound to tetrahydrofolic acid. The biochemical and nutritional properties of folacin have been the subject of many reviews. Several of the more recent ones are cited here (44–47).

METHODS AVAILABLE

Methods suitable to determine folic acid may be grouped into biological, microbiological, and chemical procedures. Chromatographic and radiometric assays for folacin are presented in the second section of this chapter.

The chick assay, first presented by O'Dell and Hogan in 1943, was the first technique used to determine what is now known as folic acid (48). The chicks were first placed on the basal diet until they became anemic; then supplements of folic acid and the test material were administered. Later, Campbell et al. developed a prophylactic method based on growth and anemia prevention for 4 weeks (49). More recent assays (50,51) have used blood and liver folacin concentrations as specific responses since growth may be affected by other diet components. Herbert and Bertino (52) reviewed the earlier bioassays.

The rat assay has not been used extensively because intestinal bacterial synthesis provides enough folacin for normal growth in the rat. Early rat assays used sulfa drugs to limit bacterial folacin synthesis and then determined the growth response to supplementation (53,54). A depletion-repletion rat bioassay based on liver folacin concentrations has recently been reported (55,56). This assay may be used with or without sulfa drugs. The rat assay requires more time and diet groups compared with the chick assay. However, rats consume less feed and many laboratories are already equipped to conduct rat studies. Additionally, the rat intestinal conjugase enzymes are more similar to other mammalian systems producing a monoglutamate end product from polyglutamate folacin digestion.

Animal assays are time-consuming and expensive. However, because of the variations in response of microorganisms to different forms of folic acid, it is often desirable to supplement microbiological data with bioassays on the animal species. Also, the methods have a definite place in studying nutritional aspects of the vitamin.

A variety of microorganisms have been used to assay for folic acid, including true bacteria, yeasts, and molds. *Lactobacillus casei* (ATCC 7469) is used to measure all folates with three or less glutamic acid residues. *Streptococcus faecalis* (ATCC 8043) was formerly the most commonly used organism until it was learned that it does not respond to methyl folates. It can also utilize pteroic acid which is not metabolically active for man. *P. cerevisiae* (*L. citrovorum*) (ATCC 8018) requires reduced folates and does not respond to methyl derivatives. When samples are assayed with all three microorganisms, the proportions of reduced, methyl, and nonmethyl folates are determined (57). Improved high-pressure chromatographic separation of folates from interfering compounds should soon make the differential assays obsolete.

The protozoan *Tetrahymena pyriformis* (*geleii*) (ATCC 30008) has been suggested as a test organism because it is able to utilize folic acid, pteroyltriglutamic acid, and pteroylheptaglutamic equally on a molar basis (58,59) and because it contains a folic acid conjugase that makes prior treatment of the samples unnecessary. The assay procedure has been described by Jukes (60) and Eigen and Shockman (25).

Bacillus coagulans, a thermophile, has also been suggested to assay for folic acid (61,62). One advantage in using this microorganism is that its high incubation temperature (55°C) eliminates the necessity for sterile technique. Also the response due to *p*-aminobenzoic acid may be overcome with 0.01% sulfanilimide. In addition, it responds to some conjugates of folic acid and some samples may be assayed without prior enzyme treatment. The main disadvantage is the possibility of a nonspecific stimulation when natural materials are used.

Folic acid has been determined quantitatively by two bioautographic methods. One involves using chromatographic separation of the folic acid compounds and subsequently detecting them in an agar plate of microorganisms. The technique is sensitive to 10^{-6} μg of folic acid (63). The other method is an adaption of the pad-plate technique for antibiotics (60). It may be used for a rapid screening of active compounds.

The chemical methods available have usually been criticized because they lack the sensitivity of microbiological assays and because other materials interfere with them. Chemical assays, however, have merit in some instances. Most have been used on purified folic acid and derivatives as assayed in pharmaceutical preparations or for studies of chemical nature.

The cleavage of pteroylglutamic acid to produce *p*-aminobenzoic acid or other related moieties is the basis of several chemical methods to determine folic acid. They have been used extensively to assay high-potency pharmaceutical products. Cleavage of the pteridine moiety is accomplished with titanous chloride, zinc (64), zinc amalgam (65), or permanganate (66) liberating *p*-aminobenzoic acid or its derivatives. These species may then be diazotized and coupled by the method of Bratton and Marshall (67) or other similar techniques (68). Absorbance of the intensely colored compound formed may be determined in either the resulting aqueous solution or, after extraction, in isobutanol. Many other compounds that are converted to aromatic amines or phenols by the reaction chosen will diazotize and interfere with the determination. Subsequent research has obviated much of this interference (66,69). Recently the cleavage products have been reexamined and not all folates are cleaved by these methods.

Another useful technique is based on measuring the fluorescence of an oxidation product of pteroylglutamic acid (2-amino-4-hydroxypteridine-6-carboxylic acid) when irradiated with a 365-nm light wave (70). It has been applied to natural extracts and is satisfactory to assay yeast. It is less satisfactory for other products because it gives results lower than those obtained by microbiological methods. A modified procedure (71) has been adapted for tetrahydrofolic acid, based on excitation at 330 nm in acid and fluorescence intensity measured at 350 nm. Concentrations of 2×10^{-4} μmoles/mL of the derivative may be measured.

Folic acid has been determined in the presence of other vitamins by the height of the waves of the polarographic spectrum in alkaline medium (72). Additional information on the older methods may be found in two excellent reviews (52,60).

ANALYTICAL METHODOLOGY

I. MICROBIOLOGICAL METHOD
(*LACTOBACILLUS CASEI* ATCC 7469)

A. Principle

See page 43.

B. Reagents

1. *Enzymatically Hydrolyzed Casein (73).*   Dissolve 8 g NaHCO$_3$ in H$_2$O to a volume of 1 L. Gradually add 60 g vitamin free casein. Adjust the pH of this solution to 8.0 with 10 N NaOH. (Do not exceed pH 8.0, because the subsequent addition of acid will precipitate large insoluble lumps.) Add 300 mg pancreatin suspended in 7 to 10 mL H$_2$O and stir 20 min. Add 2.5 mL toluene, stir another 30 min, and incubate at 37°C for 48–72 hr. (Incubation beyond 48 hr and less than 80 hr insures maximum production of peptide growth stimulants in the casein hydrolysate.) After incubation, this solution is steamed or autoclaved at 121°C for 30 min to stop the reaction and remove toluene. Cool the solution, add 10 g Celite (technical grade), and filter over a Celite bed on a Whatman No. 1 filter in a Buchner funnel. Adjust the pH of the filtrate to pH 3.7 with

approximately 60 mL glacial acetic acid. Add 12 g activated charcoal (Darco G-60), stir 10 min, and filter. Repeat the charcoal treatment three times using Celite to aid filtrations. Dilute the final filtrate to 1200 mL (1 mL = 50 mg casein) and freeze.

Dry-weight determinations should be made on small aliquots of each lot of casein digest and lots rejected that do not contain 40–50 mg/mL of solids. If large amounts of charcoal are used maximum growth of *L. casei* may be reduced (74). This procedure omits a filtration step at pH 6.0 in the original description of the hydrolysate procedure because the charcoal treatment is inefficient for the removal of folate at pH 6.0.

2. *Adenine–Guanine–Uracil Solution.*   Heat 1 g each of adenine sulfate, guanine hydrochloride, and uracil in 50 mL of 20% HCl until dissolved. Add H_2O to make 500 mL and store at room temp.

3. *Xanthine Solution.*   Dissolve 2 g xanthine in 50 mL NH_4OH with heat. Add H_2O to make 500 mL and store in the refrigerator.

4. *Acetate Buffer Solution (1.57 M, pH 4.5).*   Dissolve 18.87 g (19.8 mL) of acetic acid and 38.65 g sodium acetate in H_2O and dilute to 500 mL.

5. *Vitamin Solution.*   Dissolve 80 mg riboflavin in 320 mL sodium acetate buffer (Reagent 4) with heat. Dissolve 1.6 mg biotin in 50 mL H_2O containing 20 mg $NaHCO_3$. Dissolve 160 mg *p*-aminobenzoic acid, 320 mg pyridoxine–HCl, 32 mg thiamin–HCl, 64 mg Ca-pantothenate, and 64 mg niacin in 200 mL H_2O. Add biotin and riboflavin solutions and make up to 800 mL with H_2O.

6. *Tween 80 Solution.*   Dissolve 10 g Tween 80 in warm H_2O (45°C) and dilute to 500 mL.

7. *Salt Solution.*   Dissolve 20 g $MgSO_4 \cdot 7H_2O$, 1 g NaCl, 1 g $FeSO_4 \cdot 7H_2O$, and 1 mL concentrated HCl in H_2O and make up to 500 mL.

8. *Manganese Sulfate Solution.*   Dissolve 20 g $MnSO_4 \cdot H_2O$ in H_2O and make up to 500 mL.

9. *Basal Double-Strength Medium.*   The following quantities are based on a final dilution of 1000 mL.

Quantity	Reagent	Reagent No.
200 mL	Enzymatically hydrolyzed casein solution	1
5 mL	Adenine–guanine–uracil solution	2
5 mL	Xanthine solution	3
10 mL	Vitamin solution	5
5 mL	Tween 80 solution	6
10 mL	Salt solution	7
0.6 g	L-Asparagine hydrate	
0.5 g	L-Cysteine HCl	
40 g	Dextrose (anhydrous)	
5 mg	Glutathione, reduced	

Quantity	Reagent	Reagent No.
40 g	Sodium acetate · $3H_2O$	
1.3 g	K_2HPO_4 · $3H_2O$	
1 g	KH_2PO_4	
	Adjust pH to 6.7 $\pm$ 0.1 with NaOH	
5 mL	$MnSO_4$ solution	8
to 1000 mL	H_2O	

Mix the solutions (Reagents 1–3, 5–7) by stirring. Add the solid ingredients. Adjust the pH to 6.7 $\pm$ 0.1 with NaOH. Next add the manganese solution and dilute with H_2O to 1000 mL.

The medium is made up double strength ($2\times$) to allow the addition of sample. The $2\times$ medium is stored frozen until needed and refrigerated no longer than 1 week. If toluene is used to preserve the medium or solutions, care should be taken to remove it completely by distillation, autoclaving, or aspiration.

(a) The medium can be made up $4\times$ strength and frozen to conserve freezer space. Precipitates that form will redissolve when the medium is diluted and later autoclaved.

(b) A dry commercially prepared medium using enzymatically hydrolyzed casein is available from Difco (Code 0822). Another medium using acid-hydrolyzed casein is available from BBL. These media are usually satisfactory but vary between batches and should be tested when received. At times when commercial media are unavailable or unsatisfactory the investigator has little choice except laboratory preparation.

(c) Several investigators have published data showing that different forms of folacin do not give equal *L. casei* responses on a molar basis (75,76), whereas others have reported identical responses (17,77,78). Philips and Wright (76) published data showing the responses of *L. casei* to folic acid and 5-methyltetrahydrofolic acid were nearly identical using medium adjusted to pH 6.2 with 1 M acetic acid but not with medium having initial pH values of 6.5 or 6.8. Tizzard (79) reported improved assay results using Difco medium adjusted to pH 6.0 with lactic acid and Toennies and Frank (80) demonstrated most rapid initial *L. casei* growth in medium having an initial pH of 6.35. This lower assay pH has not been widely used but may significantly improve the results of food folacin assays.

(d) Turbidimetric *L. casei* assays are stimulated by peptides (74,81,82) that are supplied by the enzymatically hydrolyzed casein. Other basal media (BBL #11267) (83–85) have included acid-hydrolyzed casein instead. When these media are used the growth stimulants appear to be supplied by an inoculum that is grown in enriched medium and harvested in log-phase growth (85).

10. *Culture Medium for Growing Inoculum.* Dispense 2.5 mL $2\times$ medium into a series of screw cap tubes. Add 2.5 mL of a 2 ng/mL folic acid solution

in 0.05 M phosphate ascorbate buffer (Reagent 11). Loosely cap and autoclave for 15 min at 121°C. Tighten caps and incubate tubes at 37°C for 24 hr to check for sterility.

(a) This inoculum broth limits the amount of folate that may be stored by the bacteria and cause high blanks. Additionally, the lag time for growth is minimized since the bacteria are not required to adapt to a different assay medium.

11. *Phosphate–Ascorbate Buffer (0.05 M Phosphate, 0.15% Ascorbate, pH 6.1).* Dissolve 4.37 g $Na_2HPO_4 \cdot 7H_2O$, 4.65 g $NaH_2PO_4 \cdot H_2O$, and 1.5 g ascorbic acid in 1 L H_2O. Check pH and adjust, if necessary, to pH 6.1. Prepare this buffer immediately before use as the ascorbic acid is unstable for long periods at this pH.

12. *Phosphate–Ascorbate Buffer (0.1 M Phosphate, 1.0% Ascorbic Acid, pH 6.0).* Dissolve 18.96 g $Na_2HPO_4 \cdot 7H_2O$, 4.04 g $NaH_2PO_4 \cdot H_2O$, and 10 g ascorbic acid in 1 L H_2O. Add ascorbic acid immediately before use. Check pH and adjust if necessary, to pH 6.0.

13. *Phosphate–Ascorbate Buffer (0.1 M Phosphate, 1.0% Ascorbic Acid, pH 7.2).* Dissolve 8.56 g $Na_3PO_4 \cdot 12H_2O$, 20.77 g $Na_2HPO_4 \cdot 7H_2O$, and 10 g ascorbic acid in 1 L H_2O. Add ascorbic acid immediately before use. Final pH after addition of the ascorbic acid should be 7.2.

14. Stock Solution of Folic Acid (200 µg/mL). Dissolve 200 mg folic acid in 0.01 N NaOH in 20% ethanol and make up to 1 L. Dilute 1 mL to 25 mL in 0.1 N NaOH and check the concentration on the basis of molecular extinction coefficients which are $24.5 \times 10^3 E_{max}$ (mol) at 256 nm and 23.4×10^3 at 283 nm in 0.1 N NaOH (12). Divide the stock solution into aliquots and store at −20°C. This solution is stable frozen for at least 1 year.

15. *Working Standard Solution (200 ng/mL).* Dilute 1 mL of the stock solution to 1000 mL with 0.01 N NaOH in 20% ethanol and store in the refrigerator.

16. *Assay Standard Solutions (1 ng/mL and 0.1 ng/mL).* Dilute 1 mL of the working standard solution (Reagent 15) to 200 mL with phosphate-ascorbate buffer (Reagent 11). This is the high standard (1 ng/mL). Dilute the high standard 1 to 10 with the same buffer to make the low standard (0.1 ng/mL).

17. *Hog Kidney Conjugase (25).* Fresh hog kidneys are defatted and homogenized with 3 volumes of 0.32% cysteine–HCl adjusted to pH 5.4. The homogenate is autolyzed 2 hr at 37°C. It is then clarified by centrifuging 20 min at $1000 \times g$ in the cold and recentrifuged at $4000 \times g$ for 30 min. The supernatant is adjusted to pH 4.5 with 1 N HCl and treated with Dowex 1 (5 g/100 mL) for 1 hr in an ice bath to remove endogenous folate. After filtration through glass wool or centrifugation, the clear filtrate is stored at −20°C until used. This preparation can be further purified by gel filtration to remove endogenous folate (86,87).

(a) Sephadex G-25 column. Five mL of hog kidney conjugase (Reagent 17) is applied on a Sephadex G-25 column (1.5×30 cm) and this is eluted with 0.1 M acetate buffer (pH 4.8) containing 0.32% cysteine HCl. The first 17-mL fraction should be discarded. The next 10-mL fraction contains the enzyme activity that occurs as a brown band of protein material. The enzyme is excluded from the gel and appears in the void volume. Folacin enters the gel and elutes later.

18. *Chicken Pancreas.* Either fresh or dehydrated pancreas may be used. When fresh pancreas is used, grind a pancreas weighing about 4 g in a glass mortar or blend in Waring Blender. Suspend in 0.1 M phosphate buffer (pH 7.2). Prepare dried pancreas by grinding the tissues in 5 volumes of acetone. Squeeze the fine material through cheesecloth, filter, rewash with acetone, and air-dry. Grind the dry residue. The defatted powder will retain activity for several months if stored at or near 0°C. Desiccated chicken pancreas may be obtained commercially from Difco Laboratories.

(a) Purified chicken pancreas conjugase (25,88). Suspend 10 g of desiccated chicken pancreas in 300 mL 0.1 M phosphate buffer (pH 7) by stirring 1 hr at room temperature. Incubate overnight at 30°C under toluene and centrifuge. Mix the supernatant with an equal volume of 0.1 M tricalcium phosphate gel suspension (Sigma) for 30 min in an ice bath and centrifuge in the cold. Cool the upper layer below 5°C and slowly add an equal volume of ice cold ethanol with vigorous stirring. Allow the mixture to stand overnight in the cold. Centrifuge and dissolve the precipitate in 100 mL of 0.1 M phosphate buffer (pH 7) by stirring 1 hr in an ice bath. Centrifuge to remove insoluble material. Mix the supernatant with 10% by weight of Dowex 1 × 8 (chloride) for 1 hr at 0°C. Remove the Dowex by centrifugation and pour the supernatant through gauze. Store the supernatant frozen.

19. *Human Plasma Conjugase (89,29).* Outdated human plasma may be purchased from a local blood bank. Plasma containing 5000 enzyme units/mL or more is frozen in aliquots and used as needed. The enzyme activity of each batch is tested as follows.

Combine 1.0 mL of a yeast extract solution (10% Difco yeast extract in H_2O), 0.5 mL 100 mM β-mercaptoethanol, 2.5 mL acetate buffer (0.2 M, pH 4.5), and 0.9 mL H_2O. Warm the mixture to 37°C and add 0.1 mL human plasma. Incubate the mixture 1 hr at 37°C. Terminate the reaction by adding 1 mL phosphate–ascorbate buffer (0.1 M, pH 6.1, containing 2% ascorbic acid) and immediately immersing in a boiling water bath for 3 min. Use the *L. casei* microbiological assay to determine the amount of free folate in the enzyme mixture compared to a zero time blank. One unit of conjugase activity corresponds to that amount of serum or enzyme that liberates 1 ng (22.7 pmole) of folic acid in 1 hr at 37°C in the incubation mixture used.

20. *Agar Medium for Stock Culture (90).* Dissolve 4 g of Difco Bacto Yeast Extract, 2 g glucose, 2 g sodium acetate ($CH_3COONa \cdot 3H_2O$), and 6 g agar in 400 mL H_2O with heat and stirring. Dispense 10 mL into each of 40 culture tubes, cap loosely, and autoclave for 20 min at 121°C. Store in the refrigerator. The stab tubes will last several months before drying out.

(a) Bacto-*Lactobacilli* Agar from Difco may also be used.

21. *Assay Organism.*   *Lactobacillus casei* ATCC 7469 may be obtained from the American Type Culture Collection. The lyophilized bacteria are regenerated by incubating at 37°C for 18–20 hr in the inoculum broth. It may be necessary to transfer a drop of the first incubation broth to a second broth for another 18–20 hr incubation to obtain a fast-growing culture.

C. Procedure

The microbiological method described here is based on the method of Waters and Mollin (91) with additions for the extraction of food samples from Eigen and Shockman (25). Samples and solutions of folic acid should be protected from light.

1. *Preparation of Stock Culture, L. casei ATCC 7469.*   Prepare two agar stabs (Reagent 20) and incubate at 37°C for 24 hr. Reserve 1 stab unopened from which to transfer the culture the next month. Use the other stab to prepare the liquid inoculum.

2. *Preparation of Inoculum.*   Aseptically transfer the culture to 1 tube of liquid inoculum medium (Reagent 10) and incubate 16–20 hr. The morning of the assay, suspend the bacteria and transfer 0.2 mL to a second tube of inoculum medium and incubate for 6 hr at 37°C. Centrifuge the bacteria and suspend in 10 mL sterile 0.85% saline. Centrifuge and resuspend once more in 10 mL sterile saline. One drop of this suspension is used to inoculate each tube. If needed, this inoculum may be diluted further to provide sufficient inoculum for large assays.

(a) Cooperman (85) has presented an alternative inoculum preparation that should be followed if assay media based on acid hydrolyzed casein is used.

(b) Grossowicz, Waxman and Schreiber (92) have described a cryoprotected *L. casei* inoculum that may be prepared once, stored frozen in aliquots, and used directly. This may minimize one source of variation between assays. A lyophilized inoculum has also been used successfully (77).

3. *Preparation of Sample Using Conjugase.*   If the sample size is not too large the extraction can be conveniently carried out in 50-mL screw cap centrifuge tubes.

(a) Weigh out enough material to be assured of a representative sample.

(b) Add a volume of phosphate-ascorbate buffer (0.1 M phosphate, 10 g/L ascorbic acid), equal in mL to 10 or more times the dry weight of the sample in g. The buffer pH will depend on the conjugase treatment used. Use 20 or more volumes of buffer for materials high in starch such as flour.

(1) If hog kidney or human plasma conjugase is to be used, use pH 6.0 phosphate ascorbate buffer (Reagent 12). The pH optimum of these enzymes is 4.5–4.7; however, adequate activity has been found at pH 6.0 (26,31,89). Marked losses of folates, particularly 10-CHO-H_4PteGlu and H_4PteGlu, have been observed during incubation at pH 4.7 (26,93).

(2) If chicken pancreas conjugase is to be used, use pH 7.2 phosphate-ascorbate buffer (Reagent 13) (25).

The level of ascorbate used in these buffers is arbitrary. Levels of 1 g or 2 g ascorbic acid/L are adequate to protect $5\text{-}CH_3H_4PteGlu$ during autoclaving (17,20); however, as much as 10 g ascorbic acid/L does not completely protect $H_4PteGlu$ (17). Iwai (88) obtained maximal results from red blood cells using 100–150 g sodium ascorbate/L. More than 5 g ascorbic acid/L lowered radioassay values in serum (94). Excessive amounts of ascorbic acid may interfere with protein precipitation or enzyme activity and *L. casei* growth. After dilution of the extract, the final assay tubes should not contain more than 1.5 mg ascorbic acid/mL of $1 \times$ medium (95).

(c) Disperse evenly with a blender or homogenizer. Glycerol distearate, capryl alcohol, or a similar compound may be used to prevent foaming. Use of a probe homogenizer such as the Brinkman Polytron or Tek-mar Tissuemizer eliminates transfer of the sample.

(d) Heat the mixture by boiling or autoclaving for sufficient time to precipitate proteins. Large samples of 100–200 mL are autoclaved 15 min at 121°C. Small samples of 10–20 mL may be boiled 10 min in a water bath. If the material forms large lumps on heating (e.g., eggs, meat, flour), blend again to ensure a finely divided suspension.

(e) After cooling to room temperature use one of the following conjugase treatments. Chicken pancreas conjugase is the preferred enzyme where a diglutamate end product is acceptable. Hog kidney conjugase yields a monoglutamate folate but is inhibited by nucleic acids (25) and gives lower results with some plant foods (60,96). Use of human serum conjugase has been demonstrated with about 60 foods (31) but has not been widely used except in blood hemolysates.

(1) Desiccated chicken pancreas (60,96). Make a suspension of 6 mg/ml desiccated chicken pancreas in pH 7.2 phosphate-ascorbate buffer (Reagent 13). Stir 1 hr at room temperature and centrifuge. Add to the sample preparation, 3 mL chicken pancreas extract for each 1 g dry weight of sample. Add one or two drops of toluene and incubate overnight at 37°C. Prepare an enzyme blank omitting the food sample. The chicken pancreas supernatant contains approximately 20 ng folacin/mL. The folacin concentration should be determined. Preliminary experiments may establish that less pancreas extract is necessary for many types of samples.

(2) Purified hog kidney or chicken pancreas (adapted from 26,57,97). Bring the sample to known volume with H_2O, filter, or centrifuge. Combine an amount of sample extract estimated to contain 200–500 ng folacin, 0.5 mL enzyme, and buffer in a total volume of 5 mL. Use Reagent 13 (pH 7.2) for the chicken pancreas conjugase and Reagent 12 (pH 6.0) for the hog kidney conjugase. Incubate 2 hr at 37°C. Purified enzyme preparations have not been widely used in food assays. Therefore, preliminary experiments should be used to establish the optimum enzyme concentration

and incubation time. The activity of the enzyme preparation may be determined by the method of Krumdieck and Baugh (98) if the radiolabeled substrate is available or as described previously for the human plasma conjugase.

(3) Human plasma conjugase (29,31,89). Bring the sample to known volume with H_2O and filter or centrifuge. Adjust a portion of the extract to pH 4.5. Combine 5 mL of sample extract, 1 mL of 0.2 M acetate buffer (pH 4.5), 0.6 mL of 100 mM mercaptoethanol, and 0.2 mL human plasma. Add 1 drop of toluene and incubate overnight at 37°C.

(i) The authors (31) also reported good results with pH 6.0 incubation mixtues. Natural folates would be expected to be more stable at the higher pH.

(ii) Human plasma normally contains 5–15 ng folacin/mL. If the folacin contribution of the plasma is very low compared with the food source, an enzyme blank may not be necessary.

(iii) Sulfhydryl compounds are essential for activation of the plasma conjugase. The mercaptoethanol cannot be replaced by ascorbic acid.

(f) Heat the incubation mixtures in a boiling water bath or autoclave for 5 min to inactivate the enzyme and drive off the toluene.

(g) Cool mixtures. If the desiccated chicken pancreas treatment was used, bring the mixture to known volume with H_2O and filter or centrifuge.

(h) Dilute the treated extract by a factor of 10 or more to an estimated concentration of 0.4 ng/mL folacin with phosphate-ascorbate buffer (Reagent 11).

For sampling and dilution estimates, many foods contain between 0.2 and 1.2 μg folacin/gram of food (as is moisture basis). Exceptional sources such as yeast, wheat germ, liver, and spinach contain much more. Representative values for 299 foods have been compiled by Perloff and Butrum (99).

A universally satisfactory conjugase treatment for foods has not been published. It is recommended that preliminary studies be used to optimize the conjugase treatment for the range of samples to be analyzed. The desiccated chicken pancreas has been most widely used. Relatively few inhibitors have been reported and the pH for optimum enzyme activity is consistent with good folacin stability. It yields a diglutamate end product which is available to L. casei but may not be suitable for chromatographic separations. The hog kidney and serum conjugases yield a monoglutamate end product but have maximal activity of pH 4.5 where folacin is less stable. Adequate, if not maximum activity, has been reported at pH 6.0 for the latter enzymes. Many plant foods, as well as nucleic acids, appear to inhibit hog kidney conjugase. Cysteine and 2,3-dimercaptopropanol reverses the nucleic acid inhibition (25).

Crude conjugase preparations may contribute interfering substances to the food extract (26).

With some materials endogenous conjugase activity may be adequate at the proper pH. This is true of liver at pH 4.5, cabbage at pH 5.0 (30), and asparagus and spinach at pH 4.5 (100).

Additional enzyme treatments may be necessary with some types of samples. Two laboratories have reported folate adsorption to starch. Addition of an amylase source to the hog kidney conjugase treatment resulted in 10–30% higher values in cereals (101) and 100% increases in potatoes as well as quantitative recoveries of added folic acid (102). Amylase is also useful in starchy products such as flour to minimize the formation of starch gels with associated turbidity and filtration problems.

For folacin assays of milk, Cooperman and Shimizu (103) obtained optically clear extracts by first precipitating casein with rennin. Yamada (104) obtained 20 –90% higher results in milk if the sample was pretreated with 0.2% Pronase for 3 hr prior to the conjugase incubation.

Because of the diverse forms of folacin in biological materials, the recovery of internal folic acid standards cannot give complete assurance of the adequacy of extraction procedures. However, internal standards can still reveal useful information when microbiological assay inhibitors are present. For this reason, the use of internal standards is recommended when testing variations of extraction procedures.

4. *Preparation of Standard and Sample Tubes.*

(a) To duplicate 18 × 150-mm tubes add 0.0, 0.3, 0.6, 1.2, and 2.5 mL of the low working (0.1 ng/mL) standard (Reagent 16), high working standard (1.0 ng/mL) (Reagent 16), or test solutions.

(b) Add sufficient phosphate-ascorbate buffer (Reagent 11) to bring the volume in each tube to 2.5 mL.

(c) To each tube add 2.5 mL of the 2× basal medium.

(1) This assay uses a 5-mL total volume per tube. Others have used various total volumes from 2 mL to 10 mL per tube. If the volume per tube is altered, the tube size should also be altered to maintain a column of liquid with relatively anaerobic conditions at the bottom (85). The most precise portion of the response curve lies between 0.02 and 0.2 ng folic acid/mL of 1× medium.

5. *Sterilization.*

(a) Cover tubes and autoclave for 10 min at 121°C. Cool tubes to room temperature.

(1) Sheets of tin foil make convenient covers for whole racks of tubes. This simplifies the manipulations during inoculation.

(2) Other assays have been developed that eliminate this step. One is the aseptic addition method of Herbert (105,84). The other uses chloramphenicol in the medium with a chloramphenicol resistant strain of *L. casei* (106). These assays have the advantage that very labile tetrahydrofolic acid is not subjected to autoclaving with the medium. The aseptic addition method has been used successfully in several laboratories. Cooper compared both methods for serum folate and found the chloramphenicol-

adapted *L. casei* was too unstable in its growth requirements for routine reliable assays (107).

6. Inoculation.   Add one drop of the inoculum to each tube using a sterile cotton-plugged pasteur pipette.

(a) For aseptic assays the inoculum may be added to the sterile medium which is the last component added to the tubes (107).

(b) A fixed amount of inoculum can be added using an automatic pipet.

7. *Incubation.*   Incubate 18–24 hr in a well-stirred water bath at 37°C.

(a) Air cabinet incubators are not recommended. Temperatures can vary depending on the location of the assay tubes in the cabinet. Also the time required for all the tubes to reach 37°C can be as long as 2–3 hr because of the low heat capacity of air. As a result, the variance of an assay incubated in an air cabinet is significantly increased.

(b) If the sample extract contains nonfolate materials that affect the initial rate of bacterial growth, drift may appear in short-time assays. Longer incubation times may compensate for this effect on the final calculated results. In the absence of stimulatory materials, incubation times between 15 hr and 72 hr have given equivalent results (107–109).

8. *Turbidity Measurement.*   Suspend the bacteria by shaking with a Vortex mixer. Read percent transmittance or absorbance in a photometer set at any specific wave length between 540 nm and 700 nm.

(a) A stable reading is usually obtained after 30 sec in a standard photometer cell. The initial unstable reading is due to flow birefringence of the rod-shaped bacteria oriented with currents in the cell. More rapid readings may be taken on a flowing stream in an appropriate continuous flow cell (110). Alternatively, the assay may be conducted in matched assay tubes so the contents do not need to be transferred to cuvettes.

(b) A digital output of three significant figures will reduce the variability associated with reading a small analog scale.

(c) For comparison of results between laboratories, the AOAC gives procedures for standarization of photometers (111).

9. *Calculations.*

(a) Draw the standard curve for the assay by plotting percent transmittance against the log of nanograms folic acid per tube in the standard series.

(b) Determine the folic acid content of the sample series by interpolation of the percent transmittance on the standard curve.

(c) Discard values that fall on the flatter portions of the sigmoidal standard curve. This is usually less than 0.02 ng or more than 0.2 ng folic acid/mL 1× medium with half maximum growth at 0.1 ng folic acid/mL.

(d) Divide the interpolated ng/tube result by the volume of sample per tube to obtain the nanograms of folic acid per mL of sample.

(e) Average the values obtained from at least three dilutions of sample.

(1) Traditionally, values have been accepted if they agree within 10% of the mean. The ideal sample will not show any trend in the values with

increasing aliquots of sample. If the sample curves are plotted against the log of the mL of sample per tube, the curves should appear parallel to the standard curve. If the sample curve is not parallel to the standard curve and a concentration trend is apparent in the calculations, the assay is considered invalid.

In practice many extracts of natural materials produce this drift in the results but not to the extent that the drift is statistically significant using the limited data of a single extract. Such values are usually accepted even though significant drift could be demonstrated by pooling the slopes of similar samples. As a consequence, most reported values of folacin in biological materials are specific in the assay procedure used.

Some sources of drift that have been identified in folacin assays are unequal amounts of ascorbate and phosphate in the final assay tubes (109), differential response of *L. casei* to different folacin forms (75,76), presence of polyglutamate forms in the sample extract (21), and absence of peptides and other growth stimulants present in enzymatically hydro-lyzed casein and log-phase inoculum cultures (74).

(f) Calculate the folacin content of the sample as follows:

μg folacin per g sample $=$

$$\frac{(\text{Average ng/mL of extract } - \text{ conjugase blank}) \times \text{dilution factor}}{\text{g of sample } \times 1000}$$

If the conjugase enzyme contributes a significant amount of folacin, subtract the enzyme blank from the sample value.

With the increasing availability of computers, more sophisticated methods of data analysis may be used that include statistical tests of the validity of each sample and computation of confidence limits. The theory and application of these procedures has been discussed elsewhere (112–115).

II. ANIMAL ASSAYS
RAT BIOASSAY (55,116)

A. Principle

Tissue folacin stores are depleted by feeding weanling rats a low-folacin basal diet for 4 weeks and then repleted by feeding the standard or test diets for 4 weeks. Liver folacin concentration is then a function of the folacin content of the test diets. The ratio of the response slope of the test material to the standard material is used to estimate the potency of the test material. The effect of intestinal flora on liver folacin concentration is accounted for by fitting independent intercepts for the test and standard materials.

TABLE 18.3 Composition of the Rat Diet

Component	Percent
Wheat starch[a]	70.0
Vitamin-free casein[b]	20.0
Corn oil[c]	5.0
Williams-Briggs UC-1Rb Mineral mix[d]	3.5
Vitamin mix (in starch)[e]	1.0
D,L-Methionine[f]	0.5

[a]ICN Pharmaceuticals, Inc.,

[b]Teklad Test Diets,

[c]Mazola; Best Foods, CPC International, Inc.,

[d]Provides the following per kg diet: $CaCo_3$, 7.25 g; $CaHPO_4$, 11.3 g; $MnSO_4 \cdot H_2O$, 154 mg; $CuSO_4$, 13 mg; ferric citrate, 151 mg; $ZnCO_3$, 21 mg; KIO_3, 1 mg.

[e]Provides the following per kg diet: biotin, 2 mg; thiamin-HCl, 15 mg; riboflavin, 15 mg; nicotinic acid, 50 mg; pyridoxine-HCl, 15 mg; calcium panthothenate, 50 mg; menadione, 15 mg; vitamin B_{12}, 0.2 μg; choline bitartrate, 1 g; retinyl acetate, 10,000 IU; ergocalciferol, 1250 IU; dl-α-tocopherol, 50 IU.

[f]Grand Island Biologicals.

B. Equipment

1. *Male Weanling Rats.* Fisher-344 rats (CDF(F-344)/CrIBR) from Charles River Breeding Laboratories, Wilmington, Mass., have been satisfactory.

2. *Basal Diet.* The basal diet is given in Table 18.3. Allow approximately 15 g feed per rat per day. Use a source of vitamin-free casein with known low folacin content. Some sources of vitamin-free casein contain relatively high levels of folacin.

3. *Standard Diets.* Supplement the basal diets with 0, 0.2, 0.4, and 0.6 mg folic acid/kg of diet. Make 4.5-kg batches to feed 10 rats for 28 days, assuming 15 g feed intake per day and a slight excess for wastage.

4. *Test Diets.* Test materials should be substituted for starch in the basal diet on a calorie basis. A minimum of two levels of each material must be used to estimate the slope. Three levels are preferable to check the linearity of the response.

5. *Positive Control Diet.* Supplement the basal diet with 1 mg folic acid/kg of diet. This is fed to one group of extra animals from the day received to provide a comparison for normal growth and health.

C. Procedure

1. *Depletion Period.* Place weanling rats in individual cages and feed the basal diet for 4 weeks. Weigh animals twice a week to check for normal growth and health. If possible avoid housing animals in the same quarters with animals

from another supplier. Specific pathogen-free rats are immunologically naive and suseptible to respiratory infections carried by other rats. Respiratory infections are common in rats and cause decreased food consumption and weight gain.

2. *Repletion Period.* Divide animals into groups of 10 animals each such that the group mean weights and standard deviation are approximately equal. If extra animals are available, exclude the largest and smallest animals. Feed each group the assigned test or standard diet for 4 weeks. Weigh animals and record food intake twice a week.

3. *Necropsy.* At the end of the feeding period anesthetize the animals in a jar with methoxyflurane veterinary anesthetic (Metaphane, Pitman-More, Inc. Washington Crossing, NJ). Open the abdominal cavity and sever the descending aorta and hepatic artery while the heart is still beating. This allows the liver to be consistently well bled. Remove the liver, weigh, divide into three sections and freeze for later folacin analysis.

4. *Liver Analysis.* Homogenize 1 g or 2 g liver into 20 mL 0.1 M sodium acetate buffer (pH 4.5) containing 500 mg/mL ascorbic acid. Add one drop toluene, cover, and incubate overnight at 37°C. The next morning heat the homogenate 10 min in a boiling water bath and centrifuge. Dilute the supernatant to approximately 0.4 ng/mL with 0.05 M sodium phosphate buffer containing 150 mg/mL ascorbic acid (pH 6.1). Proceed with the *L. casei* microbiological assay as previously described. The livers will contain between 1 μg and 10 μg folacin/g wet weight.

D.   Calculations

Plot the response curves with liver folacin concentration on the Y ordinate versus the concentration of folacin or sample in the diet on the X abscissa. If it is suspected that variations in food intake affected the result, the folacin content of the whole liver may be plotted against the total intake of folacin or sample. Fit the responses to the equation $Y = A + BX$ using linear least squares where Y is the liver folacin, A is the intercept, B is the slope, and X is the amount of test or standard material. The ratio of $B_{test}/B_{standard}$ gives the potency of the sample. Each response has its own intercept to account for the effect of the sample on intestinal folacin synthesis by the rat. Fieller's theorem may be used to obtain the confidence limits of the potency figure (117).

Example: Data from reference (116).

$B_{test} = 0.38 \pm 0.06$ μg liver folacin/g wheat bran consumed.

$B_{standard} = 0.24 \pm 0.02$ μg liver folacin/μg folic acid consumed.

$B_{test}/B_{standard} = 1.6$ μg folacin/g bran ($1.1 < \bar{x} < 2.2$, $P = 0.95$).

1. Experience with the rat bioassay is limited because of its relatively recent publication. Further analysis of available data (118) used weighted least squares with liver weight as a co-variable and whole liver folacin as the dependent

variable (Y). In some circumstances the data fulfilled the conditions for the traditional slope ratio analysis described by Finney (115).

CHICK BIOASSAY

A. Principle

Folacin is required for normal growth and development in the chick. Day-old chicks are fed the test and standard diets for 3 weeks. Growth and tissue folacin concentrations are then a function of the folacin content of the diet.

B. Equipment

1. *Chicks.* Use day-old male chicks, 10 or 15 per diet. White Leghorn chicks have been used most frequently.

2. *Basal Diet.* Composition of the basal diet is given in Table 18.4. Allow approximately 1 kg diet per animal.

3. *Test Diets.* Test substances should be substituted on a caloric basis for glucose in the basal diet.

4. *Standard Diets.* Supplement the basal diet with 0, 0.5, 1.0, and 1.5 mg folic acid/kg diet.

TABLE 18.4 Composition of Chick Diets (119)

Ingredients	Percent
Vitamin free casein[a]	25.00
L-Arginine HCl[a]	1.50
DL-Methionine[a]	0.40
Glycine[a]	1.00
Corn oil[b]	4.00
Dextrose[a]	57.54
Vitamin mix[c,d]	1.20
Mineral mix[c,e]	6.36
Cellulose	3.00

[a]U.S. Biochemical Corp.,

[b]Mazola, Best Foods,

[c]ICN Nutritional Biochemicals,

[d]Vitamin mix provides (per kg diet): thiamin, 15 mg; riboflavin, 15 mg; niacin, 50 mg; pyridoxine, 6 mg; biotin, 0.6 mg; vitamin B_{12}, 20 μg; choline chloride, 2.0 g; calcium pantothenate, 20 mg; menadione, 1.5 mg; vitamin E, 50 units; vitamin D_3, 4500 units; vitamin A, 4500 units; anti-oxidant (butylated hydroxytoluene or ethoxyquin) 100 mg.

[e]Mineral mix provides (per kg diet): $CaHPO \cdot 2H_2O$, 18 g; $CaCO_3$, 19 g; KH_2PO_4, 14 g; $NaHCO_3$, 8.8 g; $MnSO_4 \cdot H_2O$, 0.35 g; $FeSO_4 \cdot 7H_2O$, 0.50 g; $MgSO_4$, 3.0 g; KIO_3, 0.01 g; $CuSO_4 \cdot 5H_2O$, 0.03 g; $ZnCO_3$, 0.15 g; $CoCl_2$, 1.7 mg; $NaMoO_4 \cdot 2H_2O$, 8.3 mg; Na_2SeO_4, 2.0 mg.

C. Procedure

Use 10 –15 chicks per diet, housed in heated batteries in groups of 5–10 animals
per pen. Weigh and wing band each chick initially and feed the assigned diet
for 21 days. Weigh and determine feed consumption biweekly. At the end of
the feeding period weigh each chick and kill by cervical dislocation or CO_2
asphyxiation. Remove the liver, weigh, divide into three sections, and freeze for
later folacin assay. Extract and analyze liver samples as described under the rat
bioassay.

D. Calculations

Proceed as described under the rat bioassay. Test the standard and sample
regressions for a common intercept at zero dose. If a common intercept is
obtained, the data may be analyzed as a slope-ratio assay as described by Finney
(115).

LITERATURE CITED

1. "Nomenclature Policy: Generic descriptors and trivial names for vitamins and related compounds." *J. Nutr.* **112**, 7 (1982).
2. Day, P. L., Langston, W. C., and Shukers, C. F. "Failure of nicotinic acid to prevent nutritional cytopenia in the monkey." *Proc. Soc. Exptl. Biol. Med.* **38**, 860 (1938).
3. Hogan, A. G. and Parrott, E. M. "Anemia in chicks due to vitamin deficiency." *J. Biol. Chem.* **128**, 46 (1939).
4. Stokstad, E. L. R. "Some properties of a growth factor for *Lacto-bacillus casei.*" *J. Biol. Chem.* **149**, 573 (1943).
5. Mitchell, H. K., Snell, E. E., and Williams, R. J. "The concentration of 'folic acid.' " *J. Am. Chem. Soc.* **63**, 2284 (1941).
6. Angier, R. B., Booth, J. H., Hutchings, B. L., Mowat, J. H., Semb, J., Stokstad, E. L. R., SubbaRow, Y., Waller, C. W., Northey, E. H., Seeger, D. R., Sickels, J. P., and Smith, J. M., Jr. "The structure and synthesis of the liver *L. casei* factor." *Science* **103**, 667 (1946).
7. Pfiffner, J. J., Calkins, D. G., Bloom, E. S., and O'Dell, B. L. "On the peptide nature of vitamin B$_c$ conjugate from yeast." *J. Am. Chem. Soc.* **68**, 1392 (1946).
8. Mowat, J. H., Boothe, J. H., Hutchings, B. L., Stokstad, E. L. R., Waller, C. W., Angier, R. B., Semb, J., Cosolich, D. B., and SubbaRow, Y. "The structure of the liver *L. casei* factor." *J. Am. Chem. Soc.* **7**, 14 (1948).
9. Kisliuk, R. L. "Pteroylpolyglutamates." *Mol. and Cell. Biochem.* **39**, 331 (1981).
10. Stokstad, E. L. R., Hutchings, B. L., and SubbaRow, Y. "Isolation of the liver *L. casei* factor." *Ann. N.Y. Acad. Sciences* **48**, 261 (1946).
11. Dick, M. I. B., Harrison, I. T., and Farrer, K. Y. H. "The microbiological assay of folic acid." *Austral. J. Exptl. Biol. Med. Sci.* **26**, 231 (1948).
12. Blakley, R. L. *The Biochemistry of Folic Acid and Related Pteridines.* Elsevier, New York, 92 (1969).
13. Pohland, A., Flynn, E. H., Jones, R. G., and Shire, W. "A proposed structure for folinic acid-SF, a growth factor derived from pteroylglutamic acid." *Am. Chem. Soc.* **73**, 3247 (1951).
14. Stokstad, E. L. R., Fordham, D., and DeGronigen, A. "The inactivation of pteroylglutamic acid (liver *Lactobacillus casei* Factor) by light." *J. Biol. Chem.* **167**, 877 (1947).

15. Blair, J. A. and Pearson, A. J. "Kinetics and mechanisms of the autoxidation of the 2-amino-4 hydroxy-5,6,7,8-tetra hydropteridines." *J. C. S. Perkins II* **80** (1974).

16. Blair, J. A., Pearson, A. J., and Robb, A. J. "Autoxidation of 5-methyl-5,6,7,8-tetrahydrofolic acid." *J. C. S. Perkins II* **18** 1975).

17. O'Broin, J. D., Temperley, I. J., Brown, J. P., and Scott, J. M. "Nutritional stability of various naturally occurring monoglutamate derivatives of folic acid." *Am. J. Clin. Nutr.* **28**, 438 (1975).

18. Paine-Wilson, B. and Chen, T.-S. "Thermal destruction of folacin: Effect of pH and buffer ions." *J. Food Sci.* **44**, 717 (1979).

19. Reed, L. S. and Archer, M. C. "Oxidation of tetrahydrofolic acid by air." *J. Agric. Food Chem.* **28**, 801 (1980).

20. Chen, T.-S. and Cooper, R. G. "Thermal destruction of folacin: Effect of ascorbic acid, oxygen, and temperature." *J. Food Sci.* **44**, 713 (1979).

21. Tamura, T., Shin, Y. S., Williams, M. A., and Stokstad, E. L. R. "*Lactobacillus casei* response to pteroylpolyglutamates." *Anal. Biochem.* **49**, 517 (1972).

22. Mims, V. and Laskowski, M. "Studies on vitamin B conjugase from chicken pancreas." *J. Biol. Chem.* **160**, 493 (1945).

23. Bird, O. D., Robbins, M., Vandenbelt, J. M., and Pfiffner, J. J. "Observations on vitamin B conjugase from hog kidney." *J. Biol. Chem.* **163**, 649 (1946).

24. Olson, O. E., Fager, E. E. C., Burris, R. H., and Elvehjem, C. A. "The use of a hog kidney conjugase in the assay of plant materials for folic acid." *Arch. Biochem.* **18**, 261 (1948).

25. Eigen, E. and Shockman, G. D. "Folic acid." In F. Kavanaugh, Ed., *Analytical Microbiology*, Vol. 1. Academic Press, New York, 431 (1963).

26. McMartin, K. E., Virayotha, V., and Tephly, T. R. "High pressure liquid chromatography separation and determination of rat liver folates." *Arch. Biochem. and Biophys.* **209**, 127 (1981).

27. Jagerstad, M., Lindstrand, K., and Westesson, A-K., "Hydrolysis of conjugated folic acid by pancreatic 'conjugase'." *Scand. J. Gastroenterol.* **7**, 593 (1973).

28. Reisenauer, A. M., Krumdieck, C. L., and Halsted, C. H. "Folate conjugase: Two separate activities in human jejunum." Science **198**, 196 (1977).

29. Lakshmaiah, N. and Ramasastri, B. V. "Folic acid conjugase from plasma—1. Partial purification and properties." *Internat. J. Vit. Nutr. Res.* **45**, 183 (1975).

30. Tamura, T., Buehring, K. U., and Stokstad, E. L. R. "Enzymatic Hydrolysis of pteroylpolyglutamates in cabbage." *Proc. Soc. Exptl. Biol. Med.* **141**, 1022 (1972).

31. Lakshmaiah, N. and Ramasastri, B. V. "Folic acid conjugase from plasma—3. Use of the enzyme in the estimation of folate activity in foods." *Internat. J. Vit. Nutr. Res.* **45**, 262 (1975).

32. Vilter, C. A., Spies, T. D., and Koch, M. B. "Further studies on folic acid in the treatment of macrocytopic anemia." *South. Med. J.* **38**, 781 (1945).

33. Moore, C. V., Bierbaum, O. S., Welch, A. D., and Wright, L. D. "The activity of synthetic *Lactobacillus casei* factor (folic acid) as an antipernicious anemia substance—1. Observations on four patients: Two with Addisonian pernicious anemia, one with non-tropical sprue and one with pernicious anemia of pregnancy." *J. Lab. Clin. Med.* **30**, 1056 (1945).

34. Waters, A. H. and Mollin, D. L. "The folic acid activity of serum in normal subjects and patients with megalobastic anemia." *Proc. Congr. Europ. Soc. Hematol.* **8** (332) 1961).

35. Darby, W. J. and Jones, E. "Treatment of sprue with synthetic *L. casei* factor (folic acid, vitamin M)." *Proc. Soc. Exptl. Biol. Med.* **60**, 259 (1945).

36. Sheehym, T. W., Baggs, B., Perez-Santiago, E., and Flock, M. H. "Prognosis of tropical sprue. A study of the effect of folic acid on the intestinal aspects of acute and chronic sprue." *Ann. Internat. Med.* **57**, 892 (1962).

37. Food and Nutrition Board. "*Recommended Dietary Allowances*", 9th ed. National Academy of Sciences, Washington, D.C. (1980).

38. Warren, L., Flaks, J. G., and Buchanan, J. M. "Biosynthesis of the purines—20. Integration of enzymatic transformylation reactions." *J. Biol. Chem.* **229**, 627 (1959).

39. Luzzati, D. and Guthrie, R. "Studies of a purine- or histidine-requiring mutant of *Escherichia coli.*" *J. Biol. Chem.* **216**, 1 (1955).

40. Greenberg, D. M. and Humphreys, G. K. "Biosynthesis of the thymine methyl group." *Fed. Proc.* **17**, 234 (1958).

41. McIntosh, E. N., Purko, M., and Wood, W. A. "Ketopantoate formation by a hydroxy-methylation enzyme from *Escherichia coli.*" *J. Biol. Chem.* **228**, 499 (1957).

42. Davis, B. D. "Aromatic biosynthesis—3. Role of *p*-aminobenzoic acid in the formation of vitamin B_{12}." *J. Bact.* **62**, 221 (1951).

43. Kaufman, S. "The participation of tetrahydrofolic acid in the enzyme conversion of phenylalanine to tyrosine." *Biochim. Biophys. Acta.* **27**, 428 (1958).

44. Herbert, V., Colman, N., and Jacob, E. "Folic acid and vitamin B_{12}." In R. S. Goodhart and M. E. Shils, Eds., *Modern Nutrition in Health and Disease,* 6th ed. Lea and Febiger, Philadelphia, 229 (1980).

45. Rodriguez, M. S. "A conspectus of research on folacin requirements of man." *J. Nutr.* **108**, 1983 (1978).

46. Turner, A. J. "The neurochemistry of folate: An overview." In M. Dain, L. Gram, and J. K. Penry, Eds., *Advances in Epileptology: 12th Epilepsy International Symposium.* Raven Press, New York 627 (1981).

47. National Research Council, "*Folic acid biochemistry and physiology in relation to the human nutrition requirement.*" Proceedings of a workshop on human folate requirements June 2–3, 1975. National Academy of Sciences, Washington, D.C. (1977).

48. O'Dell, B. L. and Hogan, A. G. "Additional observations on the chick anti-anemia vitamin." *J. Biol. Chem.* **149**, 323 (1943).

49. Campbell, C. J., Brown, R. A., and Emmett, A. D. "The role of crystalline vitamin B_c in the nutrition of the chick." *J. Biol. Chem.* **154**, 721 (1944).

50. Graham, D. C., Roe, D. A., and Ostertag, S. G. "Radiometric determination and chick bioassay of folacin in fortified and unfortified frozen foods." *J. Food Sci.* **45**, 47 (1980).

51. Ristow, K. A., Gregory, J. F., and Damron, B. L. "Effects of dietary fiber on the bioavailability of folic acid monoglutamate." *J. Nutr.* **112**, 750 (1982).

52. Herbert, V. and Bertino, J. R. "Folic acid." In P. Gyorgy and W. N. Pearson, Eds., *The Vitamins,* 2nd ed. Academic Press, New York, 243 (1967).

53. Day, P. L. and Trotter, J. R. "The bioassay of the vitamin M group." *Biol. Symp.* **12**, 313 (1947).

54. Asenjo, C. F., Muniz, A. I., and Quintana, M. L. "Growth response of folic acid-depleted rats to supplementation with tropical foods." *Food Research* **15**, 326 (1950).

55. Keagy, P. M. and Oace, S. M. "Development of a folacin bioassay in rats." *J. Nutr.* **112**, 87 (1982).

56. Keagy, P. M. "Integrated saturation model for tissue micronutrient concentrations applied to liver folacin." *J. Nutr.* **112**, 377 (1982).

57. Bird, O. D. and McGlohon, V. M. "Differential assays of folic acid in animal tissues." In F. Kavanagh, Ed., *Analytical Microbiology,* Vol. 2. Academic Press, New York, 409 (1972).

58. Kidder, G. W. and Dewey, V. C. "Studies on the biochemistry of *Tetrahymena*—13. B Vitamin requirements." *Arch. Biochem.* **21**, 66 (1949).

59. Dewey, V. C. and Kidder, G. W. "Factors affecting the requirement of *Tetrahymena pyriformis* (geleii) for folic acid." *J. Gen. Microbiol.* **9**, 445 (1953).

60. Jukes, T. H. "Assay of compounds with folic acid activity." In D. Glick, Ed., *Methods of Biochemical Analysis* Vol. 2. Interscience, New York, 121 (1955).

61. Baker, H., Hutner, S. H., and Sobotka, H. "Estimation of folic acid with a thermophilic bacillus." *Proc. Soc. Exptl. Biol. Med.* **89**, 210 (1955).

62. Campbell, L. L. and Sniff, E. E. "Folic acid requirement of *Bacillus coagulans.*" *J. Bact.* **78**, 267 (1959).

63. Usdin, E., Shockman, G. D., and Toennies, G. "Tetrazolium bioautography." *Appl. Microbiol.* **2**, 29 (1954).

64. Hutchings, B. L., Stokstad, E. L. R., Booth, J. H., Mowat, J. H., Waller, C. W., Angier, R. B., Semb, J., and SubbaRow, Y. "A chemical method for the determination of pteroylglutamic acid and related compounds." *J. Biol. Chem.* **168**, 705 (1947).

65. Kaselis, R. A., Leibermann, W., Seaman, W., Sickels, J. P., Sterns, E. I., and Woods, J. T. "Modified colorimetric assay of pteroylglutamic acid." *Anal. Chem.* **23**, 746 (1951).

66. Schiaffino, S. S., Webb, J. M., Loy, H. W., and Kline, O. C. "Folic acid determination involving permanganate oxidation." *J. Am. Pharm. Assoc.* **48**, 236 (1959).

67. Bratton, A. C. and Marshall, E. K. "A new coupling component for sulfanilamide determination." *J. Biol. Chem.* **128**, 437 (1939).

68. *The United States Pharmacopeia,* 17th ed. Mack Printing, Easton, Penn., 874 (1965).

69. Pelletier, O. and Campbell, J. A. "The estimation of folic acid in multivitamin-mineral preparations." *J. Pharm. Sci.* **50**, 208 (1961).

70. Allfrey, V., Teply, L. J., Geffen, C., and King, C. G. "A fluorometric method for the determination of pteroylglutamic acid." *J. Biol. Chem.* **178**, 465 (1949).

71. Uyeda, K. and Rabinowitz, J. C. "Fluorescence properties of tetrahydrofolate and related compounds." *Anal. Biochem.* **6**, 100 (1963).

72. Varela, G., Ortega, M., and Portillo, R. "Polarographic studies—14. Determination of folic acid in vitamin B complex." *Anales Real Acad. Farm.* **17**, 143 (1951).

73. Roberts, E. C. and Snell, E. E. "An improved medium for microbiological assays with *Lactobacillus casei.*" *J. Biol. Chem.* **163**, 499 (1946).

74. Clark, M. F. "Factors influencing validity and confidence limits of pantothenic acid estimation." *Anal. Chem.* **29**, 135 (1957).

75. Ruddick, J. E., Vanderstoep, J., and Richards, J. F. "Folate levels in food. A comparison of microbiological assay and radioassay methods for measuring folate." *J. Food Sci.* **43**, 1238 (1978).

76. Phillips, D. R. and Wright, J. A. "Studies on the response of *Lactobacillus casei* to different folate monoglutamates." *Brit. J. Nutr.* **49**, 183 (1982).

77. Shane, B., Tamura, T., and Stokstad, E. L. R. "Folate assay: A comparison of radioassay and microbiological methods." *Clinica Chimica Acta* **100**, 13 (1980).

78. Chen, M. F., McIntyre, P. A., and Kertcher, J. A. "Measurement of folates in human plasma and erythrocytes by a radiometric microbiologic method." *J. Nucl. Med.* **19**, 906 (1978).

79. Tizzard, J. "*L. Casei* folate assay." *N.Z.J. Med. Lab. Technol.* **33**, 85 (1979).

80. Toennies, G. and Frank, H. G. "The role of pH and buffering capacity of the medium in bacterial growth (Bacterimetric Studies 6)." *Growth* **14**, 341 (1950).

81. Koser, S. A. *Vitamin Requirements Of Bacteria and Yeasts.* Charles C. Thomas, Springfield, Il., 353, (1968).

82. Kihara, H. and Snell, E. E. "Peptides and bacterial growth—8. The nature of streptogenin." *J. Biol. Chem.* **235**, 1409 (1960).

83. Baker, H., Frank, O., and Hutner, S. H. "Simplified *Lactobacillus casei* assay for folates." In D. B. McCormick and L. D. Wright, Eds., *Methods in Enzymology,* Vol. 18. Academic Press, New York 624 (1971).

84. Scott, J. M., Ghanta, V., and Herbert, V. "Trouble free microbiologic serum and red cell folate assays." *Am. J. Med. Tech.* **40**, 125 (1974).

85. Cooperman, J. M. "Assay for folic acid activity in blood." In F. Kavanagh, Ed., *Analytical Microbiology,* Vol. 2. Academic Press, New York, 439 (1972).

86. Tamura, T., Romero, J. J., Watson, J. E., Gong, E. J., and Halsted, C. H. "Hepatic folate metabolism in the chronic alcoholic monkey." *J. Lab. Clin. Med.* **97**, 654 (1981).

87. Watson, J. and Tamura, T. *Methods of Folate Microbiological Assay.* Dept. of Nutritional Sciences, University of California, Berkeley, 94720. (Revised 1976).

88. Iwai, K., Luttner, P. M., and Toennies, G. "Blood folic acid studies." *J. Biol. Chem.* **239**, 2365 (1964).

89. Lakshmaiah, N. and Ramasastri, B. V. "Plasma folic acid conjugase." In D. B. McCormick and L. D. Wright, Eds., *Methods in Enzymology,* Vol. 66, Academic Press, New York, 670 (1980).

90. Snell, E. E. "Microbiological methods in vitamin research". In P. Gyorgy, Ed., *Vitamin Methods* Vol. 1. 1st ed. Academic Press, New York, 327 (1950).

91. Waters, A. H. and Mollin, D. L. "Studies on the folic acid activity of human serum." *J. Clin. Path.* **14**, 335 (1961).

92. Grossowicz, N., Waxman, S., and Schreiber, C. "Cryoprotected *Lactobacillus casei:* An approach to standardization of microbiological assay of folic acid in serum." *Clin. Chem.* **27**, 745 (1981).

93. Butterfield, S. and Calloway, D. H. "Folacin in wheat and selected foods." *J. Am. Dietet. Assoc.* **60**, 310 (1972).

94. Kerkay, J., Coburn, C. M., and McEvoy, D. "Effect of sodium ascorbate concentration on the stability of samples for determination of serum folate levels." *Am. J. Clin. Path.* **68**, 481 (1977).

95. Herbert, V., Fisher, B., and Koontz, B. J. "The assay and nature of folic acid activity in human serum." *J. Clin. Invest.* **40**, 81 (1961).

96. Toepfer, E. W., Zook, E. G., Orr, M. L., and Richardson, L. R. "Folic acid content of foods. Microbiological assay by standardized methods and compilation of data from the literature." USDA Handbook, No. 29. P. 16 (1951).

97. Thenen, S. W. "Folacin content of supplemental foods for pregnancy." *J. Am. Dietet. Assoc.* **80**, 237 (1982).

98. Krumdieck, C. L. and Baugh, C. M. "Radioactive assay of folic acid polyglutamate conjugase(s)." *Anal. Biochem.* **35**, 123 (1970).

99. Perloff, B. P. and Butrum, R. R. "Folacin in selected foods." *J. Am. Dietet. Assoc.* **70**, 161 (1977).

100. Leichter, J., Landymore, A. F., and Krumdieck, C. L. "Folate conjugase activity in fresh vegetables and its effect on the determination of free folate content." *Am. J. Clin. Nutr.* **32**, 92 (1979).

101. Cerna, J. and Kas, J. "Folacin in cereals and cereal products." 7th World Cereal and Bread Congress, June 28–July 2, 1982. Prague, Czechoslovakia. Abstract 265.

102. Konavalova, L. V., Andreychuk, T. V., and Stepanova, E. N. "Microbiological determination of the folic acid content in potatoes." *Vop. Pitan.* **2**, 70 (1974). (Translation TT 75-55005, USDA-OICD-IRD, Center Building 1, Hyattsville, Md 20782).

103. Cooperman, J. M. and Shimizu, N. "An improved method to assay folates in milk by a turbidmetric microbiological assay." *Anal. Letters* **12**, 1443 (1979).

104. Yamada, M. "Folate contents in milk." *Vitamins* (Japan) **53**, 221 (1979).

105. Herbert, V. "Aseptic addition method for *Lactobacillus casei* assay of folate activity in human serum." *J. Clin. Path.* **19**, 12 (1966).

106. Davis, R. E., Nicol, J., and Kelley, A. "An automated method for the measurement of folate activity." *J. Clin. Path.* **23**, 47 (1970).

107. Cooper, B. A. and Jones, E. "Superiority of simplified assay for folate with *Lactobacillus casei* ATCC 7469 over assay with chloramphenicol-adapted strain." *J. Clin. Path.* **26**, 963 (1973).

108. Slade, B. A., Harrison, J. W., and Shaw, W. "Effect of incubation time on folate values." *Am J. Clin. Path.* **61**, 74 (1974).

109. Temperley, I. J., and Horner, N. "Effect of ascorbic acid on the serum folic acid estimation." *J. Clin. Path.* **19**, 43 (1966).

110. Kavanagh, F. "Photometric Assaying." In F. Kavanagh, Ed., *Analytical Microbiology,* Vol. 2. Academic Press, New York 52 (1972).

111. Association of Official Analytical Chemists. *Official Methods of Analysis,* 13th ed. Washington, D.C. 716 (1980).

112. Hewitt, W. *Microbiological Assay. An introduction to quantitative principles and evaluation.* Academic Press, New York (1977).

113. Bliss, C. I. *The statistics of bioassay with special reference to the vitamins.* Academic Press, New York (1952).

114. Schatzki, T. F., and Keagy, P. M. "Analysis of nonlinear response in microbiological assay for folacin." *Anal. Biochem.* **65**, 204 (1975).

115. Finney, D. J. *Statistical method in biological assay,* 3rd ed. MacMillan, New York (1978).

116. Keagy, P. M. "Folacin bioavailability model applied to dietary fiber in rats." Ph.D Thesis, University of California, Berkeley (1981).

117. Zerbe, G. O. "On Fieller's theorem and the general linear model." *Am. Statistician* **32**, 103 (1978).

118. Keagy, P. M. and Oace, S. M. "Bioassay of wheat bran folacin and effect of bran and xylan on intestinal folacin synthesis in rats." *J. Nutr.* in press (1984).

119. Scott, M. L., Nesheim, M. C., and Young, R. J. *Nutrition of the Chicken.* M. L. Scott & Associates, Ithaca, New York, 496 (1969).

18 II Folacin

Chromatographic and Radiometric Assays

Jesse F. Gregory, III

SEPARATION OF FOLACIN COMPOUNDS

A. Preparative Separations

The following procedures provide a separation of folacin compounds such that individual quantitation can be performed by microbiological methods or, in the case of radiolabeled materials, by determination of radioactivity.

Paper and thin-layer chromatography have long been used for the separation of folacin compounds (1–4). These methods are useful for the rapid separation of various folacins; however, quantitation may be difficult. The use of *Lactobacillus casei* has been reported for the bioautographic detection and partial quantitation of folacin in biological materials (1). High-voltage paper electrophoresis has been shown to provide a separation of folic acid polyglutamates for characterization of synthetic products (2).

The most common method for preparative folacin separation is anion-exchange column chromatography. Diethylaminoethyl (DEAE)-cellulose was first employed by Usdin and Porath (5) for the separation of folacin monoglutamates. DEAE ion-exchange materials such as DEAE-Sephadex A-25 have been widely used for preparative separations of folacin monoglutamates in extracts of foods and other biological materials (6–12) and by numerous researchers for the routine purification of folacin compounds. DEAE-substituted ion-exchange media also have been widely used for separation of folacin polyglutamates, with retention a direct function of the glutamyl chain length for homologous folacin compounds (13–14). The oxidation state and single-carbon substituents also influence the retention properties of folacin polyglutamates (8,15), thus ion-exchange chromatograms of folacins from biological materials are very complex and often lacking in complete resolution. Cumbersome differential microbiological assays of the collected fractions are generally required for tentative identification (6,7,9,10,12,16,17). Alternative anion exchange media that have been employed for folacin separation include triethylaminoethyl (TEAE)-cellulose (18) and quaternary aminoethyl (QAE)-Sephadex A-25 (8,19–22), both of which are more strongly basic than DEAE exchangers. A volatile buffer system using triethylammonium bicarbonate has been developed for rapid purification and desalting of folacin compounds on QAE-Sephadex A-25 (20).

The separation and analysis of folacin compounds in biological materials is greatly simplified by enzymatic conversion of the folacin polyglutamates to the monoglutamyl state using a pteroyl-γ-glutamylhydrolase (conjugase), as discussed in the first section of this chapter. Selection of the appropriate enzyme is critical because complete conversion of folacin vitamers to the monoglutamate level is essential to permit an unambiguous chromatographic analysis. Conjugase preparations from chicken pancreas would be unsuitable because they yield a folacin diglutamate product, whereas mammalian kidney, liver, or plasma conjugases are capable of hydrolysis to the monoglutamate level. Conclusions from chromatographic studies of folacin compounds based on the use of chicken pancreas conjugase (6,7) are, therefore, ambiguous.

Gel filtration chromatography on low-exclusion porous materials has been shown to provide an isocratic separation of many folacin monoglutamates and polyglutamates. The chromatographic mode of separation of Sephadex G-15 and G-25 appears to involve both molecular exclusion and adsorption for folacin monoglutamates in addition to weak ionic repulsion of long-chain polyglutamates (23). As with ion exchange, oxidation state and single carbon substituents also influence folacin retention (23). Sephadex G-10 also has been used for the separation of certain folacin compounds (24), although quantitative retention data have not been reported. The parallel or sequential analysis of biological extracts on both gel filtration and ion-exchange columns permits more conclusive identification of folacin compounds than can be attained using either technique alone (8,12,16,25–29).

The biological specificity of folacin-binding proteins (FBP) recently has been applied to preparative chromatography of folacin compounds (30). Immobilization of the FBP from milk on Sepharose 4B yields a chromatographic medium that has extremely high specificity and affinity. A potential limitation of preparative chromatography with immobilized FBP is its very low affinity for 5-formyltetrahydrofolic acid (31,32). This problem presumably could be alleviated by conversion of 5-formyl to 10-formyltetrahydrofolic acid, which readily binds to FBP (33). This may be accomplished by acidification followed by neutralization (34).

As an alternative to the direct chromatographic determination of chain length of folacin polyglutamates, many researchers have employed oxidative or reductive cleavage of the C-9, N-10 bond, followed by chromatographic analysis of the resulting p-aminobenzoylglutamates (35–39). This procedure eliminates the complexity of direct analysis because it eliminates all chromatographic variables except the glutamyl chain length. Unfortunately, a large body of data was generated with these procedures which, subsequently, were shown to be ineffective in cleaving certain folacin compounds (40–41). Alternate chemical procedures for cleavage of the C-9, N-10 bond have been devised recently which permit accurate quantitation of the polyglutamyl chain length of all folacin compounds in biological materials (42–44).

An innovative electrophoretic approach to the direct determination of the chain length distribution of folacin compounds recently has been reported (45). This method is based on the formation of ternary covalent complexes of [³H]5-fluoro-2′-deoxyuridylate, thymidylate synthetase, and polyglutamates of 5,10-methylenetetrahydrofolic acid, which may be separated by polyacrylamide gel electrophoresis. Separation is a function of the net charge of the complex, which is proportional to the polyglutamate chain length. Quantitation is performed by autoradiography and densitometry. The specificity and sensitivity of the method have been demonstrated in applications to tissue folacin analysis (46) and folylpolyglutamate synthetase assays (47). Sample pretreatment procedures also permit application of the method to polyglutamates of folic acid and tetrahydrofolic acid (46).

B.   High-Performance Liquid Chromatography

A variety of separation procedures have been developed for folacin compounds using high-performance liquid chromatography (HPLC). Applications to date have been limited for food and other biological analysis because of inadequate preparative methods or a lack of sufficiently sensitive and specific detection methods. Although a gas chromatographic method has been suggested for the determination of folic acid (48), the folacin compounds are poorly suited for gas chromatographic analysis. The water-soluble nature of the folacin compounds, coupled with subtle differences in ionic properties and hydrophobicity, make the folacin compounds well suited for either ion-exchange or reverse-phase HPLC. Future research concerning HPLC applications must be directed toward sample extraction and conjugase treatment, preparative chromatography, and enhanced detectability of the folacin compounds.

Anion exchange HPLC separations of certain folacin monoglutamates were first reported by Reed and Archer (49). Although resolution of all folacin compounds could not be obtained isocratically (Figure 18.2), this procedure illustrated that rapid separations could be obtained with simple instrumentation. Gradient elution anion exchange HPLC was later reported for folacin standards and crude extracts of several foods by Clifford and Clifford (50). This procedure was inadequate for folacin quantitation because of poor chromatographic effi-

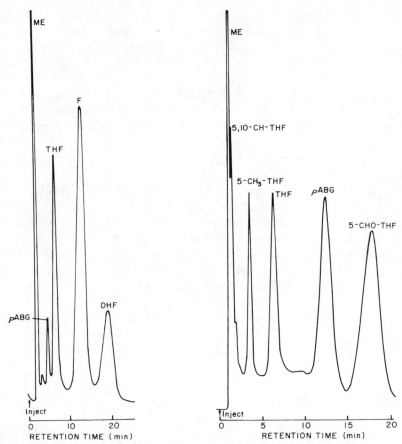

FIGURE 18–2. Isocratic separation of folacin compounds by anion exchange HPLC on Al-Pellionex-WAX. [Reprinted from Ref. (49). Copyright (1976) Elsevier Scientific Publishing Co.]A, 0.025M sodium phosphate, (pH 4.8), 1.3 ml/min, B, 0.006 M sodium phosphate, (pH 4.0), 1.2 ml/min. Mercaptoethanol (ME), p-aminobenzoyl glutamic acid (pABG), tetrahydrofolic acid (THF), folic acid (F), dihydrofolic acid (DHF), 5,10-methylenetetrahydrofolic acid (5,10-CH-THF),5-methltetrahydrofolic acid (5-CH₃-THF), and 5-formyltetrahydrofolic acid (5-CHO-THF).

ciency and uncertain peak identification. Their report that folacin polyglutamates coeluted with the monoglutamyl forms is in contrast to other ion-exchange data. Bertino and associates (51,52) developed gradient elution procedures that yielded efficient separation of various folacin polyglutamates (Figure 18.3). Adjusted retention times were related linearly to the square root of the glutamyl chain length. This procedure has been used extensively for folacin polyglutamate enzymology research (53). A similar separation of methotrexate polyglutamates also has been reported (54). Shane (55) reported a gradient elution anion-exchange method for quantitation of folacin polyglutamates in biological materials as derivatives of their *p*-aminobenzoylglutamyl cleavage products. Gradient elution anion-exchange HPLC also was utilized for quantitative analysis of folacin

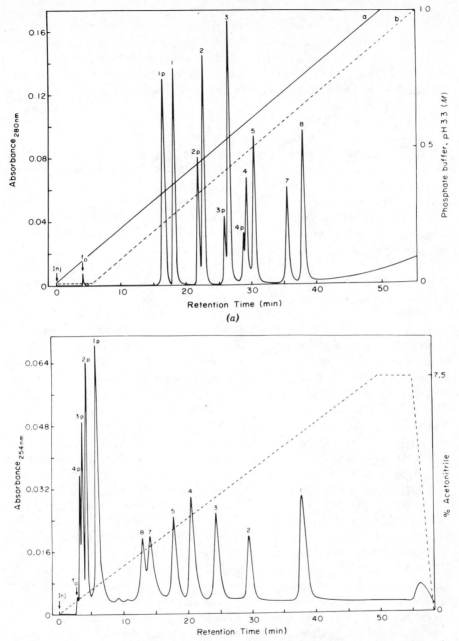

FIGURE 18–3. Anion exchange and reverse-phase HPLC. Separations of pterol - and p-amino-benzoyl oligo-γ-L-glutamates. [Reprinted from Ref. (52). Copyright (1980) Academic Press, Inc.] A, Partisil 10 SAX anion exchange column, sodium phosphate concentration gradient (0.01–1.0 M; dashed line on the chromatogram represents actual phosphate concentration at the head of the colum), B, Partisill 10 ODS-2 reverse-phase column, 0. 1 M sodium acetate buffer (pH 5.5), with 0–7.5% (v/v) acetonitrille gradient. Peaks lp, 2p, 3p, and 4p represent p-aminobenzoylmono-through tetraglutamates, while peaks 1–8 represent folic acid (pteroyl) mono-through octaglu-tamates (3–10 μG each).

477

monoglutamates in blood plasma of individuals receiving large doses of folic acid (56). The ultraviolet absorption detection was inadequate for quantitation of plasma folacin from unsupplemented subjects. Gradient elution anion exchange also has provided a convenient tool for characterizing chemical reactions of folacin vitamers (40,41).

Reverse-phase HPLC provides a wide range of parameters for manipulating folacin separations. Vitamers can be separated at neutral pH as ion pairs with cationic surfactants or in the absence of surfactants with appropriate mobile-phase polarity, ionic strength, and pH (57). Ion pair separations generally involve a mobile phase of approximately neutral pH with 15–25% methanol and 5–10 mM tetrabutylammonium phosphate for ion pairing. Isocratic (58) and methanol gradient (56,59,60) ion pair methods have been reported for folacin monoglutamate separations (Figure 18.4). As with ion exchange, resolution and efficiency are generally higher with gradient elution. Isocratic ion pair HPLC has been applied to the rapid determination of folic acid in pharmaceutical preparations (61,62) and has been employed for the separation of rat liver folacin compounds prior to microbiological assay (63). Quantitation by direct ultraviolet absorption of folacin compounds in the crude conjugase-treated rat liver extract was unsuccessful because of many interfering tissue components. Picciano and associates (64,65) developed a procedure in which folacin monoglutamate standards or food extracts were injected onto a reverse-phase column that had been equilibrated with a neutral phosphate buffer containing methanol and tetrabutylammonium phosphate. The folacin compounds were strongly retained as ion pairs. Nonretained material was immediately eluted with a neutral phosphate-perchlorate buffer, followed by separation and elution of folacin compounds using the original mobile phase (Figure 18.5). The results of limited applications to food analysis suggest that preparative chromatography or more specific detection would be required for the analysis of many biological materials (65,66).

Suppression or enhancement of the ionization of folacin functional groups by mobile-phase pH control can effectively regulate retention and separation on reverse-phase columns in the absence of ion pairing agents. Day and Gregory (67) reported an isocratic method for the separation of folacin monoglutamates using coupled octadecylsilyl and phenylsilyl columns with an acidic phosphate-acetonitrile mobile phase (Figure 18.6). Subsequent research has shown that elution with a 7.5–13% acetonitrile gradient improves resolution of tetrahydrofolic acid from the tailing ascorbate peak in this system, although isocratic conditions are suitable for many analytical and preparative applications using this procedure. A postcolumn derivatization system was devised which used $Ca(OCl)_2$ to oxidize folic acid, dihydrofolic acid, and tetrahydrofolic acid to highly fluorescent pterins, thus increasing the sensitivity and specificity of detection for these vitamers (67). The isocratic system with sequential ultraviolet absorption and oxidative fluorogenic detection has been successfully applied to the determination of folacin compounds in cabbage, liver, infant formulas, and cereals (67,68). Recent research has shown that the native fluorescence of tetrahydrofolic acid, 5-methyltetrahydrofolic acid and 5-formyltetrahydrofolic acid

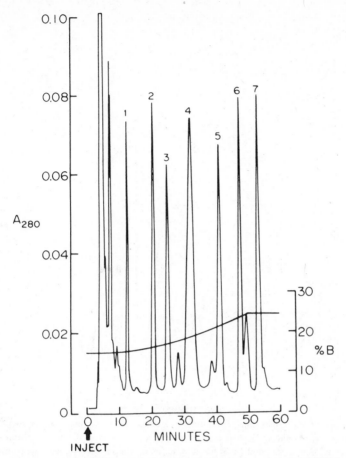

FIGURE 18–4. Separation of folacin monoglutamates by ion-pair reverse phase HPLC. μBondapak C₁₈ column; mobile phase was 10 mM tetrabutylammonium phosphate (TABP) in water, and B was a 1:1 mixture of water and 95% ethan ol ewith a final concetration of 10mM TABP. Order of elution is (1) p-aminobenzoyl glutamate acid, (2) 10-formyltetrahydrofolic acid, (3) tetrahydrofolic acid (4) 5 formyltetrahydrofolic acid, (5) dihydrofolic acid, (6) 5-methyltetrahydrofolic acid, and (7) folic acid; 3–5 nmoles each compound. [Reprinted from Ref. (60). Copyright (1981) Academic Press, Inc.]

is sufficient under these conditions to permit direct fluorometric detection, which greatly enhances the sensitivity and specificity of the method (69). Sequential detection by direct fluorescence monitoring and the postcolumn Ca(OCl)₂ oxidation system (69) permits the detection of the principal folacin vitamers encountered in foods and other biological materials (Figure 18.7). Extraction conditions were selected which yield quantitative conversion of 10-formyltetrahydrofolate to the 5-formyl isomer.

Another approach to specific and sensitive reverse-phase HPLC was reported by Lankelma et al. (70) for the electrochemical determination of 5-methyltetrahydrofolic acid in physiological fluids. A column switching valve permitted

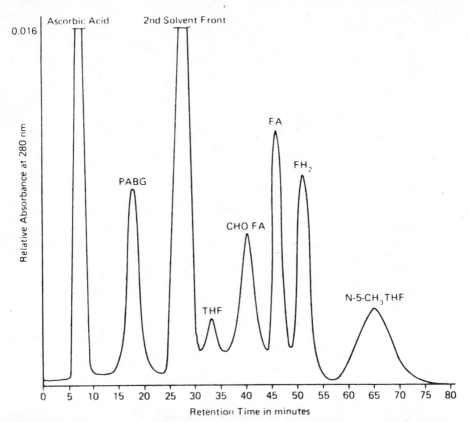

FIGURE 18.5. Stepwise ion-pair reverse-phase HPLC of folacin compounds.Two μBondapak Phenyl columns were linked in series. Columns were equilibrated in 0. 1 M potassium phosphate, (pH 7.0), with 1.2% methanol and 5 mM tetrabutylammonium phosphate, and eluted with this buffer for 6 min after sample injections. Elution of folacin cmpounds was then achieved by switching to a 0.03 M sodium perchlorate, 1.3mM potassium phosphate buffer, (pH 7.0), with 0.5% methanol. Peaks were 0.5 nmoles each of p-aminobenzoyl glutamic acid (pABG), tetrahydrofolic acid (THF), 5-formyltetrahydrofolic acid (CH-THF), folic acid (FA), dihydrofolic acid (FH₂) and 5-methyltetrahydrofolic acid (N-5-CH₃-THF). [Reprinted from Ref. (65). Copyright (1982) Elsevier Scientific Publishing Co.]

purification and concentration of samples on a precolumn prior to analytical separation and electrochemical quantitation. The use of electrochemical detectors has not yet been reported for other folacin compounds; however, it appears to be feasible. Other applications of reverse-phase HPLC for folacin analyses include separations of folacin polyglutamates by gradient elution (52; Figure 18.2B) and an isocratic system for quantitation of folic acid and pteroic acid derivatives during chemical synthesis (71). Reverse-phase HPLC also has been applied to the analysis of folacin polyglutamates in animal tissues. Eto and Krumdieck (72) have employed selective cleavage of the C-9, N-10 bond and formation of azo-dye derivatives of the resulting *p*-aminobenzoylglutamates. Reverse-phase

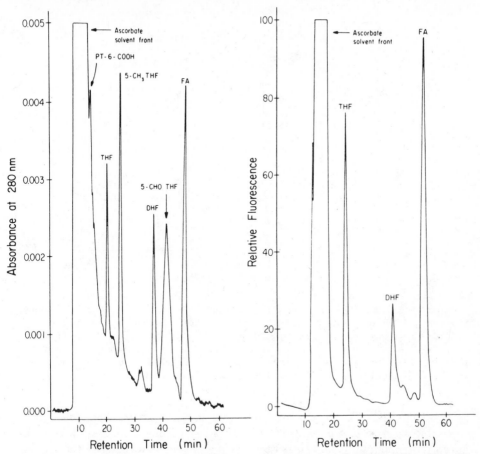

FIGURE 18.6.   Isocratic reverse-phase HPLC separation of folacin derivatives on Ulltrasphere IP and μBondapak Phenyl columns linked in series. Mobile phase was 0.33 M potassium phosphate (pH2.3) with 9.5% (v/v) acetonitrile. A. 280-nm absorption detection; B. Same as A, with postcolumn oxidation using Ca (OC1)$_2$ reagent for fluorescennce detection. Pterin-6-carboxylic acid (PT-COOH), tetrahydrofolic acid (THF), 5-methyltetrahydrofolic acid (5-CH$_3$THF), dihydrofolic acid (DHF), 5,-formyltetrahydrofolic acid (5-CHO-THF), and folic acid (FA). [Reprinted from Ref. (67). Copyright (1981) American Chemical Society.]

HPLC provided a separation according to glutamyl chain length that could be monitored by radioactivity determination in collected fractions or by direct visible absorption of unlabeled compounds. This and the similar ion-exchange procedure of Shane (55) represent a major advance in folacin polyglutamate research techniques.

In summary, HPLC methodology is currently available for the separation of various monoglutamyl folacin vitamers and for separation of intact or cleaved folacin polyglutamates according to chain length. Application of these procedures to biological materials is rapidly occurring and generally depends on optimization of sample extract purification and folacin detection methods for the particular

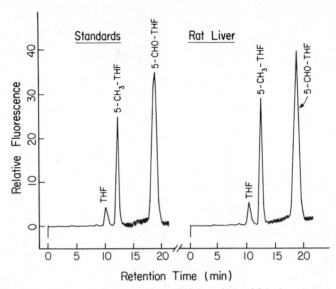

FIGURE 18.7. Chromatograms of reverse-phase HPLC analysis of folacin standards and rat liver folacin compounds using a μBondapak Phenyl column. Mobile phase was 0.033 M potassium phosphate (pH 2.3) with a 7.2–11,0% (v/v) acetonitrile g4adient (15-min linear progam). Detection was direct fluorescence monitoring: 290-nm excitation, 357-nm emission. Standards: tetrahydrofolate (THF, 0.163 nmles), 5-methyl-tetrahydrofolate (5pCH₃pTHF,0.110 nmoles), and 5-formyltetrahydrofolate (5-CHO-THF, 0.105 nmoles), Detection sensitivity was increased at 13.5 min. [Reprinted from Ret. (69). Copyrig ht (1984) Journal of Nutrition, American Institute of Nutrition.]

analysis required. The rapid separations and high chromatographic efficiency attainable by HPLC will facilitate the analysis of unlabeled or radiolabeled folacin compounds in biological research that previously required the use of much slower preparative ion-exchange methods.

FOLACIN RADIOASSAY PROCEDURES

The discovery and characterization of FBPs quickly led to the development of ligand-binding radioassays for folacin compounds. These radioassays permit a sensitive, rapid, and specific determination of many folacin compounds and provide an alternative to microbiological assays in certain applications. The greatest emphasis in radioassay methodology has been in blood plasma analysis, although these methods have been partially evaluated for the analysis of foods and other biological materials. Radiometric assays can be performed with readily obtained reagents or with commercially available assay kits.

Most radiometric assay procedures are based on competition between radiolabeled and unlabeled folacin compounds for a FBP, that is, as a competitive binding assay (31,73–91). Quantitation is performed by determination of radioactivity associated with the soluble binding protein after adsorption and removal of unbound folacin compounds. A sequential binding procedure has been developed that involves the incubation of unlabeled folacin with the binding protein prior to the addition of the labeled compound (31). Sequential binding yields very high sensitivity but has no real advantage over competitive binding methods in most applications. Radioimmunoassays have been developed that use an antiserum produced with a folic acid conjugate of methylated serum albumin (92,93). The radioimmunoassays are highly specific for folic acid and are unsuitable for the quantitation of other folacin vitamers. The production and analytical use of antibodies that would respond uniformly to the broader class of folacin compounds has not been examined.

Variables involved in selection of a suitable competitive binding radioassay procedure include: (1) type of radiolabeled folacin, (2) folacin compound used as a standard, (3) pH of the reaction mixture, (4) source of the FBP, and (5) method of adsorption of unbound folacin. Tritiated folic acid is commercially available at high specific activity. Folic acid derivatives that are labeled with γ-emitting nuclides (^{75}Se or ^{125}I) are available, which permit quantitation of the radioassay by γ-counting. FBPs used in folacin radioassays have included those from milk and milk fractions* (31,73–80,82,83,85,86,88–91,95), porcine blood plasma (84), porcine kidney (81), and intact bacterial cells (74). The selection of the binder source (various milk preparations or kidney folacin binding protein) has been left to the discretion of the user in a recent method description (89). Methods of separation of protein-bound from free folacin have been based largely on the use of purified charcoal mixed ("coated") with albumin (32,81,86,88), hemoglobin (75–78,80,83), or dextrans (79,82,84,85). Dextran or albumin charcoal mixtures provide equivalent adsorption in the experience of the author, whereas Waxman and Schreiber (87) reported that hemoglobin charcoal mixtures are somewhat more effective. The efficacy of adsorbent mixtures has been studied in detail by Zettner and Duly (94). Small DEAE-Sephadex (90) or Sephadex G-25 columns (95) have been employed as an alternative to charcoal adsorption methods.

The unlabeled folacin compound selected for radioassay calibration must be stable and have an affinity for the binding protein that is comparable to that of the folacin in the sample. Many procedures have been based on *dl*-5-methyltetrahydrofolic acid as a standard because the *l*-isomer is the principal folacin derivative in plasma (31,75–82,84,85,88,89,91). Folic acid, which is more stable than 5-methyltetrahydrofolic acid, cannot be used as an accurate standard in assays run at pH 7.2–8.0 because of its greater affinity for the FBP than that of 5-methyltetrahydrofolic acid (96). Folic acid is preferable as a standard in assays run at pH 9.3 because of its greater stability and equivalent binding affinity (96). Radioassays of folacin in foods fortified with folic acid would also require the use of folic acid standards and pH 9.3 buffering. Waxman and Schreiber (89) evaluated the merits of pH 7.4 and 9.3 assays and concluded that

---

* It is important to recognize that, although commercial crystalline bovine β-lactoglobulin has been widely used as a folacin binder, the actual FBP is present as a contaminant in these preparations and is distinctly different from β-lactoglobulin.

pH 9.3 assays for plasma folate are susceptible to error from variation in binding affinity if the pH deviates from the desired 9.3.

Many of the initial radiometric procedures for the determination of folacin in plasma exhibited variable correlation with *L. casei* methods because of inherent variation in the folacin-binding capacity of plasma (78,97). Dunn and Foster (78) observed that denaturation of plasma proteins by heating at 100°C for 15 min at pH 10.5 released endogenous plasma folacin from binding proteins and, thus, improved the accuracy of the assay. Similar heat treatments and a recent "no-boil" method (91) have been widely used and permit quantitation of total plasma folacin irrespective of the plasma folacin-binding capacity. These treatments also have the effect of denaturing the unsaturated (free) FBP, which would eliminate its potential for interference in the radioassay. Longo and Herbert (32) suggested that bovine skim milk may contain a "releasing factor" that would eliminate the need for a preliminary heat treatment. This has not been substantiated, and they subsequently recommended a heat treatment for serum preparation in radioassays (98).

A major advantage of radioassay methodology over the bacterial growth methods is its lack of sensitivity to antibiotics in biological samples. The FBPs employed generally have little affinity for folacin analogs and oxidation products, which yields a high degree of radioassay specificity (31,32,75,77,83). The antifolate drug methotrexate has been reported to interfere with radioassays at levels attained in plasma following high-dose chemotherapy (99,100). Waxman and Schreiber have reported that pH 7.4 radioassays are less susceptible to methotrexate interference than those run at pH 9.3 (89).

Several commercial assay kits have been examined for their response to various folacin vitamers and their correlation with microbiological assays. Shane et al. (32) found that oxidation state, stereochemical form, one-carbon substituent, and glutamyl chain length influenced the molar response of folacin compounds to a variable degree among the assay kits. One kit that used a porcine plasma FBP and a *dl*-5-methyltetrahydrofolic acid standard was shown to yield erroneous results because of a lack of affinity of the binding protein for the unnatural *d*-isomer of the calibration standard. Although careful standardization can justify the use of radioassay methods for plasma folacin assay, the variable response of the radioassays as a function of folacin vitamer chemistry indicates that application of these methods to foods, other plant and animal tissue extracts, and fluids such as erythrocyte hemolysates may yield tenuous results. Data suggesting questionable accuracy of several radioassays for erythrocyte folacin have been reported (96,97), however other radioassay methods for erythrocyte folacin determination have been shown to be adequate (32,89). Several reports have indicated that certain radioassay kits provide suitable clinical diagnostic data for plasma folacin (101–104).

Applications of radioassay methodology to the analysis of foods and other biological tissues have been limited and not conclusive. Tigner and Roe (105) employed a competitive binding radioassay (pH 9.3) for the analysis of rat tissues.

Direct comparisons with *L. casei* assays yielded results that strongly supported the accuracy of the radiometric procedure. This radioassay also yielded results that correlated closely with *L. casei* values for folacin in a variety of frozen foods (106). Reingold et al. (66) reported that the pH 9.3 radioassay yielded results that were higher than those obtained with *L. casei* for folacin in selected infant foods. Klein and Kuo (107) also reported higher radioassay values for spinach products than those obtained with *L. casei*. Gregory et al. (68) reported variable agreement between radioassay, reverse-phase HPLC, and *L. casei* methods that was dependent upon the particular food analyzed. Potential interference by folic acid oxidation products in the radioassay of fortified foods was shown to be insignificant, while the low response to 5-formyltetrahydrofolic acid would result in an underestimation of folacin in biological materials that underwent a conversion of the 10-formyl to the 5-formyltetrahydrofolate isomer during extraction (Figure 18.8). The results of these studies indicate that further research and careful validation for each type of sample are required before widespread use of the folacin radioassay for many biological materials would be justified.

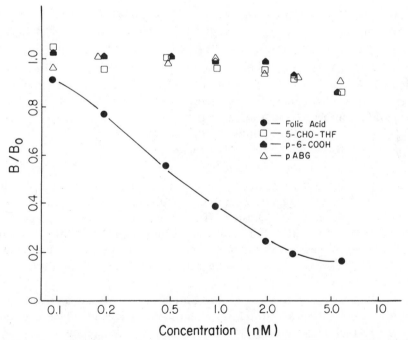

FIGURE 18.8. Binding curves for selected folacin derivatives in radio assay with milk folacin binding protein at pH 9.3. Abbreviations: B=observed ³H- folic acid bound, B_0=³H folic acid bound in absence of unlabelled test compound. [Reprinted form Ref. (68). Copyright (1982) Institute of Food Technologists.]

ANALYTICAL METHODOLOGY

I. DETERMINATION OF FOLIC ACID IN FORTIFIED CEREAL AND INFANT FORMULA PRODUCTS BY REVERSE-PHASE HPLC

A. Principle

This method is based on isocratic reverse-phase separation of folic acid from other extracted compounds, followed by its quantification by sequential ultraviolet absorption and fluorogenic postcolumn derivatization detection methods (67). Fluorescence detection is based on postcolumn flow-injection cleavage of folic acid to pterin derivatives using $Ca(OCl)_2$ as an oxidant. Tetrahydro- and dihydrofolic acid also can be determined by this fluorometric procedure, whereas substituted reduced vitamers do not yield a significant fluorescent response. Applications of reverse-phase HPLC to the determination of naturally occurring folacin vitamers are discussed elsewhere (69).

B. Equipment

1. *HPLC System Comparable To the Following*:
   (a) Altex Model 110A pump.
   (b) Rheodyne Model 7120 injection valve with $100 \mu l$ sample loop. Octadecylsilyl guard column cartridge, 4.6 mm $\times$ 3 cm (Brownlee Labs, Inc.).
   (c) Analytical column. Ultrasphere IP (4.6 mm $\times$ 25 cm; Altex Scientific), μBondapak C_{18} (3.9 mm $\times$ 30 cm; Waters Associates), or μBondapak Phenyl (3.9 mm $\times$ 30 cm; Waters Associates), each of which has been found to provide satisfactory separations. The use of two columns in series, which is routinely employed for complex mixtures of folacin compounds (67), is not required for the determination of folic acid.
   (d) Ultraviolet absorption detector, 280 nm (Model 153, Altex Scientific).
   (e) Postcolumn derivatization system. Immediately after the UV detector, the $Ca(OCl)_2$ oxidant reagent is metered into the column eluate via a three-way manifold (Dionex) using a Technicon AutoAnalyzer® proportioning pump or a Milton Roy Mini Pump at 0.23 mL/min. The combined eluate-reagent stream is passed through a 10-m Teflon delay coil (0.8 mm i.d.) in a 60°C water bath for about a 2-min delay before entering the fluorescence detector.
   (f) Fluorescence detector. Fluoro-Monitor from American Instrument Co., or equivalent with a 70 μL flow cell, General Electric Blacklight lamp (Model F4T4-BL), a Corning 7-65 excitation filter, and a Wratten 2-A emission filter.
   (g) Recorder. Linear Instrument Co. Model 385 dual channel recorder or equivalent.
2. *Refrigerated centrifuge.*

3. *Syringe Filter.* With 0.45-μm pore size nylon membrane (Rainin Instrument Co.) for sample filtration.

4. *Filtration Apparatus.* For mobile-phase buffer with 0.45-μm pore size membrane (Gelman Instrument Co.).

C. Reagents

1. *Mobile Phase Buffer.* 0.033 M potassium phosphate (pH 2.3) containing 12% (v/v) acetonitrile. Transfer 4.6 mL (0.066 mole) of concentrated H_3PO_4, 240 mL acetonitrile, and approximately 1600 mL of deionized H_2O to a 2-L beaker. Adjust to pH 2.3 by dropwise addition of 6 N KOH. Dilute to volume in a 2-L volumetric flask. Filter through 0.45-μm membrane and degas by sonication under vacuum (water aspiration) for 5 min immediately prior to use.

2. *Extraction Buffer.* 0.1 M potassium phosphate (pH 7.0) containing 0.25% (w/v) sodium ascorbate.

3. *$Ca(OCl)_2$ Postcolumn Reagent.* 0.005% (w/v) HTH dry chlorine (Olin Co.) in 0.1 M K_2HPO_4 and 0.2 M NaCl. Prepare an intermediate solution of 0.1% (w/v) HTH dry chlorine in H_2O, then dilute 1:20 with a solution of 0.105 M K_2HPO_4 and 0.21 M NaCl. This reagent is stable for 3 days.

4. *Folic Acid Standard.* Dissolve 20 mg folic acid (Sigma Chemical Co.) in 3 mL of 5% (w/v) K_2HPO_4 in a 200-mL volumetric flask, then dilute to volume with the pH 7.0 phosphate-ascorbate buffer (Reagent 2). Prepare a working standard at an approximate concentration of 0.1 mg/mL by appropriate dilution with this buffer. Both ultraviolet absorption and fluorescence detectors yield a linear response over a wide folic acid concentration range.

D. Procedure

1. *Cereal Extraction* Homogenize a 10 g sample with 100 mL of pH 7.0 phosphate-ascorbate buffer (Reagent 2) in a Waring Blender for 1 min at high speed. Centrifuge for 15 min at $10,000 \times g$.

2. *Infant Formula Extraction.* Dilute 20 mL of a liquid sample or suitably diluted dry product with an equal volume of the pH 7.0 phosphate-ascorbate buffer (Reagent 2). Add 6 N HCl.

3. *HPLC Analysis.* Flush the methanol storage solvent from the HPLC system by pumping deionized H_2O (filtered through 0.45-μm membrane), followed by the mobile-phase buffer. Allow approximately 20 min for column equilibration. Prior to shutting off the HPLC system, flush with filtered H_2O, then methanol.

Because of variation between columns, preliminary experiments are required to determine the proper flow rate and mobile-phase acetonitrile concentration to provide a retention time for folic acid of approximately 15 min. Typical conditions used for Ultrasphere IP, μBondapak C_{18}, and μBondapak Phenyl columns are a mobile phase with 12% acetonitrile and a flow rate of 1.0 mL/min. Inject samples and standards using a filled loop technique for maximum precision. Calculate sample folic acid concentration relative to the fluorescence peak height or area of the standard.

II.   DETERMINATION OF TOTAL FOLACIN BY COMPETITIVE BINDING RADIOASSAY

A.   Principle

The method reported here is a competitive binding radioassay, which is based on the pH 9.3 assay reported by Longo and Herbert (32,98) and is described by Herbert on page 525. It provides an accurate assessment of plasma folacin, and its utility for the analysis of rat tissues and certain foods has been demonstrated (105,106). The radioassay has been reported to yield results that are significantly higher than the *L. casei* assay for spinach (107) and cabbage (68). Although Waxman and Schreiber have pointed out several advantages of pH 7.4 assays over pH 9.3 methods (89), the pH 9.3 method is recommended here for greater accuracy when applied to materials which may contain folacin vitamers other than 5-methyltetrahydrofolic acid.

B.   Equipment

1. *Clinical Centrifuge.*
2. *Boiling Water Bath.*
3. *Liquid Scintillation Spectrometer.*
4. *Disposable Plastic Screw-Capped Conical 10-mL Centrifuge Tubes.*

C.   Reagents

1. *Lysine Buffer pH 9.3*   To prepare 1000 mL, place 9.13 g (0.05 mole) L-lysine HCl and 1.0 g gelatin (Type II from swine skin; Sigma) in 800 mL of H₂O. Heat in a boiling water bath until the gelatin dissolves, then cool under running tap water. Add 5 g sodium ascorbate, adjust to pH 9.3 by dropwise addition of 6 N NaOH, then dilute to volume in a 1000-mL volumetric flask. Store at 2–4°C for no more than 1 week.

2. *Tritiated Folic Acid Working Solution.*   Prepare a working ³H-labeled folic acid solution of approximately 2.5 ng/mL (0.243 μCi/mL) from commercially obtained [3′,5′,7,9-³H]folic acid (Amersham Corporation, 43 Ci/mmole, 1 mCi/mL, typically 85–90% radiochemical purity). Mix 15 μL of the undiluted [³H]folic acid solution and 50 mL of the pH 9.3 lysine buffer; store at −20°C in disposable plastic tubes in 2.5-mL portions.

3. *Folic Acid Working Standards.*   Prepare a 100 μg/mL solution of folic acid by dissolving 20 mg of folic acid (Sigma Chemical Co.) in 4 mL of 5%

(w/v) K_2HPO_4 and diluting to 200 mL with H_2O. Dilute 100 μL of this solution to 100 mL with the pH 9.3 lysine buffer to yield a 100 ng/mL intermediate standard. Working standards of 1, 2, 5, 10, 20, 30, and 50 ng/mL are prepared by diluting 0.1 mL through 5.0 mL of the intermediate solution to 10 mL with the pH 9.3 lysine buffer. These standards are stable at 2–4°C for several weeks or for months at -20°C if protected from light.

4. *Folacin-Binding Protein Solution.* Nonfat dry milk, skim milk, or whey protein concentrate products are all suitable for folacin-binding radioassay use (32,105). A binding curve must be run to determine the dilution that will yield the desired 50–60% binding of [³H]folic acid in the absence of unlabeled folic acid. Suitably diluted solutions are stable for several weeks at 2–4°C. Binders prepared using commercial whey protein concentrate (e.g., Hi-Protal-50; Tetroid Co.) may be stored for months as a 100-mg/mL stock solution at -20°C without appreciable loss of binding capacity.

5. *Dextran-Charcoal Adsorbent.* Suspend 2 g activated charcoal (Darco G-60; Fisher Scientific Co.) and 0.2 g dextran (mean mol. wt. 40,000; Sigma Chemical Co.) in cold H_2O. Keep on ice and agitate by magnetic stirring immediately before use. Prepare fresh daily.

6. *Liquid Scintillation Cocktail.* Any commercially available cocktail that is compatible with aqueous samples may be used.

D. Procedures

1. *Milk Protein Binding Curve.* The milk product to be used as a folacin binder in the assay must be screened to determine the suitable working dilution. Prepare serial dilutions of the milk product (10-fold to undiluted for skim milk; 10–100 mg/mL for nonfat dry milk; 5–50 mg/mL for whey protein concentrate). Determine the binding capacity of the milk protein for [³H]folic acid in the absence of added unlabeled folacin as shown in the assay protocol for milk binder control in Table 18.5. The appropriate dilution to be used in the assay is that which binds 50–60% of the total folate radioactivity.

2. *Plasma Samples.* To eliminate the unsaturated plasma FBP level as a potential variable in the assay, the procedure described incorporates a heat denaturation step for all samples and standards (78,98). The heat treatment can be omitted if preliminary experiments show a low and consistent level of unsaturated FBP, as may be the case in the quantitation of animal bioassays for biologically available folacin. It should be recognized that the heat treatment may cause a slight underestimation of plasma folacin because of the greater thermal stability of the folic acid standards than that of the 5-methyltetrahydrofolic acid present in plasma (85).

The assay protocol for plasma is outlined in Table 18.5. Following mixing of the blanks, standards, and plasma samples with the pH 9.3 lysine buffer, cap all tubes and heat in a boiling water bath for 15 min. Upon cooling, add the diluted milk binder and incubate at ambient temperature for 30 min in the dark.

TABLE 18.5   Protocol for Folacin Radioassay.*

	Lysine Buffer	Standard or Sample	Labeled ^{3}H-folic Acid	Milk Binder	Dextran-Charcoal
Total [^{3}H]Folic acid (total radiolabeled)	1.4	0	0.1	0	0
Supernatant control (blank)	1.0	0	0.1	0	0.4
Milk binder control	0.9	0	0.1	0.1	0.4
Standards (folic acid, unlabeled)	0.8	0.1 (1.0–50 ng/mL)	0.1	0.1	0.4
Samples (serum, hemolysate, or food extract)	0.8	0.1	0.1	0.1	0.4

*Volumes are in milliliters; all samples were run in duplicate. The sequence of additions is described in the text.

Add the dextran-charcoal adsorbent, mix well, incubate at least 10 min at ambient temperature, then centrifuge at 1,500 × g for 10 min. Pipette 1.0 mL of the supernatant into a 20-mL scintillation vial, add 10 mL of Amersham PCS cocktail or other suitable medium. Mix well and count for at least 3 min in a liquid scintillation spectrometer. A preliminary experiment must be performed to determine whether corrections for variations in counting efficiency between samples and standards are required.

3. *Foods, Plant, and Animal Tissues.*   Extract milk products and infant formulas as described for the HPLC procedure. Perform the radioassay as described for plasma, including the heat treatment to denature the FBP in the sample extract.

Extract fresh and frozen liver by homogenizing with three volumes of 0.1 M potassium acetate buffer (pH 4.5) containing 1.0% (w/v) sodium ascorbate, followed by a 2-hr autolysis period at 37°C. Heat the homogenates in a boiling water bath for 5–10 min, cool in an ice bath, then centrifuge at 10,000 × g for 15 min at 2°C. Other foods, plant, and animal tissues are normally extracted by homogenizing in 3 volumes of 0.1 M potassium phosphate buffer (pH 7.0) containing 1.0% (w/v) sodium ascorbate. Heat in a boiling water bath for 5–10 min, cool, then centrifuge for 15 min at 10,000 × g. Heat treatments used for the extraction of animal tissues should be as short as is required to achieve a clear supernatant following centrifugation. This is to minimize the spontaneous conversion of 10-formyltetrahydrofolic acid to the 5-formyl isomer (69), which does not respond in the radioassay (68). Preliminary experiments to determine the effect of conjugase treatments on radioassay response are recommended for the determination of naturally occurring folacin. All extracts should be diluted as needed in the pH 9.3 lysine buffer. Perform the radioassay as outlined in Table 18.5

Recovery determination should be performed periodically by adding a known concentration of folic acid to the sample prior to homogenization.

E. Calculation of Results

The percentage of ^{3}H-labeled folic acid bound is calculated as $(A/A_0) \times 100\%$, where A = counts per minute (cpm) in the standard or sample tubes minus the cpm in the supernatant control, and A_0 = cpm in the total [^{3}H]folic acid tubes minus the cpm in the supernatant control. All cpm data must be corrected for counting efficiency if significant differences in efficiency are observed between samples and standards. The "supernatant control" represents the amount of radioactivity that is not bound to the charcoal; it is almost entirely due to degradation of the labeled folate.

The standard curve is plotted as log percent bound [^{3}H]folic acid vs. log concentration of standards (ng/mL or pmoles/mL). Alternatively, 1/percent bound vs. concentration can be plotted. The sample concentration is interpolated from the standard curve.

LITERATURE CITED

1. Eigen, E. and Shockman, G. D. "The Folic Acid Group." In F. Kavanaugh, Ed., *Analytical Microbiology*, Academic Press, New York, 431–488 (1963).

2. Godwin, H. A., Rosenberg, I. H., Ferenz, C. R., Jacobs, P. M., and Meinehofer, J. "The synthesis of biologically active pteroyloligo-γ-L-glutamates (folic acid conjugates). Evaluation of [^{3}H]pteroylheptaglutamate for metabolic studies." *J. Biol. Chem.* **247**, 2266 (1972).

3. Brown, J. P., Davidson, G. E., and Scott, J. M. "Thin-layer chromatography of pteroylglutamates and related compounds. Application to transport and metabolism of reduced folates in blood." *J. Chromatogr.* **79**, 195 (1973).

4. Scott, J. M. "Thin-layer Chromatography of Pteroylmonoglutamates and Related Compounds." In D. B. McCormick and L. D. Wright, Eds., *Methods in Enzymology*, Vol. 66. Academic Press, New York, 437–443 (1980).

5. Usdin, E. and Porath, J. "Separation of folic acid and derivatives by electrophoresis and anion exchange chromatography." *Arkiv. Kemi.* **2**, 41 (1957).

6. Butterworth, C. E., Santini, R., and Frommeyer, W. B. "The pteroylglutamate components of American diets as determined by chromatographic fractionation." *J. Clin. Invest.* **42**, 1929 (1963).

7. Santini, R., Brewster, C., and Butterworth, C. E. "The distribution of folic acid active compounds in individual foods." *Am. J. Clin. Nutr.* **14**, 205 (1964).

8. Buehring, K. U., Tamura, T., and Stokstad, E. L. R. "Folate coenzymes of *Lactobacillus casei* and *Streptococcus faecalis.*" *J. Biol. Chem.* **249**, 1081 (1974).

9. Bird, O. D., McGlohon, V. M., and Vaitkus, J. W. "Naturally occurring folates in the blood and liver of the rat." *Anal. Biochem.* **12**, 18 (1965).

10. Noronha, J. M. and Silverman, M. "Distribution of folic acid derivatives in natural materials. I. Chicken liver folates." *J. Biol. Chem.* **237**, 3299 (1962).

11. Thenen, S. W. and Stokstad, E. L. R. "Effect of methionine on specific folate coenzyme pools in vitamin B-12 deficient and supplemented rats." *J. Nutr.* **103**, 363 (1973).

12. Shin, Y. S., Kim, E. S., Watson, J. E., and Stokstad, E. L. R. "Studies of folic acid compounds in nature. IV. Folic acid compounds in soybeans and cow milk." *Can. J. Biochem.* **53**, 338 (1975).

13. Baugh, C. M. and Krumdieck, C. L. "Naturally occurring folates." *Ann. N.Y. Acad. Sci.* **186**, 7 (1971).

14. Krumdieck, C. L. and Baugh, C. M. "The solid-phase synthesis of polyglutamates of folic acid." *Biochem.* **8**, 1568 (1969).

15 Uyeda, K. and Rabinowitz, J. C. "Fluorescence properties of tetrahydrofolate and related compounds." *Anal. Biochem.* **6**, 100 (1963).

16. Brody, T., Watson, J. E., and Stokstad, E. L. R. "Folate pentaglutamate and folate hexaglutamate mediated one-carbon metabolism." *Biochem.* **21**, 276 (1982).

17. Rao, K. N. and Noronha, J. M. "A general method for characterizing naturally occurring folate compounds, illustrated by characterizing Torula yeast (*Candida utilis*) folates." *Anal. Biochem.* **88**, 128 (1978).

18. Usdin, E. "Blood folic acid studies. IV. Chromatographic resolution of folic acid-active substances obtained from blood." *J. Biol. Chem.* **234**, 2373 (1959).

19. Chan, M. M.-S. and Stokstad, E. L. R. "Metabolic responses of folic acid and related compounds to thyroxine in rats." *Biochim. Biophys. Acta* **632**, 244 (1980).

20. Parker, D. J., Wu, T.-F., and Wood, H. G. "Total synthesis of acetate from CO_2: Methyl-tetrahydrofolate, an intermediate, and a procedure for separation of the folates." *J. Bacteriol.* **108**, 770 (1971).

21. Chan, C., Shin, Y. S., and Stokstad, E. L. R. "Studies of folic acid compounds in nature.— 3. Folic acid compounds in cabbage." *Can. J. Biochem.* **51**, 1617 (1973).

22. Reed, B. and Scott, J. M. "Identification of the Intracellular Folate Coenzymes of Different Cell Types." In D. B. McCormick and L. D. Wright, Eds., *Methods in Enzymology.* Vol. 66. Academic Press, New York, 501–507 (1980).

23. Shin, Y. S., Buehring, K. U. and Stokstad, E. L. R. "Separation of folic acid compounds by gel chromatography on Sephadex G-15 and G-25." *J. Chromatogr.* **124**, 53 (1976).

24. Kas, J. and Cerna, J. "Chromatography of folates on Sephadex G-10." *J. Chromatogr.* **124**, 53 (1976).

25. Shin, Y. S., Williams, M. A., and Stokstad, E. L. R. "Identification of folic acid compounds in rat liver." *Biochem. Biophys. Res. Commun.* **47**, 35 (1972).

26. Batra, K. K., Wagner, J. R., and Stokstad, E. L. R. "Identification of folate coenzymes in romaine lettuce." *Fed. Proc.* **32**, 928 (1973).

27. Shin, Y. S., Buehring, K.U., and Stokstad, E. L. R. "Studies of folate compounds in nature. Folate compounds in rat kidney and red blood cells." *Arch. Biochem. Biophys.* **163**, 221 (1974).

28. Tamura, T., Shin, Y. S., Buehring, K. U., and Stokstad, E. L. R. "The availability of folates in man: Effect of orange juice supplement on intestinal conjugase." *Brit. J. Haematol.* **32**, 123 (1976).

29. Conner, M. J. and Blair, J. A. "The identification of the folate conjugates found in rat liver 48h after the administration of radioactively labelled folate tracers." *Biochem. J.* **186**, 235 (1980).

30. Selhub, J., Ahmad, O., and Rosenberg, I. H. "Preparation and Use of Affinity Colums with Bovine Milk Folate-Binding Protein (FBP) Covalently Linked to Sepharose 4B." In D. B. McCormick and L. D. Wright, Eds., *Methods in Enzymology,* Vol. 66. Academic Press New York, 686–690 (1980).

31. Rothenberg, S. P., DaCosta, M., and Rosenberg, Z. "A radioassay for serum folate: Use of a two-phase sequential-incubation ligand-binding system." *New Engl. J. Med.* **286**, 1335 (1972).

32. Longo, D. L. and Herbert, V. "Radioassay for serum and red cell folate." *J. Lab. Clin. Med.* **87**, 138 (1976).

33. Shane, B., Tamura, T., and Stockstad, E. L. R. "Folate assay: a comparison of radioassay and microbiological methods." *Clin. Chim. Acta* **100**, 13 (1980).

34. Robinson, D. R. "The Nonenzymatic Hydrolysis of N^5, N^{10}-Methenyltetrahydrofolic Acid and Related Reactions." In D. B. McCormick and L. D. Wright, Eds., *Methods in Enzymology,* Vol 18B. Academic Press, New York, 716–725 (1971).

35. Houlihan, C. M. and Scott, J. M. "The identification of pteroylpentaglutamate as the major folate derivative in rat liver and the demonstration of its synthesis from exogenous [³H]pteroylglutamate." *Biochem. Biophys. Res. Commun.* **48**, 1675 (1972).

36. Brown, J. P., Davidson, G. E., and Scott, J. M. "The identification of the forms of folate found in the liver, kidney, and intestine of the monkey, and their biosynthesis from exogenous pteroylglutamate (folic acid)." *Biochim. Biophys. Acta* **343**, 78 (1974).

37. Baugh, C. M., Braverman, E., and Nair, M. G. "The identification of poly-γ-glutamyl chain lengths in bacterial folates." *Biochem.* **13**, 4952 (1974).

38. Scott, J. M. "Folate Polyglutamate Chain Length of Mammalian and Bacterial Cells." In *Folic Acid: Biochemistry and Physiology in Relation to the Human Nutrition Requirement.* National Academy of Sciences, Washington, D.C., 43–55 (1977).

39. Tyerman, M. J., Watson, J. E., Shane, B., Schultz, D. E., and Stokstad, E. L. R. "Identification of glutamate chain lengths of endogenous folylpoly-γ-glutamates in rat tissues." *Biochim. Biophys. Acta* **497**, 234 (1977).

40. Maruyama, T., Shiota, T., and Krumdieck, C. L. "The oxidative cleavage of folates. A critical study." *Anal. Biochem.* **84**, 277 (1978).

41. Lewis, G. P. and Rowe, P. B. "Oxidative and reductive cleavage of folates—a critical appraisal." *Anal. Biochem.* **93**, 91 (1979).

42. Baugh, C. M., Braverman, E. B., Nair, M. G., Horne, D. W., Briggs, W. T., and Wagner, C. "The peracid cleavage of 5-methyltetrahydrofolic acid at the C^9-N^{10} bridge." *Anal. Biochem.* **92**, 366 (1979).

43. Eto, I. and Krumdieck, C. L. "Determination of three different pools of reduced one-carbon-substituted folates—1. A study of the fundamental chemical reactions." *Anal. Biochem.* **109**, 167 (1980).

44. Foo, S. K., Cichowicz, D. J., and Shane, B. "Cleavage of naturally occurring folates to unsubstituted p-aminobenzoylpoly-γ-glutamates." *Anal. Biochem.* **107**, 109 (1980).

45. Priest, D. G., Happel, K. K., and Doig, M. T. "Electrophoretic identification of poly-γ-glutamate chain-lengths of 5,10-methylenetetrahydrofolate using thymidylate synthetase complexes." *J. Biochem. Biophys. Methods* **3**, 201 (1980).

46. Priest, D. G., Happel, K. K., Magnum, M., Bednarek, J. M., Doig, M. T., and Baugh, C. M. "Tissue folylpolyglutamate chain-length characterization by electrophoresis as thymidylate synthetase-fluorodeoxyuridylate ternary complexes." *Anal. Biochem.* **115**, 163 (1981).

47. Priest, D. G., Doig, M. T., Bednarek, J. M., McGuire, J. J., and Bertino, J. R. "Electrophoretic assay of folylpolyglutamate synthetase activity." *J. Biochem. Biophys. Methods* **5**, 273 (1981). *Methods* **5**, 273 (1981).

48. Seifert, R. M. "An approach to the chemical analysis of folic acid: Gas chromatography of a degradation product from synthetic folic acid samples." *J. Sci. Food Agric.* **25**, 1509 (1974).

49. Reed, L. S. and Archer, M. C. "Separation of folic acid derivatives by high-performance liquid chromatography." *J. Chromatogr.* **121**, 100 (1976).

50. Clifford, C. K. and Clifford, A. J. "High pressure liquid chromatographic analysis of food for folates." *J. Assoc. Offic. Anal. Chem.* **60**, 1248 (1977).

51. Stout, R. W., Cashmore, A. R., Coward, J. K., Horvath, C. G., and Bertino, J. R. "Separation of substituted pteroyl monoglutamates and pteroyl oligo-γ-L-glutamates by high pressure liquid chromatography." *Anal. Biochem.* **71**, 119 (1976).

52. Cashmore, A. R., Dreyer, R. M., Horvath, C., Knipe, J. O., Coward, J. K., and Bertino, J. R. "Separation of Pteroyl-oligo-γ-L-glutamates by High-performance Liquid Chromatography." In D. B. McCormick and L. D. Wright, Eds., *Methods in Enzymology,* Vol. 66. Academic Press, New York, 459–468 (1980).

53. McGuire, J. J., Hsieh, P., Coward, J. K., and Bertino, J. R. "Enzymatic synthesis of folylpolyglutamates. Characterization of the reaction and its products." *J. Biol. Chem.* **255**, 5776 (1980).

54. Jolivet, J. and Schilsky, R. L. "High-pressure liquid chromatography analysis of methotrexate polyglutamates in cultured human breast cancer cells." *Biochem. Pharmacol.* **30**, 1387 (1981).

55. Shane, B. "High performance liquid chromatography of folates: Identification of poly-γ-glutamate chain lengths of labeled and unlabeled folates." *Am. J. Clin. Nutr.* **35**, 599 (1982).

56. Chapman, S. K., Greene, B. C., and Streiff, R. R. "A study of serum folate by high-performance ion-exchange and ion-pair partition chromatography." *J. Chromatogr.* **145**, 302 (1978).

57. Horvath, H., Melander, W., and Molnar, I. "Liquid chromatography of ionogenic substances with nonpolar stationary phases." *Anal. Chem.* **49**, 142 (1977).

58. Branfman, A. R. and McComish, M. "Rapid separation of folic acid derivatives by paired-ion high-performance liquid chromatography." *J. Chromatogr.* **151**, 87 (1978).

59. Allen, B. A. and Newman, R. A. "High-performance liquid chromatographic separation of clinically important folic acid derivatives using ion-pair chromatography." *J. Chromatogr.* **190**, 241 (1980).

60. Horne, D. W., Briggs, W. T., and Wagner, C. "High-pressure liquid chromatographic separation of the naturally occurring folic acid monoglutamate derivatives." *Anal Biochem.* **116**, 393 (1981).

61. McSharry, W. O. and Mahr, F. P. "High-pressure liquid chromatographic assay of folic acid: A collaborative study." *J. Pharm. Sci.* **68**, 241 (1979).

62. Holcomb, I. J. and Fusari, S. A. "Liquid chromatographic determination of folic acid in multivitamin-mineral preparations." *Anal. Chem.* **53**, 607 (1981).

63. McMartin, K. E., Vivayotha, V., and Tephly, T. R. "High-pressure liquid chromatography separation of rat liver folates." *Arch. Biochem. Biophys.* **209**, 127 (1981).

64. Reingold, R. M., Picciano, M. F., and Perkins, E. G. "Separation of folate derivatives by *in situ* paired-ion high-pressure liquid chromatography." *J. Chromatogr.* **190**, 237 (1980).

65. Reingold, R. N. and Picciano, M. F. "Two improved high-performance liquid chromatographic separations of biologically significant forms of folate." *J. Chromatogr.* **234**, 171 (1982).

66. Reingold, R. N., Picciano, M. F., and Perkins, E. G. "Identification of folate forms in selected infant foods." *Fed. Proc.* **39**, 656 (1980).

67. Day, B. P. and Gregory, J. F. "Determination of folacin derivatives in selected foods by high-performance liquid chromatography. *J. Agr. Food Chem.* **29**, 374 (1981).

68. Gregory, J. F., Day, B. P. F., and Ristow, K. A. "Comparison of high performance liquid chromatographic, radiometric, and *Lactobacillus casei* methods for determination of folacin in selected foods." *J. Food Sci.* **47**, 1568 (1982).

69. Gregory, J. F., Sartain D. B., and Day, B. P. F. "Fluorometric determination of folacin in biological materials using high performance liquid chromatography." *J. Nutr.* **114**, 341 (1984).

70. Lankelma, J., Vander Kleijn, E., and Jansen, M. J. Th. "Determination of 5-methyltetrahydrofolic acid in plasma and spinal fluid by high-performance liquid chromatography, using on-column concentration and electrochemical detection." *J. Chromatogr.* **182**, 35 (1980).

71. Temple, C., Rose, J. D., and Montgomery, J. A. "Chemical conversion of folic acid to pteroic acid." *J. Org. Chem.* **46**, 3666 (1981).

72. Eto, I. and Krumdieck, C. L. "Determination of three different pools of reduced one-carbon-substituted folates—3. Reversed-phase high-performance liquid chromatography of the azo dye derivatives of *p*-aminobenzoylpoly-γ-glutamates and its application to the study of unlabeled endogenous pteroylpolyglutamates of rat liver." *Anal. Biochem.* **120**, 323 (1982).

73. Metz, J., Zalusky, R., and Herbert, V. "Folic acid binding by serum and milk." *Am. J. Clin. Nutr.* **21**, 289 (1968).

74. McCall, M. S., White, J. D., and Frenkel, E. P. "Bacteria as specific binding agents for an isotopic assay of serum folate." *Proc. Soc. Exptl. Biol. Med.* **134**, 536 (1970).

75. Waxman, S., Schreiber, C., and Herbert, V. "Radioisotopic assay for measurement of serum folate levels." *Blood* **38**, 219 (1971).

76. Archibald, E. L., Mincey, E. K., and Morrison, R. T. "Estimation of serum folate levels by competitive protein binding assay." *Clin. Biochem.* **5**, 232 (1972).

77. Waxman, S. and Schreiber, C. "Measurement of serum folate levels and serum folic acid-binding protein by ³H-PGA radioassay." *Blood* **42**, 281 (1973).

78. Dunn, R. T. and Foster, L. B. "Radioassay of serum folate." *Clin. Chem.* **19**, 1101 (1973).

79. Mincey, E. K., Wilcox, E., and Morrison, R. T. "Estimation of serum and red cell folate by a simple radiometric technique." *Clin. Biochem.* **6**, 274 (1973).

80. Tajuddin, M. and Gardyna, H. A. "Radioassay of serum folate, with use of a serum blank and nondialyzed milk as folate binder." *Clin. Chem.* **19**, 125 (1973).

81. Kamen, B. A. and Caston, J. D. "Direct radiochemical assay for serum folate: Competition between ³H-folic acid and 5-methyltetrahydrofolic acid for a folate binder." *J. Lab. Clin. Med.* **83**, 164 (1974).

82. Shaw, W., Slade, B. A., Harrison, J. W., and Nino, H. V. "Assay of serum folate: Difference in serum folate values obtained by *L. casei* bioassay and competitive protein-binding radioassay." *Clin. Biochem.* **7**, 165 (1974).

83. Schreiber, C. and Waxman, S. "Measurement of red cell folate levels by ³H-pteroylglutamic acid (³H-PteGlu) radioassay." *Brit. J. Haematol.* **27**, 551 (1974).

84. Mantzos, J. "Radioassay of serum folate with use of pig plasma folate binders." **Acta Haematol. 54**, 289 (1975).

85. Mitchell, G. A., Pochron, S. P., Smutny, P. V., and Guity, R. "Decreased radioassay values for folate after serum extraction when pterolyglutamic acid standards are used." *Clin. Chem.* **22**, 647 (1976).

86. Rudzki, Z., Nazuruk, M., and Kimber, R. J. "The clinical value of the radioassay of serum folate." *J. Lab. Clin. Med.* **87**, 859 (1976).

87. Waxman, S. and Schreiber, C. "Measurement of Serum Folate Levels: Current Status of Radioassay Methodology." In *Folic Acid: Biochemistry and Physiology in Relation to the Human Nutrition Requirement.* National Academy of Sciences, Washington, D.C., 98–109 (1977).

88. Waxman, S., Schreiber, C., Rose, M., Johnson, I., Sheppard, R., Sumbler, K., Keen, A., and Guilford, H. "Measurement of serum folate by ⁷⁵Se-selenofolate radioassay." *Am. J. Clin. Pathol.* **70**, 359 (1978).

89. Waxman, S. and Schreiber, C. "Determination of Folate by Use of Radioactive Folate and Binding Proteins." In D. B. McCormick and L. D. Wright, Eds., *Methods in Enzymology.* Vol. 66. Academic Press, New York, 468–483 (1980).

90. Farina, P. R. and Grattan, J. A. "Radioiodinated pteroyltyrosine: A novel analog for folate radioassay." *Anal. Biochem.* **113**, 124 (1981).

91. Theobald, R. A., Batchelder, M., and Sturgeon, M. F. "Evaluation of pteroylglutamic acid and *N*-5-methyltetrahydrofolic acid reference standards in a new "no-boil" radioassay for serum folate." *Clin. Chem.* **27**, 553 (1981).

92. DaCosta, M. and Rothenberg, S. P. "Identification of an immunoreactive folate in serum extracts by radioimmunoassay." *Brit. J. Hematol.* **21**, 121 (1971).

93. Hendel, J. "Radioimmunoassay for pteroylglutamic acid." *Clin. Chem.* **27**, 701 (1981).

94. Zettner, A. and Duly, P. E. "Relative efficacy of separation of "free" and "bound" [3′,5′-³H] pteroylglutamate by charcoal coated with various materials." *Clin. Chem.* **21**, 1927 (1975).

95. Mantzos, J., Gyftaki, E., Alevizou-Terzaki, V., Manesis, E., and Malamos, B. "Determination of serum folates by the use of competitive binding protein: Preliminary studies." *Jahrestag. Ges. Nuclearmed. Antwerpen,* **68** (1971).

96. Givas, J. K. and Gutcho, S. "pH dependence of the binding of folates to milk binder in radioassay of folates." *Clin. Chem.* **21**, 427 (1975).

97. Eichner, E. R., Paine, C. J., Dickson, V. L., and Hargrove, M. D. "Clinical and laboratory observations on serum folate-binding protein." *Blood* **46**, 559 (1975).

98. Colman, N., Longo, D. L., and Herbert, V. "Folate radioassay and crude milk binder." *Blood* **48**, 626 (1976).

99. Lindemans, J., Van Kapel, J., and Abels, J. "Evaluation of a radioassay for serum folate and the effects of ascorbate and methotrexate." *Clin. Chim. Acta* **65**, 15 (1975).

100. Carmel, R. "Effects of antineoplastic drugs on *Lactobacillus casei* and radioisotopic assays from serum folate" *Am. J. Clin. Pathol.* **69**, 137 (1978).

101. McGown, E. L., Lewis, C. M., Dong, M. H., and Sauberlich, J. E. "Results with commercial radioassay kits compared with microbiological assay of folate in serum and whole-blood." *Clin. Chem.* **24**, 2186 (1978).

102. Laso, F. J., Celada, A., Busset, R., and Garcia, B. "Interet clinique du dosage de l'acide folique par radio-essai." *Schweiz. Med. Wschr.* **108**, 1393 (1978).

103. Waddell, C. C., Domstad, P. A., Pircher, F. J., Lerner, S. R., Brown, J. A., and Lawhorn, B. K. "Serum folate levels. Comparison of microbiologic assay and radioisotope kit methods." *Am. J. Clin. Pathol.* **66**, 746 (1976).

104. Johnson, I., Guilford, H., and Rose, M. "Measurement of serum folate: Experience with ^{75}Se-selenofolate radioassay." *J. Clin. Pathol.* **30**, 645 (1977).

105. Tigner, J. and Roe, D. A. "Tissue folacin stores in rats measured by radioassay." *Proc. Soc. Exptl. Biol. Med.* **160**, 445 (1979).

106. Graham, D. C., Roe, D. A., and Ostertag, S. G. "Radiometric determination and chick bioassay of folacin in fortified and unfortified frozen foods." *J. Food Sci.* **45**, 47 (1980).

107. Klein, B. P. and Kuo, C. H. "Comparison of microbiological and radiometric assays for determining total folacin in spinach." *J. Food Sci.* **46**, 552 (1981).

19 Vitamin B$_{12}$

Henry B. Chin

GENERAL CONSIDERATIONS

Vitamin B$_{12}$ is a member of a group of compounds collectively known as cobalamins. The structure of vitamin B$_{12}$ is shown in Figure 19.1. Chemically, the molecule is composed of a central cobalt atom coordinated by a nearly planar porphyrin-like group called corrin. In the case of vitamin B$_{12}$, the axial coordination sites are occupied by a base, dimethylbenzimidazole, and a cyano group. Although cyanocobalamin is officially termed vitamin B$_{12}$, the molecule is actually an artifact of the isolation and extraction process. The predominant form of the cobalamins found in most biological materials is coenzyme B$_{12}$ (Figure 19.2). In the coenzyme, the axial cyanide group is replaced by an adenine nucleoside connected by a cobalt-carbon. Other cobalamins are also known, for example, methyl-(CH$_3$), hydroxo-(OH), nitrito-(NO$_2$), and sulfito-(HSO$_3$) in which other moieties substitute for the cyano or adenosine group. Other compounds containing bases different from dimethylybenzimidazole are known and are termed B$_{12}$ analogs.

The therapeutic effect of raw liver in the treatment of pernicious anemia provided the impetus for the isolation and characterization of the responsible compound. The isolation of the compound was independently reported in 1948 by Rickes et al. (1) and Smith (2). The eventual elucidation of the structure of the materials as cyanocobalamin by Hodgkin (3–6) was significant in that this was the largest structure to be determined by X-ray crystallography to that time. Hodgkin received the Nobel Price in Chemistry for this work. In 1960, Barker et al. (7) reported the isolation of coenzyme B$_{12}$. The coenzyme was shown to contain an adenine nucleoside in place of the cyanide moiety. The X-

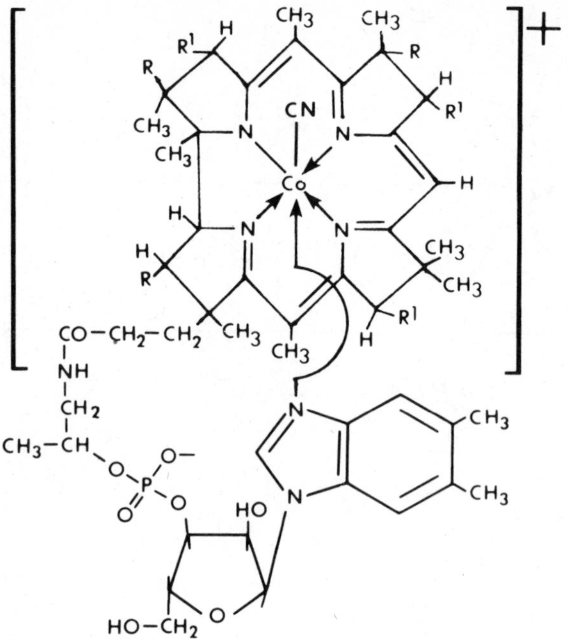

FIGURE 19.1 The structure of cyanocobalamin (R $=$ CH$_2$CONH$_2$ R^1 $=$ CH$_2$ CH$_2$ CONH$_2$). Mol. wt. $=$ 1355.42.

ray analysis of the structure was undertaken by Lenhert and Hodgkin (8,9) and they reported in 1961 that the nucleoside was linked to the cobalamin by a cobalt-carbon. This was a remarkable discovery in that it was the first demonstration of a stable cobalt–carbon bond (10).

The cobalt–carbon bond in coenzyme B$_{12}$ is unusual in that it can be reversably broken and reformed. The ability of the molecule to function in isomerization reactions, such as the conversion of lysine to 2,5-diamino hexanoate (11–13) by amino group migration, in the conversion of ethanolamine to acetaldehyde and ammonia (14–16) and in methyl transfer reactions (10) lies in the reactivity of the cobalt–carbon bond.

Coenzyme B$_{12}$ is unstable toward light and acid and base hydrolysis (17). The first reaction that takes place is the cleavage of cobalt–carbon bond. In the absence of a stabilizer, such as cyanide, the molecule will undergo further degradation. In the presence of cyanide or sulfite, the corresponding substituted cobalamins are formed. Cyanocobalamin is relatively stable.

Cyanocobalamin occurs as a tasteless, odorless red crystalline powder or as red needle-like crystals. It is very hydroscopic in its anhydrous state but moisture can be removed at 105°C under reduced pressure. It has a solubility in water at 25°C of 1.25 g/100 mL and is soluble in alcohols, phenols, and other polar compounds with hydroxy groups, for example, ethylene diol, but is insoluble in most other organic solvents. The crystals do not melt before decomposing. The

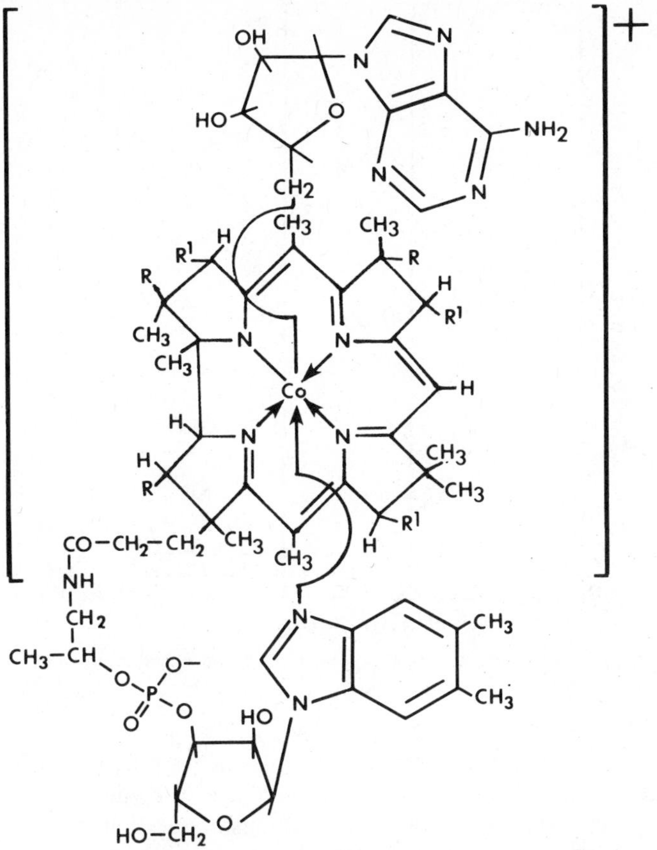

FIGURE 19.2 The structure of coenzyme B_{12}. The cobalt–carbon bond length is $2.05 \pm 0.05°$ A. The ability of the nucleoside to rotate about the cobalt–carbon bond is hindered by interaction with groups attached to the corrin ring.

ultraviolet and visible absorption spectra of cyanocobalamin shown in Figure 19.3 have maxima at 278, 361, and 550 nm.

The predominant forms of cobalamins found in foods are coenzyme B_{12} and hydroxocobalamin (18). It is believed that the binding of the coenzyme to proteins present in foods protects the molecule from chemical attack. Although there was some question of the stability of vitamin B_{12} in the presence of other food components, notably ascorbic acid (19), Marcus et al. (20) and Newmark et al. (21) report no effect by added ascorbic acid.

Vitamin B_{12} in foods is stable during heating and thermal processing. Although there is one report (22) of losses during cooking and thermal processing ranging up to 75%, other workers (23–25) report losses amounting, in the worst case, to only 27%. The vitamin is lost through leaching into the cooking liquid or drippings.

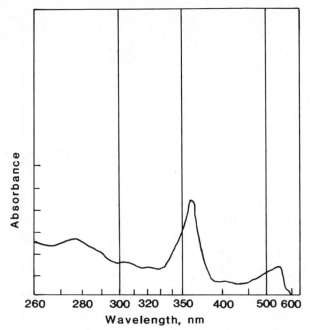

FIGURE 19.3   The absorption spectrum of cyanocobalamin in water.

Herbert et al. (26), using radioassay techniques with specially prepared binding proteins, demonstrated that a substantial portion of the vitamin B$_{12}$ in vitamin preparations is attributable to vitamin B$_{12}$ analogs of questionable health benefit.

METHODS AVAILABLE

Anodic stripping voltametry (27) and differential pulse polarography (28) have been described for cyanocobalamin and other cobalamin derivatives. The $E_{1/2}$ for the reduction of vitamin B$_{12}$ was reported to be $-1.12V$ (vs. SCE) (29) and peaks in the reduction of hydroxocobalamin (B$_{12a}$) were reported at $-0.12V$ and $-0.92V$ (vs. SCE) in 0.2 M phosphate buffer (28). Although these methods offer the promise of great sensitivity, the presence of interferences (28) limits their usefulness.

Thin-layer chromatography (18,30,31,32,33) and open-column chromatography (34,35) have been applied to both the direct assay of cobalamins and to the fractionation and removal of interfering substances from sample extracts prior to microbiological or radioassay. The direct assay relying on spectrophotometric or visual detection is limited to high-potency materials.

For the determination of vitamin B$_{12}$ in dry feeds, atomic absorption spectrophotometry of cobalt has been proposed following extraction of the sample and absorption of the cobalamins onto charcoal. Inorganic forms of cobalt are removed by chelation with EDTA and washing with water. The method has a sensitivity of approximately 2 μg vitamin B_{12}/g (36).

Cyanocobalamin can be determined by spectrophotometric measurement at 550 nm (37).

Recently, several procedures employing high-pressure liquid chromatography (HPLC) to separate and identify cobalamins have been described. The cobalamins are separated on either a reverse-phase column (38–40), or on an Aminex A-6 cation exchange column (41). These procedures, employing UV detection, have a detection limit of 10–20 μg/mL.

The methods that have been proven to have the greatest applicability are the microbiological and radioassays. The Association of Official Analytical Chemists (42) and the United States Pharmacopeia (43) recommend *Lactobacillus leichmannii* (ATCC 7830) as the assay organism, whereas the British Analytical Methods Committee (44) recommends the use of the protozoa *Ochromonas malhamensis*. Reviews by Voigt and Eitenmiller (45) and Shaw and Bissell (46) show that *O. malhamensis* has greater specificity for cobalamins than *L. leichmannii* and more closely approximates the clinical activity of the cobalamins. In particular, the B_{12}-sparing ability of deoxyribosides toward *L. leichmannii* is of concern in materials, such as fermentation broths, where they may be present in substantial amounts. The contribution of deoxyribosides and other noncobalamins to the growth of *L. leichmanni* can be determined and corrected for in the assay by adjusting the pH of extracts to 12 and autoclaving to 30 min at 121°C (21). This procedure destroys vitamin B_{12}. Microbiological activity remaining can be taken as noncobalamin growth factors for the organism. Less than 20% of the vitamin B_{12} activity in diet samples is due to noncobalamins. In most food samples and in serum, this is not a significant consideration since little deoxyribosides are present and the organism is 4000-fold less responsive to this material compared to the cobalamins. In a direct comparison of the two organisms (47), samples of food with vitamin B_{12} contents ranging from 0.2 to 116 μg/100 g were assayed following uniform extraction procedures. The results from the two assay organisms were in general agreement, although statistically significant higher results were found using *O. malhamensis*. For use in routine assays, the longer incubation time (3–4 days) required for *O. malhamensis* compared with *L. leichmannii* (1–2 days) recommends the latter organism especially if samples are known to be devoid of substances capable of nonspecific stimulation of the organism.

Other organism that have been employed include *Lactobacillus lactis* (46), *Euglena gracilis* (48), and *Escherichia coli* (18). *L. lactis* is similar to *L. Leichmannii* in that it responds to deoxyribosides, but vitamin B_{12} is not required for growth under anaerobic conditions. *E. coli* is the least specific of the organisms, having no natural requirement for vitamin B_{12}. *E. gracilis* is stimulated by serum and blood but it has been used in the analysis of foods (48).

Although the use of radioassay techniques has been widespread in clinical laboratories in the analysis of serum, its application to other materials has been delayed. The earlier radioassay procedure (35) was limited chiefly to high-potency materials and was not a true radioisotope dilution technique as the term is currently defined. The radioassay procedure of Bacher et al. (35) is truly a spectrophotometric assay using a radioactive "tracer" added to the sample to determine extraction efficiency. Radioisotope dilution, first described by Lau et al. (49), employs competitive binding between endogenous vitamin B$_{12}$ in serum and added radioactive vitamin B$_{12}$ to an intrinsic factor. Since the number of binding sites is dependent upon the limited amount of intrinsic factor added, the amount of bound radioactive B$_{12}$ is inversely related to the amount of endogenous vitamin B$_{12}$ in the serum. In the procedure of Lau et al. (49) the unbound cobalamins are absorbed onto albumin-coated charcoal and removed by centrifugation, and the activity in the supernatant is determined. The application of commercial kits for the radioisotope dilution assay of clinical samples to food samples has been examined by several workers. Newmark et al. (21) report that the results from the RID assay are highly dependent upon the extraction procedure employed. Richardson et al. (50) extracted the cobalamins using pH 4.6 buffer containing sodium cyanide and heating in a boiling water bath for 30 min. They speculated that differences found between the results by microbiological assay and RID were due to the requirement for a more rigorous extraction of cobalamins for the RID procedures. Casey et al. (51) in a later report showed that when samples were extracted by the AOAC procedure, the results of RID and microbiological assays were comparable. Marcus et al. (20) demonstrated a dependency of the radioassay procedures on the presence of cyanide, although the AOAC extraction procedure that does not employ cyanide gave results comparable with the British procedure that incorporates cyanide. To remove possible interfering proteins, Beck (52) partitioned extracts containing cyanocobalamins into benzyl alcohol and later back extracted the cyanocobalamin into water.

ANALYTICAL METHODOLOGY

I.   EXTRACTION PROCEDURES

The validity of the assay results for all except the animal feeding studies is dependent upon the complete extraction of cobalamins from the sample and the quantitative recovery of vitamin activity. Early it was recognized that to quantitatively recover the cobalamins, the extraction medium had to incorporate a stabilizing agent such as sodium metabisulfite or sodium cyanide. In light of the predominance of coenzyme B$_{12}$ as the major form of vitamin B$_{12}$ found in foods, it is reasonable to expect an enhancement in the recovery of vitamin activity when cyanide is present in the extraction media and available to convert the cobalamins into the more stable cyanocobalamin. In the presence of metabisulfite, it is possible that sulfitocobalamin is formed.

The AOAC (42) recommends autoclaving samples in an acidic buffer with sodium metabisulfite. Skeggs (53) has suggested an extracting solution incorporating sodium cyanide to effect complete extraction and stabilization of the cobalamins. The British Analytical Methods Committee recommends a cyanide extraction at a pH of 4.6–5 (44). Shenoy and Ramasarma (54) have used enzymatic digestion with papain followed by stabilization of the released cobalamins with potassium cyanide. Direct comparisons of the extraction procedures are difficult to make since many workers vary concentrations of reagents and extraction time and temperature on the basis of previous experiences. However, Skeggs (53) has indicated that the direct cyanide extraction compares favorably with the papain digestion procedure and Voigt et al. (55) have shown that enzymatic treatment of some materials may produce noncobalamin substances capable of stimulating the growth of *L. leichmannii*. Newmark et al. (21) and Marcus et al. (20) in comparing the efficacy of the AOAC and British extraction methods showed that the AOAC procedure gave slightly higher or comparable results. The results reported by Marcus et al. indicate that a minimum concentration of potassium cyanide in the final solution of 100 $\mu g/g$ is required for maximal stabilization of the cobalamins.

In the radioassay methods, the methods of extraction have been particularly controversial. Skeggs (53) and Newmark (21) suggested that some discrepancies in assay results could be attributable to the failure of the extraction procedure to convert all of the cobalamins to cyanocobalamins against which the protein binding is compared. However, Casey et al. (51) using the AOAC extraction, which does not incorporate cyanide, find comparable vitamin B_{12} contents in foods when assayed using a commercial radioisotope dilution assay kit and when assayed microbiologically. Their conclusion was that the more rigorous AOAC extraction stabilizes and quantitively extracts the cobalamins.

II.   MICROBIOLOGICAL METHOD
LACTOBACILLUS LEICHMANNII ATCC 7830

A.   Principle

See page 43.

B.   Equipment

See page 50.

C.   Reagents

Reagents 27, 28, 29, and 33, which are needed for this method, are listed on page 57. In addition, the following reagents are required for the analysis of vitamin B_{12}:

38. *Extracting Solution.*   To each 100 mL of H_2O add 1.3 g Na_2HPO_4, 1.2 g citric acid, and 1.0 g $Na_2S_2O_5$.

39. *Vitamin B_{12} Stock Solution (100 ng/mL).*   Accurately weigh 10 mg USP cyanocobalamin reference standard. Dissolve in 25% ethanol and dilute to 500

mL with additional 25% ethanol. Dilute 5 mL of this solution in 1 L. This stock solution contains 100 ng B$_{12}$/mL. Store in dark at 10°C.

40. Vitamin B$_{12}$ Intermediate Solution (1 ng/mL). Dilute 10 mL of stock solution to 1 L with 25% ethanol. Store in dark at 10°C.

41. Vitamin B$_{12}$ Working Solution (0.025 ng/mL). Dilute 5 mL of Intermediate Solution to 200 mL with H$_2$O. Prepare fresh for each assay.

D. Procedure

The procedure that is described is basically that recommended by AOAC (42).

1. *Precautions for the Assay of Vitamin B$_{12}$.* The precautions for the assay of vitamin B$_{12}$ are necessitated by three factors. First, some microorganisms are capable of producing vitamin B$_{12}$. Thus, equipment needs to be cleaned and autoclaved and reagents should avoid contact with materials that may harbor cobalamin-producing organisms. This may preclude the use of rubber stoppers and deionized water since microorganisms can grow on the ion-exchange materials and the stoppers are difficult to sterilize. Second, vitamin B$_{12}$ is a large molecule that binds well to various materials. Thus, glassware must be meticulously cleaned prior to each use. An acid wash followed by 13 rinsings with H$_2$O followed by two rinsings with H$_2$O was recommended by Skeggs (53). Although most commercial detergents may contain ingredients making them unsuitable for use in cleaning glassware for the assay of vitamin B$_{12}$, a cleaning solution composed of reagent-grade sodium lauryl sulfate can be used, followed by thorough rinsing. Third, minute quantities of vitamin B$_{12}$ are being measured. Concentrations in food samples are typically 1–10 μg/g and concentrations in the assay solution are 0.01–0.03 ng/mL (10–30 parts/trillion). Thus, contamination from utensils and handling are important considerations.

2. *Preparation of Stock Culture, Lactobacillus leichmannii, ATCC 7830.* Prepare the stock culture as described on page 57 using Reagent 29.

3. Preparation of Inoculum. Make a transfer of cells from the stock culture of *L. leichmannii* into 10 mL of liquid culture medium (Reagent 28, page 57). Incubate 6–24 hr at 37°C. Centrifuge and decant the supernatant. Aseptically resuspend the cells in 10 mL of saline solution (Reagent 33, page 57). Centrifuge and decant the supernatant. Repeat the washing twice more. Resuspend cells in 10 mL of saline solution (Reagent 33, page 57) and dilute an aliquot to 10 mL with saline solution to give a solution that is barely cloudy to the eye. This final solution is the inoculum.

4. *Extraction of Samples.*

(a) To each gram of sample add at least 25 mL of extracting solution. Homogenize the mixture using a Polytron Homogenizer (Brinkman Instruments) or equivalent equipment incorporating mechanical and ultrasonic action.

(b) Autoclave the mixture 10 min at 121°C and cool. If lumping occurs, mix until particles are evenly dispersed.

(c) Dilute the mixture with H_2O to a measured volume and let undissolved particles settle. Decant, filter, or centrifuge to obtain an aliquot of clear solution. Add H_2O and adjust the solution to pH 6.0. Add additional H_2O to dilute vitamin to a concentration approximating that of the standard solution. Excess metabisulfite may interfere with the test organism. It is advisable that the assay solution contain less than 0.03 mg $Na_2S_2O_5$/mL.

5. *Special Sample Preparations.* Although the above described extraction procedure appears to give complete extractions of the cobalamins from most samples, alternative procedures have been suggested for specific materials that the reader may wish to employ in special circumstances.

(a) Sodium Cyanide Extraction. See page 507.

(b) Enzymatic Extraction (54). Mix 1 g of sample with 50 mL of H_2O and 0.5 mL of a 0.5% aqueous suspension of papain, and incubate at 60°C for 1 hr. Add 1 mL of 5% sodium metabisulfite, steam 5 min. Cool, dilute to volume, and filter. 10 mg KCN and one drop of 1 N HCl may be substituted for the sodium metabisulfite and may be added prior to incubation at 60°C.

6. *Preparation of Standard Tubes.*

(a) To duplicate series of eight tubes, add 0 (for uninoculated blanks), 0 (for inoculated blank), 0.5 , 1.0, 1.5, 2.0, 3.0, 4.0, and 5.0 mL vitamin B_{12} working standard (Reagent 41).

(b) Add H_2O to bring volume to 5 mL.

(c) Add 5 mL assay medium (Reagent 27).

7. *Preparation of Assay Tubes.*

(a) To triplicate series of five tubes add 1, 2, 3, 4, and 5 mL of sample extract.

(b) Add H_2O to bring volume to 5 ml.

(c) Add 5 ml assay medium (Reagent 27).

8. *Sterilization.*

(a) Cap the tubes and steam for 10 min or autoclave at 121°C for 7 min. Cool rapidly.

9. Inoculation and Incubation. Inoculate tubes except uninoculated blanks with one drop of inoculum. Incubate at 37°C. Incubate up to 40 hr for turbidimetric measurements and up to 72 hr for titrimetric measurements.

10. *Turbidimetric Reading.*

(a) Tubes not to be read immediately should be placed in a refrigerator to retard further growth.

(b) Using a vortex mixer, resuspend the cells in the tubes and transfer an aliquot to a cuvette. Set the spectrophotometer to 620 nm and adjust the instrument to 100% T with an uninoculated blank. If the inoculated blank shows a reading of less than 90% T, the assay should be discarded.

(c) Reset to 100% using the inoculated blank and read the transmittance of the remaining tubes. Disregard results of the assay if the transmittance of the 5 mL of standard solution is less than expected.

11. *Titration.*

(a) Tubes not to be read immediately should be placed in a refrigerator to retard further production of acid.

(b) Titrate the contents of each tube with 0.1 N NaOH using bromothymol blue indicator or to pH 6.8. Disregard assay results if response of inoculated blank is 1.5 mL more than uninoculated blank. The 5-mL level of standard should require 8–12 mL.

12. *Calculation.*

(a) Average the replicate values for each level of standard and unknown.

(b) Plot a standard curve from the values at each level of standard.

(c) By reference to the standard curve, determine the amount of vitamin B_{12} present in the assay tubes. Divide the vitamin B_{12} content by the volume of assay solution added to the tube. The assay is valid when the concentration of the vitamin shows no dependence on the volume of assay solution used. The results in terms of ng/mL from each level of assay solution are averaged.

(c) The vitamin B_{12} content of the sample is calculated by:

$$\mu g / 100 \text{ g} = \frac{\mu g/mL}{\text{wt. of sample}} \times \frac{\text{dilution factor}}{10}$$

III.   MICROBIOLOGICAL METHOD
        OCHROMONAS MALHAMENSIS ATCC 11532

The method described is that recommended by the British Analytical Methods Committee (44).

A.   Principle

The principle upon which the method is based is identical to that for the bacterial assay. *Ochromonas malhamensis* has a more animal-like specificity in its response to cobalamins.

B.   Equipment

The equipment required for the *O. malhamensis* assay is similar to that for the *L. leichmannii* assay except for the need of a rotary shaker to be used during the incubation of the samples.

C.   Reagents

1. *Sodium Cyanide, 1%.*   Dissolve 1 g NaCN in 75 mL H_2O and dilute to 100 mL.

2. 1N Hydrochloric Acid.

3. *Vitamin B$_{12}$ Stock Solution (100 ng/mL).*   Refer to *L. leichmannii* assay.

4. *Vitamin B$_{12}$ Working Solution (0.2 ng/mL).*   Dilute 1 mL of vitamin B$_{12}$ Stock Solution to 500 mL with H$_2$O.

5. *Assay Medium.*   Bacto-B$_{12}$ *Ochromonas* Medium (Difco Laboratories) or equivalent.

D. Procedure

1. *Preparation of Stock Culture, Ochromonas malhamensis, ATCC 11532.* Dilute 1 mL of Vitamin B$_{12}$ Stock Solution (100 ng/mL) to 400 mL with H$_2$O. Add to 100 mL of assay medium. Dispense 10-mL aliquots of this enriched medium into 50-mL Erlenmeyer flasks and autoclave for 10 min at 121°C. Transfer the organism into this medium at 4–5-day intervals and incubate at 27– 30°C, 1 ft below a 60 W tubular tungsten filament lamp. The organism is transferred by taking 0.5 mL of the current growth to a flask of sterile medium. The parent culture should be dense and yellow-brown at the time of subculturing.

2. *Preparation of Inoculum.*   Dilute a 5-day stock culture 10-fold with sterile assay medium, and inoculate with 0.5 mL of this diluted culture. Alternatively one drop of the undiluted 5-day culture may be used as the inoculum.

3. *General Sample Preparation.*   The assay is designed to determine vitamin B$_{12}$ as the cyanocobalamin and is subjected to elevated temperatures for complete conversion.

(a) Weigh 1 g sample into a 125-mL Erlenmeyer flask; add 30 mL H$_2$O and 0.05–0.5 mL freshly prepared 1% aq NaCN. Mix and adjust pH to 4.6–5.0 with 1 N HCl. Let stand 30 min at room temperature with occasional shaking and readjustment of pH, if necessary.

(1) For other sample sizes, use proportionate amounts of reagents.

(2) The amount of NaCN added depends on the amount of vitamin B$_{12}$ as it frees the bound vitamin and changes it to the cyano form. Final concentration of NaCN in assay medium should not exceed 10 μg/mL.

(b) Place flask in boiling water bath 30 min, cool, transfer to 100-mL volumetric flask, and dilute to volume with H$_2$O. Sample is now diluted 1:100.

(c) Clarify by centrifugation and dilute 50 mL of clear liquid to approximately 0.2 ng/mL.

(i) Starchy samples may be further clarified by treating with Taka-diastase.

(d) To illustrate dilution further, assume the sample contains 40 μg/g.

(1) Pipette 1 mL of 1:100 dilution to a glass-stoppered 250-mL graduated cylinder. Make up to exactly 200 mL with H$_2$O and shake vigorously. Sample is then diluted 1:20,000.

(2) Pipette 10 mL of 1:20,000 dilution into a 100-mL graduated cylinder and make to volume with H$_2$O. Shake vigorously to insure adequate mixing. Sample is then diluted 1:200,000 and our theoretical sample is so

dispersed that each mL contains 0.2 ng vitamin B_{12}. That amount of vitamin B_{12} is near the middle of the assay range.

(e) Where estimates of the amount of vitamin B_{12} cannot be made, several dilutions should be assayed. All dilutions are to be made using suitable volumetric procedures.

4. *Specific Sample Preparation.*

(a) Gut Mucosa.   Refer to the enzymatic extraction described in the *L. leichmannii* procedure [Section D.5(b)].

5. *Preparation of Assay Tubes.*

(a) Add 0.5, 1, 2, and 4 mL of vitamin B_{12} working solution to a quadruplicate set of 19×150-mm test tubes.

(b) Add 0.5, 1, 2, and 4 mL of sample extract to an identical set of test tubes.

(c) Bring volumes to 4 mL with H_2O and add 1 mL of basal medium. Add 4 mL H_2O and 1 mL basal medium to five test tubes.

(d) Plug tubes and autoclave 10 min at 121°C.

6. *Inoculation and Incubation.*

(a) Cool tubes in water bath after removal from autoclave.

(b) Inoculate each tube except one of the five blank tubes with one drop of inoculum.

(c) Place on shaker in the dark and incubate at 29–30°C for 72 hr.

7. *Turbidimetric Reading.*

(a) After incubation, place all tubes in an autoclave or steam chamber 10 min to kill organisms. Add 5 mL H_2O, if necessary, and shake well prior to reading in a spectrophotometer at 540 nm.

(b) Place the uninoculated blank to read 100% T or 0.0 A. The four inoculated blanks should read no more than 90% T or 0.05 A.

(c) Read standard and assay tubes using uninoculated blank at 100% T.

8. *Calculation.*   See page 62.

9. *Special Precautions.*   See page 504.

IV.   RADIOISOTOPE DILUTION METHOD

Radioisotope dilution (RID) methods for the determination of vitamin B_{12} have undergone rapid development over the past 20 years. This period has seen the initial efforts of a few workers in the elucidation of the principles of such assays lead to the development of commercial RID kits for use in clinical laboratories. Accordingly, the experimental parameters and analytical reagents have undergone a process of refinement as researchers attempt to find those conditions giving the most reproducible and valid assay results. Variables introduced by the various researchers include the measurement of absorbed versus free labeled vitamin B_{12} and the use of various absorbents and binding proteins.

Some of the reagents used in the commercial kits are of a proprietary nature. Thus, it is difficult to choose a single procedure as being the method of choice.

The method described below is based upon the RID procedure of Lau et al (49). The binding protein solutions and coated charcoal solutions are those of Lau et al. The extraction and assay procedures are those described by Casey et al (51). The scintillation liquid, as is noted, is from Bennick and Ono (25). This procedure is described because the reagents are readily available in the United States, it is not dependent upon the continued manufacture of a commercial kit, and it incorporates the standard AOAC extraction method.

A.   Principle

This method is similar to that described for blood serum. Exogeneous radioactive labeled (^{57}Co) vitamin B_{12} and cobalamins that have been extracted from the sample, competitively bind to a glycoprotein (intrinsic factor). Radioactive vitamin B_{12} and endogeneous cobalamins will bind to the intrinsic factor (IF) in proportion to their relative concentrations, with the concentration of the IF as the limiting factor. Free cobalamins are separated from IF-bound cobalamins by absorption onto treated charcoal and the amount of free labeled vitamin B_{12} is determined. The concentration of vitamin B_{12} in the sample is determined from a standard curve comparing radioactivity recovered with standard amounts of vitamin B_{12}.

B.   Equipment

1. *Gamma counter (Beckman LSC-100 Liquid Scintillation Counter).*
2. *Centrifuge.*
3. *Vortex Mixer.*
4. *Heating Bath.*
5. *Reaction Tubes, 12 × 75 mm polypropylene.*
6. *Polytron Homogenizer (Brinkmann Instruments).*

C.   Reagents

1. *Extracting Solution.*   The same extractant as for the *L. leichmannii* microbiological assay (Reagent 38) can be used.

2. *Phosphate Buffer (pH 7.0).*   Dissolve 9.1 g KH_2HPO_4 and 18.9 g Na_2HPO_4 in H_2O and dilute to 1 L.

3. *Binding Protein Stock Solution.*   Dissolve 100 mg National Formulary Intrinsic Factor (RIA Products, Inc.) in 100 mL 0.9% saline. Store solution at 4°C; it is stable for about 30 days.

4. *Binding Protein Working Solution.*   Dilute 1 mL binding protein stock solution to 100 mL with 0.9% saline.

(a) Dilution of binding solution should be determined as described on page 523. Approximately 60–80% of the added ^{57}Co vitamin B$_{12}$ (500 pg) should be bound by the amount of IF used.

5. *Hemoglobin-Coated Charcoal.* Mix 1 g hemoglobin powder (Sigma) in 200 mL H$_2$O with an equal amount (200 mL) 5% aqueous suspension of Norit "A" charcoal.

6. ^{57}Co *Vitamin B$_{12}$ (Cyanocobalamin) Solution.* Prepare a solution containing 1 ng ^{57}Co vitamin B$_{12}$/mL by making a serial dilution of a stock solution containing a weighed amount of ^{57}Co vitamin B$_{12}$ (100–300 μCi/μg, Amersham Corp.). This solution is stable for 3 months when stored at 5°C (Lau et. al. (49)).

7. *Vitamin B$_{12}$ Stock Solution (100 ng/mL).* See Reagent 39, page 503.

8. *Vitamin B$_{12}$ Intermediate Solution (1 ng/mL).* Dilute 1 mL stock solution to 100 mL with saline (Reagent 10).

9. *Vitamin B$_{12}$ Working Standards.* Pipette 0-, 2-, 4-, 8-, 20-, or 100-mL aliquots of intermediate solution into 100-mL volumetric flasks and dilute to volume with saline. These standards contain 0, 20, 40, 80, 200, or 1000 pg vitamin B$_{12}$/mL, respectively. Prepare working standards daily.

(a) Standard dilutions may need to be adjusted depending on samples. Sample values should fall in the mid range of the standard curve.

10. *Saline Solution (0.9%).* Dissolve 8.8 g NaCl in H$_2$O and dilute to 1 L.

The radioassay reagents are also available in kits from Bio-Rad Laboratories, or RIA Products, Inc.

D. Procedure

1. *Extraction.*

(a) Weigh sample (about 20 g) containing approximately 70–90 ng vitamin B$_{12}$ into flask with 50 mL extracting solution (Reagent 38, page 993). Homogenize with Polytron Homogenizer.

(1) Meat samples can also be extracted with 0.07 M acetic acid–sodium acetate buffer (pH 4.6) containing KCN to convert released B$_{12}$ to the more stable cyanocobalamin form. Further enzymatic and/or heat treatment might be required to complete the B$_{12}$ extraction (25).

(2) Beck (52) extracted B$_{12}$ from fish with NaNO$_2$ and NaCN in H$_2$O (0.5/0.2/100, w/w/v), pH adjusted to 4.0. Oily filtrates were extracted with petroleum ether to remove fatty material. Further clean-up of the extract was obtained by extracting the cyanocobalamin in benzyl alcohol followed by re-extracting into H$_2$O after the addition of chloroform.

(b) Autoclave samples at 121°C for 10 min. Cool to room temp and dilute to 100 mL with phosphate buffer (pH 7.0) (Reagent 2).

(c) Mix well and filter through Whatman No. 2 paper.

2. *Radioassay.* The protocol is shown in Table 19.1.

(a) Pipette 0.5 mL filtrate or working standards into duplicate tubes containing 1.5 mL saline solution (reagent 10). Blanks for standard and filtrate are prepared as shown in Table 19.1

(b) Add 0.5 mL ^{57}Co vitamin B_{12} solution (Reagent 6) to each tube and mix with Vortex mixer.

(c) Add 0.5 mL binding protein (IF) solution (Reagent 4) to each tube and mix with Vortex mixer.

(d) Add 2 mL hemoglobin coated charcoal (Reagent 5), mix with Vortex mixer, and centrifuge at 3000 rpm for 15 min.

(e) Decant and count the radioactivity in the supernatant.

(1) The original procedure of Lau et al. (49) did not use a scintillation cocktail.

(2) Bennink and Ono (52) use a scintillation cocktail composed of 667 mL toluene, 337 mL Triton X-199, 6 g 2,5-diphenyloxazole, and 200 mg 1,4-di-2-(phenyloxazoly)benzene. Other appropriate scintillation fluids compatible with aqueous samples (e.g., Ready Solve GP, Beckman) may be used. Add 5 mL scintillation cocktail to 1 mL supernatant for counting.

E.   Calculation of Results

1. Prepare a standard curve by plotting the ln (cpm standard minus cpm standard blank) versus ln pg vitamin B_{12} per tube.

(a) The binder control is used as a check on binding efficiency.

2. Obtain the vitamin B_{12} content of the filtrate directly from the standard curve ln (cpm sample filtrate minus cpm filtrate blank) or by calculation from the regression equation of the standard curve.

3. Calculate the concentration of vitamin B_{12} in the samples by the following equation:

$$\text{pg vitamin } B_{12}/100 \text{ g} = \frac{2 \times C \times 100}{W} \times 100$$

TABLE 19.1   Protocol for Vitamin B_{12} Radioassay.*

	Saline	Standard or Sample	^{57}Co Vit B_{12}	IF Binder	Hemoglobin- Coated Charcoal
Standard blank	2.5	0	0.5	0	2
Standard (vitamin B_{12})	1.5	0.5	0.5	0.5	2
Filtrate blank	2.0	0.5	0.5	0	2
Sample filtrate	1.5	0.5	0.5	0.5	2
Binder control	2.0	0	0.5	0.5	2

*Volumes are in mL; all samples are run in duplicate.

where C = pg vitamin B$_{12}$ determined from standard curve and W = weight of sample extracted.

LITERATURE CITED

1. Rickes, E. L, Brink, N. G., Koniusky, F. R., Wood, T. R., and Folkers, K. "Crystalline vitamin B$_{12}$." *Science* **107**, 396 (1948).

2. Smith, E. L. "Purification of anti-pernicious anemia factors from liver." *Nature* **161**, 638 (1948).

3. Hodgkin, D. C., Kamper, J., MacKay, M., Pickworth, J., Trueblood, K. N., and White, J. G. "Structure of vitamin B$_{12}$." *Nature* **172**, 64 (1956).

4. White, J. G. "3. The crystal structure analysis of the air-dried B$_{12}$ crystals." *Proc. Roy. Soc.* **A266**, 440 (1962).

5. Hodgkin, D. C., Lindsey, J., MacKay, M., and Trueblood, K. N. "The structure of vitamin B$_{12}$—4. The x-ray analysis of air-dried crystals of B$_{12}$." *Proc. Roy. Soc.* **A266**, 475 (1962).

6. Brink-Shoemaker, C., Cruickshank, D. W. J., Hodgkin, D. C., Kamper, M. J., and Pilling, D. "The structure of vitamin B$_{12}$—6. The structure of vitamin B$_{12}$ grown from and immersed in water." *Proc. Roy. Soc.* **A278**, 1 (1964).

7. Barker, H. A., Smyth, R. D., Weissbach, H., Munch-Peterson, A., Toohey, J. I., Ladd, J. N., Volcani, B. E., and Wilson, R. M. "Assay, purification and properties of the adenylcobamide coenzyme." *J. Biol. Chem.* **235**, 181 (1960).

8. Lenhert, P. G. and Hodgkin, D. C. "Structure of the 5,6-dimethylbenzimidazolyl cobamide coenzyme." *Nature* **192**, 937 (1961).

9. Lenhert, P. G. "The structure of vitamin B$_{12}$—7. The x-ray analysis of the vitamin B$_{12}$ coenzyme." *Proc. Roy. Soc.* **A303**, 45 (1968).

10. Schrauzer, G. N. "Organocobalt chemistry of vitamin B$_{12}$ model compounds (cobaloximes)." *Acc. Chem. Res.* **1**, 97 (1968).

11. Morley, C. G. D. and Stadtman, T. C. "Studies on the fermentation of Dα-lysine. Purification and properties of an adenosine triphosphate regulated B$_{12}$-coenzyme dependent Dα-lysine mutase complex from *Clostridium stricklandii.*" *Biochem.* **9**, 48 (1970).

12. Tsai, L. and Stadtman, T. C. "Anaerobic degradation of lysine—4. Cobamide coenzyme-dependent migration of an amino group from carbon 6 of β-lysine (3,6-diaminohexanoate) to carbon 5 forming a new naturally occurring amino acid, 3,5-diaminohexanoate." *Arch. Biochem. Biophys.* **125**, 210 (1968).

13. Stadtman, T. C. and Renz, P. "Anaerobic degradation of lysine—5. Some properties of the cobamide coenzyme-dependent β-lysine mutase of *Clostridium stricklandii.*" *Arch. Biochem. Biophys.* **125**, 226 (1968).

14. Hull, W. E., Mauck, L., and Babior, B. M. "Mechanism of action of ethanolamine-lyase, an adenosyl cobalamin-dependent enzyme." *J. Biol. Chem.* **250**, 8023 (1975).

15. Mauck, L., Hull, W. E., and Babior, B. M. "Interaction between ethanolamine ammonia-lyase and methyl cobalamin." *J. Biol. Chem.* **250**, 8997 (1975).

16. Schrauzer, G. N. and Stadlbauer, E. A. "Ethanolamine ammonia-lyase: Inactivation of the holoenzyme by N$_2$O and the mechanism of action of coenzyme B$_{12}$." *Bioinorg. Chem.* **4**, 185 (1975).

17. Hogenkamp, H. P. C. "The chemistry of cobalamins and related compounds." In B. M. Babior, Ed., *Cobalamin: Biochemistry Pathophysiology.* Wiley, New York, 21–73 (1975).

18. Farquharson, J. and Adams, J. F. "The forms of vitamin B$_{12}$ in foods." *Brit. J. Nutr.* **36**, 127 (1976).

19. Herbert, V. and Jacob, S. E. "Destruction of vitamin B$_{12}$ by ascorbic acid." *J. Am. Med. Assoc.* **230**, 241 (1974).

20. Marcus, M., Prabhudesai, M., and Wassef, S. "Stability of vitamin B_{12} in the presence of ascorbic acid in food and serum: Restoration by cyanide of apparent loss." *Am. J. Clin. Nutr.* **33**, 137 (1980).

21. Newmark, H. L., Scheiner, J., Marcus, M., and Prabhudesai, M. "Stability of vitamin B_{12} in the presence of ascorbic acid." *Am. J. Clin. Nutr.* **29**, 645 (1976).

22. Hozova, B. and Sorman L. "Microbiological determination of vitamin B_{12} in heat-treated foods." *Prumsyl Potravin* **29**, 496 (1978). [*Food Sci. Tech. Abstr.* **11**, S1799 (1979).]

23. Yamaguchi, K. and Hayashi, J. "Effects of various cooking methods on vitamin B_{12}—2. Influence of heating procedures (2)." *Japanese J. Nutr.* **31**, 26 (1973).

24. Grasbeck, R. and Salonen, E. -M. "Vitamin B_{12}." *Prog. Food Sci. Nutr.* **2**, 193 (1976).

25. Bennink, M. R. and Ono, K. "Vitamin B_{12}, E and D content of raw and cooked beef." *J. Food Sci.* **47**, 1786 (1982).

26. Herbert, V., Drivas, G., Foscaldi, R., Manusselis, C., Colman, N., Kanazawa, S., Das, K., Gelernt, M., Herzlich, B., and Jennings, J. "Multivitamin/mineral food supplements containing vitamin B_{12} may also contain analogues of vitamin B_{12}." *New Engl. J. Med.* **307**, 255 (1982).

27. Duca, A. and Diaburici, M. "Voltammetric behavior of some derivatives of vitamin B_{12}." *Bule. Inst. Politch. Iasi* **23**, (Sect. 2) 1 (1977). [*Anal. Abstr.* **35**, 4E30 (1978).]

28. Youssefi, M. and Birke, R. L. "Determination of sulfide and thiols in the presence of vitamin B_{12a} by pulse polarography." *Anal. Chem.* **49**, 1380 (1977).

29. Diehl, H., Sealock, R. R., and Morrison, J. I. "The polarography of vitamin B_{12}." *Iowa State Coll., J. Sci.* **24**, 433 (1950).

30. Kazakevich, I. and Vecher, A. S. "Identification of certain cobalamins and quantitative determination of cyanocobalamin by thin-layer chromatographic methods." *Vesti Akad. Navuk BSSR, Ser. Viyal. Navuk* **22** (1977). [*Anal. Abstr.* **34**, 3D197 (1978).]

31. Thielemann, H. "Limits of identification of cyanocobalamin on various sorption layers." *Sci. Pharm.* **45**, 315 (1977).

32. Chiang, H. C., Lin, Y., and Wu, Y. C. "Polyamide-silica gel thin-layer chromatography of water soluble vitamins." *J. Chromatogr.* **45**, 161 (1969).

33. Thielemann, H. "Thin-layer chromatographic separation and identification of constituents of the multivitamin preparation Summavit 10." *Pharmazie* **35**, 125 (1980).

34. Castro, A., Cid, A., Buschbaum, P. A., and Clark, L. "New radioassay for serum vitamin B_{12} determination using chicken serum as binder and anion-exchange-resin column separation." *Res. Commun. Chem. Pathol. Pharmacol.* **24**, 583 (1979).

35. Bacher, F. A., Boley, A. E., and Shonk, C. E. "Radioactive tracer assay for vitamin B_{12} and other cobalamins in complex mixtures." *Anal. Chem.* **26**, 1146 (1954).

36. Whitlock, L. L., Melton, J. R., and Billings, T. J. "Determination of vitamin B_{12} in dry feeds by atomic absorption spectophotometry." *J. Assoc. Off. Anal. Chem.* **59**, 580 (1976).

37. Chanda, R. and Dey, N. K. "Spectrophotometric assay of cyanocobalamin and adulterant in thiamine plus pyridoxine plus cyanocobalamin injectable preparations." *J. Inst. Chem.* (India) **51**, 21 (1979).

38. Hattori, T., Asakawa, N., Ueyama, M., Shinoda, A., and Miyake, Y. "Deparation of vitamin B_{12} analogues by high-pressure liquid chromatography." *Yakugaku Zasshi* **100**, 386 (1980). [*Anal. Abstr.* **39**, 6D255 (1980).]

39. Mowot, D., Delepone, B., Boisseau, J., and Gayot, G. "Total separation of cobalamins and of coenzyme B_{12} by high-pressure liquid chromatrography." *Ann. Pharm. Fr.* **37**, 235 (1979). [*Anal. Abstr.* **38**, 4E41 (1980).]

40. Pellerin, F., Letavernier, J. F., and Chanon, N. "Identification of cobalamins by high-pressure liquid chromatography." *Ann. Pharm. Fr.* **35**, 9 (1977). [*Anal. Abstr.* **34**, 6D191 (1978).]

41. Shugart, L. "Identification of fluorescent derivatives of adenosylmethionine and related analogues with high-pressure liquid chromatography." *J. Chromatogr.* **174**, 250 (1979).

42. Association of Official Analytical Chemists. *Official Methods of Analysis*, 13th ed. Washington, D.C., 761 (1980).

43. *The United States Pharmacopeia*, 19th ed. U.S. Mack Printing, Easton, Penn., 613 (1975).

44. Analytical Methods Committee. "The estimation of vitamin B$_{12}$." *Analyst* **81**, 132 (1956).

45. Voigt, M. N. and Eitenmiller, R. R. "Comparative review of the thiochrome, microbial and protozoan analyses of B-vitamins." *J. Food Protection* **41**, 730 (1978).

46. Shaw, W. H. C. and Bissell, C. J. "The determination of vitamin B$_{12}$. A critical review." *Analyst* **85**, 389 (1960).

47. Lichtenstein, H., Beloian, A., and Reynolds, H. "Comparative vitamin B$_{12}$ assay of foods of animal origin by *Lactobacillus leichmannii* and *Ochromonas malhamensis*." *J. Agri. Food Chem.* **7**, 771 (1959).

48. Adams, J. F., McEwan, F., and Wilson, A. "The vitamin B$_{12}$ content of meals and items of diet." *Brit. J. Nutr.* **29**, 65 (1973).

49. Lau, K. S., Gottlieb, C., Wasserman, L. R., and Herbert, V. "Measurement of serum vitamin B$_{12}$ level using radioisotope dilution and coated charcoal." *Blood* **26**, 202 (1965).

50. Richardson, P. J., Favell, D. J., Gridley, G. C., and Jones, G. H. "Application of a commercial radioassay test kit to the determination of vitamin B$_{12}$ in food." *Analyst* **103**, 865 (1978).

51. Casey, P. J., Speckman, K. R., Ebert, F. J., and Hobbs., W. E. "Radioisotope dilution technique for determination of vitamin B$_{12}$ in foods." *J. Assoc. Off. Anal. Chem.* **65**, 85 (1982).

52. Beck, R. A. "Comparison of two radioassay methods for cyanocobalamin in seafoods." *J. Food Sci.* **44**, 1077 (1979).

53. Skeggs, H. R. "Vitamin B$_{12}$." In P. Gyorgy and R. S. Harris, Eds., *The Vitamins*, Vol. 7, 2nd ed. Academic Press, New York, 277–302 (1967).

54. Shenoy, K. G. and Ramasarma, G. D. "Extraction procedure and determination of the vitamin B$_{12}$ content of some animal livers." *Arch. Biochem. Biophys.* **51**, 374 (1954).

55. Voigt, M. N., Eitenmiller, R. R., and Ware, G. O. "Comparison of protozoan and conventional methods of vitamin analysis." *J. Food Sci.* **44**, 729 (1979).

20 Vitamin B_{12} and Folacin Radioassays in Blood Serum

Victor Herbert and Neville Colman

GENERAL CONSIDERATIONS

Isotope-dilution assays are methods used for quantitative measurement of a specific component in a mixture. There are several types of isotope-dilution methods (1,2), but all require separation of a portion of that component in a pure state, and eliminate the need for complete quantitative recovery of the compound. In such an assay, a known quantity of a radioactively labeled pure form of a compound with a measured initial specific activity is added to a sample containing an unknown quantity of the same component in unlabeled form. After the addition, some portion of the pure compound can be isolated from the mixture and the unknown quantity is determined from the amount of dilution of the specific activity of the labeled form. For this procedure, only the initial and final specific activities and the weight of the labeled pure form added are needed.

A variant of isotope-dilution assay which does not require chemical purification has been termed "competitive inhibition assay," "saturation analysis," "radioassay," and when limited to antigen-antibody reactions, "radioimmunoassay," which is a subset of radioassays. This method, in which quantitative assay of an unknown amount of chemical was made by using dilution of the

515

unknown quantity with a known quantity of the same chemical, was first used by Landsteiner (3). In his system, colorless antigen (unknown) was mixed with yellow antigen (labeled known), a portion of the mixture was precipitated with a small known quantity of antibody capable of binding only a fraction of the antigen present, and the amount of color remaining in the supernatant was compared with a control consisting of the colored antigen only. This concept was applied by Herbert (4) to the radioassay of vitamin B_{12}, and Yalow and Berson (5) applied it to the first radioimmunoassay, that of insulin. For this elegant work, Yalow received half the 1977 Nobel Prize in Medicine (Berson having unfortunately died several years before the award), with the other half being shared by Shally and Guillemin. From these studies, and subsequent ones, it is clear that radioisotope-dilution assays for any agent can be developed whenever the following conditions are met: [1] the agent to be measured is available in isotopic or other labeled form and the specific activity of this agent is known; [2] a binder exists with a reproducible capacity to bind the agent and can be uniformly distributed through mixing, and [3] a method is available for separating the free from the bound agent after achieving equilibrium. It is assumed that tracer, agent to be measured, and binder behave the same chemically during the assay of both the unknowns and the controls. The separation can be carried out in any number of ways, including column and paper chromatography, ultrafiltration, paper electrophoresis, exhaustive dialysis, and precipitation. The simplest procedure is so-called "instant dialysis" with coated charcoal. Assays using this technique have been developed for vitamin B_{12} (6) and folic acid (7), and both vitamins can be simultaneously radioassayed (8–10).

A competitive inhibition radioassay measures numbers of molecules only when the unknowns and tracer are identical in affinity for the binder; they all measure the relative affinity of a large mixture of unknown ligands and known radioactive tracer for a small number of binding sites. Hydroxocobalamin or folate triglutamate, or other molecules with high binding affinity in the unknown solution, may "read" the same as two or more molecules of the competing lower binding affinity tracer cyanocobalamin or pteroylglutamic acid (11,12) because of preferential uptake. Results recorded as quantities of cyanocobalamin or folate really mean "the unknown contains competitive binding affinity equal to that of such-and-such a number of tracer cyanocobalamin or pteroylglutamic acid molecules."

Special Considerations for Vitamin B₁₂ Radioassays

Serum "vitamin B_{12}" consists of the sum of "true B_{12}" (i.e., hydroxocobalamin and other cobalamins biologically active for humans), designated B_{12} in Figure 20.1, plus the serum content of other corrinoids (i.e., molecules that have the heme-like corrin nucleus of cobalamin, but differ from cobalamin in part of the rest of their structure), designated A (analogs) (13–19). Pure intrinsic factor (IF) binds only cobalamins, whereas R-binders bind all corrinoids (cobalamin + analogs) (18). The R-binders are the rapid-electrophoretic-mobility B_{12} binders ubiquitous in body fluids, including saliva, serum, cerebrospinal fluid, bile, and

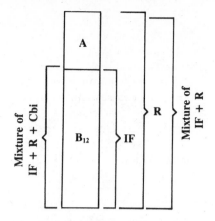

A = Analogues (i.e., cobalamins plus
    all other corrinoids)

B_{12} = Cobalamins (biologically active B_{12})

Cbi = Cobinamide (a corrinoid)

IF = Intrinsic factor

R = R-binders

FIGURE 20.1 Schematic depiction of binding of corrinoids to intrinsic factor (IF) and R-binder.

urine. The IF apparently binds to both ends of the cobalamin molecule, whereas R appears to attach only to the corrin end. The brackets in Figure 20.1 identify the portion of total serum corrinoids bound by different commercially available B_{12} radioassay binders. The mixture (IF + R + X Cbi) binds more than just true B_{12} and therefore more of the total corrinoid than pure IF does when the amount (X) of pre-added cobinamide exceeds the cobalamin-binding capacity of the mixture by about 100-fold. If the excess reaches 1000-fold, there will be some binding of analogs to IF despite its specificity for cobalamins, and the mixture will therefore bind a little less of the true B_{12}. Because of the specificity of the IF portion for cobalamin, the mixture (IF + R) may bind somewhat less than the amount of total corrinoids that are bound by R alone.

Kolhouse and colleagues (13) suggested the use of intrinsic factor concentrates (which are impure intrinsic factor contaminated with R-binder), with the binder blocked by preincubation with analog (such as cobinamide) as an alternative to using pure intrinsic factor. This is satisfactory, but such preparations can yield a little higher results for true cobalamin than with pure intrinsic factor, depending on the amount of blocker added, just as results for total corrinoids with un-blocked impure intrinsic factor are a little lower than those with pure R-binder.

Any binder may be selected for serum B_{12} radioassays, if the following guide-lines are used: (1) know what binder is being used; (2) report to the clinician what is being measured (e.g., cobalamin or cobalamin plus analogs) and what binder was used; (3) enjoin the clinician that if the laboratory result disagrees with clinical judgment, clinical judgment should be followed; (4) do other studies, such as the dU suppression test, *vide infra*, and repeat the B_{12} assay by another method (20) when the laboratory and clinic conflict.

Confusion arises when results reported as "serum vitamin B$_{12}$ levels" are actually serum total corrinoid levels rather than serum cobalamins, but the normal range given with the report is for cobalamins, rather than total corrinoids (13,16,19). For maximum reliability, each laboratory should develop its own normal range for whatever "serum B$_{12}$" assay(s) it uses; the range of normal determined in a different laboratory should not be used because minor variations in methodology, such as pH (21,22), may produce major differences in the test results. As vitamin B$_{12}$ deficiency develops, both total corrinoids and cobalamin levels fall. The noncobalamin corrinoid component of the total corrinoids stays the same or falls (21,24), except in conditions such as liver disease (21,22).

Measurement of serum total corrinoids appears to be as reliable a test as is the measurement of cobalamin alone (16,17,21–23), because the rank order within each test is generally unchanged. False results may be obtained with either test under certain conditions (4,13,16,25,26). In general, vitamin B$_{12}$ deficiency should be suspected when the level is < 250 pg total corrinoids/mL serum or < 150 pg cobalamin/mL serum, but the particular levels differ in various laboratories. For example, R-binder may measure less noncobalamin corrinoids at pH 2 than at pH 9.3 (22), so the lower limit of normal may be 200 at pH 2, but 250 at pH 9. The serum B$_{12}$ assay developed by Lau et al. (27) provides a reliable measure of vitamin B$_{12}$ deficiency. Other workers also have noted that the sum of true cobalamin plus analogs falls as B$_{12}$ deficiency develops. Using the R-binder in the serum radioassay for total corrinoids, values below a cutoff point of 250 pg/mL serum suggest B$_{12}$ deficiency, while there is a lower cutoff point (approximately 150 pg/mL) in the assay with IF (14,23,28).

Reports that radioassays using R-binder give "erroneously normal results" in patients with vitamin B$_{12}$ deficiency usually are due to setting the cutoff point for suspected deficiency too low. Thus, if a laboratory is measuring total corrinoids by radioassay using R-binder, and arbitrarily sets the lower limit of normal at 200 pg/mL whereas their methodology actually produces a higher normal limit of 250–300 pg/mL, some patients with vitamin B$_{12}$ deficiency and total serum corrinoids of 200–300 pg/mL might erroneously be diagnosed as not B$_{12}$ deficient (16). The general rule, since the first microbiological assay of serum vitamin B$_{12}$ three decades ago, remains valid: If there is megaloblastosis and some damage to myelin, the patient has vitamin B$_{12}$ deficiency and should be treated with vitamin B$_{12}$ regardless of what the serum B$_{12}$ results may be.

Blood serum may contain analogs derived from eating animal products raised on feed supplemented with vitamins and minerals that were capable of damaging the B$_{12}$ molecule (29). Using pure IF as cobalamin binder and salivary R as total corrinoid binder, such analogs were found in multivitamin/mineral supplements taken daily by about 100 million Americans (30–32). Nutrients that have been known since the 1950s to be capable of damaging vitamin B$_{12}$ when present in large amounts include thiamin and nicotinamide, vitamin C and copper, vitamin E, and iron, although, when present in smaller amounts, iron and copper may be protective (33–35). Vitamin B$_{12}$ is protected against destruction in the oxidized (Co^{3+}) state, is more easily destroyed in the reduced state (Co^{+}), and is protected against destruction by agents such as cyanide and dithiothreitol (33–35).

If the patient has a myeloproliferative disorder or liver disease, the serum B_{12} level may be normal by any assay, despite severe tissue B_{12} deficiency (21). In such instances, where serum B_{12} levels do not reflect low tissue vitamin status because of abnormalities in serum-binding proteins or antibodies, the dU suppression test will accurately measure tissue status (36).

In the presence of liver disease or myeloproliferative disorders, large quantities of B_{12}-binding proteins may be released into the serum (37,39). These proteins may bind vitamin B_{12} irreversibly, resulting in a normal (or elevated) serum vitamin B_{12} level, despite tissue depletion and biochemical deficiency of the vitamin (39).

During the progress of pregnancy, the serum vitamin B_{12} level tends to fall and serum vitamin B_{12}-binding capacity tends to rise (37). This phenomenon appears to be physiologically analogous to the fall in serum iron and rise in iron-binding capacity in pregnancy.

Recent work suggests that microbiological assays using *Lactobacillus leichmannii* (40) or *Euglena gracilis* (40 a) to measure vitamin B_{12} may give erroneously high values for pharmaceutical products, because the microorganisms grow on B_{12} analogs that are not cobalamins. High-performance liquid chromatography confirms that more than 98% of the microbiological assayable "vitamin B_{12}" is not the true vitamin, but noncobalamin corrinoids recognized by differential radioassays (i.e., radioassays that use either IF binder which identifies only cobalamins, or R-binders for total corrinoids). The differential radioassays, therefore, separate true cobalamins from noncobalamin corrinoids, whereas microbiological assays cannot distinguish some of these compounds.

METHODS AVAILABLE

Because "vitamin B_{12}" in serum is attached to a binding protein, the first step in assay of the vitamin is to free it from its binder. One way to do so is to heat it in 0.25 N HCl for 15 min at 100°C; another way is to raise the pH to approximately 13 (27,39,41–43). Such high pH can destroy the binder unless carried out for only a few seconds (44), although Gräsbeck et al. (45), the first to dissociate B_{12} from binders by using high pH, were able to preserve binder in the system. The free "vitamin B_{12}" is then mixed with a known amount of radioactive vitamin B_{12}. The mixture is combined with a binder (or carrier) of a known fixed maximal capacity to bind approximately two-thirds of the amount of radioactive "B_{12}" previously added to the unknown sample. This is shown in Figure 20.2 where National Formulary Intrinsic Factor (NFIF) was used. NFIF is a mixture of IF and R, and therefore measures total corrinoids. The carrier will "biopsy" the pool of mixed radioactive and nonradioactive B_{12} (Figure 20.2) by taking out a piece of that pool equal to the binding capacity of the carrier. It is necessary that the binding be reproducible from tube to tube. Once some B_{12} is attached to the carrier, it yields a complex with a molecular weight greatly in excess of B_{12} alone and some free B_{12}. The free and bound B_{12} can be separated by any modality capable of separating large molecules from small.

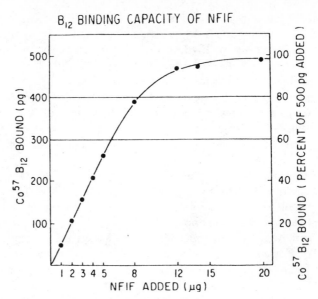

FIGURE 20.2 Typical binding curve for National Formulary Intrinsic Factor concentrate (NFIF) with ^{57}Co-B$_{12}$.

Separation may be carried out by any of many different modalities, ranging from precipitation to dialysis, through DEAE to solid-phase separating columns, or glass beads to which intrinsic factor is covalently bound (46–51). Batch separation with coated charcoal has been found to be simple and reproducible (27,52). The coated charcoal concept is shown in Figure 20.3. Solid-phase systems with irreversibly attached B$_{12}$ binders are also simple and reproducible with controls for the possibility that B$_{12}$ can attach to nonspecific binding sites on the solid phase or in the solution and go undetected (52,54). In a recent comparison of pure intrinsic factor assay for B$_{12}$ in serum using coated charcoal versus glass beads, we found glass beads gave unsatisfactorily higher results (25).

Another alternative to separating free from bound radioactive ligand (when the ligand emits low-energy photons) is the use of radiation-absorbing particles, such as tungsten powder or bismuth oxide, bound to the particles of coated charcoal or bound to an antibody in a double-antibody assay (55). The bismuth absorbs (attenuates) the radiation from the free or antibody-bound radioligand, making it unnecessary to separate physically free from bound, since now only that portion of the radioligand not bound to bismuth-charcoal or bismuth-antibody is measurable. This technique was designated internal sample attenuator counting (ISAC) by its developer; it eliminates both centrifugation and removal of supernatant (55).

Although it has not been found to be necessary to use either cyanide or albumin to stabilize assays, others have found these additions desirable (56,57). Workers who have attempted to set up radioassay for vitamin B$_{12}$ from the

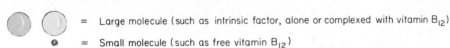

= Large molecule (such as intrinsic factor, alone or complexed with vitamin B_{12})

= Small molecule (such as free vitamin B_{12})

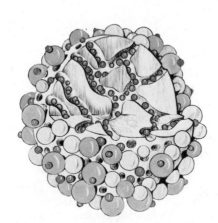

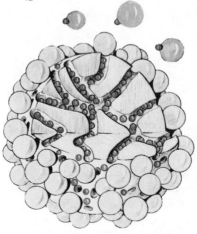

Uncoated charcoal particle adsorbs large and small molecules on its surface. Molecules small enough to get thru its pores are adsorbed on the walls of its channels.

Charcoal particle pre-saturated with large molecules can only adsorb small molecules. (They go thru its pores and are adsorbed on the walls of its channels.)

Charcoal non-specifically adsorbs many large and small molecules. Large molecules (such as intrinsic factor and serum proteins) cannot get into charcoal particle channels thru small pores, and thus are adsorbed only on outer surface and walls of larger channels.

FIGURE 20.3   The coated-charcoal absorption concept.

literature alone have often experienced difficulty; such difficulty usually is overcome after a visit to any laboratory successfully doing these assays by any of the many modifications of the basic methodology.

Many good commercial kits are now available for determination of serum "B_{12}" by radioassay. Some kits are labeled as "vitamin B_{12}" when in fact they assay total corrinoids (the sum of vitamin B_{12} and B_{12} analogs in serum). Other kits assay cobalamin (vitamin B_{12}) alone. The best kits are those that contain the necessary reagents to offer the customer the option of assaying cobalamin alone or total corrinoids, or both. The National Council on Clinical Laboratory Standards (NCCLS) has provided guidelines for evaluating B_{12} (cobalamin) assays (58). It has been noted that no-boil assays may have problems related to interference from high levels of endogenous cobalamin-binding protein in the serum of patients with myeloproliferature disorders or anti-intrinsic factor antibodies in serum (15,53,54). However, these are not problems in no-boil assays that do not use intrinsic factor or other exogenous binders (54).

Folate radioassays are reviewed by Gregory in Chapter 18. The principles and methodology are similar to those described for vitamin B$_{12}$. The radioassay for folacin has been used most successfully for determination of blood folates, and less successfully for other tissue extracts and foods. A number of commercial kits are available for folacin radioassays.

ANALYTICAL METHODOLOGY

I. VITAMIN B$_{12}$ RADIOASSAY

A. Principle

The determination of vitamin B$_{12}$ by radioassay is a competitive inhibition assay based on the isotope-dilution principle, in which the binder used is impure hog intrinsic factor concentrate containing R binder. Hemoglobin-coated charcoal is used to separate free and bound B$_{12}$ as described by Lau et al. (27). As for any serum B$_{12}$ array, the mean and standard deviation for normal subjects should be determined after log transformation, to correct for skewness of raw data toward higher values.

B. Reagents

1. *Hemoglobin Solution.*
    (a) Wash discarded human red blood cells twice with 0.9% saline.
    (b) Hemolyze cells with an equal volume of H$_2$O, followed by adding one-half volume of toluene.
    (c) Shake mixture vigorously for 5 min, then centrifuge 15 min at 3000 rpm.
    (d) Discard the two top layers, consisting of toluene and cell debris, and pass the bottom layer, which is the hemoglobin, through Whatman No. 1 filter paper to yield a clear red filtrate.
    (e) Determine the hemoglobin content of the filtrate in the conventional manner and adjust the hemoglobin concentration with H$_2$O to 10 g/100 mL (6).
2. *Hemoglobin-Coated Charcoal.*
    (a) Add 5 g Norit A to a flask containing 100 mL H$_2$O.
    (b) To another flask, add 0.25 g hemoglobin solution and H$_2$O to a final volume of 100 mL.
    (c) Pour the hemoglobin into the charcoal solution and swirl for 10 sec.
        (1) The preferred charcoal coat for vitamin B$_{12}$ radioassay is hemoglobin. However, albumin or dextran may also be used (27).
        (2) Uncoated charcoal may be effective when small amounts are used relative to the amount of plasma, because the plasma proteins coat the

charcoal. As a rule, charcoal is fully coated when the weight of the protein exceeds 10% of the weight of the charcoal (50).

3. *National Formulary Intrinsic Factor (NFIF) Binder.* (Hog intrinsic factor concentrate containing R binder.)

(a) Prepare a stock solution of 100 mg NFIF in 100 mL 0.9% saline. This may be stored at $-20°C$ for up to 1 year.

(b) Bring 1 mL stock solution to 100 mL with saline for the working solution. This solution may be stored frozen or at 5°C.

(1) This solution has a binding capacity of approximately 800 pg vitamin B_{12}/mL. The binding capacity of the NFIF solution should be determined prior to use.

(2) Other binders, including saliva, serum from patients with chronic myelogenous leukemia, and chicken serum have been used (59–63). Regardless of what binder is used, its capacity to bind B_{12} should be determined.

4. *Vitamin B_{12} Standard.* Dilute cyanocobalamin standard to a concentration of 1 μg/mL.

5. *^{57}Co Vitamin B_{12}.* Dilute ^{57}Co vitamin B_{12} to 1 μg/mL. Standardization of $^{57}Co\ B_{12}$ is done by adding equal amounts of radioactive and unlabeled forms and measuring the fall in binding capacity of NFIF. A 50% fall should be observed if concentrations are equal. The quantity needed to bind about 60% of the radioactive B_{12} is then known (27).

C. Procedure

1. *Binding Curve for NFIF.*

(a) Set up a series of test tubes in duplicate.

(b) Put no binder in the first, one unit of binder (e.g., 0.5 mL) in the second, two units of binder in the third, and so on until there is a series of 10–15 tubes with sequentially increasing amounts of binder.

(c) Add an identical amount of $^{57}Co\ B_{12}$ to each tube. For blood serum assays, 500 pg falls in the middle of the normal range, and so that amount should be used.

(d) Briefly agitate the tubes and incubate them for 30 min at room temperature or 37°C, so that association of B_{12} and IF goes to completion.

(e) Separate free vitamin from bound using 2.0 mL coated charcoal and count the radioactivity in the supernatant or in the precipitate using a scintillation counter.

(f) From the data, construct a curve (Figure 20.4). On the curve, determine the point where it begins to break (represented by the upper horizontal line). Move downward from that break point approximately one-quarter to one-third of the way down toward the baseline (represented by the lower horizontal line). This point represents the standard amount of that particular batch of binder which may be used.

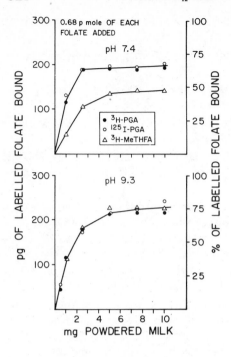

FIGURE 20.4 Milk binding curves for [^{3}H]+PGS, [^{125}I]+PGS, and [^{3}H]+MeTHFA at pH 7.4 and 9.3.

(1) The binder stock solution may be dispensed in tubes in quantities sufficient for 1 day's assays and frozen at −20°C. For each assay, thaw one tube; discard any binder not used that day. Repeated thawing and freezing decrease the binding capacity.

2. *The Protocol For the Radioassay Is Shown In Table 20.1.* All assays are run in duplicate.

TABLE 20.1   Assay Protocol for Vitamin B$_{12}$ in Serum

				Sequence of Addition			
Sample	0.9% Saline (mL)	Unknown Serum (mL)	0.25N HCl (mL)	^{57}Co B$_{12}$ (1 μg/mL) (mL)	NFIF (mL)	0.9% Saline (mL)	Coated Charcoal (mL)
Unknown Serum	1.5	0.5	0.5	0.5	0.5	0	2.0
Supernatant control (serum)^a	1.5	0.5	0.5	0.5	0	0.5	2.0
NFIF control^b	2.0	0	0.5	0.5	0.5	0	2.0
Supernatant control (NFIF)^a	2.0	0	0.5	0.5	0	0.5	2.0

^{a}The supernatant controls should contain less than 1% of the added radioactivity since the ^{57}Co B$_{12}$ is not bound by the NFIF and is adsorbed on the charcoal.

^{b}The ^{57}Co B$_{12}$ binding capacity of the NFIF can be checked with this sample.

(a) Set up a series of 10-mL test tubes.

(b) Add 0.5 mL unknown serum to 1.5 mL 0.9% saline for unknown serum and serum supernatant control tubes. The tubes for NFIF control and NFIF supernatant control contain 2.0 mL saline.

(c) Add 0.5 mL 0.25 N HCl to each tube.

(d) Cap tubes with cotton wool, and heat in a boiling water bath for 15 min and then cool with tap water.

(e) Add 0.5 mL ^{57}Co B$_{12}$ to each tube and mix for 10 sec.

(f) Add 0.5 mL NFIF to unknown serum and NFIF control, and 0.5 mL saline to the supernatant control.

(g) Mix contents thoroughly, and add 2 mL coated charcoal.

(h) Centrifuge tubes at 3000 rpm for 15 min and decant supernatant into counting tubes.

D. Calculation

Subtract the counts per minute (cpm) for the supernatant controls (serum and NFIF) from the unknown and NFIF tubes, respectively, to obtain net counts. Calculate the serum B$_{12}$ levels from the following formula:

$$\text{pg B}_{12}/\text{mL serum} = \frac{1}{n} \times \text{pg } ^{57}\text{Co B}_{12} \left[\frac{B}{B^1} - 1 \right]$$

where n = mL of serum assayed;
$\quad\quad\quad B$ = net cpm of NFIF control;
$\quad\quad\quad B^1$ = net cpm of unknown serum.

II. FOLACIN RADIOASSAY

A. Principle

The determination of folacin by a radiometric assay is based on the isotope-dilution principle and is a competitive binding radioassay using liquid or dry skim milk as binder (64, 65). Its use has been reported by numerous workers and is described in detail by Longo and Herbert (7). The application to food samples is given by Gregory on page 488.

B. Reagents

1. *0.05 M Lysine Hydrochloride–Gelatin–Sodium Azide Buffer (pH 9.3)*. Dissolve 4.54 g L-lysine HCl, 500 mg sodium azide, and 500 mg gelatin in 450 mL H$_2$O. Heat to 70–80°C in a boiling water bath to dissolve the gelatin. Cool to room temperature and adjust pH to 9.3 with 6 N NaOH, and dilute to a final

volume of 500 mL with H$_2$O. Store refrigerated at 4°C, and bring to room temperature before use. This is stable for 2 months.

(a) Since pH is critical and must be 9.3 $\pm$ 0.05, it should be checked and adjusted just prior to each assay.

(b) This buffer differs from the pH 9.3 buffer in the assay of Givas and Gutcho (8,9) in that it does not contain ascorbate, which is necessary only if samples are to be heated. In this situation, add 2.5 g sodium ascorbate prior to adjustment of pH to 9.3.

(c) Addition of serum should not change the pH of the buffer.

2. *Pteroylglutamic Acid (PGA) Standards.* Prepare a 100 μg/mL PGA solution by weighing 10 mg crystalline PGA into a folate-free 100-mL beaker; add approximately 20 mL 0.1 M NaOH to dissolve PGA. Adjust pH to 7 with 0.1 M HCl. Quantitatively transfer solution to a 100-mL volumetric flask and bring to volume with H$_2$O. This solution can be frozen at -20°C in small aliquots in aluminum foil-covered test tubes, and is stable for months. Prior to an assay, thaw, remove aliquot for standard, and refreeze remainder. Prepare working standards containing 1, 2, 5, 10, and 20 ng PGA/mL by making serial dilutions of the 100 μg/mL standard with lysine buffer (Reagent 1).

(a) Dilute 50 μL PGA standard (100 μg/mL) to 5 mL. Dilute 100 μL of 1 μg/mL solution to 5 mL with lysine buffer (Reagent 1) to give 20 ng/mL. Dilute 2 mL of 20 ng/mL to 4 mL to give 10 ng/mL, and so on.

(b) An intermediate standard containing 100 ng/ml can be prepared by diluting 100 μL of the 100 μg/mL standard to 100 mL. Prepare working standards by diluting 0.1, 0.2, 0.5, 1.0, and 2.0 mL of the intermediate solution (100 ng/mL) to 10 mL with the lysine buffer (Reagent 1).

(c) An intermediate standard containing 10 ng/mL can be prepared by diluting 10 μL of the 100 μg/mL standard to 100 mL. Appropriate aliquots can be taken to provide directly the amounts of PGA needed for the standard curve.

(d) The diluted working standards are stable for over 1 month if kept at 4°C in aluminum foil wrapped tubes or brown bottles to protect from light.

(e) Each time new standards are prepared, a standard curve should be run parallel with old standards for comparison.

(f) The purity of the PGA can be monitored by paper and thin-layer chromatography (63).

3. *Radioactive Labeled PGA.* Either [^{3}H]PGA or [^{125}I]PGA can be used.

(a) [^{3}H]PGA (Tritiated PGA). Dilute liquid or powdered [^{3}H]PGA (33mCi/μmole, or similar specific activity, Becton Dickinson Immunodiagnostics or Amersham/Searle) with lysine buffer (Reagent 1) to a concentration of 2 to 4 ng [^{3}H]PGA/mL (0.2–0.4 ng/100 μL).

(1) If 100 μL of this solution gives more than 6000–8000 cpm, unlabeled PGA may be used to decrease the specific activity.

(2) [^{3}H]PGA is stable for months if stored at -20°C. The working

dilutions can be kept at 4°C in small brown bottles or foil-wrapped tubes and are stable for months.

(b) [^{125}I]PGA (Monoiodinated monotyramide of PGA). Dilute the stock [^{125}I]PGA solution (Diagnostic Biochemistry or Smith Kline Instruments), which generally contains 1 μCi/mL in 2-mercaptoethanol, 1:5 to 1:10 with lysine buffer (Reagent 1).

(1) The diluted [^{125}I]PGA yields 5500–8000 cpm in a gamma counter (Packard Autogamma Scintillation Spectrometer). The supernate control varies from 450–1500 cpm.

(2) The undiluted [^{125}I]PGA is stable at −20°C for weeks. The dilutions should be prepared for the day's work from the original material as received, since this isotope is not as stable in dilution as the [^{3}H]PGA.

(3) About 0.01–0.02 μCi [^{125}I]PGA binds to milk at pH 9.3 as though it contains 0.2–0.4 ng PGA. The amount of [^{125}I]PGA equivalent to 0.2–0.4 ng PGA is determined by one of the following methods.

(i) Using [^{3}H]PGA. Construct a milk-binding curve (see Procedure and Figure 20.4) at pH 9.3 using 0.3 ng [^{3}H]PGA in a 100 μL volume. The quantity of milk that binds approximately 50% of the tracer can be determined from this curve. Prepare a series of three test tubes containing this amount of milk (100 μL volume). Incubate with 100 μL [^{125}I]PGA in three different arbitrary dilutions (1:5, 1:7.5, 1:10). The tube which has approximately 50% of its charcoal adsorbable radioactivity bound is assumed to contain the equivalent of 0.3 ng PGA and is the quantity of [^{125}I]PGA then used in the radioassay.

(ii) Using [^{125}I]PGA. Determine the degree of degradation as described in (4), below. If the net counts of undegraded [^{125}I]PGA are at least 6000 cpm, construct a milk binding curve as for [^{3}H]PGA (see Procedure and Figure 20.4). The quantity of milk that binds approximately 50% of the undegraded [^{125}I]PGA is then used in the radioassay.

If it is desired, the amount of PGA present in the undegraded [^{125}I]PGA can be determined by constructing a standard curve on logit-log paper, using five concentrations of unlabeled PGA premixed with the [^{125}I]PGA. The quantity of radioactive PGA is presumed to be equal to the quantity of nonradioactive PGA which inhibits 50% of the binding of radioactive PGA to milk. This is based on the assumption that the radioactive and nonradioactive PGA bind equally to the milk.

The standard curve with [^{125}I]PGA should have a slope such that the values in the range of 1–5 ng folate/mL serum can be easily discerned. This requires that not more than 95% of trace binding occur with 50 μL of the 1 ng/mL PGA standard. These requirements are met when the radioactive PGA contains less than 400 pg PGA/100 μL. The absolute quantity of [^{125}I]PGA is not important if these conditions are met.

TABLE 20.2   Assay Protocol for Folacin in Serum

Sample (Tube Number)	Lysine Butter (mL)	Standard or Unknown (50 µL)	Radioisotope (µL)	Milk Binder (µL)	Coated Charcoal (mL)
			Sequence of Addition		
Total radioactive folate (1,2)	1.4	0	100	0	0
Supernate control (3,4)	1	0		0	0.4
Standard curve (5,6)	0.9	0		100	
(7,8)	0.8	1 ng PGA/mL			
(9,10)		2 ng PGA/mL			
(11,12)		5 ng PGA/mL			
(13,14)		10 ng PGA/mL			
(15,16)		20 ng PGA/mL			
Unknown serum (17,18)		50 µL serum			
Unknown hemolysate (19,20)		50 µL hemolysate (1:20 dilution)			

(4) Determine the radioactivity of 100 µL of a 1:10 dilution of each new lot of [^{125}I]PGA both before and after adsorption onto 5 mg (0.5 mL) coated charcoal at pH 9.3. The radioactivity not removed by the coated charcoal is assumed to be degraded [^{125}I]PGA (64). This degradation control is performed in each assay (supernate control, Table 20.2).

4. *Milk Binder.*   Liquid or powdered skim milk can be used as binder, although the folate-binding capacity of instant milk powder may be less reliably reproducible from batch to batch than that of liquid skim milk (65). The milk binder in liquid skim milk is stable for about 1 month when stored at 4°C, when purchased within 1 week of pasteurization. One-half pint will last for as many assays as can be done in 1 month. Binders prepared from commercial whey proteins may also be used, but it should be noted that the folate binder is not the β-lactoglobulin fraction (66).

5. *Coated Charcoal.*   Prepare albumin-coated charcoal by mixing equal volumes of 2.5% (w/w) solution of Norit A neutral charcoal in 0.9% (w/v) saline with 1.75% (w/w) solution of salt-poor human albumin. For dextran-coated charcoal, suspend 2 g activated charcoal (e.g., Darco G-60) and 0.2 g dextran in cold H$_2$O. Prepare hemoglobin coated charcoal as described for vitamin B$_{12}$ radioassay. Any of the three charcoal adsorbents can be used and should be prepared daily.

C.   Procedure

1. *Binding Curve.*   The quantity of milk used in the assay should provide maximum binding with linear kinetics; that is, binding of PGA should be pro-

portional to binder concentration. To ascertain the level which is sufficient to bind 50–60% of the labeled PGA, construct a binding curve for each new batch of milk. Incubate a fixed amount of labeled folate (0.3 ng) for 30 min at room temperature with increasing quantities of milk (e.g., undiluted to 10-fold dilution for skim milk; 10–100 mg/mL for nonfat dry milk; 5–50 mg/mL for whey protein concentrate). Dilute the milk with lysine buffer (Reagent 1) prior to use in the assay. Follow the protocol in Table 20.2 and the procedure below for separating unbound folate and measuring radioactivity.

(a) The amount of each batch of milk binder selected should be sufficient to bind approximately 50–60% of the radioactively labeled PGA as shown in a typical binding curve (Figure 20.4) for [³H]PGA, [¹²⁵I]PGA and [³H]methyltetrahydrofolic acid (MeTHFA) at pH 9.3. The quantity chosen should be below that point on the curve where the ascending limb ceases to be a straight line.

(1) At pH 9.3, [³H]MeTHFA binds as well as [¹²⁵I]PGA and [³H]PGA, as long as relatively low levels of folate are present with increasing (but always large) amounts of binder.

(2) Although in a single batch of milk the binding stays constant for approximately a month, the milk should not be diluted to the assay concentration until immediately prior to use; any leftover milk should be discarded. This is because a "releasing factor" in bovine milk which releases folate from plasma protein is destroyed more rapidly in diluted milk at pH 9.3 (7).

2. *Assay Protocol for Determining Serum Folate Levels.*

(a) The assay protocol is given in Table 20.2.

(1) The procedure used is essentially identical to that of Gutcho and Mansbach (9) except that they used purified milk binder, and freed the serum folate from endogenous binder by heat.

(b) Number sufficient tubes (12 × 75 mm polypropylene or glass) for controls, duplicates of the standard PGA dilutions, and serum samples.

(c) Pipette 1.4 mL lysine buffer (Reagent 1) into the tubes 1 and 2, 1 mL into the next 2, 0.9 mL into the next 2, and 0.8 mL into remaining tubes.

(d) Deliver 50 μL (Eppendorf pipette) of the standards (see Reagent 2) as indicated in Table 20.2, into each standard tube. The first four tubes are controls and do not have added standard or binder.

(e) Deliver 50 μL of serum or hemolyzate into duplicate sample tubes. Assays can be carried out using 20–100 μL samples if the alteration in sample volume is compensated for by alteration in buffer volume.

(1) To eliminate possibility of plasma-binding protein in the serum, a heating step may be used at this point (8,9). In this case, heat tubes 15 min in a boiling water bath, then cool in cold water bath.

(f) With an Eppendorf pipette, deliver 100 μL of radioactive folate (containing the equivalent of 2–4 ng PGA/mL) into each tube and vortex or mix by hand.

(g) Pipette 100 µL milk binder (appropriate concentration to give 50–60% binding of tracer) into each tube, except the first four, and vortex each tube.

(h) Incubate all tubes for 30 min at room temp in the dark.

(i) Agitate the coated charcoal suspension by vortexing or with a magnetic stirrer 10 min prior to the end of the incubation. After the 30 min incubation period, pipette 0.4 mL of the well-mixed charcoal suspension into all tubes except 1 and 2, and vortex.

(1) The charcoal used may be albumin-, dextran-, or hemoglobin-coated. If hemoglobin-coated charcoal is used, add 0.5 mL.

(j) Centrifuge tubes at 1,500 $\times g$ for 10 min.

(k) When using [^{3}H]PGA, decant the supernate into liquid scintillation counting vials containing 10 mL Instagel (Packard Instruments) or other scintillation cocktail capable of solubilizing 1.5 mL aqueous samples. Vortex gently until the solution clears and count in a liquid scintillation counter (e.g., Packard or Beckman Instruments). When using [^{125}I]PGA, decant the supernate into tubes and count directly in a gamma counter.

D. Calculation

The average cpm in duplicate tubes 1 and 2 represent the total amount of radioactive folate added to each tube. Tubes 3 and 4 represent the cpm not adsorbed by coated charcoal, due mainly to degraded radioactive folate. Since this radioactivity is not available to the milk binder, it is subtracted from each tube (supernate control). Tubes 5 and 6 reflect the amount of radiofolate the milk can bind (i.e., B_0, binding of radiofolate in presence of zero unlabeled folate). This amount should be 50–60% of the total cpm minus the supernate control.

Tubes 7 to 16 are duplicates of the five concentrations of unlabeled PGA that compete with the labeled PGA for the binding sites. The greater the con-

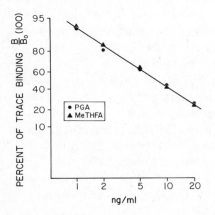

FIGURE 20.5   Standard curve for folacin radioassay.

centration of cold PGA in the standards (or samples), the greater is the competition for binding sites, and thus, the lower the number of counts bound. The number of cpm bound is B (minus the supernate control).

Draw a standard curve by plotting the percentage of B_0 cpm bound at each concentration of unlabeled PGA, i.e., B/B_0 versus concentration of standards (unlabeled PGA), on logit-log paper (1×3 cycle log-log paper). A typical standard curve is illustrated in Figure 20.5.

The folate level of a particular serum sample is determined by finding the B/B_0 of its supernate on the standard curve and interpolating to a concentration on the x axis.

LITERATURE CITED

1. Kamen, M. D. *Isotopic Tracers in Biology,* 3rd ed. Academic Press, New York, 176 (1957).

2. Overman, R. T. and Clark, H. M. *Radioisotope Techniques.* McGraw-Hill, New York (1960).

3. Landsteiner, K. *The Specificity of Serological Reactions.* Harvard University Press, Cambridge, Mass. (1945).

4. Herbert, V. "Studies on the role of intrinsic factor in vitamin B_{12} absorption, transport and storage." *Amer. J. Clin. Nutr.* **7,** 433 (1959).

5. Yalow, R. S. and Berson, S. A. "Immunoassay of endogenous plasma insulin in man." *J. Clin. Invest.* **39,** 433 (1960).

6. Lau, K.-S., Gottlieb, C., Wasserman, L. R., and Herbert, V. "Measurement of serum vitamin B_{12} level using radioisotope dilution and coated charcoal." *Blood* **26,** 202 (1965).

7. Longo, D. L. and Herbert, V. "Radioassay for serum and red cell folate." *J. Lab. Clin. Med.* **87,** 138 (1976).

8. Givas, J. and Gutcho, S. "pH dependence of the binding of folates to milk binder in radioassays of folates." *Clin. Chem.* **21,** 427 (1975).

9. Gutcho, S. and Mansbach, L. "Simultaneous radioassay of serum vitamin B_{12} and folic acid." *Clin. Chem.* **23,** 1609 (1977).

10. Jacob, E., Colman, N., and Herbert, V. "Evaluation of simultaneous radioassay for two vitamins: Folate and vitamin B_{12}." *Clin. Res.* **25,** 537A (1977).

11. Herbert, V. and Colman, N. "Hydroxocobalamin (OH-B_{12}) 'reads' higher than cyanocobalamin (CN-B_{12}) in radioassays using R binder, but not in radioassays using pure intrinsic factor (IF) as binder." *Fed. Proc.* **38,** 796 (1980).

12. Colman, N. and Herbert, V. "Cerebrospinal fluid (CSF) folate levels are much higher by radioassay than by microbiologic assay." *Clin. Res.* **28,** 491A (1980).

13. Kolhouse, J. F., Kondo, H., Allen, N. C., Podell, E., and Allen, R. H. "Cobalamin analogues are present in human plasma and can mask cobalamin deficiency because current radioisotope dilution assays are not specific for true cobalamin." *New Engl. J. Med.* **299,** 785 (1978).

14. Muir, M. and Chanarin, I. "Absorption of cobalamins from serum by intrinsic factor (IF) and B_{12}-binding protein (R) attached to polyacrylamide beads. Evidence for cobalamin analogues and their effect in a B_{12}-assay system." *Blood* **58** (Suppl. 1), 39 (1981).

15. Allen, R. H. "Clinical role and current status of serum cobalamin (vitamin B_{12}) assays." *Ligand Quart.* **4**(3), 37 (1981).

16. Herbert, V., Colman, N., Palat, D., Manusselis, C., Drivas, G., Block, E., Akerkar, A., Weaver, D., and Frenkel, E. "Is there a 'gold standard' for human serum vitamin B_{12} assay?" Submitted to *Brit. J. Haemat.*

17. Waldenlind, L., Lamminpaeae, K., and Sundblad, L. Y. "Determination of total and true cobalamin with the SimulTRAC® assay." *Scand. J. Clin. Lab. Invest.* **42**, 225 (1982).

18. Gottlieb, C. W., Retief, F. P., and Herbert, V. "Blockade of vitamin B$_{12}$-binding sites in gastric juice, serum and saliva by analogues and derivatives of vitamin B$_{12}$ and by antibody to intrinsic factor." *Biochim. Biophys. Acta.* **145,** 560 (1967).

19. Cooper, B. A. and Whitehead, V. M. "Evidence that some patients with pernicious anemia are not recognized by radiodilution assay for cobalamin in serum." *N. Engl. J. Med.* **299,** 816 (1978).

20. Donaldson, R. B., Jr. " 'Serum B$_{12}$' and the diagnosis of cobalamin deficiency." *N. Engl. J. Med.* **299,** 827 (1978).

21. Herbert, V. "B$_{12}$ and folate deficiency." In B. Rothfeld, Ed., *Nuclear Medicine in Vitro.* Lippincott, Philadelphia (1983).

22. Herbert, V., Landau, L., Bash, R., Grosberg, S., and Colman, N. "Ability of megadoses of vitamin C to destroy vitamin B$_{12}$ and cobinamide and to reduce absorption of vitamin B$_{12}$ (with a note on B$_{12}$ radioassays)." In B. Zagalak and W. Freidrich, Eds., *Vitamin B$_{12}$: Proceedings of the Third European Symposium on Vitamin B$_{12}$ and Intrinsic Factor.* Walter de Gruyter, New York, 1069 (1979).

23. Cooper, B., Frenkel, E. P., Colman, N., Herbert, V., Akerkar, A., Block, E., and Weaver, D. "Multi-laboratory evaluation of 'serum vitamin B$_{12}$ level' measured by radioassay for 'total B$_{12}$' vs. 'true cobalamin' vs. microbiologic assay with *Euglena gracilis.*" *Clin. Chem.* **25**(6), 1136 (1979).

24. Chanarin, I. and Muir, M. "Demonstration of vitamin B$_{12}$ analogues in human sera not detected by microbiologic assay." *Brit. J. Haemat.* **51,** 171 (1982).

25. Altz-Smith, M., Miller, R. K., Cornwell, P. E., Butterworth, C. E., and Herbert, V. "Low serum vitamin B$_{12}$ levels in rheumatoid arthritis." *Arthritis and Rheumatism* **25** (Suppl. 4), S116 (1982).

26. Herbert, V. and Colman, N. "Evidence humans may use some analogues of B$_{12}$ as cobalamins (B$_{12}$): Pure intrinsic factor (IF) radioassay may 'diagnose' clinical B$_{12}$ deficiency where it does not exist." *Clin. Res.* **29**(2), 571A (1981).

27. Lau, K.-S., Gottlieb, C., Wasserman, L. R., and Herbert, V. "Measurement of serum vitamin B$_{12}$ level using radioisotope dilution and coated charcoal." *Blood* **26,** 202 (1965).

28. Mollin, D. L., Hoffbrand, A. V., Ward, P. G., and Lewis, S. M. "Interlaboratory comparison of serum vitamin B$_{12}$ assay." *J. Clin. Pathol.* **33,** 243 (1980).

29. Allen, R. H. "Cobalamin (Cb1, vitamin B$_{12}$) analogues." *Proc., 18th Congr. Int. Soc. Hematol.,* Montreal, (August 16–22), 53 (1980).

30. Herbert, V., Drivas, G., Foscaldi, R., and Manusselis, C. "Are multivitamin/mineral preparations with vitamin B$_{12}$ harmless? They may degrade some B$_{12}$ to analogs." *Clin. Res.* **29**(3), 673A (1981).

31. Herbert, V., Drivas, G., Foscaldi, R., Manusselis, C., Colman, N., Kanazawa, S., Das, K., Gelernt, M., Herzlich, B., and Jennings, J. "Multivitamin/mineral food supplements containing vitamin B$_{12}$ may also contain analogues of B$_{12}$." *New Engl. J. Med.* **307,** 255 (1982).

32. Kondo, H., Binder, M. J., Kolhouse, J. F., Smythe, W. R., Podell, E. R., and Allen, R. H. "Presence and formation of cobalamin analogues in multivitamin/mineral pills." *J. Clin. Invest.* **70,** 889 (1982).

33. Pratt, J. M. *Inorganic Chemistry of Vitamin B$_{12}$.* Academic Press, New York (1972).

34. Hogenkamp, H. P. C. "The interaction between vitamin B$_{12}$ and vitamin C." *Am. J. Clin. Nutr.* **33** 1 (1980).

35. Herbert, V. "Vitamin B$_{12}$." *Am. J. Clin. Nutr.* **34,** 971 (1981).

36. Herbert, V. "NCCLS Task Force Review: Vitamin B$_{12}$ radioassay methods: The dU suppression test—What is it?" *Ligand Quart.* **2**(2), 11 (1979).

37. Jacob, E., Baker, S. J., and Herbert, V. "Vitamin B_{12}-binding proteins." *Physiol. Rev.* **60**, 918 (1980).

38. Carmel, R. "Cobalamin-binding proteins of man." *Contemporary Hematology/Oncology.* Plenum Press, New York, 79 (1981).

39. Chanarin, I. *The Megaloblastic Anemias.* Blackwell, New York (1979).

40. Herbert, V. and Drivas, G. "Spirulina and vitamin B_{12}." *J. Amer. Med. Assoc.* **248**, 3096 (1982).

40a. Herbert, V., Drivas, G., Chu, M., Levitt, D., Cooper, B.: Differential radioassays better measure cobalamin content of vitamins and "health foods" than do microbiologic assays. Some products sold to vegetarians as rich vitamin B-12 sources are not. The official United States Pharmacopeia (U.S.P.) method (*L. leichmannii*) and *E. gracilis* assay as "vitamin B-12" non-cobalamin corrinoids. *Blood* **62** (Suppl 1), 37A (1983).

41. Newmark, P. A., Green, R. and Mollin, D. L. "A comparison of the properties of chicken serum with other vitamin B_{12} binding proteins used in radioisotope dilution methods for measuring vitamin B_{12} concentrations." *Br. J. Haematol.* **25**, 359 (1973).

42. Houts, T. M. and Carney, J. A. "Radioassay for cobalamin (vitamin B_{12}) requiring no pretreatment of serum." *Clin. Chem.* **27**, 263 (1981).

43. Ithakissios, D. S., Kubiatowitz, D. O., and Wicks, J. H. "Room temperature radioassay for B_{12} with oyster toadfish (*Opsanus tau*) serum as binder." *Clin. Chem.* **26**, 323 (1980).

44. Herbert, V., Manusselis, C., Drivas, G., and Temperley, D. "Noncompetitive radioassay of human serum vitamin B_{12} (cobalamin) and total corrinoids (cobalamin + analogs of B_{12}), based on instant alkali dissociation of B_{12}-transcobalamin complexes without damaging transcobalamins." *Clin. Res.* **30**(2), 560A (1982).

45. Grasbeck, R., Stenman, U.-H., Puutula, L., and Visuri, K. "A procedure for detaching bound vitamin B_{12} from its transport protein." *Biochim. Biophys. Acta.* **148**, 292 (1968).

46. Zalusky, R. and Herbert, V. "Isotope dilution methods using coated charcoal." In R. L., Hayes, F. A. Goswitz, and B. E. P. Murphy, Eds., *Radioisotopes in Medicine: In Vitro Studies.* U.S. Atomic Energy Commission, Division of Technical Information (June), 395 (1968).

47. Colman, N. "Technological factors affecting use of radioassays in the assessment of the nutritional anemias." *Ligand Quart.* **4**(3), 31 (1981).

48. Rothenberg, S. P. "Assay of serum vitamin B_{12} concentration using Co^{57} B_{12} and intrinsic factor." *Proc. Soc. Exper. Biol.* **108**, 45 (1961).

49. Friedner, S., Josephson, B., and Levin K. "Vitamin B_{12} determination by means of radio-isotopic dilution and ultrafiltration." *Clin. Chim. Acta* **24**, 171 (1969).

50. Frenkel, E. P., Keller, S., and McCall, M. S. "Radioisotopic assay of serum vitamin B_{12} with the use of DEAE cellulose." *J. Lab. Clin. Med.* **68**, 510 (1966).

51. Wide, L. and Killander, A. "A radioabsorbent technique for the assay of serum vitamin B_{12}." *Scand. J. Clin. Lab. Invest.* **27**, 130 (1966).

52. Gottlieb, C., Lau, K.-S., Wasserman, L. R., and Herbert, V. "Rapid charcoal assay for intrinsic factor (IF), gastric juice unsaturated B_{12} binding capacity, antibody to IF, and serum unsaturated B_{12} binding capacity." *Blood* **25**, 875 (1965).

53. Zucker, R. M., Podell, E., and Allen, R. H. "Multiple problems with current no-boil assays for serum cobalamin." *Ligand Quart.* **4**(3), 52 (1981).

54. Zucker, R. M., Podell, E. R., and Allen, R. H. "The authors' reply." *Ligand Quart.* **4**(3), 62 (1981).

55. Thorell, J. I. "Internal sample attenuator counting (ISAC). A new technique for separating and measuring bound and free activity in radioimmunoassays." *Clin. Chem.* **27**, 1969 (1981).

56. Liu, Y. K. and Sullivan, L. W. "An improved radioisotope dilution assay for serum vitamin B_{12} using hemoglobin-coated charcoal." *Blood* **39**, 426 (1972).

57. Hillman, R. S., Oakes, M., and Finholt, C. "Hemoglobin-coated charcoal radioassay for

serum vitamin B$_{12}$. A simple modification to improve intrinsic factor reliability." *Blood* **34,** 385 (1969).

58. *National Committee for Clinical Laboratory Standards: Guidelines for Evaluation a B$_{12}$ (Cobalamin) Assay.* NCCLS, Villanova, Penn. (1980).

59. Herbert, V., Gottlieb, C. W., and Lau, K.-S. "Hemoglobin-coated charcoal assay for serum vitamin B$_{12}$." *Blood* **28,** 130 (1966).

60. Carmel, R. and Coltman, C. A., Jr. "Radioassay for serum vitamin B$_{12}$ with the use of saliva as the vitamin B$_{12}$ binder." *J. Lab. Clin. Med.* **74,** 967 (1969).

61. Rothenberg, S. P. "A radioassay for serum B$_{12}$ using unsaturated transcobalamin I as the B$_{12}$ binding protein." *Blood* **31,** 44 (1968).

62. Lau, K.-S. "Radioassay of serum B$_{12}$ using chicken serum." Manual of Procedures, Nutritional Anaemia Research Laboratory Training Course, March 25–April 5, 1968, Department of Pathology, University of Malaya, Kuala Lumpur. (Financed by USPHS Grant Am 11048 to Dr. V. Herbert.)

63. Green, R., Newmark, P. A., Musso, A. M., and Mollin, D. L. "The use of chicken serum for measurement of serum vitamin B$_{12}$ concentration by radioisotope dilution: Description of method and comparison with microbiological assay results." *Br. J. Haemat.* **27,** 507 (1974).

64. Herbert, V. and Bertino, J. "Folic acid." In P. Gyorgy and W. N. Pearson, Eds., *The Vitamins: Chemistry, Physiology, Pathology, Methods, Vol. 7,* 2nd ed. Academic Press, New York, 243 (1967).

65. Waxman, S., Schreiber, C., and Herbert, V. "Radioisotopic assay for measurement of serum folate levels." *Blood* **38,** 219 (1971).

66. Colman, N. "Laboratory assessment of folate status." *Clin. Lab. Med.* **1,** 775 (1982).

21 Biotin

J. Scheiner

GENERAL CONSIDERATIONS

Biotin (vitamin H, egg white injury factor, coenzyme R, Bios II B), one of the most active biological substances known, is found in minute amounts in every living cell. Interest in the nutritional, biochemical, and clinical role of biotin was generated by studies which demonstrated that feeding a diet either low in biotin or, more frequently, using a diet with raw egg white added produced biotin deficiency in the rat, chick, poult, pig, monkey, man and other animal species (1–7). The chick and poult, however, require an outside source of biotin, even when egg white is replaced by other proteins. Diets containing sulfonamides also produced biotin deficiency in the rat (8,9).

The effectiveness of egg white in producing biotin deficiency is due to the presence of the glycoprotein avidin, which forms a complex with biotin that renders the biotin unavailable to the host. Avidin also forms tight complexes when biotin is the prosthetic group of an enzyme, resulting in loss of enzyme activity (10). The biotin-binding capacity is present not only in the egg whites but also in the egg yolks of avian species and the turtle (11). Avidin is heat-labile. Prolonged heating of egg white denatures the avidin and destroys its biotin-binding capacity. Another biotin-binding protein similar to avidin, strep-tavidin, is produced by Streptomycetes (12,13).

Biotin deficiency produces dermatitis and perosis in chicks and poults (14–16); alopecia, seborrheic skin changes, spasticity of the hind legs and cracks in the feet of pigs (2). The activities of the biotin-dependent enzymes are also decreased (17). These enzymes are involved in carboxylation, transcarboxylation, and decarboxylation reactions, and function in the vitally important metabolic processes of glucose and fat synthesis (10,17,18). Among the most important enzymes are pyruvate carboxylase which catalyzes the conversion of pyruvate to oxalacetate; acetyl-coenzyme A (CoA) carboxylase, which catalyzes the conversion of acetyl-CoA to malonyl-CoA; and propionyl-CoA carboxylase, which converts propionyl-CoA to methyl malonyl-CoA (17).

Until 1966, biotin deficiency seemed merely a laboratory curiosity with no commercial significance, even though a number of investigators had reported biotin deficiency in poults fed rations containing components suitable for commercial feeds. It was generally believed that the combination of biotin in the feed ingredients plus the biotin produced in the intestine by bacteria supplied sufficient biotin to meet the poult's requirement. However, starting in 1966, a number of reports on biotin deficiency in commercial flocks appeared in the literature (19). Apparent biotin deficiencies in swine under commercial conditions were also reported (19). This increase in biotin deficiency has led to the development of methods for the assessment of nutritional status (17) and fortification of chicken, turkey, and swine feeds with biotin.

In humans, infant seborrheic dermatitis and the related Leiner's disease are biotin responsive (20). Biotin deficiency has been reported in individuals during prolonged total parenteral nutrition (21,22). Biotin administration has successfully controlled multiple carboxylase deficiency even in an unborn infant (23–26). It has been suggested that diseases related to biotin metabolism may be more common than previously thought (27).

The naturally occurring isomer, *d*-biotin, has twice the activity of *dl*-biotin for all microorganisms and animals. The *l*-form is biologically inactive. Reviews and original papers offer further details on the chemistry and biological specificity of biotin derivatives for microorganisms and animals (28–34).

Some of the important properties of biotin are given in the following table (35,36).

Empirical formula	$C_{10} H_{16} O_3 N_2 S$
Optical rotation $[\alpha]_D^{22}$	$+92°$ (0.1 N NaOH)
Melting point	230–232°C (decomposition)
Molecular weight	244.31
Solubility	
H_2O	Slightly soluble
Ethyl alcohol 95%	Slightly soluble
Ethyl ether	Insoluble
Acetone	Insoluble
Chloroform	Insoluble
Ethyl acetate	Insoluble

Concentrated aqueous solutions of biotin can be obtained by neutralizing the free acid with the equivalent amount of an alkali. Biotin is quite stable to moderate acid treatment but is rather unstable to alkali or strong acid. Rancid fats (37) and chlorine (38) inactivate biotin. Crystalline biotin is not affected by ethylene oxide (39). Aqueous solutions at pH 4–9 are stable at 100°C. Oxidizing agents such as hydrogen peroxide or potassium permanganate destroy it.

Modifying the biotin molecule produces compounds with biological activities different from the parent compound. The structures of some of the more important compounds are shown in Figure 21.1.

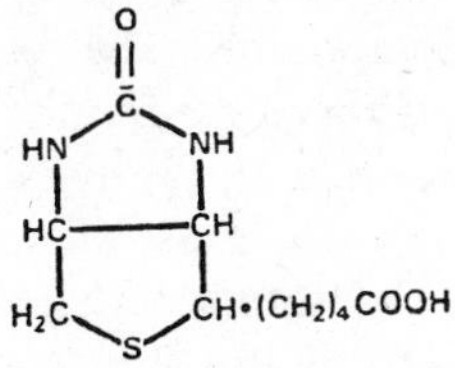

Biotin

Hexahydro-2-oxo-1-H-thieno [3,4-d-]
imidazole-4-pentanoic acid

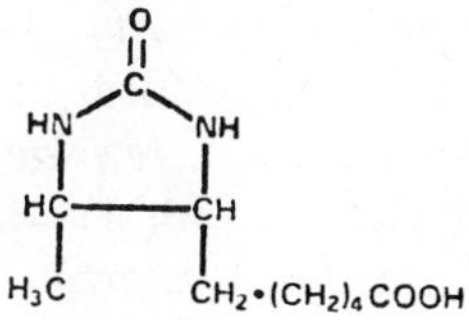

Dethiobiotin

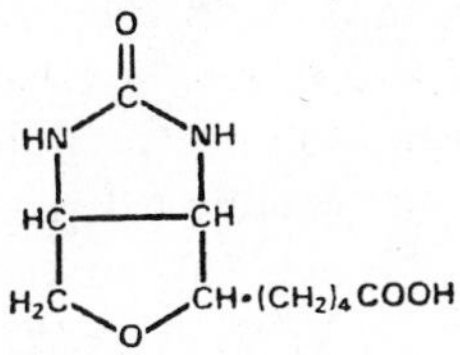

Oxybiotin
(O-heterobiotin)

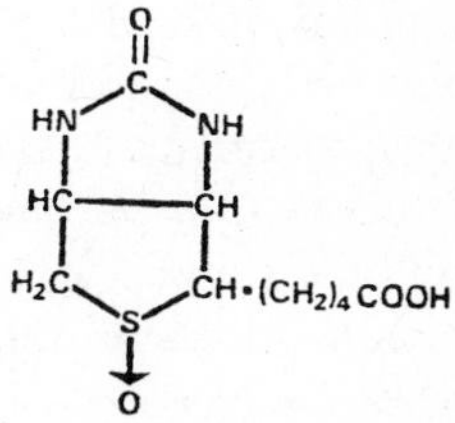

Biotin
Sulfoxide

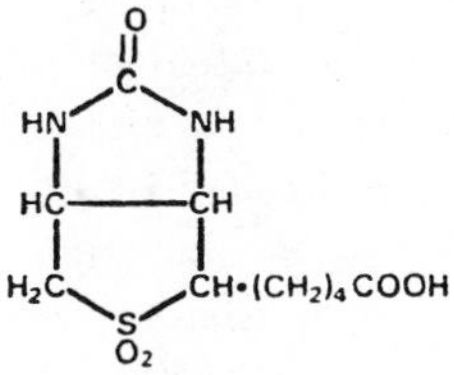

Biotin Sulfone

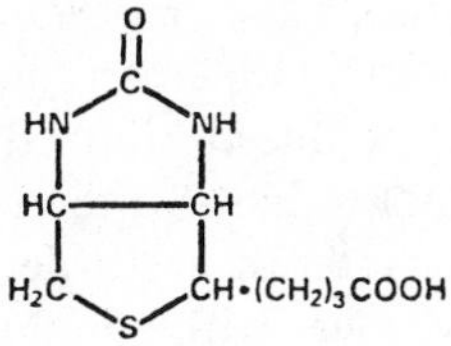

Norbiotin

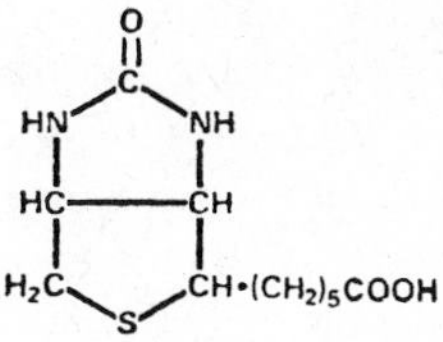

Homobiotin

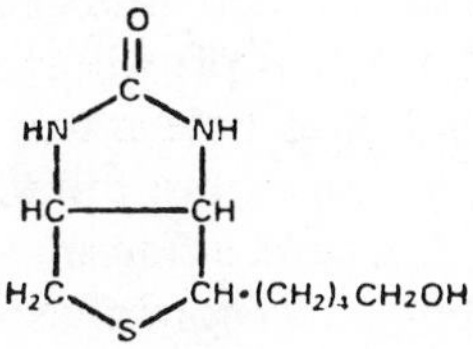

Biotinol

FIGURE 21.1 Biotin and related compounds.

Removing the sulfur atom yields dethiobiotin which may replace biotin in the nutrition of certain microorganisms, for example, *Saccharomyces cerevisiae, Neurospora crassa,* and *Escherichia coli*; act as an antibiotin (i.e., may inhibit growth in the presence of biotin) for other microorganisms, such as *Lactobacillus casei*; or have no biotin or antibiotin effect, such as *Lactobacillus plantarum* (40,41). Some strains of microorganisms produce dethiobiotin (42,43). Microorganisms that use dethiobiotin in place of biotin apparently convert it to biotin (44–46). The replacement of the sulfur atom with an oxygen or carbon atom produces biologically active compounds. The oxygen analog, *d,l*-oxybiotin (*O*-heterobiotin), can replace biotin for *S. cerevisiae, L. plantarum,* and *L. casei* but is inactive for *Streptococcus faecalis*. The activity of oxybiotin relative to biotin varies from organism to organism (47,48). The carbon analog, *d,l*-carbobiotin, has about 15% of the growth promoting activity of *d*-biotin (49).

In those organisms where oxybiotin and carbobiotin possess growth-promoting activity, the compounds are used per se. The activity of oxybiotin and carbobiotin indicate that the stereochemical configuration of the molecule has a direct bearing on the activity of biotin. Biotin *l*-sulfoxide, an oxidation product of biotin, was isolated from *Aspergillus niger* filtrate. The *l*-sulfoxide has 100% activity for *A. niger*, as compared with *d*-biotin, but negligible activity in supporting growth of *S. cerevisiae, L. plantarum,* and *L. casei*. Its optical isomer the *d*-sulfoxide is as active as biotin in promoting growth of *S. cerevisiae* and *L. plantarum* but shows no detectable activity toward *L. casei* (50,51). Biotin sulfone, a higher oxidation product, partially replaces biotin in *S. cerevisiae* and *E. coli* whereas it inhibits the growth of *L. casei* and *L. plantarum* (52).

Homologs of biotin and biotin sulfone show antibiotin activity for some yeasts and bacteria; other yeasts can utilize the biotin homologs (nor-biotin and homobiotin) as sources of biotin (53,54). With the exception of oxybiotin, which has 3–17% the activity of biotin, none of the above analogs has significant biotin activity in animals. On the other hand, biotinol, the alcohol analog of biotin, does not replace biotin in the nutrition of microorganisms but is fully as effective as *d*-biotin in curing egg white-induced biotin deficiency in the rat (55). Both man and the rat convert biotinol to biotin after an oral or intramuscular administration. Other compounds of interest are α-dehydrobiotin, α-methyldethiobiotin, and α-methylbiotin, substances with antibiotin activity produced by streptomyces (56,57).

In nature, biotin is present in conjugated or bound form where the vitamin is attached to a carrier. The carrier can vary from a simple amino acid, as in biocytin (Figure 21.2), to complex higher-molecular-weight compounds such as peptides and proteins (18,58,59). Complete liberation of biotin from these bound forms requires hydrolysis with acid at elevated temperatures. Less drastic hydrolysis is required to liberate biotin from products of plant origin than from products of animal origin. Negligible amounts are liberated by autolysis but enzymatic liberation may be satisfactory in some cases (1,60–62). A higher percentage of free biotin is usually found in substances of plant origin than in substances of animal origin (19,63).

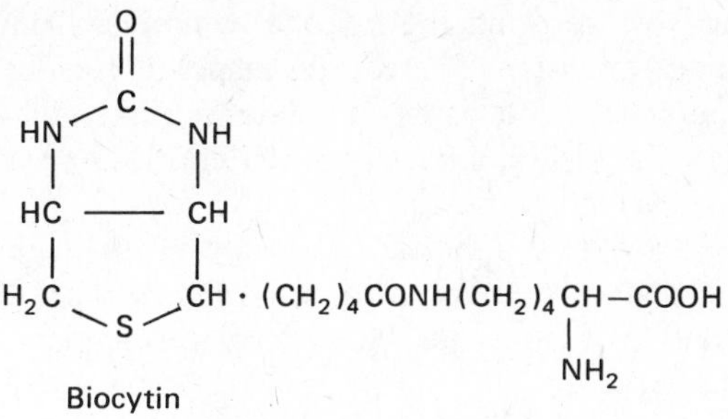

FIGURE 21.2 Biocytin.

In general, the values obtained by microbiological assay after acid hydrolysis are in agreement with values obtained by the chick assay. However, the biotin content of certain feed ingredients (barley, wheat, oats, milo, and fish meals) is considerably higher by microbiological assay, indicating that part of the biotin in these ingredients is unavailable to the chick (64–66).

Certain unsaturated fatty acids, lipids (e.g., lecithin) and other substances replace biotin for growth of certain microorganisms (67–75). On the other hand, lysolecithin, which differs from lecithin in that it does not contain an unsaturated fatty acid, inhibits the growth of L. casei in the presence of suboptimal amounts of biotin in the medium. This inhibitory effect is counteracted by increasing the quantity of biotin (76). Further information on biotin is available in an excellent review by Gyorgy and Langer (77).

METHODS AVAILABLE

The methods available for the determination of biotin are microbiological, biological, chemical, and enzymatic. The microbiological methods are very sensitive and widely applicable. Biological assays using either chicks or rats are time-consuming, require large numbers of animals for accuracy, and are costly to run in terms of manpower, space, and cost of animals and their diet. Chemical assays vary widely in sensitivity and are in many cases nonspecific. The enzymatic assay requires further investigation and standardization.

The microbiological method is commonly used for the determination of biotin. A variety of organisms have been employed, including the bacteria L. casei (78,79), L. plantarum, formerly known as L. arabinosus (17,80), and Clostridium butylicum (63); the yeast S. cerevisiae (81); the mold N. crassa (82); and the protozoan Ochromonas danica (83). The L. casei method has the drawbacks that some of the constituents are very time consuming in preparation and the organism is subject to nonspecific stimulation by small amounts of fatty materials and other natural substances. The Clostridium butylicum assay requires anaerobic conditions and does not have any advantages to warrant the effort required to produce suitable growth conditions. In the Neurospora assay, the response to biotin is determined by weighing the mycelia, a time-consuming operation requiring a great deal of precision. *S. cerevisiae* responds to substances other than the intact biotin molecule and assays of natural materials are therefore not necessarily specific. The *Ochromonas* assay requires 3–5 days incubation prior to reading the assay turbidimetrically.

The method used by most laboratories today is the *L. plantarum* (ATCC 8014) assay. The growth requirements of *L. plantarum* are less complex than those of *L. casei* and as a consequence, this microorganism is less subject to nonspecific stimulation.

Direct assay of some soluble natural products, especially those originating from the autolysis of actively metabolizing material, with *L. plantarum* yields lower results than with *L. casei*. These differences disappear after hydrolysis with acid. Recent studies have demonstrated the presence in *L. casei* of an enzyme biotinidase, which releases biotin from biocytin and other small biotin complexes (84). The absence of this enzyme in *L. plantarum* (85) explains the lower assay results with this organism. Agar plate assays for biotin are less sensitive and more inaccurate than tube assays (86–88).

Ultramicro methods employing *L. plantarum* and *S. cerevisiae* for the determination of biotin in histochemical and cytochemical studies have been reported (89–91). One approach which requires 1/500 to 1/1000 the sample size of the macroassay depends on measurement of light absorbance of bacterial suspensions in microcuvettes. *L. plantarum* results were more consistent and lower than results obtained with *S. cerevisiae*. In a unique approach, a microscopic microbiological assay capable of determining 10^{-15} g was developed where submicro droplets of the incubation mixture were employed under oil. The bacterial growth is measured by light scatter.

Biological assays with animals do not require pretreatment of the samples and they measure the amount of biotin available to the animal. Both the chick and the rat are used for the assay of biotin (5,92–94). Biotin deficiency in the chick is produced by feeding a diet low in biotin whereas in the rat the diet must contain avidin. Chick assays are less erratic than rat assays, less costly to run, and are the preferred assay.

Isotope dilution assays are based on the competition between radioactive biotin and nonradioactive biotin for the binding site of avidin (95,96). The method is sensitive, analyzing 1–10 ng of biotin, but has only been applied to a very limited number of natural products. Both *L. plantarum* and isotope dilution values were given in one report (96). Agreement between the two methods was good for a poultry feed and an antibiotic. However, the radioassay values for two wheat samples were approximately 20% and 55% higher than the microbiological assay value. As the biotin in wheat is only partially available as shown by chick assay, the higher radioassay values for wheat suggest that isotope dilution assays are not ready for general use.

The fluorometric assay (97) based on the quenching of tryptophan fluorescence by biotin is a relatively sensitive assay, analyzing as little as 20 ng. The method cannot be applied to biological materials because of their high tryptophan content.

Early thin-layer chromatographic procedures were both insensitive and subject to large errors (98,99). Improved accuracy and reproducibility was claimed by measuring the in situ reflectance of a spot visualized by spraying with 4-dimethylaminocinnamaldehyde (100).

Colorimetric assays for biotin employ the reaction of *p*-dimethylaminocinnamaldehyde with biotin (101); or the determination of the iodine formed by the reduction of iodate when the sulfur atom is oxidized to sulfone (102). These procedures require very high biotin levels and their usage is limited to high potency solid and liquid preparations.

A gas-liquid chromatography procedure was developed for the determination of biotin in agricultural premixes and injectable pharmaceutical preparations (103). The method involves the injection of the biotin silyl ester equivalent to 5 μg *d*-biotin in 5 μL and is too insensitive for assay of most pharmaceutical products.

An interesting biochemical approach utilizes the enzymatic binding of the biotin in situ to the pyruvate carboxylase apoprotein of the biotin-deficient yeast and the subsequent estimate of pyruvate carboxylase activity by a $^{14}CO_2$ fixation method (104). The assay has a sensitivity comparable to microbiological assays but values for five natural materials by the enzymatic method averaged 55% of values for the same extracts obtained by a yeast plate assay. The most serious disadvantage of the method is its sensitivity to interference by some property or factor of the samples tested.

ANALYTICAL METHODOLOGY MICROBIOLOGICAL METHOD
(*LACTOBACILLUS PLANTARUM*, ATCC 8014)

A. Principle

See page 43.

B. Equipment

See page 50.

C. Reagents

Reagents 1, 2, 3, 4, 5, 6, 7, 8, 9, 28, 29, 33, 34, 35, 36, and 37 on pages 51–58 are required. In addition, the following reagents will be needed for this method:

38. *6 N Sulfuric Acid.* If a considerable number of samples are to be assayed for biotin, a relatively large volume of the extractant should be prepared. To prepare 9 L of 6 N H_2SO_4, add 1500 mL concentrated H_2SO_4 slowly and with stirring to about 7 L H_2O. After cooling make to 9 L with H_2O.

39. *2 N Sulfuric Acid.*   Add 500 mL concentrated H_2SO_4 slowly and with stirring to about 7 L H_2O. After cooling, make to 9 L with H_2O.

40. *20% Sodium Hydroxide.*   To 40 g NaOH pellets add 160 mL H_2O and stir until dissolved. This solution is used to neutralize the acid used in extraction of the samples.

41. *Working Biotin Standard.*   Dilute 5 mL of the biotin stock solution (Reagent 6) to 250 mL with 50% ethyl alcohol (stock solution 2). Dilute 5 mL stock solution 2 to 500 mL with 50% ethyl alcohol (stock solution 3). Prepare the working standard every day by diluting 5 mL stock solution 3 to 250 mL with H_2O. This working standard contains 0.2 ng/mL.

42. *Basal Medium for Biotin Assay.*   Add 1 mL each of calcium pantothenate (Reagent 5) and niacin (Reagent 7) stock solutions to 500 mL of the basal medium stock solution (Reagent 9). Mix. The medium may be prepared in advance and kept frozen at −20°C. If 2 L are prepared, place 500–700 mL in 1000-mL suction flasks and use as needed. The medium can be thawed (in the dark) and refrozen at least once. Commercially prepared dehydrated biotin-free assay medium of similar composition is available (Difco) and can be used for the assay of pharmaceuticals and many natural materials. As some lot-to-lot variation may occur, each lot of medium should be tested for utility prior to routine use.

D.   Procedure

The general comments made in Section D of Chapter 3 regarding microbiological procedures pertain to biotin analysis as well.

1. *Preparation of Stock Culture L. plantarum (ATCC 8014).*   Stock cultures are prepared by the stab inoculation of Bacto-Lactobacilli Agar (Reagent 29) or Bacto-Micro Assay Culture Agar (Difco). Incubate at 35–37°C for 24–48 hr and store tubes under refrigeration. The culture should be transferred at 2–4-week intervals for maintenance. Fresh stab cultures less than 1 week old are used for inoculum preparation.

2. *Preparation of Inoculum.*   Transfer cells from stock cultures to sterile tubes containing 10 mL of Bacto-Lactobacilli Broth (Reagent 28) or Bacto-Micro Inoculum Broth (Difco). Incubate overnight at 35–37°C. Under aseptic conditions, centrifuge culture and decant supernatant. Wash cells with 10-mL portions of sterile 0.9% NaCl solution (Reagent 33). Cells should be washed at least one time. The cells are resuspended in 10 mL sterile 0.9% NaCl solution. The cell suspension is then diluted 1:100 with 0.9% NaCl solution. One drop of the dilution is used to inoculate each of the assay tubes.

3. *Preparation of Samples.*   Materials of plant origin are extracted with 2 N H_2SO_4, those of animal origin with 6 N H_2SO_4 and mixtures (e.g., feed of mixed composition) with 2 N H_2SO_4

(a) Weigh or pipette sufficient material to contain approximately 200 ng of biotin into a 50-mL Erlenmeyer flask.

(1) In choosing the quantity of material to be extracted, the degree of homogeneity with respect to biotin should be considered. Samples smaller than 1–2 g should be avoided, if possible. For high-potency samples (e.g., liver) the samples may need to be diluted considerably to permit assay of the biotin content [see Section D.3(e)].

(b) Add 25 mL of H_2SO_4 of appropriate normality and thoroughly mix.

(1) No universal procedure is in use for liberating biotin from natural materials. Autolysis of the samples and enzymatic hydrolysis (Takadiastase and papain) may result in considerable liberation of biotin from some samples, but often fail to release as much biotin as is obtained by acid treatment. Reports indicate that some biotin is destroyed when 6 N H_2SO_4 is used for certain samples, particularly from plant sources. Alternative procedures used 0.5 N, 1 N, 2 N, 3 N, or 4 N H_2SO_4. It may be necessary to study the stability of biotin to the hydrolytic procedure, particularly where previous studies with the products tested have not been conducted. Experiments on this subject that may be useful are included in the bibliography (19, 60, 61, 78, 80, 105–107).

(2) Do not use HCl in place of H_2SO_4 as HCl may inactivate biotin (108).

(c) Autoclave the mixture at 121°C (15 psi) for 2 hr.

(1) The length of time recommended may need to be shortened if preliminary studies indicate that biotin destruction occurs under these conditions. Subsequent experimentation may reveal that ½–1 hr would be more satisfactory.

(d) Cool, transfer to a 100-mL volumetric flask, make to volume, and filter if necessary.

(e) Dilute a 10-mL aliquot to 60–70 mL with H_2O in a 100-mL beaker and neutralize with 20% NaOH to pH 6.8 (pH meter or bromothymol blue outside indicator). Dilute to 100 mL in a volumetric flask.

(1) If the quantity of biotin in the original sample differs widely from 200 ng, it will be necessary to dilute accordingly so that the final solution contains approximately 0.2 ng/mL.

(2) The use of two steps in the dilution procedure rather than diluting originally to 1 L permits changes in the final dilutions without having to rehydrolyze the sample in case the potency is much less than expected.

(3) The effects of the lipid constituents of the sample on the validity of the biotin assay (see General Considerations) are largely or completely eliminated as a result of the following factors:

(i) Filtration of the acid extracts [Section D.3(d)] will remove a large portion of the lipid constituents.

(ii) The high sensitivity of the assay necessitates great dilution of the sample which will reduce the effects of the lipids on stimulating growth of the organism. Approximately 100 μg of oleic acid per tube in a biotin-deficient medium will elicit a growth response (71). It is conceivable, however, that occasional low-potency samples high in fat containing oleic acid and other biotin-active lipids might present some difficulties. A few simple tests conducted by filtering the samples at pH 4.5 or by ether extraction of the samples will demonstrate whether lipid contamination is invalidating the biotin assay results. It has been found, for example, that with egg samples, filtration at an acid pH may be insufficient to remove interfering lipids and that it may be necessary to extract these samples with ether.

Pharmaceuticals and premixes are extracted as below.

(a) Solutions. Dilute in H_2O.

(b) Suspensions where biotin is not in solution. Pipette an aliquot into volumetric flask, add H_2O until flask is approximately half full, add a few drops 1 N NaOH until alkaline, shake well, bring to volume. Subdilute to assay range.

(c) Tablets or capsules. Homogenize in 0.1 N NaOH, transfer quantitatively to a volumetric flask, bring to volume. Subdilute to assay range.

(d) Premixes (109). For potencies up to 1 g/lb. Place 5 g sample in 1-L flask. Add 50 mL 0.1 N NaOH and 250 mL H_2O. Swirl flask vigorously at first and then every 5 min over a period of 20–30 min. Bring to volume. Subdilute to assay range. If the concentration of NaOH in the final dilution is 6×10^{-5} N or less no pH adjustment is necessary.

For potencies greater than 1 g/lb extract with 300 mL 0.1 N NaOH as above.

4. *Preparation of Standard Tubes.*

(a) To duplicate tubes add 0.0-, 0.5-, 1.0-, 1.5-, 2.0-, 2.5-, 3.0-, 4.0-, and 5.0-mL volumes of the working biotin standard solution (0.2 ng/mL, Reagent 41). For turbidimetric assays, add an additional 0.0 mL tube which is not inoculated. This tube is used to set the instrument to 100% transmittance.

(b) Add H_2O to a final volume of 5.0 mL in each tube.

(c) To each tube, add 5.0 mL of the biotin medium (Reagent 42).

(1) See page 542.

5. *Preparation of Assay Tubes.*

(a) To duplicate tubes add 1.0-, 2.0-, and 3.0-mL aliquots of the test solution.

(1) More levels of test solution may be advantageous. The use of different levels permits evaluation of the validity of the assay over a range of biotin concentrations within the limits of the standard curve.

(2) Where the approximate potency of the sample is not known, it may be desirable to add the test solution over a greater range of concentration (i.e., 0.1-, 0.5-, 1.0-, 2.0-, 3.0-, 4.0-, and 5.0-mL) where 7 tubes

are used per sample. Appropriate dilutions can then be made for subsequent assays.

(b) Add H_2O to a volume of 5.0 mL in each tube.

(c) Add 5.0 mL of the biotin basal medium to each tube.

6. *Sterilization.* See page 59.

7. *Inoculation and Incubation.* See page 59.

8. *Titration or Turbidimetric Measurement.* After incubation stop growth by heating at 100°C for 10 min in the autoclave. See page 60.

Frequently, satisfactory results can be obtained turbidimetrically for colored samples by adding a tube containing 5 mL of sample that is not inoculated and using it as a color blank. The correction is feasible if the color blank is less than 10% of the total reading (expressed as absorbance) and no significant change in color occurs during incubation. A comparision of results by titrimetric and turbidimetric assays of the same final dilution will indicate the practicality of using the turbidimetric method. The use of a color blank is illustrated in [Section D.9(b)] below.

9. *Calculation.*

(a) Titrimetric.

(1) Draw a standard curve for the assay by plotting mL 0.1 N NaOH used in titrating the standard tubes against nanograms of biotin per tube in the standard series.

(2) Determine the biotin content of the tubes in the unknown series by interpolation of the titer values on the standard curve.

(3) Discard any values that show more than 1 ng or less than 0.1 ng of biotin per tube. Calculate the biotin content of each mL of test solution for each of the duplicate sets of tubes.

(4) Calculate the biotin content of the test material from the average of the values for 1 mL of test solution, obtained from at least three sets of these tubes which do not vary by more than 10% from the average, using the following formula:

$$\text{ng/g} = \frac{\text{mean ng/mL}}{\text{wt. of sample}} \times \text{volume} \times \text{dilution factor}$$

(b) Turbidimetric.

(1) Mix the contents of each tube well, transfer the contents to an appropriate tube or cuvette, place in the spectrophotometer, colorimeter, or turbidimeter and read the transmittance when the steady state is reached (usually within 30 sec). Set the instrument at 100% *T* with the uninoculated blank and read the standard and samples.

(2) If the inoculated blank shows a reading of 90% *T* or below, discard the assay.

(3) Draw a standard curve for the assay by plotting the transmittance of the standard tubes against nanograms of biotin per tube in the standard series.

(i) Frequently a straight-line relationship is obtained over most of the curve by plotting the logarithm of transmittance against the concentration. This is easily accomplished by using semilogarithmic graph paper.

(4) To correct for color, convert the transmittance reading for each level of the sample and the color blank to the corresponding absorbance (A).

(5) Subtract a proportionate amount of the color blank for each level of sample; for example, subtract one-fifth the color blank for the 1-mL level, two-fifths for the 2-mL level, etc.

(6) Convert the corrected A back to transmittance and determine the biotin content of each tube by interpolation of the corrected transmittances on the standard curve.

(7) Continue as in Section D.9(a)(3) and (4). A typical example of the calculation of results of a titrimetric and turbidimetric assay on a colored solution using the same final standard and sample dilution follows:

Titrimetric Assay Standard Curve Series

Standard (mL)	ng Biotin per Tube	0.1 N NaOH (duplicate tubes) (mL)	
0.0	0.0	1.6	1.6
0.5	0.1	5.5	5.9
1.0	0.2	7.8	7.6
1.5	0.3	8.8	8.9
2.0	0.4	9.9	9.9
2.5	0.5	10.3	10.5
3.0	0.6	11.0	11.0
4.0	0.8	11.6	11.7
5.0	1.0	12.2	12.2

Unknown Test Series

Five g of animal feed were diluted to 250 mL following hydrolysis. After filtration, a 4-mL portion was neutralized and diluted to 100 mL, 1-, 2-, 3-, 4-, and 5-mL portions were tested as described in the procedure.

Titrimetric Assay

Sample (mL)	0.1 N NaOH (mL)	ng Biotin per Tube	ng Biotin per mL
1.0	6.8	0.15	0.150
1.0	6.6	0.14	0.140
2.0	8.9	0.31	0.155
2.0	8.8	0.30	0.150
3.0	10.1	0.43	0.143
3.0	10.1	0.43	0.143
4.0	10.8	0.56	0.140
4.0	10.9	0.58	0.145
5.0	11.5	0.75	0.150
5.0	11.5	0.75	0.150
			av. 0.147

The values in column 3 were found by interpolation of the values shown in column 2 on a standard curve.

Sample calculation

$$\frac{0.147 \times 100}{4 \text{ mL}} \times \frac{250}{5} = 184 \text{ ng/g}$$

Turbidimetric Assay Standard Curve Series

Standard (mL)	ng Biotin per Tube	Transmittance (mV)	
0.0 (uninoc.)	0.0	1000	997
0.0 (inoc.)	0.0	944	954
0.5	0.1	768	752
1.0	0.2	676	670
1.5	0.3	578	591
2.0	0.4	492	492
2.5	0.5	445	434
3.0	0.6	398	386
4.0	0.8	309	314
5.0	1.0	236	228

Unknown Test Series.

Same as above.

Turbidimetric Assay

Aliquot (mL)	T^a	A^b	Blank (Bl)	A-Bl	T	ng Biotin per Tube	ng Biotin per mL
1.0	727	0.13847	0.00772	0.13075	740	0.120	0.120
1.0	740	0.13077	0.00772	0.12305	753	0.110	0.110[c]
2.0	574	0.24109	0.01544	0.22565	595	0.290	0.145
2.0	587	0.23137	0.01544	0.21593	608	0.278	0.139
3.0	482	0.31696	0.02315	0.29381	508	0.417	0.139
3.0	483	0.31606	0.02315	0.29291	509	0.408	0.136
4.0	409	0.38828	0.03087	0.35741	439	0.520	0.130
4.0	414	0.38300	0.03087	0.35213	444	0.510	0.128
5.0	335	0.47496	0.03859	0.43637	366	0.659	0.132
5.0	334	0.47626	0.03859	0.43767	365	0.660	0.132
5.0(uninoc)	915	0.03859					av. 0.133

[a] in millivolts.
[b] Absorbance.
[c] Outside $\pm 10\%$ limit therefore not included in calculation.

The values in column 7 were found by interpolation of the values shown in column 6 on a standard curve.

Sample calculation

$$\frac{0.133 \times 100}{4} \times \frac{250}{5} = 1.66 \text{ ng/g}$$

LITERATURE CITED

1. Hertz, R. "Biotin and the avidin-biotin complex." *Physiol. Rev.* **26**, 479 (1944).

2. Cunha, T. J., Lindley, D. C., and Ensminger, M. E. "Biotin deficiency syndrome in pigs fed dessicated egg white." *J. Animal Sci.* **5**, 219 (1946).

3. Waisman, H. A. and Elvehjem, C. A. "Acute and chronic biotin deficiencies in the monkey (*Macacca mulatta*)." *J. Nutr.* **26**, 361 (1943).

4. Hegsted, D. M., Oleson, J. J., Mills, R. C., Elvehjem, C. A., and Hart, E. B. "Studies on a dermatitis in chicks distinct from pantothenic acid deficiency." *J. Nutr.* **20**, 599 (1940).

5. Ansbacher, S. and Landy, M. "Biotin and scaly dermatitis of the chick." *Proc. Soc. Exptl. Biol. Med.* **48**, 3 (1941).

6. Patrick, H., Boucher, R. V., Dutcher, R. A., and Knandel, H. C. "Biotin and prevention of dermatitis in turkey poults." *Proc. Soc. Exptl. Biol. Med.* **48**, 456 (1941).

7. Sydenstricker, V. P., Singal, S. A., Briggs, A. P., DeVaughn, N. M., and Isbell, H. "Observations on the egg white injury in man." *J. Am. Med. Assoc.* **118**, 1199 (1942).

8. Nielsen, E. and Elvehjem, C. A. "The growth promoting effect of folic acid and biotin in rats fed succinylsulfathiazole." *J. Biol. Chem.* **145**, 713 (1942).

9. Daft, F. S., Ashburn, L. L., and Sebrell, W. H. "Biotin deficiency and other changes in rats given sulfanilylguanidine or succinylsulfathiazole in purified diets." *Science* **96**, 321 (1942).

10. Moss, J. and Lane, M. D. "The biotin-dependent enzymes." *Adv. in Enzymol.* **35**, 321 (1971).

11. Korpela, J. K., Kulomaa, M. S., Elo, H. A., and Tuohimaa, P. J. "Biotin-binding protein in eggs of oviparous vertebrates." *Experimentia* **37**, 1065 (1981).

12. Tausig, F. and Wolf, F. J. "Streptavidin—a substance with avidin-like properties produced by microorganisms." *Biochem. Biophys. Res. Commun.* **14**, 205 (1964).

13. Chaiet, L. and Wolf, F. J. "The properties of Streptavidin, a biotin-binding protein produced by Streptomycetes." *Arch. Biochem. Biophys.* **106**, 1 (1964).

14. Patrick, H., Boucher, R. V., Dutcher, R. A., and Knandel, H. C. "The nutritional significance of biotin in chick and poult nutrition." *Poultry Sci.* **21**, 476 (1942).

15. Marusich, W. L., Ogrinz, E. F., Brand, M., and Mitrovic, M. "Induction, prevention and therapy of biotin deficiency in turkey poults on semi-purified and commercial-type rations." *Poultry Sci.* **49**, 412 (1970).

16. Dobson, D. C. "Biotin requirement of turkey poults." *Poultry Sci.* **49**, 546 (1970).

17. Whitehead, C. C. "The assessment of biotin status in man and animals." *Proc. Nutr. Soc.* **40**, 165 (1981).

18. Wood, H. G. and Barden, R. E. "Biotin enzymes." *Ann. Rev. Biochem.* **46**, 385 (1977).

19. Scheiner, J. and DeRitter, E. "Biotin content of feedstuffs" *J. Agric. Food Chem.*, **23**, 1157 (1975).

20. Svejcar, J. and Homolka, J. "Experimental experiences with biotin in babies." *Ann. Paediat.* **174**, 175 (1950).

21. Mock, D. M., deLorimer, A. A., Liebman, W. M., Sweetman, L., and Baker, H. "Biotin deficiency: An unusual complication of parenteral alimentation." *N. Engl. J. Med.* **304**, 820 (1981).

22. Bozian, R. C., Moussavian, N., and Piepmeyer, J. L. "Biotin deficiency during prolonged home total parenteral nutrition (TPN)." *Clin. Res.* **29**, 622A (1981).

23. Munnich, A., Saudubray, J. M., Carré, G., Coudé, F. X., Ogier, H., Charpentier, C., and Frézal, J. "Defective biotin absorption in multiple carboxylase deficiency." *Lancet* **2**, 263 (1981).

24. Thoene, J., Baker, H., Yoshino, M., and Sweetman, L. "Biotin-responsive carboxylase deficiency associated with subnormal plasma and urinary biotin." *N. Engl. J. Med.* **304**, 817 (1981).

25. Baumgartner, R., Suormala, T., Wick, H., Bachmann, C., and Jaggi, K. H. "Biotin dependency causing multiple carboxylase deficiency in vivo." *Pediatr. Res.* **15**, 1189 (1981).

26. Roth, K. S., Yang, W., Allan, L., Saunders, M., Gravel, R. A., and Dakshinamurti, K. "Prenatal administration of biotin in biotin responsive multiple carboxylase deficiency." *Pediatr. Res.* **16**, 126 (1982).

27. Tanaka, K. "New light on biotin deficiency." *N. Engl. J. Med.* **304**, 839 (1981).

28. Melville, D. B. "The chemistry of biotin." *Vitamins and Hormones* **2**, 29 (1944).

29. Luckey, T. D., Moore, P. R., and Elvehjem, C. A. "A differential microbiological assay for *O*-heterobiotin." *Proc. Soc. Exptl. Biol. Med.* **61**, 97 (1946).

30. Hofmann, K. and Winnick, T. "The determination of oxybiotin in the presence of biotin." *J. Biol. Chem.* **160**, 449 (1945).

31. Hofmann, K., Winnick, T., and Axelrod, A. E. "The use of Raney's nickel in a differential assay for oxybiotin and biotin." *J. Biol. Chem.* **169**, 191 (1947).

32. Emerson, G. A. "The biological activity of biotin and related compounds." *J. Biol. Chem.* **157**, 127 (1945).

33. Stokes, J. L. and Gunness, M. "Microbiological activity of synthetic biotin, its optical isomers, and related compounds." *J. Biol. Chem.* **157**, 121 (1945).

34. Perlman, D. "Desthiobiotin and *O*-heterobiotin as growth factors for 'normal' and 'degenerate' strains of *Clostridia.*" *Arch. Biochem.* **16**, 79 (1948).

35. du Vigneaud, V. *The Biological Action of the Vitamins.* The University of Chicago Press, 144 (1942).

36. *Biotin 'Roche,'* rev. ed. Hoffmann-LaRoche, Nutley, N.J., 5 (1956).

37. Pavcek, P. L. and Shull, G. M. "Inactivation of biotin by rancid fats." *J. Biol. Chem.* **146**, 351 (1942).

38. Harrison, J. S. and Miller, E. J. "The inactivation of biotin by chlorine." *Analyst* **74**, 463 (1949).

39. Bakerman, H., Romine, M., Schricker, J. A., Takahashi, S. M., and Mickelsen, O. "Stability of certain B vitamins exposed to ethylene oxide in the presence of choline chloride." *J. Agric. Food Chem.* **4**, 956 (1956).

40. Melville, D. B., Dittmer, K., Brown, G. B., and du Vigneaud, V. "Desthiobiotin." *Science* **98**, 497 (1943).

41. Lilly, V. G. and Leonian, L. H. "The antibiotin effect of desthiobiotin." *Science* **99**, 205 (1944).

42. Tsuboi, T., Sekijo, C., Yoshimura, Y., and Shoji, O. "Studies in production of biotin by microorganisms, Part III." *Agric. Biol. Chem.* **31**, 1135 (1967).

43. Izumi, Y., Kano, Y., Inagaki, K., Kawase, N., Tani, Y., and Yamada, H. "Characterization of biotin biosynthetic enzymes of *Bacillus sphaericus.* A desthiobiotin producing bacterum." *Agric. Biol. Chem.* **45**, 1983 (1981).

44. Dittmer, K., Melville, D. B., and du Vigneaud, V. "The possible synthesis of biotin from desthiobiotin by yeast and the anti-biotin effect of desthiobiotin for *L. casei*." *Science* **99**, 203 (1944).

45. Leonian, L. H. and Lilly, V. G. "Conversion of desthiobiotin into biotin or biotin-like substances by some microorganisms." *J. Bact.* **49**, 291 (1945).

46. Tatum, E. L. "Desthiobiotin in the biosynthesis of biotin." *J. Biol. Chem.* **160**, 455 (1945).

47. Rubin, S. H., Flower, D., Rosen, F., and Drekter, L. "The biological activity of *O*-hetero-biotin." *Arch. Biochem.* **8**, 79 (1945).

48. Winnick, T., Hofmann, K., Pilgrim, F. J., and Axelrod, A. E. "The microbiological activity of *dl*-oxybiotin and related compounds." *J. Biol. Chem.* **161**, 405 (1945).

49. Wormser, H. C., Israsena, S., Meiling, M. S., Williams, C., and Perlman, D. "Synthesis and growth-promoting activity of *dl*-cis-hexahydro-4-(4-carboxy,butyl)-2-cyclopentimidazolone; Carbobiotin." *J. Pharm. Sci.* **61**, 1168 (1972).

50. Wright, L. D., Cresson, E. L., Valiant, J., Wolf, D. E., and Folkers, K. "Biotin L-sulfoxide—3. The characterization of biotin L-sufoxide from a microbiological source." *J. Am. Chem. Soc.* **76**, 4163 (1954).

51. Melville, D. B., Genghof, D. S., and Lu, J. M. "Biological properties of biotin D- and L-sulfoxides." *J. Biol. Chem.* **208**, 503 (1954).

52. Wright, L. D. "The microbiological determination of biotin." *Biological Symposia* **12**, 290 (1947).

53. Rubin, S. H. and Scheiner, J. "Antibiotin effect of homologs of biotin and biotin sulfone." *Arch. Biochem.* **23**, 400 (1949).

54. Belcher, M. R. and Lichstein, H. C. "Growth promotion and antibiotin effect of homobiotin and norbiotin." *J. Bact.* **58**, 579 (1949).

55. Drekter, L., Scheiner, J., DeRitter, E., and Rubin, S. H. "Utilization of *d*-biotinol by microorganisms, the rat and human." *Proc. Soc. Exptl. Biol. Med.* **78**, 381 (1951).

56. Hanka, L. J., Bergy, M. E., and Kelly, R. B. "Naturally occurring anti-metabolite antibiotic related to biotin." *Science* **154**, 1667 (1966).

57. Hanka, L. J., Martin, D. G., and Reineke, L. M. "Two new antimetabolites of biotin:α-methyldethiobiotion and α-methylbiotin." *Antimicrob. Agents Chemother.* **1**, 135 (1972).

58. Wright, L. D., Cresson, E. L., Skeggs, H. R., Wood, T. R., Peck, R. L., Wolf, D. E., and Folkers, K. "Biocytin, a naturally-occuring complex of biotin." *J. Am. Chem. Soc.* **72**, 1048 (1950).

59. Wright, L. D., Cresson, E. L., Skeggs, H. R., Peck, R. L., Wolf, D. E., Wood, T. R., Valiant, J., and Folkers, K. "The elucidation of biocytin," *Science* **114**, 635 (1951).

60. Thompson, R. C., Eakin, R. E., and Williams, R. J. "The extraction of biotin from tissues." *Science* **94**, 589 (1941).

61. Bowden, J. P. and Peterson, W. H. "Release of free and bound forms of biotin from proteins." *J. Biol. Chem.* **178**, 533 (1949).

62. Chang, W. S. and Peterson, W. H. "Purification of bound forms of biotin." *J. Biol. Chem.* **193**, 587 (1951).

63. Lampen, J. O., Bahler, G. P., and Peterson, W. H. "The occurrence of free and bound biotin." *J. Nutr.* **23**, 11 (1942).

64. Wagstaff, R. K., Dobson, D. C., and Anderson, J. O. "Available biotin content of barley." *Poultry Sci.* **40**, 503 (1961).

65. Anderson, J. O. "Studies on the need for supplemental biotin in chick rations." *Poultry Sci.* **49**, 569 (1970).

66. Frigg, M. "Bio-availability of biotin in cereals." *Poultry Sci.* **55**, 2310 (1976).

67. Williams, V. R. and Fieger, E. A. "Growth stimulants for the microbiological assay of biotin." *Ind. Eng. Chem., Anal. Ed.* **17**, 127 (1945).

68. Williams, V. R. "Growth stimulants in the *Lactobacillus arabinosus* biotin assay." *J. Biol. Chem.* **159**, 237 (1945).

69. Trager, W. "A fat-soluble material from plasma having the biological activities of biotin." *Proc. Soc. Exptl. Biol. Med.* **64**, 129 (1947).

70. Axelrod, A. E., Hofmann, K., and Daubert, B. F. "The biotin activity of a vaccenic acid fraction." *J. Biol. Chem.* **169**, 761 (1947).

71. Williams, V. R. and Fieger, E. A. "Further studies on lipide stimulation of *Lactobacillus casei.*" *J. Biol. Chem.* **170**, 399 (1947).

72. Williams, W. L., Broquist, H. P., and Snell, E. E. "Oleic acid and related compounds as growth factors for lactic acid bacteria." *J. Biol. Chem.* **170**, 619 (1947).

73. Trager, W. "Further studies on a fat-soluble material from plasma having biotin activity." *J. Biol. Chem.* **176**, 133 (1948).

74. Shull, G. M., Thoma, R. W., and Peterson, W. H. "Amino acid and unsaturated fatty acid requirements of *Clostridium sporogenes.*" *Arch. Biochem.* **20**, 227 (1949).

75. Hodson, A. Z. "Oleic acid interference in the *Neurospora crassa* assay for biotin." *J. Biol. Chem.* **179**, 49 (1949).

76. Trager, W. "The effects of lysolecithin on the growth of *Lactobacillus casei* in relation to biotin, pantothenic acid and fat-soluble materials with biotin activity." *J. Bact.* **56**, 195 (1948).

77. Gyorgy, P. and Langer, B. "Biotin—Chemistry." In W. H. Sebrell, and R. S. Harris, Eds., *The Vitamins*, Vol. 2, 2nd ed. Academic Press, New York, 263 (1968).

78. Shull, G. M., Hutchings, B. L., and Peterson, W. H. "A microbiological assay for biotin." *J. Biol. Chem.* **142**, 913 (1942).

79. Shull, G. M. and Peterson, W. H. "Improvements in the *Lactobacillus casei* assay for biotin." *J. Biol. Chem.* **151**, 201 (1943).

80. Wright, L. D. and Skeggs, H. R. "Determination of biotin with *Lactobacillus arabinosus.*" *Proc. Soc. Exptl. Biol. Med.* **56**, 95 (1944).

81. Hertz, R. "Modification of the yeast-growth assay method for biotin." *Proc. Soc. Exptl. Biol. Med.* **52**, 15 (1943).

82. Hodson, A. Z. "The use of *Neurospora* for the determination of choline and biotin in milk products." *J. Biol. Chem.* **157**, 383 (1945).

83. Baker, H., Frank, O., Matovitch, V. B., Pasher, I., Aaronson, S., Hutner, S. H., and Sobotka, H. "A new assay method for biotin in blood, serum, urine and tissues." *Anal. Biochem.* **3**, 31 (1962).

84. Knappe, J., Brummer, W., and Biederbick, K. "Reinigung und Eigenschaften der Biotinidase aus Schweinenieren und *Lactobacillus casei.*" *Biochem. Z.* **338**, 599 (1963).

85. Koivusalo, M., Elorriaga, C., Kaziro, Y., and Ochoa, S. "Bacterial biotinidase." *J. Biol. Chem.* **238**, 1038 (1963).

86. Genghof, D. S., Partridge, C. W. H., and Carpenter, F. H. "An agar plate assay for biotin." *Arch. Biochem.* **17**, 413 (1948).

87. Morris, S. and Jones, A. "A plate assay technique for biotin, nicotinic acid and pantothenic acid." *Analyst* **78**, 15 (1953).

88. Jones, A. "The plate assays of vitamins of the B-group." *Analyst* **79**, 586 (1954).

89. Glick, D., Lichstein, H. C., Ferguson, R. B., and Twedt, R. M. "Studies in histochemistry— 53. Microbiological assay in quantitative histo-and cytochemistry." *Proc. Soc. Exptl. Biol. Med.* **99**, 660 (1958).

90. Ferguson, R. B., Lichstein, H. C., and Glick, D. "Studies in histochemistry—56. Microbiological determination of biotin in microgram amounts of tissue." *Arch. Biochem. Biophys.* **89**, 31 (1960).

91. Glick, D. and Ferguson, R. B. "Histochemistry Studies in-67. Microscopic microbiological assay. Determination of biotin to 10–15 gram." *Proc. Soc. Exptl. Biol. Med.* **109**, 811 (1962).

92. Hegsted, D. M., Oleson, J. J., Mills, R. C., Elvehjem, C. A., and Hart, E. B. "Studies on a dermatitis in chicks distinct from pantothenic acid deficiency." *J. Nutr.* **20**, 599 (1940).

93. Rubin, S. H., Drekter, L., and Moyer, E. H. "Biological activity of synthetic *d,l*-desthiobiotin." *Proc. Soc. Exptl. Biol. Med.* **58**, 352 (1945).

94. Axelrod, A. E., Pilgrim, F. J., and Hofmann, K. "The activity of *dl*-oxybiotin for the rat." *J. Biol. Chem.* **163**, 191 (1946).

95. Dakshinamurti, K., Landman, A. D., Ramamurti, L., and Constable, R. J. "Isotope dilution assay for biotin." *Anal. Biochem.* **61**, 225 (1974).

96. Hood, R. L. "A radiochemical assay for biotin in biological materials." *J. Sci. Food Agric.* **26**, 1847 (1975).

97. Lin, H. J. and Kirsch, J. F. "A sensitive fluorometric assay for avidin and biotin." *Anal. Biochem.* **81**, 442 (1977).

98. Bolliger, H. R. and Konig, A. "Vitamins including carotenoids, chlorophylls and biologically active quinones." In E. Stahl, Ed., *Thin Layer Chromatography; A Laboratory Handbook,* 2nd ed., Springer-Verlag, New York, 306–307 (1969).

99. Nuttall, R. T. and Bush, B. "The detection of ten components of a multi-vitamin preparation by chromatographic methods." *Analyst* **96**, 875 (1972).

100. Groningsson, K. and Jansson, L. "TLC determination of biotin in a lyophilized multivitamin preparation." *J. Pharm. Sci.* **68**, 364 (1979).

101. Tsuda, T. "Colorimetric determination of *d*-biotin." *Ann. Sankyo Res. Lab.* **20**, 65 (1968).

102. Plinton, C., Mahn, F. P., Hawrylyshyn, M., Venturella, V. S., and Senkowski, B. Z. "Colorimetric determination of biotin." *J. Pharm. Sci.* **58**, 875 (1969).

103. Viswanathan, V., Mahn, F. P., Venturella, V. S., and Senkowski, B. Z. "Gas-liquid chromatography of *d*-biotin." *J. Pharm. Sci.* **59**, 400 (1970).

104. Haarasilta, S. "Enzymatic determination of biotin." *Anal. Biochem.* **87**, 306 (1978).

105. Snell, E. E., Eakin, R. E., and Williams, R. J. "A quantitative test for biotin, its occurrence and properties." *J. Am. Chem. Soc.* **62**, 175 (1940).

106. Schweigert, B. S., Nielsen, E., McIntire, J. M., and Elvehjem, C. A. "Biotin content of meat and meat products." *J. Nutr.* **26**, 65 (1943).

107. Cheldelin, V. H., Eppright, M. A., Snell, E. E., and Guirard, B. M. "Enzymatic liberation of B-vitamins from plant and animal tissues." University of Texas Press, Publication No. 4237, Austin, 15 (1942).

108. Axelrod, A. E. and Hofmann, K. "The inactivation of biotin by hydrochloric acid," *J. Biol. Chem.* **187**, 23 (1950).

109. Scheiner, J. "Extraction of added biotin from animal feed premixes." *J. Assoc. Off. Anal. Chem.* **49**, 882 (1966).

22 Choline

Paul B. Venugopal

GENERAL CONSIDERATIONS

Choline (Ch), known in the past as neurine, is a quarternary ammonium compound: (β-hydroxyethyl) trimethyl ammonium hydroxide. Choline has been an established dietary essential since 1932 and is required in relatively large quantities when compared to other vitamins. It is necessary for normal growth, bone metabolism, lipid metabolism, egg production, prevention of fatty livers, and perosis. Choline biogenesis in plant and animal tissues appears to be universal and this confers a unique status on the vitamin. However, in some species such as growing chicken and turkey, choline requirements can surpass the body's capacity for *de novo* synthesis and so choline is a dietary supplement in the feeds.

A. Physical Properties

Choline is a colorless viscid liquid, crystallized with great difficulty by drying over P_2O_5 under high vacuum; its melting and boiling points are not well defined. The molecular weight is 121.18. Choline is soluble in water, absolute methanol and ethanol, aqueous formic acid, formaldehyde, acetone, and acetonitrile. It is sparingly soluble in chloroform, dry acetone and wet ether, and is insoluble in dry ether, petroleum ether, toluene, and carbon tetrachloride. Mixtures of aqueous formic acid and acetone, aqueous perchloric acid and trichloracetic acid solutions have been used to solubilize and extract choline and acetylcholine (ACh) from plant material and animal tissues. Dilute aqueous solutions of choline are stable whereas concentrated solutions are not, especially when heated to 100°C. On heating, anhydrous choline decomposes mostly into trimethylamine

TABLE 22.1 Total Choline Content of Foods

Animal Sources

Sample		Choline[a]	Sample		Choline[a]	Sample		Choline[a]
Beef:	Liver	5.1	Veal:	Liver	5.66	Hog:	Liver	4.79
	Kidney	2.62		Kidney	3.02		Kidney	2.49
	Brain	4.1		Leg	1.02		Brain	3.25
	Heart	1.7		Shoulder	0.93		Heart	2.0
	Tongue	1.08		Stew meat	0.96		Tongue	1.19
	Round steak	0.68		Cooked stew	1.42		Pancreas	2.85
	Rib roast	0.71		Rib roast	0.98		Shoulder	0.83
							Chops	0.67
							Ham	1.2
							Cooked ham	1.22
Chicken:	Liver	2.97	Lamb:	Kidney	3.12	Processed Meats:	Bologna	0.60
	Kidney	1.94		Shoulder	1.03		Frankfurter	0.57
	Heart	2.05		Chops	0.76		Canadian bacon	0.8
	Egg whole	5.04		Leg	0.84		Liver sausage	2.31
	Egg yolk	14.78		Stew meat	0.79			
	Egg white	0.19		Cooked stew	1.22			
Dairy:	Whole milk, fresh	0.13	Fish:	Fish meal	2.85			
				Trout muscle	0.75			
	dry powder	1.38						
	Skim milk, fresh	0.35						
	dry powder	1.38						
	Cheddar cheese	0.41						

556

Plant Sources

Cereal Grains

Wheat:			Corn:			Rice:		
	Whole	0.8		Yellow	0.32		Whole	0.97
	Germ	3.52		Germ	1.39		Parboiled	0.85
	Defatted germ	3.67		Yellow meal	0.32		Bran	1.47
	Bran	1.24		White meal	0.08–0.36		Germ	2.6
	Flours	0.52–0.6					Polishings	0.99
Oats:	Whole	0.81	Barley:	Whole	1.08			
	Rolled	1.31		White bread	1.63–1.81			

Nuts and Legumes

Peanuts	1.41		Cowpeas		2.23
Pecans	0.43		Black-eyed peas		1.71
Mungbeans	1.81		Cotton seed		
Soybeans				meal	2.93
	mature	2.95		kernel	2.59
	green	2.61	Peanut meal		1.96
Lentils	1.93		Soybean meal		2.99
Garbanzos	2.12		Peanut butter		1.26

Vegetables

Spinach	2.06		Carrots	0.82
Green cabbage	2.18		Turnips	0.81
Asparagus	1.11		Sweet potatoes	0.3
Irish potatoes	0.92			

Samples are fresh and not dried. Data collected from: Engel (4), McIntire et al. (5), Glick (6), Kirk (7), and Hardinge and Crooke (8).
[a] mg/g fresh food.

and glycol and lesser amounts of dimethylaminoethanol and dimethyl vinyl-amine.

B.   Chemical Properties

The strongly alkaline choline forms salts with organic and inorganic acids. The most common salts are chloride and dihydrogen citrate. The aqueous solutions of these salts are stable and neutral to litmus; choline chloride is soluble in alcohol, whereas the citrate is not. Commercially available synthetic choline and choline derivatives are produced from trimethylamine and ethylene cholorohy-drin or ethylenedioxide.

Choline and ACh are quantitatively precipitated as reineckate, enneaiodide, and other complexes such as choline phosphotungstate, choline cadmium chlo-ride, and choline uranium salt. Both choline and ACh are strongly hydrophilic and form ion pairs with hydrophobic counter ions such as dipicrylamine or hexanitrodiphenylamine, and these ion pair complexes can be extracted by or-ganic solvents such as methylene dichloride (1); this procedure is a selective isolation for these compounds when present in microquantities in biological material. Another selective isolation is a liquid cation exchange procedure using sodium tetraphenylboron and 3-hepatanone (2) or sodium tetraphenylboron and butene-nitrile (3).

C.   Occurrence

Choline occurs widely in nature. Glandular meats or organ tissues, brain, and egg yolk are the richest animal sources, and germs of cereals, legumes, and defatted oil seed meals are the best plant sources. The total choline content of some food products are presented in Table 22.1, compiled from various published sources (4–8). To convert these values to choline chloride, these must be mul-tiplied by the factor 1.15.

D.   Biological Functions

Choline is distributed in biological material as free choline, as ACh and as phosphoryl choline in complex phospholipids such as lecithins, sphingomyelins and lipoproteins (Figure 22.1). In the animal body, free choline is present in all tissues (high in liver and kidney), ACh and sphingomyelin in brain and nerve tissues, and bound phosphatidyl choline in lipoproteins and in all living cell membranes, and in body fluids such as blood, lymph, saliva, bile, semen, etc. Plant materials contain free choline and phosphatidyl choline. The major func-tions of choline in the body are:

  1.   source of biologically labile methyl groups for transmethylation reactions;
  2.   precursor of ACh, essential in the transmission of nerve impulses; and
  3.   vital constituent of phosphatidyl choline which is essential for cell mem-

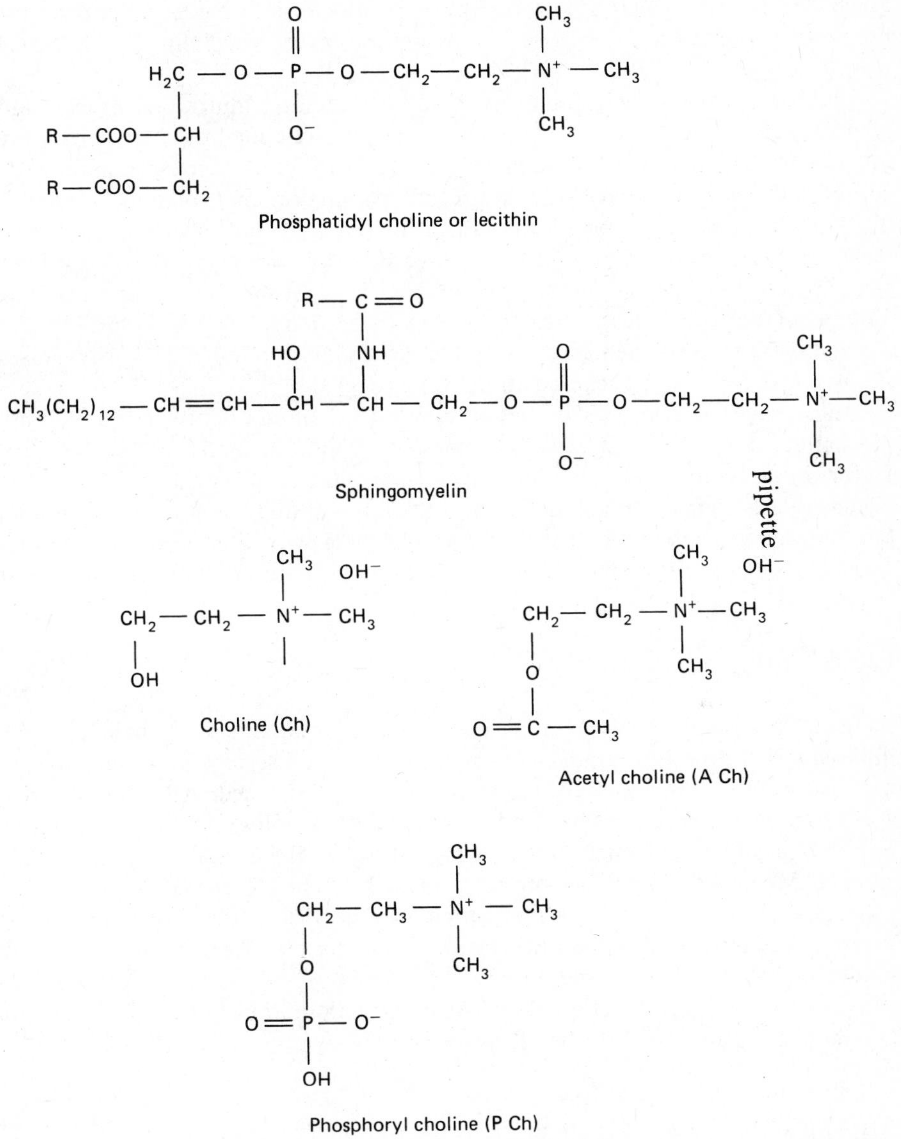
Phosphatidyl choline or lecithin
Sphingomyelin
pipette
Choline (Ch)
Acetyl choline (A Ch)
Phosphoryl choline (P Ch)

FIGURE 22.1 Structures of choline compounds.

brane structure and permeability, and for lipoproteins in the transport of fat-soluble substances.

Since choline is involved both directly and indirectly in biologic functions, it is not possible to define or standardize vitamin activity for choline in the usual terms.

Choline deficiency in mammals is manifested as fatty infiltration of liver and hemorrhagic kidney damage, produced mainly by choline-free diets, which are also deficient in methionine, vitamin B_{12}, and folacin. Under certain experimental conditions, choline metabolism is affected by intakes of protein, cholesterol, alcohol, the type of carbohydrate and fat in the diet, and environmental temperature. Grown on the same diet, rats raised in cold temperatures do not have the choline deficiency symptoms seen in rats raised at laboratory temperatures. Young animals with less efficient or impaired choline *de novo* synthesis are susceptible to choline deficiency. Choline deficiency in poultry primarily causes perosis, a tendon defect leading to deformed legs.

An average American daily diet is reported to contain between 400–900 mg of choline, due to widespread occurrence of choline in foods; other accessory factors directly involved in choline biosynthesis also occur in the foods. Clinical evidence of a dietary choline deficiency in human adults has not been found so far. However, in children raised on formula diets with limited intakes of methionine, vitamin B_{12}, and folacin, choline could become a dietary factor of importance.

E.   Sample Preparation

Some of the common food materials encountered for choline assay include: meat, milk, and fish products; grains and grain products; oil seeds and oil seed meals; and vegetables. Dry materials are ground up and extracted. All these samples should be refrigerated to prevent microbial growth. Choline is quite stable under normal conditions but microbial growth will utilize the available choline in the sample. Meat, milk, and fish products must be kept frozen. Milk samples at room temperature lose all choline content within 48 hr. For choline and ACh determinations in microquantities from animal tissues, fresh tissues collected immediately following the sacrifice must be quickly frozen in liquid nitrogen or acetone-dry ice and processed forthwith for extraction. Poultry feeds that contain choline supplements should be refrigerated.

METHODS AVAILABLE

Available assay methods for free and bound choline can be classified under four groups: chemical, biochemical, microbiological, and physiological, and these methods were extensively reviewed (9–12). Extraction procedures also differ depending upon the analytical method, choline content of the material, hydrolysis, and pH control.

A. Chemical Methods

1. *Gravimetry.*   Following extraction from the food material, choline is precipitated from the extraction medium as periodide or enneaiodide (13,14), phosphotungstate (15), choline cadmium chloride complex (16), choline uranium complex (17), or reineckate complex (18); these complexes are determined gravimetrically. When low choline content results in insufficient yield, the metals in these complexes are analyzed to determine the choline content (e.g., mercury in mercury-choline complex) (19).

2. *Spectrophotometry and Colorimetry.*   The periodide precipitation method had been modified to selectively precipitate choline and the choline enneaiodide is dissolved in ethylene dichloride and is measured spectrophotometrically at 365 nm with a sensitivity of 5 μg of choline (14). Choline and ACh present in microquantities in biological tissues are extracted as dipicrylamine ion pairs and separated by liquid-liquid chromatography in microcolumns as picrate ion pairs. Finally ACh is measured at 420 nm as dipicrylamine ion pair and choline as picrate at 375 nm; 1–10 μg levels can be measured (1).

In an aqueous alkaline solution, hydroxylamine converts ACh into acetyl hydroxamic acid; the latter reacts with $FeCl_3$ to a reddish-brown complex salt, which can be measured colorimetrically at 546 nm. The procedure suggested by Hestrin (20) has been modified for microquantities of ACh using paper chromatographic separation and densitometry (21).

The choline reineckate complex is soluble in acetone and the pink color is measured spectrophotometrically at 526 nm. This method has been modified for a number of specific applications and for semimicroquantities of choline (22–25). This colorimetric procedure is extensively employed for foods and feeds and will be described in detail.

3. *Fluorometry.*   The active acetyl group in ACh readily undergoes hydrazinolysis, to form acetyl hydrazide. Salicylaldehyde reacts with this acetyl hydrazide to form intensely fluorescent acetylhydrazyl salicylhydrazone which can be measured at 370/475 nm in a spectrophotofluorimeter. Fellmann (26) developed this procedure to measure 0.5 nmoles of ACh from tissues and this will be described in detail for ACh assay.

4. *Gas Chromatography.*   Demethylation products from either the pyrolysis of choline and ACh halides or from N-demethylation of ACh by sodium benzene thiolate are quantified by chromatography separation on suitable columns such as Pennwalt 223 packing or a mixture of 0.5% OV 101 and 5% DDTS on Gas Chrom Q or 10% Poly A 135 on Gas Chrom Q, and so on. The pyrolysis procedure was developed by Green and Szilagyi (27) and the N-demethylation procedure by Jenden and Hanin (28). The sensitivity of the pyrolysis method is 2 ng and for N-demethylation, it is 2 ng for ACh and 12 ng for choline.

B. Biochemical Methods

Enzymes such as acetyl choline esterase (E.C.3.1.1.7), choline acetyl transferase (E.C.2.3.1.6), and choline phosphokinase (E.C.2.7.7.32), which react with choline and ACh, are utilized in the biochemical assays; both acetate and choline moieties are determined. Radioisotope-labeled cofactors are used; these radioassays are sensitive but time consuming. These enzyme reactions are coupled to other enzyme reactions that utilize nicotinamide-adenine dinucleotides (NADH). The fluorescent property of NADH is used to indirectly determine choline and ACh. These biochemical methods are applicable to biological tissues and fluids.

1. *Enzymic Radioassay.*

(a) ACh $\xrightarrow{\text{acetyl choline esterase}}$ acetate + choline

(b) Choline + acetyl CoA $\xrightarrow[\text{transferase}]{\text{choline acetyl}}$ ACh + CoA

(c) Choline + ATP $\xrightarrow[\text{Mg}^{2+}]{\text{choline phosphokinase}}$ phosphoryl choline + ADP

Both choline and ACh isolated from tissues are separated by electrophoresis and ACh is hydrolyzed by ACh esterase. Choline is then acetylated with [^{14}C]acetyl coenzyme A, and the labeled ACh is again separated by electrophoresis and counted (29).

Choline is phosphorylated with [^{32}P]ATP using choline phosphokinase, and the phosphorylated choline is isolated by ion-exchange chromatography (Amberlite CG400) and the radioactivity counted (3,30,31). Nanogram quantities of both choline and ACh can be assayed following delicate isolation procedures. These radioassays are time consuming and tedious and involve sophisticated equipment and purification of the enzymes involved.

2. *Fluorimetric Assays.*

These assays measure the reduced NADH, which is involved in enzyme reactions associated with either the phosphorylation of choline or acetylation of coenzyme A with the acetate from ACh.

(a) Measurement of NADH production

(1) Acetate + CoA $\xrightarrow[\text{ATP, K}^+, \text{Mg}^{2+}]{\text{acetyl CoA synthetase}}$ acetyl CoA + AMP + PP$_i$

(2) Malate + NAD$^+$ $\xrightarrow{\text{malate dehydrogenase}}$ oxaloacetate + NADH

(3) Oxaloacetate + acetyl CoA $\xrightarrow[\text{enzyme}]{\text{citrate condensing}}$ CoA + citrate

(4) ACh $\xrightarrow{\text{ACh esterase}}$ acetate + choline

The preceding reactions are carried out by treating the assay mixture of suitable buffers, malate, CoA, NAD$^+$, malate dehydrogenase (E.C.1.1.1.37), and citrate condensing enzyme (E.C.4.1.3.7), and sample tissue extract with enzymes acetyl-CoA synthetase (E.C.6.2.1.1.) and ACh esterase. Production of reduced nucleotide (NADH) stoichiometrically with ACh present in the sample is measured fluorimetrically (32). This procedure can be adapted to spectrophotometry by measuring the absorbance at 340 nm. The fluorimetry range covers 1–80 nmoles of ACh and spectrophotometry covers 50–200 nmoles of ACh and the reproducibility is $\pm 5\%$.

(b) Measurement of NADH disappearance

(1) $\text{ACh} \xrightarrow{\text{ACh esterase}} \text{acetate} + \text{choline}$

(2) $\text{Choline} + \text{ATP} \xrightarrow[\text{Mg}^{2+}]{\text{choline phosphokinase}} \text{phosphoryl choline} + \text{ADP}$

(3) $\text{ADP} + \text{phosphoenolpyruvate} \xrightarrow[\text{K}^+, \text{Mg}^{2+}]{\text{pyruvate kinase}} \text{ATP} + \text{pyruvate}$

(4) $\text{Pyruvate} + \text{NADH} \xrightarrow{\text{lactate dehydrogenase}} \text{lactate} + \text{NAD}^+$

The preceding reactions are carried out in the NADH-linked fluorimetric assay for both choline and ACh (33). The assay mixture containing suitable buffers and the sample tissue extract is treated with ATP, NADH, phosphoenolpyruvate, pyruvate kinase (E.C.2.7.1.40), lactate dehydrogenase (E.C.1.1.1.27), and hexokinase (E.C.2.7.1.1.). The reaction mixture is temperature-equilibrated prior to reagent addition so that any contaminants such as ADP, pyruvate, and glucose can react and be depleted. Choline phosphokinase is then added and the change is fluorescence level due to choline, (or disappearance of NADH) is recorded. Acetyl cholinesterase is then added and the change in fluorescence due to ACh is measured. This procedure can be adapted to spectrophotometry. With highly purified choline phosphokinase, it is possible to measure 1 nmole or less of choline. Thin tissue slices of brain could be used for the assay without any isolation procedures.

Both of these methods are specific and sensitive and could be used routinely.

C. Microbiological Methods

Microbial assays for choline measure the growth response of mutant strains of the mold *Neurospora crassa* (strains 34486 and 47904). The dry weight of the mycelium is the assay criterion. This assay for total choline in natural products, originally developed by Horowitz and Beadle (34), has been modified and used for milk products (35) and for plasma and urine (36). Since these mutants also respond to analogs, derivatives, and precursors of choline such as methylaminoethanol, dimethyl amino ethanol, ACh, phosphoryl choline, ethyl substituted cholines, and methionine, the assay sample should be free of these compounds.

The assay sample is autoclaved with 3% sulfuric acid for 2 hr, to liberate choline from its bound forms and then neutralized with barium hydroxide. Choline, methionine, and other interfering materials present in this hydrolysate are absorbed on a Permutit column, from which choline is eluted with 5% sodium chloride. Aliquots of this eluate and standard choline solutions are added to the basal culture medium in suitable flasks and sterilized. The flasks are then aseptically inoculated with the culture of *Neurospora crassa* (ATCC no. 9277) and incubated for three days at 25°C. The mycelium from each flask is removed, dried, and weighed.

Choline content of the sample is determined by reference to a standard growth-response curve, which is obtained by plotting the dry weights of mycelia against standard amounts of choline.

Choline values determined on different amounts of the sample eluate usually agree within 10%; chemical and microbial assays on the same sample show fairly similar values. Though time consuming, the assay is specific and is applicable to foods with appreciable choline content.

D. Physiological Methods

Classical biological assay methods such as growth response in experimental animals fed choline-deficient diets are not feasible for choline. Even the determination of labile methyl groups by comparing the degree of prevention of renal pathology, in experimental animals on a methyl-deficient diet, by test material and by choline, is not practical, because of the *de novo* synthesis of methyl groups. Folic acid and cobalamine influence this *de novo* synthesis.

The pharmacological action of ACh on tissues is used for the assay of choline and ACh. These procedures were discussed by Fiesen (37). In the past, rectus abdominis muscle of frog and the isolated intestine of the rabbit were used; other muscle tissues used in the above assay are hamster stomach strip (38), longitudinal muscle slices of Japanese medical leech (39), and clam heart muscle (40). These methods are not applicable for choline assay in food material due to interfering substances such as potassium, histamine, and other physiologically active compounds.

A radioimmunoassay for ACh was developed by preparing an ACh-like immunogen and using it in the production of antibodies specific for ACh (41). Application of this assay for ACh and choline in food material is feasible with suitable adaptations.

ANALYTICAL METHODOLOGY

I.   REINECKATE METHOD FOR TOTAL CHOLINE

A. Principle

Potassium or ammonium reineckate (ammonium tetrathiocyanodiammonochromate, $NH_4[CR(NH_3)_2(SCN)_4]$) reacts quantitatively with choline to form a red precipitate. The choline reineckate complex is soluble in acetone; this pink to bright red acetone solution absorbs light at 526 nm and the absorption is proportional to choline concentration. Quantities of the order of 0.3 mg choline can be estimated. A standard curve is necessary to determine the choline content of the sample. The original gravimetric method of Kapfhammer and Bischoff (18) with subsequent modifications was adapted by Lim and Schall (25) for the assay of total choline in feeds and foods.

B. Equipment

1. *Extraction Apparatus of the Goldfisch or Similar Type.* With capacity for 10–12 simultaneous extractions.

2. *Adsorbent Columns.* Approximately 25 cm long and 7.5-mm i.d. with a reservoir of 50-mL capacity at the top and a constricted drain tip at the bottom. Place a plug of glass wool at the bottom and fill the column to a height of 18 cm with Florisil. Wash with methanol. Connect a flexible tube with a pinchcock to the drain tip. Maintain methanol in the column until used.

3. *Rack To Support the Adsorbent Columns.*

4. *Spectrophotometer.* Or photoelectric colorimeter with filter to measure light transmission at 526 nm.

5. *Spectrophotometer Cuvets.*

C. Reagents

These reagents are stable and may be stored.

1. *Methanol.* Reagent grade.

2. *Chloroform.* Reagent grade.

3. *Methyl Acetate.* Reagent grade, methanol free.

4. *Glacial Acetic Acid.*

5. *Barium Hydroxide.* Reagent grade.

6. *Florisil.* Activated at 650°C (Floridin Co.).

7. *Acetic Acid–Methanol Mixture.* Mix 10 mL glacial acetic acid and 80 mL acetone.

8. *Aqueous Acetone.* 10% acetone in H_2O, by volume.

9. *Choline Stock Solution.* Dissolve 5.7613 g anhydrous choline chloride in H_2O and dilute to 100 mL. Keep refrigerated. Choline chloride is hygroscopic and should be weighed with care.

The following reagents should be prepared daily:

10. *Extractant.* Saturate 100 mL methanol by adding 4–5 g anhydrous $Ba(OH)_2$ and shaking for 10 min. Add 10 mL chloroform, mix, and decant to remove excess $Ba(OH)_2$.

11. *Choline Working Standard.* Dilute 2 mL choline chloride stock solution to 100 mL with H_2O; this standard solution contains 1 mg choline/mL.

12. *Ammonium Reineckate Solution.* Prepare a saturated solution by shak-

ing 2–3 g ammonium reineckate in 100 mL H_2O for 10 min. Filter to remove excess reineckate.

D. Procedure

1. *Extraction.*

(a) Weigh and transfer an adequate amount of sample (estimated to contain 5–50 mg choline) into a Goldfisch thimble. Add 30 mL extractant (Reagent 10) and reflux for 4 hr.

(1) The "high" setting on the extractor is adequate for this refluxing (2–4 drops/sec).

(b) Cool and filter into 100-mL volumetric flask. Use 5–10-mL portions of acetic acid–methanol (Reagent 7) to wash the thimble and the contents and to transfer and to wash the suspended material. Collect all the washings in the flask; check the pH and adjust to pH 6 with glacial acetic acid, if necessary. Dilute to volume with methanol and mix.

(1) Both free and bound choline in most samples of foods and feeds can be extracted by this procedure. For the assay of free choline, the sample extraction can be reduced to 1 hr and $Ba(OH)_2$ omitted from the extractant.

(c) Mild acid hydrolysis is required for the complete extraction of total choline from certain samples of plant origin that may contain choline xanthate and other choline salts. The extractant is an equal mixture of 1 N HCl and methanol (v/v). Weigh an adequate amount of sample containing 5–50 mg choline into a 250-mL wide-mouth Erlenmeyer flask. Add 50–60 mL of acid extractant, cover the mouth of the flask with a funnel to minimize evaporation, and heat on a steam bath for 3 hr. Use glass beads or boiling chips to prevent bumping during the extraction. After the digestion has started, check and adjust the pH to pH 3–4 with HCl, if it becomes necessary. Cool, filter into a 100-mL volumetric flask and dilute to volume with methanol.

2. *Purification.*

(a) Transfer an aliquot of the extract (estimated to contain 2–4 mg choline) to the Florisil adsorbent column. Remove the flexible tubing from the draining tip and allow the aliquot to pass into the column. Rinse down the reservoir with 5 mL methanol (Reagent 1) and again with 10 mL methanol.

(1) Chlorophyll contaminant, if any, will show on the column as a green band of color.

(b) Wash down the column with two 10-mL portions of methylacetate (Reagent 3) to remove the green color. Wait for each portion to enter the column bed before adding the next portion. Pass 10 mL cold 10% aqueous acetone through the column followed by 5 mL ammonium reineckate (Reagent 12). Wash finally with 10-mL portions of glacial acetic acid, until the column is clear.

(c) Elute the reddish pink band of choline reineckate with 10 mL of 100%

reagent-grade acetone; wait until the pink color reaches the tip of the column and then collect the eluate in a 10-mL volumetric flask. Dilute to volume with acetone.

(d) Transfer 1.0-, 2.0-, 3.0-, and 5.0-mL aliquots of the freshly made working standard choline solution (Reagent 11) to prepared Florisil adsorbent columns. Treat these standards as described above for the sample and collect the eluates in different flasks.

3. *Spectrofluorometry.*

(a) Set the spectrofluorometer at 370 nm excitation and 475 nm emission with the slit open at 8 nm band, after a 30-min warmup of the instrument. The slit may be adjusted later for required sensitivity. With the shutter closed, adjust dark current and zero controls to zero reading.

(b) Read the absorbancy of the standard choline reineckate solutions and prepare the standard curve by plotting absorbance versus concentration.

(c) Read the absorbancy of the eluted sample choline reineckate and determine its concentration from the standard curve.

4. *Calculation.*

mg choline/100 g sample

$$= \text{mg choline from standard curve} \times \frac{100}{\text{mL aliquot}} \times \frac{100}{\text{g sample}}$$

II.   FLUORIMETRIC METHOD FOR ACETYLCHOLINE

A.   Principle

ACh, absorbed on a cation-exchange resin, is allowed to react with hydrazine, forming acetyl hydrazide. Choline remains bound on the resin, while the acetylhydrazide is eluted with HCl. This hydrazide reacts with salicylaldehyde to form intensely fluorescent acetylhydrazyl salicylhydrazone. The fluorescence, which is proportional to the concentration of ACh, can be measured at 370/475 nm in a spectrophotofluorometer. A standard curve is necessary to determine the ACh content of the sample. The assay procedure is sensitive enough to detect as little as 0.5 nmole (0.08 μg) of ACh. Fellman (19) developed this procedure for ACh assay in animal tissues (Figure 22.2).

B.   Equipment

1. *TenBroek Homogenizer.*
2. *Sorvall Refrigerated Centrifuge.*
3. *Standard Chromatography Tubes.*   1 × 25 cm with a 15-mL reservoir at the top and draining tip at the bottom.
4. *Racks To Support Chromatography Columns.*
5. *Centrifuge Tubes 15 mL, 30 mL.*

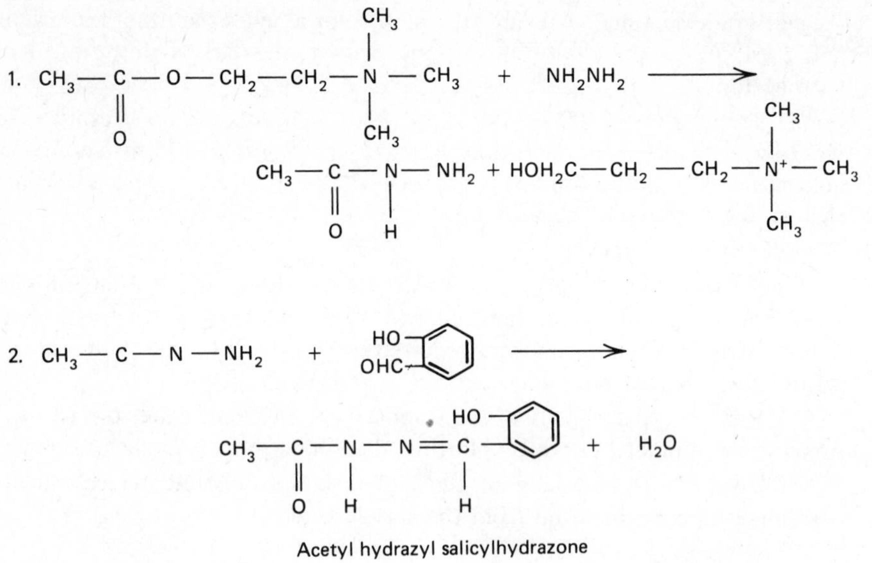

1. $CH_3-\underset{\underset{O}{\|}}{C}-O-CH_2-CH_2-\underset{\underset{CH_3}{|}}{\overset{\overset{CH_3}{|}}{N}}-CH_3$ + NH_2NH_2 ⟶

$CH_3-\underset{\underset{O}{\|}}{C}-\underset{\underset{H}{|}}{N}-NH_2$ + $HOH_2C-CH_2-CH_2-\underset{\underset{CH_3}{|}}{\overset{\overset{CH_3}{|}}{N^+}}-CH_3$

2. $CH_3-C-N-NH_2$ + (HO, OHC on benzene ring) ⟶

$CH_3-\underset{\underset{O}{\|}}{C}-\underset{\underset{H}{|}}{N}-N=\underset{\underset{H}{|}}{C}-$ (HO on benzene ring) + H_2O

Acetyl hydrazyl salicylhydrazone

FIGURE 22.2 Reaction for fluorimetric determination of acetylcholine.

6. *Aminco-Bowmann Spectrophotofluorometer.*
7. *Cuvets for the Fluorometer.*

C. Reagents

These reagents are stable:

1. *3 M Sodium Chloride.* Dissolve 702 g NaCl in 4 L H_2O.
2. *4 N Sodium Hydroxide.* Dissolve 200 g NaOH in 1 L H_2O.
3. *2 N Hydrochloric Acid.* Add 166 mL of HCl to 834 mL H_2O to make 1 L.
4. *0.07 N Hydrochloric Acid.* Add 5.8 mL of concentrated HCl to 994.2 mL H_2O to make 1 L.
5. *Potassium Iodide–Iodine Solution.* Dissolve 2.5 g KI and 5.0 g iodine in 50 mL H_2O. Remove undissolved iodine by centrifugation.
6. *Bio Rex 70 Resin–Sodium Form 50–100 Mesh (Bio Rad Laboratories).* Three pounds of resin are processed and kept stored. Wash the resin with H_2O several times in a large beaker and allow it to settle. Remove very small particles that do not settle along with the wash H_2O. Treat the resin with alkali and acid in succession as follows: Stir the resin in H_2O in the large beaker and adjust to pH 10 with 5 N NaOH, using a pH meter. Allow the resin to settle and decant the supernatant and wash the resin three times with H_2O. Adjust to pH 1 with 2 N HCl and rinse once with H_2O. Repeat this alkali-acid treatment three times. Then adjust to pH 8 with 0.5 N NaOH. Transfer the resin to tall beaker or

column and rinse with 3 M NaCl using 4 L/lb of resin. Finally, wash the resin with H_2O repeatedly till the final rinse is free of chloride.

(a) Addition of $AgNO_3$ solution to the rinse acidified with dilute HNO_3 should result in a clear solution.

(b) To prepare the resin column, transfer the resin to a 1×25-cm chromatography tube to a height of 4 cm after laying a loose plug of glass wool at the draining end. Attach flexible tubing with a pinchcock to the draining tip. Keep the column moist with water by keeping 2 mL H_2O on the top of the resin column when it is not in use.

7. *Ethyl Ether.*

8. *Acetone.*

9. *Dimethyl Formamide.* Spectroscopy grade.

These reagents may be prepared weekly:

10. *ACh Iodide Stock Solution.* Weight accurately 4.19 mg ACh iodide and dissolve in 100 mL of H_2O. This contains 2.5 mg ACh/100 mL or 25 μg/mL. Keep refrigerated.

11. *0.01 M Tetramethyl Ammonium Bromide.* Dissolve 15.4 mg tetramethyl ammonium bromide in 10 mL H_2O and store refrigerated.

12. *0.2 M Potassium Borohydride.* Dissolve 108 mg KBH_4 in 10 mL dimethyl formamide. If turbid, the solution should be centrifuged and the clear supernatant removed and stored.

These reagents should be prepared daily:

13. *2 M Hydrazine.* Dissolve 0.64 mL analytical grade or redistilled hydrazine in 10 mL H_2O.

14. *4% Salicylaldehyde.* Dissolve 0.2 mL salicylaldehyde in 5 mL dimethyl formamide; transfer to a brown bottle and store in refrigerator.

15. *10% Trichloracetic Acid.* Dissolve 10 g trichloracetic acid in H_2O to make a final volume of 100 mL.

16. *ACh Working Standard.* Dilute 2 mL ACh iodide stock solution to 100 mL; 1 mL contains 0.5 μg of ACh.

D. Procedure

1. *Extraction.*

(a) Remove the specific sample tissue as quickly as possible, weigh, and homogenize it in 9 volumes of fresh cold 10% trichloroacetic acid (Reagent 15) in a TenBroek Homogenizer.

(1) The sample should be kept frozen in dry ice–acetone during the rapid transfer to the laboratory.

(b) Centrifuge this homogenate at 12,000 $\times$ g for 15 min at 0°C and use the supernatant for ACh assay. Dilute an aliquot to 10 mL for the assay. This sample should contain at least 0.5 nmole or 0.08 μg of ACh.

2. *Purification and Assay.*

(a) To the 10-mL assay sample in a centrifuge tube, add 0.1 mL of 0.01 M tetramethylammonium bromide (Reagent 11) and then 0.4 mL of potassium iodide–iodine (Reagent 5) solution. Mix well and cool in ice for 20 min. Centrifuge at 0°C for 5 min at 12,000 × g to sediment the ACh iodide. Discard the supernatant and add 5 mL of anhydrous ethyl ether to dissolve the sediment by stirring. Add 5 mL of H$_2$O, mix thoroughly, and allow the iodine-containing ether layer to separate. Decant and discard the ether layer. Repeat the ether-extracting procedure three times, discarding the ether layer every time. Place the sample in a 47°C water bath for 5 min to remove the residual ether and bubble compressed air gently through the solution for 1 min to get rid of traces of ether. Remove from the water bath and cool.

(b) Transfer the 5-mL aqueous solution to the resin column in the chromatography tube. Add 20 mL H$_2$O to the top of the resin column without disturbing, and pass H$_2$O as a rinse through the column. Do not allow the column to run dry. Carefully add 0.15 mL 2 M hydrazine (Reagent 13) to the top of the column. After exactly 2 min elute with 7 mL 0.07 N HCl (Reagent 4). Discard the first 2 ml of the eluate and collect the remaining 5 ml.

(c) Transfer 1.0-, 2.0-, 3.0-, 4.0-, and 5.0-mL aliquots of the freshly made working standard (Reagent 16) and 5 mL H$_2$O (water blank) into separate tubes and treat these standards with anhydrous ethyl ether. Continue the procedure as described above for the sample.

(d) Add 0.1 mL 4% salicylaldehyde solution (Reagent 14) to the 5-mL eluates of water blank, standards, and sample and incubate at 37°C for 30 min.

(e) Following incubation, add 0.1 mL 0.2 M KBH$_4$ (Reagent 12) to the tubes of water blank, standards, and sample. Mix and wait 8 min. Add 0.15 mL 2 N NaOH (Reagent 3), mix well, and read immediately in an Aminco-Bowman Spectrophotofluorometer.

3. *Spectrofluorometry.*

(a) Set the spectrofluorometer at 370 nm excitation and 475 nm emission with the slit open at 8 nm band, after a 30-min warmup of the instrument. The slit may be adjusted later for required sensitivity. With the shutter closed, adjust dark current and zero controls to zero reading.

(b) With the slit adjusted for maximum sensitivity, quickly read the fluorescence of the standard solutions, starting with the most concentrated standard. Read the water blank and then the sample.

4. *Calculation.*

(a) Plot a standard curve using the readings of the standards after subtracting the water blank and determine the ACh concentration of the eluate from the standard curve.

μg ACh/100 g sample

$$= \mu\text{g ACh from standard curve} \times \frac{10}{\text{mL aliquot}} \times \frac{100}{\text{g sample}}$$

(1) *Precaution*: Impurities in hydrazine will give high blank values; if need be, redistill hydrazide before use. Extra care should be taken in redistilling this reactive chemical.

(2) Although not necessary, it is advantageous to determine the elution pattern of the batch of resin used by running 12–15 nmoles or 1.96–2.4 μg of acetyl-[1-^{14}C]-choline through the assay procedure described above, and count the radioactivity of 1-mL aliquote of 7 mL eluate of the acetyl hydrazide. The elution pattern changes very little; the first 2 mL do not contain radioactivity whereas the last 5 mL contain the most radioactivity.

LITERATURE CITED

1. Eksborg, S. and Persson, B. A. "Acetyl choline in rat brain after selective isolation by ion pair extraction and micro column separation." *Acta Pharmacentica Suecica* **8**, 205 (1971).

2. Fonnum, F. "Radiochemical micro assays for the determination of choline acetyl transferase and acetyl cholinesterase activities." *Biochem. J.* **115**, 469 (1969).

3. Goldberg, A. M. and McCaman, R. E. "The determination of pico-mole amounts of acetyl choline in mammalian brain." *J. Neurochem.* **20**, 1 (1973).

4. Engel, R. W. "The choline content of animal and plant products." *J. Nutr.* **25**, 441 (1943).

5. McIntire, J. M., Schweigert, B. S., and Elvehjem, C. A. "The choline and pyridoxine content of meats." *J. Nutr.* **28**, 219 (1944).

6. Glick, D. "Choline content of pure varieties of wheat, oats, barley, flax, soybeans and milled fractions of wheat." *Cereal Chem.* **22**, 95 (1945).

7. Kirk, M. C. "The nutritive value of rice and its products." *Ark. Agr. Exptl. Station Bull.* **589** (1957).

8. Hardinge, M. G. and Crooke, H. "Lesser known vitamins in foods." *J. Am. Dietet. Assoc.* **38**, 240 (1961).

9. Wilson, J. and Lorenz, K. "Biotin and choline in foods: Nutritional importance and methods of analysis—A review." *Food Chem.* **4**, 115 (1979).

10. Hanin, I. (Ed.) *Choline and Acetylcholine: Handbook of Chemical Assay Methods.* Raven Press, New York (1974).

11. Griffith, W. H. and Nyc, J. F. "Choline." In W. H. Sebrell and R. S. Harris, Eds., *The Vitamins, Chemistry, Physiology, Methods,* Vol. 2. Academic Press, New York, 2 (1971).

12. Engel, R. W. and Ackerman, C. J. "Chemical estimation of choline." In D. Glick, Ed., *Methods of Biochemical Analysis,* Vol. 1. Interscience, New York, 285 (1954).

13. Sharpe, J. S. "Choline as a precursor of guanidine: Decrease in the amount of choline of the hen egg during incubation." *Biochem. J.* **17**, 41 (1923).

14. Smits, G. "Modification of the periodide method for the determination of choline." *Biochim. Biophys. Acta* **26**, 424 (1957).

15. Gakenheimer, W. C. and Reguera, R. M. "An assay for choline chloride in pharmaceutical products." *J. Am. Pharm. Assn.* **35**, 311 (1946).

16. Wachsmuth, H. "New general reagent for alkaloids: Qualitative and quantitative applications." *Bull Soc. Chim. Belg.* **35**, 311 (1946).

17. Soye, C. Sur la formation du complex $[(NO_3)_2 \ UO_2C_5H_{15}O_2N]^n$ *Compt. Rend.* **231**, 349 (1950).

18. Kapfhammer, J. and Bischoff, C. "Acetyl cholin und cholin aus tierischen Organen. 1. Mitteilung-Darstellung aus Rinderblut." *Z. Physiol. Chem.* **191**, 179 (1930).

19. Eagle, E. "The choline content of biological fluids." *J. Lab. Clin. Med.* **27**, 103 (1941).

20. Hestrin, S. "The reaction of acetyl choline and other carboxylic acid derivatives with hydroxylamine and its analytical applications." *J. Biol. Chem.* **180**, 249 (1949).

21. Schumacher, H. and Ehl, R. "Quantitative photometry detection of esters of choline." In Hanin, Ed., *Choline and Acetyl Choline: Handbook of Chemical Assay Methods.* Raven Press, New York, 195 (1974).

22. Engel, R. W. "Modified methods for the chemical and biological determination of choline." *J. Biol. Chem.* **144**, 701 (1942).

23. Glick, D. "Concerning the reineckate method for the determination of choline." *J. Biol. Chem.* **156**, 643 (1944).

24. Ackerman, C. J. and Salmon, W. D. "A simplified and specific method for estimation of choline." *Anal. Biochem.* **1**, 327 (1960).

25. Linn, F. and Schall, E. D. "Determination of choline in feeds." *J. Assoc. Off. Agric. Chem.* **47**, 501 (1964).

26. Fellman, J. H. "A chemical method for the determination of acetyl choline; its application in a study of presynaptic release and choline acetyltransferase activity." *J. Neurochem.* **16**, 135 (1969).

27. Green, J. P. and Szilagyi, P. I. A. "Measurement of acetyl choline by pyrolysis gas chromatography." In I. Hanin, Ed., *Choline and Acetyl Choline: Handbook of Chemical Assay Methods.* Raven Press, New York, 151 (1974).

28. Jenden, D. J. and Hanin, I. "Gas chromatographic micro estimation of choline and acetyl choline after N-demethylation by sodium benzenethiolate." In I. Hanin, Ed., *Choline and Acetyl Choline: Handbook of Chemical Assay Methods.* Raven Press, New York, 135 (1974).

29. Saelens, J. K., Allen, M. P., and Simke, J. P. "Determination of acetyl choline and choline by an enzymatic assay." *Archives Internationales de Pharmacodynamic et de Therape* **186**, 279 (1970).

30. Schuberth, J., Sparf, B., and Sundwall, A. Determination of choline. In E. Heilbronn and A. Winter, Eds., *Symposium on the Effect of Drugs on Cholinergic Mechanisms in the Central Nervous System.* Skokloster, Almquist and Wiksell, Stockholm, 15 (1970).

31. Reid, W. D., Haubrich, D. R., and Krishna, G. "Enzymic radioassay for acetyl choline and choline in brain." *Anal. Biochem.* **42**, 390 (1971).

32. O'Neill, J. J. and Sakamoto, T. "Enzymatic fluorometric determination of acetyl choline in biological extracts." *J. Neurochem.* **17**, 1451 (1970).

33. Browning, E. T. and Brostrom, M. A. "NADH-linked fluorometric enzyme assay for acetyl choline and choline." In I. Hanin, Ed., *Choline and Acetyl Choline: Handbook of Chemical Assay Methods.* Raven Press, New York, 109 (1974).

34. Horowitz, N. H. and Beadle, G. W. "A microbiological method for the determination of choline by the use of a mutant of Neurospora." *J. Biol. Chem.* **150**, 325 (1943).

35. Hodson, A. Z. "The use of *neurospora* for the determination of choline and biotin in milk products." *J. Biol. Chem.* **157**, 383 (1945).

36. Luecke, R. W. and Pearson, P. B. "The microbiological determination of choline in plasma and urine." *J. Biol. Chem.* **153**, 259 (1944).

37. Friesen, A. J. D. "Measurements of acetyl choline." In E. E. Daniel and D. M. Patton, Eds., *Methods in Pharmacology—3. Smooth Muscle.* Plenum Press, New York, 623 (1975).

38. Vapaatalo, H. and Linden, I. B. "Superfused hamster stomach strip—a sensitive bioassay for acetyl choline." *Naunyn-Schmiedberg's Arch. Parmacol.* **297** (Suppl. II) (1977).

39. Kadota, K. and Nagata, M. "Bioassay of acetyl choline with thin muscle strips of Japanese medical leach and frog." *Japan. J. Pharmacol.* **27** (Suppl.) (1977).

40. Cottrell, G. A., Powell, B., and Stanton, M. "Simple method for measuring a picogram of acetyl choline using the clam (*Mya arenaria*) heart." *Brit. J. Pharmacol.* **40**, 866 (1970).

41. Spector, S., Felix, A., Semenuk, G., and Finberg, J. P. M. "Development of a specific radio immunoassay for acetyl choline." *J. Neurochem.* **30**, 685 (1978).

ABBREVIATIONS

The following list of abbreviations is limited to those most frequently cited throughout this book. Any abbreviations not listed below are properly identified in the chapter in which they are used.

Abbreviation	Word
A	absorbance(s)
aq	aqueous
atm.	atmosphere, atmospheric
AUFS	Absorption Units Full Scale
C	degrees Celsius (Centigrade)
cm	centimeter(s)
cpm	counts per minute
diam	diameter
e.g.	for example
F	degrees Fahrenheit ($^\circ C = (5/9) \times (^\circ F - 32)$)
fl oz	fluid ounce(s) (29.57 mL)
ft	foot (30.48 cm)
g	gram(s)
g	gravity (in centrfg)
gal.	gallon(s) (3.785 L)
GLC	gas-liquid chromatography
H_2O	water, distilled and/or deionized
HPLC	high-performance liquid chromatography
hr	hour(s)
ht	height
i.d.	inner diameter (or dimension)
in	inch(es) (2.54 cm)
kg	kilogram(s)

L	liter(s)
lb	pound(s) (453.6 g)
liq	liquid
m	meter(s); milli--as prefix
M	molar (as applied to concn), not molal
max	maximum
mg	milligram(s)
min	minute(s)
mL	milliliter(s)
mm	millimeter(s)
N	normal (as applied to concn extraction; equations, normality of titrating reagent
ng	nanogram (10^{-6}g)
nm	nanometer (10^{-9}m); formerly μ
No.	number
o.d.	outer diameter
oz	ounce(s) (28.35 g)
p	pico (10^{-12}) as prefix
ppb	parts per billion ($1/10^9$)
ppm	parts per million ($1/10^6$)
psi	pounds per square inch (absolute)
psig	pounds per square inch gage (atmospheric pressure $= 0$)
pt	pint(s) (473 ml)
qt	quart(s) (946 ml)
rpm	revolutions per minute
sec	second(s)
sq	square
std dev	standard deviation
T	transmittance
temp	temperature
TLC	thin-layer chromatography
USP	United States Pharmacopeial Convention
UV	ultraviolet
v/v	both components measured by volume
vol	volume; also volumetric when used with flask
w/w	both components measured by weight
wt	weight
λ	wavelength in nm
μg	microgram(s) (10^{-6}g)

μl	microliter(s) (10^{-6}l)
μm	micrometer(s) (10^{-6}m; formerly μ
'	foot (feet) ($1' = 30.48$ cm)
"	inch(es) ($1'' = 2.54$ cm)
/	per
%	percent (parts per 100); percentage
>	more than; greater than; above; exceeds (use with numbers only)
<	less than; under; below (use with numbers only)
$\geq$	not more than; not greater than; equal to or less than
$\leq$	not less than; equal to or greater than; equal to or more than; at least

MANUFACTURERS AND SUPPLIERS

The following list of manufacturers and suppliers is limited to those that are cited specifically in the text. In no way does the listing constitute product endorsement or approval. Its compilation constitutes merely a convenience to the readers. Products from other sources may serve equally well provided proper testing demonstrates them to be satisfactory.

Ace Glass Inc., 1430 N. W. Blvd., Vineland, NJ 08360.

Altex Division, Beckman Instruments, Inc., 1716 Fourth St., Berkeley, CA 94710.

Alltech Associates, Inc., 2051 Waukegan Rd., Deerfield, IL 60015.

Amersham Corp., 2636 S. Clearbrook Dr., Arlington Heights, IL 60005.

American Instrument Co., 185 Port Reading Ave., Port Reading, NJ 07064

American Type Culture Collection, 12301 Parklawn Dr., Rockville, MD 20852.

Amicon Corp., 21 Hartwell Ave., Lexington, MA 02173.

Aminco, see SLM Instruments, Inc.

Analabs, Inc., 80 Republic Dr., North Haven, CT 06472.

Applied Science, 2051 Waukegan Rd., Deerfield, IL 60015.

Bausch & Lomb, Instrument and Systems Division, 42 East Ave., Rochester, NY 14603.

BBL Microbiological Systems, Box 243 Cockeysville, MD 21030

Beckman Instruments, Inc., Box C-19600, Irvine, CA 92713.

Becton-Dickinson Immunodiagnostic, Hyson, Wescott & Dunning, Charles & Chase Sts., Baltimore, MD 21201.

Becton-Dickinson, Labware, 1950 Williams Dr., Oxnard, CA 93030.

Bio-Rad Laboratories, 2200 Wright Ave., Richmond, CA 94804.

Bio-Serv, Inc., Box BS, Frenchtown, NJ 08825.

Boehringer Monnheim Biochemicals, Box 50816, Indianapolis, IN 46250.

Brinkman Instruments, Cantiague Rd., Westbury, NY 11590.

B. Brown Instruments, Grandview Dr., South San Francisco, CA 94080.

Brownlee Labs, Inc., 2045 Martin, Santa Clara, CA 95050.

Burdick & Jackson Laboratories, Inc., Hoffmann-LaRoche, Inc., 1953 S. Harvey St., Muskegon, MI 49442.

Burrell Corp., 2223 Fifth Ave., Pittsburgh, PA 15219.

Calbiochem-Behring Corp., American Hoechst Corp., Box 12087, San Diego, CA 92112.

Charles River Breeding Laboratories, Inc., 251 Ballardvale St., Wilmington, MA 01887.

Corning Glass Works, Science Products, Corning, NY 14831.

Crawford Fitting Co., 29500 Solon Rd., Solon, OH 44139.

Diagnostic Biochemistry, 10457 H Roselle St., San Diego, CA 92121.

Diagnostic Products Corp., 5700 W. 96th St., Los Angeles, CA 90045.

Difco Laboratories, Box 1058 A, Detroit, MI 48232.

Dionex Corp., 1228 Titan Way, Sunnyvale, CA 94086.

E.I. DuPont de Nemours & Co., Wilmington, DE 19898.

Fisher Scientific Company, 711 Forbes Ave., Pittsburgh, PA 15219.

Eastman Kodak Company, Kodak Laboratory and Specialty Chemicals, Rochester, NY 14650.

Elanco Products Co., Division of Eli Lilly & Co., Box 1750, Indianapolis, IN 46206.

Floridin Co., 3 Penn Center, Pittsburgh, PA 15235.

Gelman Sciences, Inc., 600 S. Wagner Rd., Ann Arbor, MI 48106.

Glenco Scientific Inc., 2802 White Oak Dr., Houston, TX 77007.

Grand Island Biologicals, Grand Island, NY 14072.

Haake Buchler Instruments, Inc., 244 Saddle River Rd., Box 549, Saddle Brook, NJ 07662.

Hamilton Co., Box 17500, Reno, NV 89510.

Hewlett-Packard, Co., 1501 Page Mill Rd., Palo Alto, CA 94304.

Hoffmann-LaRoche, Nutley, NJ 07110.

Humphrey Products, Box 2008, Kalamazoo, MI 49003.

ICN Nutritional Biochemicals, 26201 Miles Rd., Cleveland, OH 44128.

ICN Pharmaceuticals, Inc., Life Sciences Group, 26201 Miles Rd., Cleveland, OH 44128.

Kipp & Zonen, 390 Central Ave., Bohemia, NY 11716.

Kontes, Spruce St., Box 729, Vineland, NJ 08360.

Kratos-Schoeffel Instruments, 24 Broker St., Westwood, NJ 07675.

LDC/Milton Roy, Box 10235, Riviera Beach, FL 33404.

Lab-Glass, Northwest Blvd., Vineland, NJ 08360.

Linear Instruments Corp., 500 Edison Way, Reno, NV 89502.

Mallinckrodt, Inc., 675 McDonnell Blvd., Box 5840, St. Louis, MO 63134.

Matheson, 30 Sea View Dr., Secaucas, NJ 07630

MER Chromatographic, 2423 - D Old Middlefield Way, Mountain View, CA 94040.

E. Merck & Co., Inc., Box 2000, Rahway, NJ 07056.

Miles Laboratories, Inc., Research Products Division, Box 2000, Elkhart, IN 46515.

Millipore Corp., Bedford, MA 01730.

Nupro Co., 4800 E. 345th St., Willoughby, OH 44094.

Packard Instrument Co., Inc., 2200 Warrenville Rd., Downers Grove, IL 60515.

Penn Airbourne Products, Co., 950 Industrial Blvd., Southhampton, PA 18960.

Penntube Plastics, Holley St. & Madison Ave., Clifton Heights, PA 19018.

Perkin-Elmer, Analytical Instruments, Main Avenue, Norwalk, CT 06856.

Pfaltz and Bauer, Inc., 375 Fairfield Ave., Stamford, CT 06902.

Pharmacia Fine Chemicals, 800 Centennial Ave., Piscataway, NJ 08854.

Picker Corp. 595 Miner Rd., Highland Heights, OH 44143.

Preiser Scientific Inc., 900 MacCorkle Ave. S.W., Charleston, WV 25322.

Rainin Instrument Co., Mack Rd., Woburn, MA 01801.

Read Plastics, 12331 Wilkins Ave., Rockville, MD 20852.

Rheodyne, Inc., Box 996, Cotati, CA 94928.

RIA Products Inc., 411 Waverly Oaks Rd., Box 914, Waltham, MA 02154.

Scientific Products, 1430 Waukegan Rd., McGaw Park, IL 60085.

Searle Analytical, Inc., 2000 Nuclear Dr., Des Plaines, IL 60018.

(The) Separations Group, Box 867, 16695 Spruce, Hesperia, CA 92345.

Shimadzu Scientific Instruments, Inc., 9147 Red Branch Rd., Columbia, MD 21045.

Sigma Chemical Co., Box 14508, St. Louis, MO 63178.

SLM Instruments, Inc./American Instrument Co., 810 W. Anthony Dr., Urbana, IL 61801.

Smith Kline Corp., Diagnostics Division, Box 61947, Sunnyvale, CA 94086.

Supelco Inc., Supelco Park, Bellefonte, PA 16823

Technicon Industrial Systems, 511 Benedict Ave., Tarrytown, NY 10591.

Teklad Test Diets, Box 4220, 2826 Latham Dr., Madison, WI 53711.

Tekmar Co., Box 37202, Cincinnati, OH 45222.

Turner Designs, 2247 Old Riddlefield Way, Mountain View, CA 94043.

Ultra-Violet Products, Inc., 5114 N. Walnut Grove Ave., San Gabriel, CA 91776.

United States Pharmacopeial Convention, Inc., 12601 Twin Brook Parkway, Rockville, MD 20852.

U. S. Biochemical Corp., Box 22400, Cleveland, OH 44122.

Valco Instruments Co., Inc., Box 55603, Houston, TX 77255.

VWR Scientific, Box 3200, San Francisco, CA 94119.

Waters Associates, 34 Maple St., Milford, CT 01757.

Whatman, Inc., 9 Bridewell Pl., Clifton, NJ 07014.

Wheaton Scientific, 1000 N. Tenth St., Millville, NJ 08332.

Index